Neurosurgery Update I

Neurosurgery Update I

Diagnosis, Operative Technique, and Neuro-Oncology

Editors

Robert H. Wilkins, M.D.
Professor and Chief
Division of Neurosurgery
Duke University Medical Center
Durham, North Carolina

Setti S. Rengachary, M.D.
Professor and Chief
Section of Neurological Surgery
University of Missouri at Kansas City School
of Medicine
Kansas City, Missouri

McGraw-Hill, Inc.
Health Professions Division
New York St. Louis San Francisco Colorado Springs Auckland
Bogotá Caracas Hamburg Lisbon London Madrid Mexico
Milan Montreal New Delhi Paris San Juan São Paulo
Singapore Sydney Tokyo Toronto

Neurosurgery Update I

1234567890 HALHAL 9876543210

ISBN 0-07-079828-1

This book was set in Plantin by York Graphic Services, Inc.; the editors were Sally Barhydt, Edward Bolger, and Mariapaz Ramos-Englis; the production supervisor was Annette Mayeski. Halliday Lithograph Corporation was printer and binder.

Library of Congress Cataloging-in-Publication Data

Neurosurgery update I / [edited by] Robert H. Wilkins, Setti S.
  Rengachary.
      p.   ca.
    ISBN 0-07-079828-1
    1. Nervous system—Surgery.   I. Wilkins, Robert H.
  II. Rengachary, Setti S.   III. Title: Neurosurgery update I.
    [DNLM: 1. Nervous System—surgery.   WL 366 N49524]
  RD593.N4193 1990
  617.4'8—dc20
  DNLM/DLC
  for Library of Congress   90-5624
                                              CIP

NEUROSURGERY UPDATE
is dedicated to
innovative neurosurgeons throughout the world.

CONTENTS

CONTRIBUTORS

Numbers in brackets refer to the contributors' chapters.

Rune Aaslid, Ph.D.
Research Associate Professor, Department of Neurological Surgery, University of Washington School of Medicine, Seattle, Washington [9]

Mark J. Alberts, M.D.
Assistant Professor, Division of Neurology, Duke University Medical Center, Durham, North Carolina [22]

Ossama Al-Mefty, M.D.
Professor of Neurosurgery, University of Mississippi Medical Center, Jackson, Mississippi [43]

Robert E. Anderson, B.S.
Research Associate, Department of Neurologic Surgery, Mayo Medical School, Rochester, Minnesota [27]

Arthur G. Arand, M.D.
Resident, Department of Neurosurgery, University of Cincinnati Medical Center, Cincinnati, Ohio [16]

Russell J. Asleson, M.D.
Instructor, Department of Radiology, Medical College of Wisconsin, Milwaukee, Wisconsin [4]

Sarah M. Beale, M.D.
Fellow, Division of Neuroradiology, Case Western Reserve University School of Medicine, Cleveland, Ohio [2]

Darell D. Bigner, M.D., Ph.D.
Edwin L., Jr., and Lucille Finch Jones Cancer Research Professor of Pathology (Neuropathology), Duke University Medical Center, Durham, North Carolina [26]

Sandra H. Bigner, M.D.
Professor, Department of Pathology, Duke University Medical Center, Durham, North Carolina [26]

Russell A. Blinder, M.D.
Assistant Professor, Department of Radiology, Duke University Medical Center, Durham, North Carolina [6]

Derald E. Brackmann, M.D.
Clinical Professor of Otolaryngology, University of Southern California School of Medicine, Los Angeles, California [36]

Jeffrey N. Bruce, M.D.
Resident, Department of Neurological Surgery, College of Physicians & Surgeons of Columbia University, New York, New York [41]

Guy L. Clifton, M.D.
Associate Professor, Division of Neurosurgery, Medical College of Virginia, Richmond, Virginia [20]

James N. Davis, M.D.
Professor of Medicine (Neurology), Pharmacology, and Neurobiology, Duke University Medical Center, Durham, North Carolina [21]

Evandro de Oliveira, M.D.
Clinical Associate Professor, Department of Neurological Surgery, University of Florida College of Medicine, Gainesville, Florida [47]

Jacques E. Dion, M.D.
Assistant Professor, Department of Radiological Sciences, University of California, Los Angeles Medical Center, Los Angeles, California [12]

William T. Djang, M.D.
Wake Radiology Consultants, Raleigh, North Carolina [6]

Gary R. Duckwiler, M.D.
Assistant Professor, Department of Radiological Sciences, University of California, Los Angeles Medical Center, Los Angeles, California [12]

Jonathan J. Dutton, M.D., Ph.D.
Associate Professor, Department of Ophthalmology, Duke University Medical Center, Durham, North Carolina [11]

Peter Dyck, M.D.
Clinical Professor of Neurosurgery, University of Southern California School of Medicine, Los Angeles, California [3]

Michael J. Ebersold, M.D.
Associate Professor, Department of Neurologic Surgery, Mayo Medical School, Rochester, Minnesota [50]

Joseph C. Farmer, Jr., M.D.
Associate Professor, Division of Otolaryngology, Duke University Medical Center, Durham, North Carolina [15]

Michael R. Fetell, M.D.
Clinical Associate Professor, Department of Neurology, College of Physicians & Surgeons of Columbia University, New York, New York [41]

Herbert E. Fuchs, M.D., Ph.D.
Resident, Division of Neurosurgery, Duke University Medical Center, Durham, North Carolina [26]

Alberto A. Gabbai, M.D.
Associate Professor of Neurology, University of São Paulo, São Paulo, Brazil [24]

Manning M. Goldsmith, M.D.
Former Assistant Professor, Department of Otolaryngology-Head and Neck Surgery, The Johns Hopkins University School of Medicine, Baltimore, Maryland [34]

Larry B. Goldstein, M.D.
Assistant Professor of Medicine (Neurology), Duke University Medical Center, Durham, North Carolina [21]

Linda Gray, M.D.
Assistant Professor, Department of Radiology, Duke University Medical Center, Durham, North Carolina [6]

John R. Green, M.D.
Senior Consultant, Barrow Neurological Institute, Phoenix, Arizona [1]

Barton L. Guthrie, M.D.
Assistant Professor, Department of Neurological Surgery, George Washington University Medical Center, Washington, District of Columbia [50]

Griffith R. Harsh IV, M.D.
Assistant Professor, Department of Neurological Surgery, School of Medicine, University of California, San Francisco, San Francisco, California [46]

Victor M. Haughton, M.D.
Professor of Radiology and Biophysics, Medical College of Wisconsin, Milwaukee, Wisconsin [4]

William E. Hitselberger, M.D.
Neurosurgeon, Otologic Medical Group, Inc., Los Angeles, California [35]

Fred H. Hochberg, M.D.
Attending Neurologist, Massachusetts General Hospital, Boston, Massachusetts [24]

William F. House, M.D.
Clinical Professor of Otolaryngology, University of Southern California School of Medicine, Los Angeles, California [35]

Ian T. Jackson, M.B., Ch.B.
Director, Institute of Craniofacial and Reconstructive Surgery, Providence Hospital, Southfield, Michigan [29]

Michael E. Johns, M.D.
Andelot Professor and Chairman, Department of Otolaryngology-Head and Neck Surgery, The Johns Hopkins University School of Medicine, Baltimore, Maryland [34]

Andrew B. Kaufman, M.D.
Associate Clinical Professor of Surgery, University of Missouri at Kansas City School of Medicine, Kansas City, Missouri [10]

Wayne M. Koch, M.D.
Assistant Professor, Department of Otolaryngology-Head and Neck Surgery, The Johns Hopkins University School of Medicine, Baltimore, Maryland [31]

Walter Kucharczyk, M.D.
Assistant Professor, Department of Radiology, University of Toronto, Toronto, Ontario [5]

Edward R. Laws, Jr., M.D.
Professor and Chairman, Department of Neurological Surgery, George Washington University Medical Center, Washington, District of Columbia [27]

Don M. Long, M.D., Ph.D.
Professor and Director, Department of Neurosurgery, The Johns Hopkins University School of Medicine, Baltimore, Maryland [28]

Roger Lowlicht, M.S., D.D.S.
Assistant Clinical Professor, Section of Otolaryngology, Yale University School of Medicine, New Haven, Connecticut [33]

Pedro Lylyk, M.D.
Clinical Instructor, Department of Radiological Sciences, University of California, Los Angeles Medical Center, Los Angeles, California [12]

Leonard I. Malis, M.D.
Professor and Chairman, Department of Neurosurgery, The School of Medicine of the City University of New York, New York, New York [42]

Paul C. McAfee, M.D.
Associate Professor, Department of Orthopedic Surgery, The Johns Hopkins University School of Medicine, Baltimore, Maryland [34]

Paul C. McCormick, M.D.
Assistant Professor, Department of Neurological Surgery, College of Physicians & Surgeons of Columbia University, New York, New York [38]

John T. McElveen, Jr., M.D.
Assistant Professor, Division of Otolaryngology, Duke University Medical Center, Durham, North Carolina [35, 44]

Arnold H. Menezes, M.D.
Professor and Vice-Chairman, Division of Neurosurgery, University of Iowa College of Medicine, Iowa City, Iowa [32]

Kenneth D. Miller, Jr., M.D.
Clinical Associate Professor of Radiology, Tulane University School of Medicine, New Orleans, Louisiana [8]

Michael T. Modic, M.D.
Professor of Radiology and Neurosurgery, Case Western Reserve University School of Medicine, Cleveland, Ohio [2]

Aage R. Møller, Ph.D.
Professor of Neurological Surgery, University of Pittsburgh School of Medicine, Pittsburgh, Pennsylvania [14]

Robert A. Morantz, M.D.
Clinical Professor of Neurosurgery and of Radiation Oncology, University of Kansas School of Medicine; Director, Brain Tumor Institute of Kansas City, Kansas City, Missouri [25]

David W. Newell, M.D.
Assistant Professor of Neurological Surgery, University of Washington School of Medicine, Seattle, Washington [9]

Robert G. Ojemann, M.D.
Visiting Neurosurgeon, Massachusetts General Hospital, Boston, Massachusetts [45]

Michio Ono, M.D.
Research Fellow, Department of Neurological Surgery, University of Florida College of Medicine, Gainesville, Florida [40]

Roger J. Packer, M.D.
Professor of Neurology, University of Pennsylvania School of Medicine, Philadelphia, Pennsylvania [48]

Roy A. Patchell, M.D.
Assistant Professor of Neurosurgery and Neurology, University of Kentucky, Albert B. Chandler Medical Center, Lexington, Kentucky [51]

Richard D. Penn, M.D.
Professor of Neurosurgery, Rush Medical College, Chicago, Illinois [13]

Kalmon D. Post, M.D.
Professor and Vice-Chairman, Department of Neurological Surgery, College of Physicians & Surgeons of Columbia University, New York, New York [38]

John C. Price, M.D.
Associate Professor, Department of Otolaryngology-Head and Neck Surgery, The Johns Hopkins University School of Medicine, Baltimore, Maryland [31]

Charles E. Rawlings III, M.D.
Former Resident, Division of Neurosurgery, Duke University Medical Center, Durham, North Carolina [19]

Setti S. Rengachary, M.D.
Professor and Chief, Section of Neurological Surgery, University of Missouri at Kansas City School of Medicine, Kansas City, Missouri [49]

Albert L. Rhoton, Jr., M.D.
R.D. Keene Family Professor and Chairman, Department of Neurological Surgery, University of Florida College of Medicine, Gainesville, Florida [39, 40, 47]

Allen D. Roses, M.D.
Jefferson-Pilot Corporation Professor of Neurobiology and Neurology, Duke University Medical Center, Durham, North Carolina [22]

Eugene Rossitch, Jr., M.D.
Resident, Division of Neurosurgery, Duke University Medical Center, Durham, North Carolina [17]

Richard Anthony Ruiz, M.D.
Instructor, Section of Otolaryngology, Yale University School of Medicine, New Haven, Connecticut [33]

H. Earl Ruley, Ph.D.
Associate Professor, Department of Biology and Center for Cancer Research, Massachusetts Institute of Technology, Cambridge, Massachusetts [23]

Clarence T. Sasaki, M.D.
Oshe Professor and Chairman, Section of Otolaryngology, Yale University School of Medicine, New Haven, Connecticut [33]

Raymond Sawaya, M.D.
Associate Professor, Department of Neurosurgery, University of Cincinnati Medical Center, Cincinnati, Ohio [16]

Bernd Scheithauer, M.D.
Professor of Pathology, Mayo Medical School, Rochester, Minnesota [50]

Henry H. Schmidek, M.D.
Vice-Chairman, Department of Neurosurgery, Henry Ford Neurosurgical Institute, Detroit, Michigan [23]

Luis Schut, M.D.
Professor of Neurosurgery, University of Pennsylvania School of Medicine, Philadelphia, Pennsylvania [48]

Laligam N. Sekhar, M.D.
Associate Professor, Department of Neurological Surgery, University of Pittsburgh School of Medicine, Pittsburgh, Pennsylvania [30, 37]

Chandra Nath Sen, M.D.
Assistant Professor, Department of Neurological Surgery, University of Pittsburgh School of Medicine, Pittsburgh, Pennsylvania [30, 37]

Clough Shelton, M.D.
Clinical Assistant Professor of Otolaryngology, University of Southern California School of Medicine, Los Angeles, California [35]

Roger M. L. Smith, M.B., Ch.B.
Fellow, Department of Radiology, University of Toronto, Toronto, Ontario [5]

Bennett M. Stein, M.D.
Byron Stookey Professor of Neurological Surgery, College of Physicians & Surgeons of Columbia University, New York, New York [41]

Leslie N. Sutton, M.D.
Associate Professor of Neurosurgery, University of Pennsylvania School of Medicine, Philadelphia, Pennsylvania [48]

Hope Turner, R.N., M.S.
Research Associate, Division of Neurosurgery, Medical College of Virginia, Richmond, Virginia [20]

Fernando Viñuela, M.D.
Director, Endovascular Therapy Service, Department of Radiological Sciences, University of California, Los Angeles Medical Center, Los Angeles, California [12]

Victor Waluch, Ph.D., M.D.
Clinical Professor of Radiology, University of Southern California School of Medicine, Los Angeles, California [3]

Robert E. Wharen, Jr., M.D.
Neurologic Surgery, Mayo Clinic Jacksonville, Jacksonville, Florida [27]

Robert H. Wilkins, M.D.
Professor and Chief, Division of Neurosurgery, Duke University Medical Center, Durham, North Carolina [17, 19]

Charles B. Wilson, M.D.
Tong-Po Kan Professor and Chairman, Department of Neurological Surgery, School of Medicine, University of California, San Francisco, San Francisco, California [46]

H. Richard Winn, M.D.
Professor and Chairman, Department of Neurological Surgery, University of Washington School of Medicine, Seattle, Washington [9]

Fremont P. Wirth, M.D.
Neurological Institute of Savannah, Savannah, Georgia [18]

Byron Young, M.D.
Johnston-Wright Chair of Surgery, University of Kentucky, Albert B. Chandler Medical Center, Lexington, Kentucky [51]

Michael R. Zalutsky, Ph.D.
Associate Professor of Radiology, Duke University Medical Center, Durham, North Carolina [26]

Robert A. Zimmerman, M.D.
Professor of Radiology, University of Pennsylvania School of Medicine, Philadelphia, Pennsylvania [7]

FOREWORD

One of the most important problems encountered on a daily basis by the neurosurgeon in community practice, the neurosurgeon in an academic department, the neurosurgical resident, the medical student interested in neurosurgery, and the physician in an allied discipline is the need to keep up to date with the knowledge that that individual must have to give the best care to his or her patients. Sources of information include weekly and monthly journals, books, postgraduate lecture courses, practical instructional courses, individual lectures, hospital rounds, medical society meetings, discussions with colleagues, audio and video tapes, computer simulations of clinical problems, and computer searches for specific topics. All have a role, and the physician must decide how best to manage the precious time available for ongoing education.

Of particular importance to the neurosurgeon is the immediate availability of a concise summary of the important aspects of a clinical problem containing the relevant information of both new and old knowledge. This need was met in 1985 when Dr. Robert H. Wilkins and Dr. Setti S. Rengachary edited the three-volume textbook, *Neurosurgery*, containing 352 chapters. What make this such an outstanding reference source, to which I have referred many times, are the wide range of subjects covered, the emphasis that the editors place on presenting established as well as evolving techniques, the selection of authors for their knowledge and expertise, the balance of basic and clinical sciences, the pre-

sentation of subjects such as neuropathology and neuroradiology in conjunction with the related clinical subject, the careful selection of pertinent references, the inclusion of historical aspects of neurosurgery, the discussion of practical subjects needed by the neurosurgeon, and the fact that the two editors are active practicing neurosurgeons who understand the needs of their colleagues.

Five years later most of the information in *Neurosurgery* is still current. However, a massive amount of new information has developed. The authors have successfully edited two companion works, or updates, which essentially follow the same basic format as *Neurosurgery* and digest this new information into a form that is easily accessed. The *Neurosurgery Updates* provide concise summaries on new diagnostic studies, new and refined surgical techniques, advances in basic science that relate to the neurosurgeon, advances in medical, radiologic, and surgical therapy related to neurosurgical problems, and some uncommon disorders not covered in the original text. In addition, the history of cerebral and spinal localization is reviewed.

These five volumes will provide the neurosurgeon with immediate access to a concise presentation on almost any problem or question that will be encountered in the daily practice of neurosurgery.

Robert G. Ojemann, M.D.
Boston, Massachusetts

PREFACE

The explosion of new knowledge since the publication, in 1985, of the three-volume work *Neurosurgery* has stimulated us to bring this work up to date. Because so much material in those three volumes is still current, however, a formal second edition seemed premature. We have decided to address new developments in our field with two companion volumes, or *Updates*, the second of which will be published in late 1990.

The enthusiastic response to the first edition of *Neurosurgery* has encouraged us to follow essentially the same format in *Neurosurgery Update I: Diagnosis, Operative Technique, and Neuro-Oncology*. We perceive that two areas have made significant strides since the original publication—magnetic resonance imaging and techniques in the management of tumors involving the base of the skull. Most of this volume is devoted to these two areas. However, in planning for the present work, we carefully reviewed the progress made in every area of neurosurgery and its allied fields and tried to incorporate every new development of significance to neurosurgeons. In addition, some rare or uncommon lesions of the nervous system such as histiocytosis X, paraganglioma of the cauda equina, and pituitary carcinoma, which were not part of the previous volumes, are included in *Neurosurgery Update* for completeness.

Neurosurgery Update, as was true of *Neurosurgery*, would not have been possible without the enthusiastic response from the contributors who shared their expertise. We sincerely thank all of them, and especially Robert G. Ojemann, M.D., who also prepared the Foreword. We express our appreciation of J. Dereck Jeffers, Sally J. Barhydt, and Mariapaz R. Englis of the Health Professions Division at McGraw-Hill for their work in the preparation of this volume. We thank Gloria K. Wilkins for her tireless secretarial efforts and Elizabeth Adams for checking the accuracy of all of the references at the Duke Medical Center Library. Finally, we thank our wives and children for their devotion and support.

Robert H. Wilkins, M.D.
Setti S. Rengachary, M.D.

Neurosurgery Update I

Diagnosis, Operative Technique,
and Neuro-Oncology

1

The Concept of Cerebral and Spinal Localization and the Beginnings of Neurological Surgery

John R. Green

The beginnings of our knowledge about the brain and spinal cord are first recorded in the Edwin Smith surgical papyrus, the most complete treatise on surgery of all antiquity.[3] This is a compilation of ancient manuscripts believed to have been written about 1700 B.C.—a summation of the knowledge of the Egyptian counselor to the Pharaoh Zoser, Imhotep, and his disciples. Professor JH Breasted of the University of Chicago published in facsimile hieroglyphic transliteration a translation and commentary on the Edwin Smith surgical papyrus. The papyrus was not discovered until 1862, but Breasted has commented, if the work of Imhotep and his followers had been known as early as the writings of Hippocrates and his disciples, the title "Father of Medicine" might properly have been considered for Imhotep.

The brain is mentioned for the first time in history. Paralysis of the bladder and intestines is noted to occur with lesions of the spinal cord. Diagnosis and treatment of 48 injured patients are described, as are phenomena following severe cranial and spinal injuries.

The slow progression from ancient views about brain structure and function to contemporary knowledge of anatomy and physiology is outlined in Tables 1-1 to 1-7. The beginnings of cerebral localization, neurology, and neurological surgery were established more than a century ago by many investigators in many different countries.[21] A hundred years ago, our predecessors inquired whether motor function, general sensation, mental activity, and vision were localized to specific regions of the brain, but they did not probe in any detail into the submodalities of these functions.

TABLE 1-1 Ancient Views of Brain Function[21]

1. Primitive peoples: Unknown.
2. Egyptian (3000–1000 B.C.): Phenomena following severe cranial and spinal injuries described. Respiration believed to be the carrier of every vital function.
3. Homeric (1000 B.C.): Life thought to reside in the breath. The seat of the soul was conceived to be in the diaphragm.
4. Greek:
   a. Pythagoras (580–489 B.C.): Placed the rational soul in the brain.
   b. Alcmaeon (500 B.C.): Brain, not diaphragm or heart, was the seat of senses and center of intellect.
   c. Hippocrates (460–377 B.C.): Brain considered as the most powerful organ of the body, seat of pleasures and sorrow, and messenger of consciousness and movement.
   d. Plato (428–348 B.C.): Immortal human soul in brain; mortal soul in torso; heart, source of blood.
   e. Aristotle (384–322 B.C.): Liver, mirror of soul; heart, seat of emotions; brain, to cool blood.
   f. Herophilus (300 B.C.): Brain, center of nervous system; described four ventricles; differentiated nerves from tendons; divided nerves into motor and sensory.
   g. Erasistratos (290 B.C.): Greater complexity of brain of man associated with his higher intelligence.

The discussion on the subject of localization of function in the cerebral cortex that occurred at a meeting of the International Medical Congress in London in 1881 marked a milestone in our knowledge of the subject.[38] Goltz of Strasbourg confronted Ferrier of London. Goltz argued against specific cerebral localization because precise ablations of the cerebral cortex in Goltz's animal model showed restitution of function and because general rather than specific residual disabilities resulted after cerebral lesions in his dog model. Ferrier argued in favor of cerebral localization of specific brain functions. Ferrier's monkeys demonstrated without question that localized lesions could produce loss of specific motor, sensory, or visual functions (Fig. 1-1). A council appointed by the congress, recognizing species differences, ruled in favor in Ferrier. The work of the localizationists

TABLE 1-2 Cerebral Localization: Sixteen Centuries A.D.[21]

1. Galen (A.D. 130–200): Brain, center for motion and sensation; body, instrument of the soul; disproved that voice comes from heart; disproved that heart is seat of intelligence and will.
2. Posidonius of Byzantium (4th century): Began the ventricular doctrine of seat of soul and of mental functions.
3. Nemusius of Syria (390): Frontal ventricles: imagination, psychical spirits, and sense organs; middle part of brain: intellect, divining dreams, and prognostication; hinder brain: memory and its vital spirit.
4. Avicenna (980–1037): Elaborated on the ventricular doctrine of psychological functions; no interest in cerebral cortex; great interest in white matter, ventricles, and subcortical connections.
5. Andreas Vesalius (1514–1564): Father of anatomy, began modern biological science; detailed account of the ventricles; denounced localization of mental functions in the ventricles.
6. Ambroise Paré (1510–1590): Described symptoms and signs of increased intracranial pressure and surgical treatment.

TABLE 1-3 Cerebral Localization: Seventeenth and Eighteenth Centuries[21]

1. William Harvey (1578–1657): Discovered the circulation of blood; introduced experimental physiology; no new information on cerebral localization.
2. René Descartes (1596–1650): Localized seat of soul in pineal gland.
3. Thomas Willis (1621–1675): Cerebrum controls voluntary movements and sensation; cerebellum controls involuntary movements such as the heart and lungs; corpus striatum, receives all sensations and is seat of sensus communis; corpus callosum, where imagination takes place; cerebral cortex, where memories are stored.[12]
4. John Locke (1630–1704): Like Willis, rejected "innate ideas" of Descartes; concept of the mind as a blank tablet; softened the rigid separation of mind and body; stimulated anatomists and physiologists to consider a connection.
5. Giovanni Battista Morgagni (1682–1771): Introduced anatomic thinking into pathology; localized pathological lesions in definite organs; described most of the pathological lesions with which we are familiar today; chapter "On Diseases of the Head," structural link between lesions and syndromes.
6. Albrecht van Heller (1708–1777): Denied that any one part of cerebrum controls motion; all portions of central nervous system are equal; opposed location of the soul in the central nervous system.

TABLE 1-4 Cerebral Localization: Early Nineteenth Century[21]

1. Franz Josef Gall (1758–1828): First to draw widespread attention to the cerebral convolutions and their functions.[18]
2. Julien Jean Legallois (1770–1814): Earliest precise localization of functions in brain; discovery of respiratory center in medulla (1811).
3. Luigi Rolando (1773–1831): One of first to study effects of electrical current on the brain of animals; suggested movements.
4. Charles Bell (1774–1842): Established that nerves of special senses are traceable from specific areas of the brain to their end organs, and that spinal nerves carry sensory functions in posterior roots and motor functions in anterior roots.
5. Francois Magendie (1783–1855): Independently and more completely verified "Bell's Law"; described foramen of Magendie.
6. Pierre Flourens (1794–1867): Pioneered technique of precise extirpation of cerebral cortex in pigeons, rabbits, dogs; concluded that nervous system formed a single system, making him a strong opponent of localization.
7. Jean Baptiste Bouillaud (1796–1875): Brain role in movements, intelligence, and volition; speech localization is in the anterior lobes.
8. Robert Bentley Todd (1825): Mentation, voluntary movement, and emotions are functions of the cerebral cortex, corpus striatum, and upper midbrain, respectively.
9. Herbert Spencer (1855): Described developmental levels of human intellect; suggested that brain must have localized functions; profound influence on John Hughlings Jackson.
10. Rudolf Virchow (1858): Established cell as central unit in pathology, finally destroying ancient "humoral" pathology.

TABLE 1-5 Early Anatomical Studies of Cerebral Localization[21]

1. Gennari (1782) and Vic d'Azyr (1786): Described the white line in cerebral cortex near the calcarine fissure.
2. JGF Baillarger (1840): Intimate connections between white and gray matter of the cerebral cortex were discovered; ushered in modern conceptions of cortical function.
3. Louis Pierre Gratiolet (1854): Modern description of the cerebral convolutions and nomenclature.
4. Theodor Meynert (1867–68): First detailed histological study of cerebral cortex; cortex as a complex center for all cerebral processes because of "association" fibers and the "radiations of Meynert" between the cortex and the basal ganglia.

and of the antilocalizationists has continued, resulting in our current, more moderate concepts.

The British School

Following John Hughlings Jackson (Fig. 1-2),[29,41] WR Gowers[20] (Jackson's former registrar) asked the following advanced questions concerning the localization and etiology of epileptic seizures as early as 1881:

1. What is the seat of the discharge which thus produces the symptoms of the fit?
2. Is the seat of the discharge the seat of the disease?
3. How far does such discharge explain the symptoms of the attack?
4. What is the nature of the morbid change which causes the discharge?

TABLE 1-6 Cerebral Localization: Later Nineteenth Century[21]

1. Pierre Paul Broca (1824–1880)[4,39]: Confirmed the principle of localization, finding the third frontal convolution as the one which presents the most extensive loss of substance in cases of "aphemia," "the convolution of Broca" (Ferrier) (1861).
2. John Hughlings Jackson (1835–1911)[41]: Nervous system is sensory-motor machine with many coordinated centers; suggested probability of motor centers within the territory of the middle cerebral artery, but less precise and circumscribed than Broca and Wernicke thought; postulated three evolutionary levels of sensory-motor mechanisms—lowest in spinal cord, medulla and brain stem, middle being the rolandic level, and highest in the prefrontal lobes.
3. Jean Martin Charcot (1825–1893): Brain is not a homogeneous organ but an association of different areas, each having different functions; first to show cortical topography of human brain lesions that cause motor dysfunction and the degeneration of the pyramidal tracts.
4. Carl Wernicke (1848–1904): Published first comprehensive account of the achievements in cerebral localization (1881–1883); his theory of the nature of aphasia placed the auditory center in the first temporal convolution and the conceptual basis of articulated speech in Broca's area.

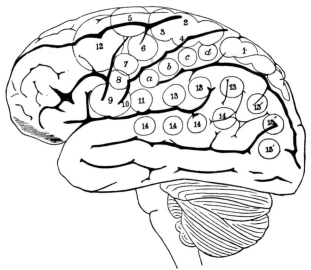

Figure 1-1 Ferrier's cortical map, 1876. (From Clarke and O'Malley.[6]) (1) Center for movements of the opposite leg and foot as are concerned in locomotion. (2) (3) (4) Centers for various complex movements of arms and legs, as in climbing and swimming. (5) Center for extension forward of arm and hand, as in putting forth hand to touch something in front. (6) Center for movements of hand and forearm, in which biceps is particularly engaged; supination of hand and flexion of forearm. (7) (8) Centers for the elevators and depressors of the angles of the mouth, respectively. (9) (10) Center for movements of lips and tongue, as in articulation; disease causes aphasia; generally known as "Broca's convolution." (11) Center of the platysma; retraction of angle of mouth. (12) Center for lateral movement of the head and eyes, with elevation of the eyelids and dilation of the pupil. (a) (b) (c) (d) Centers for movement of the head and wrist. (13) (13′) Center of vision; supramarginal lobule and angular gyrus. (14) Center of hearing; superior temporosphenoidal convolution. The center of smell is situated in the subiculum cornu Ammonis. The center of taste is near the center of smell but not defined. The center of touch is in the hippocampal region.

The next member of the British school to extend investigations, with electrical stimulation on the motor area of the rhesus monkey, was Victor Horsley (1857–1916)[24,26–28] of the University College Hospital, London. Horsley carried out similar experiments on cortical localization in the orangutan and in human beings. He joined the staff of the National Hospital, Queen Square, London, in 1886, when he did his first operation there for focal epilepsy associated with a meningocortical cicatrix. Contemporary knowledge of localization of cortical function was limited. Horsley's accurate scientific methods confirmed the deductions made by Jackson from his study of epilepsy. Horsley, because of his work, has been termed the "Founder of Modern Neurological Surgery." Horsley and his associates published pioneer-

TABLE 1-7 Neurophysiological Studies of Cerebral Localization[21]

1. Edward Hitzig (1838–1907) and Gustav Theodor Fritsch (1838–1927): Started a new era in the concept of cerebral localization in 1870, crudely mapped out the motor part of the cerebral cortex of dogs by electrical stimulation; also concluded that individual psychological functions were in circumscribed centers of the cerebral cortex.[16]
2. David Ferrier (1843–1928)[13,14]: Confirmed the findings of Hitzig and Fritsch in the monkey, and put to experimental proof the views of Hughlings Jackson on the pathology of epilepsy, chorea, and hemiplegia; developed a map of cortical functions of the monkey brain and transferred them to a diagram of the human brain in 1876 (Fig. 1-1).
3. Herman Munk (1839–1912): Criticized, corrected, and extended the work of Ferrier; his contributions to visual neurophysiology are classic.
4. Friedrich Leopold Goltz (1834–1902): Through experiments on dogs, was able to show circumscribed functional areas of the cerebral cortex, isolated by electrical stimulation, their function confirmed by operative ablation, leaving no severe (permanent) deficits of movement, sensation, or intellect; an important pioneer in the modern holistic theory of cortical function; took the unwarranted step of applying the findings of his dogs to the physiology of the monkey and human brain.

ing contributions about cerebral localization and surgery (Fig. 1-3).

The third British series of experiments on cortical localization were those conducted by Charles Sherrington (1857–1952), the "Father of Modern Neurophysiology" (Fig. 1-4).

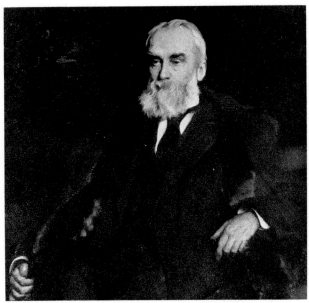

Figure 1-2 John Hughlings Jackson (1835–1911), one of the founders of cerebral localization and of neurology. Courtesy of the Williams and Wilkins Co., Baltimore. (From Holmes G, The National Hospital, Queen Square, 1860–1948. London, Livingstone, 1954.)

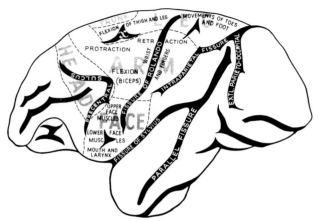

Figure 1-3 Horsley's cortical map, 1888. Somatotopic representation of the motor cortex of the monkey (external surface) published by Horsley and Schäfer in 1888. Courtesy of the Royal Society of London. (From Horsley V, Schäfer EA: A record of experiments upon the functions of the cerebral cortex. *Philos Trans R Soc Lond* 179B:1–45, 1888.)

in association with ASF Grünbaum (1869–1921). Like Ferrier, Sherrington and Grünbaum transferred the results from their primate investigations to the human brain, mainly because of the latter's evolutionary proximity to the brain of higher primates.[5,6] Sherrington collaborated in the proceedings of the council that investigated the evidence and laboratory animals in the Goltz-Ferrier dispute of 1881. He spent 1 year with Goltz in Strasbourg and parted with a gift of three monkeys to Goltz. According to historians, Goltz suspected Sherrington's motive was to suggest repetition of Ferrier's experiments on cerebral localization with higher species of experimental animals instead of using dogs.

Among their 300 publications, Sherrington and his colleagues contributed a number related to cerebral localization. By the end of the nineteenth century, the work of Grünbaum and Sherrington had established separation of the motor area in the prerolandic zone and the sensory area in the postrolandic zone in higher primates. They employed unipolar faradic current from an inductorium that allowed finer localization than would have been possible with the usual bipolar electrode. Sherrington's associates, Sharpey-Schäfer and Brown, did the first detailed study of the temporal lobe cortex in 1888, noting that ablation did not alter auditory function, as had been reported by Ferrier, but caused a profound mental change in some of their monkeys, an observation that was not appreciated at the time. Sherrington's classic, *The Integrative Action of the Nervous System*, first published in 1906 and again in 1947, defined reciprocal innervation, the synapse, and the function of the motor cortex.[40]

Structure and Function

At the beginning of this past century, there were differences of opinion regarding whether there was discrete localization of function in the cerebral cortex or whether function was the general responsibility of the whole cortex or the whole nervous system.[22]

Neuron and Nerve Network Controversy

Camillo Golgi, with his silver staining technique, discovered previously invisible nerve structures and connections, leading him to become the most influential proponent of the nerve network doctrine in 1883. Wilhelm His's equally brilliant studies of nervous tissue in 1887 led him to conclude that all nerve connections were indirect or arose secondarily, opposing Golgi's network theory. His's concept was one of independence of nerve units. August Forel independently confirmed the work of His in 1887, as did Santiago Ramon y Cajal in 1888, and HWG von Waldeyer-Hartz in 1891. Waldeyer applied the term *neuron* to the independent nerve unit, and this concept of nerve tissue became known as the neuron doctrine—suggesting a possible anatomic basis for localization of function. Cajal, more than anyone else, was instrumental in establishing that the neuron theory was not a theory but a fact. The Nobel laureates in physiology or medicine in 1906 were Golgi and Cajal.

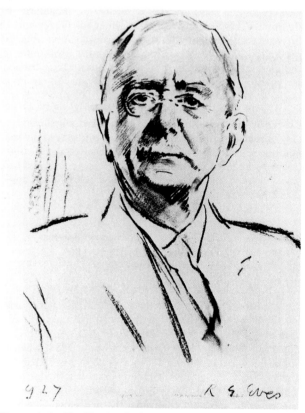

Figure 1-4 Sir Charles S. Sherrington (1857–1952), "Father of Modern Neurophysiology." (From Haymaker W, Schiller F: The founders of neurology. Springfield, IL, Charles C Thomas, 1970.)

Correlation of Structure and Function

The first detailed histological study of the cerebral cortex (in 1867 and 1868) by Theodore Meynert, of Austria, referred to the possible association of cell morphology and function. For Meynert the cerebral cortex was a complex center for all cerebral processes because it was connected with other structures and parts of itself by means of projection, commissural, and association fibers. Paul Emil Flechsig, of Leipzig, applied his method of myelogenesis to the brain in 1893. His work was based on the fact that the nerve fibers in the different parts of the nervous system of the developing human fetus and infant receive their myelin sheath at different stages of growth. He identified groups of fibers and their dependent cortical areas in a chronological sequence of development; function was possible only when myelinization was complete. He isolated projection areas, motor or sensory, that were dependent upon fibers that matured early, chiefly before birth, and neighboring association areas, controlling intellectual functions, fibers which matured after birth. This was an outstanding contribution to the history of cortical localization because his basic divisions into motor, sensory, and association were correct even though many of his conclusions have been disproved.

Alfred W Campbell, Sherrington's associate, made one of the first and most adequate comparative studies of the cytoarchitecture of the anthropoid cerebral cortex with correlation of histology and function in 1903. Based upon Grünbaum's and Sherrington's studies of human and anthropoid brains, further work was published in 1905. Campbell's approach was factual, was without speculation, and contained excellent drawings. Campbell pointed out the deficiency in all brain maps, i.e., the artist's inability to show parts of the buried cortex. He believed that the histologist must follow the clinician and physiologist in the study of cortical function in order to obtain more accurate information about the extent and limits of differentiated areas.

Oskar and Cecile Vogt, of Berlin, contended that every recognizable difference in cortical structure represented a functional variation. Their work was more extensive than that of the other workers in the field but was accepted by few. The Vogts inspired Brodmann to specialize in cytoarchitectonics and were collaborators with Otfrid Foerster. They dominated the field of cytoarchitectonic cortical localization in the first decades of the twentieth century. They parceled the cerebral cortex to extremes (over 100 zones). Their results couldn't be duplicated, and they applied their results in animals to human beings.

Korbinian Brodmann was Flechsig's contemporary and Campbell's counterpart in the field of cytoarchitectonics. He was strongly influenced by Alzheimer and by the Vogts. He aimed at correlation between cortical form and functions to substantiate the theory of localization within the cortex. His concept of increasing differentiation during evolution has been amply confirmed. He identified 52 cortical areas, grouped into 11 histological regions. The numbering of Brodmann's areas on cortical maps, first published in 1909, is still widely used.

C von Economo and GN Koskinas brought cytoarchitectonics to an acceptable standard in 1925, dissipating some of the confusion resulting from the Vogts' plethora of cortical areas. Von Economo and Koskinas's massive treatise on cortical cytoarchitectonics reduced the emphasis on functional correlations.

The Antilocalizationists

Friedrich Leopold Goltz was one of the earliest and best known opponents of cortical localization, based on his observations of functional recovery following cortical ablation experiments in dogs, reported in 1881. Later in life, he was willing to accept some of the evidence of the localizationists, being termed a "half-localizationist" by Brodmann in 1911. He thus reached a position closer to the one held today than did his contemporaries. He anticipated some of the concepts of Lashley and the holistic theory of total brain function. Goltz's unwarranted step of applying the physiology of the dog brain to the physiology of the human brain was his major error.

Constantin von Monakow also objected to the parceling of the cerebral cortex by the localizationists. He introduced concepts which made neurology a truly biological science. He summarized his idea of diaschisis in 1911. Diaschisis was considered to represent, in association with other forms of shock, a bridge between nervous phenomena, localized and unlocalized. Immediate symptoms were thought to be an unreliable guide to the functions of a destroyed cortical area because diaschisis produced transient effects at a distance by diminishing or abolishing function. His monograph on cerebral localization in 1914 emphasized that the cerebral cortex functioned by an interplay of many parts, not by the activity of circumscribed areas. To von Monakow, the time factor was essential in the analysis and interpretation of cortical localization, and "chronological layers" rather than spatial ones formed as the brain developed.

Karl S Lashley, American psychologist, based his opinions on physiological ablations in animals and on learning techniques in animals and humans. He was the most important proponent of the controversial holistic theory of cerebral functions. Lashley's theory of functional equivalence of the cerebral cortex supported Goltz's conclusions. He believed that the cerebral cortex acts in an integrated fashion and that there is integration between it and all parts of the brain. He and his colleague, G Clark, regarded architectonic charts as meaningless.

Perspective

One hundred years following the Discussion on the Function of the Cortex Cerebri that took place at the International Medical Congress in London, a meeting was held in Oxford on the same topic on the morning of August 4, 1981. The doctrine of cerebral localization (i.e., that different parts of the cortex normally perform different specialized functions) was not doubted, but there was no unanimity about how to separate or count the number of parts of the cortex or their functions, or about common characteristics of the functions of different parts. The extreme positions of the localizationists and antilocalizationists had mellowed. What emerged from that meeting was an agreement to continue studying cortical function, encompassing the diverse roles of the different parts to explain the plasticity that must underlie the restitution of function that so impressed early antilocalizationists.

The Beginnings of Neurological Surgery

The advances in neurological localization and the addition of aseptic surgery made possible the beginnings of neurological surgery.[30] Surgery in the pre-Listerian era, when there was a paucity of knowledge about brain functions, and wounds of any type became infected, was particularly discouraging. In the 1860s Semmelweiss brought asepsis to obstetrics and Lister[33,34] initiated antisepsis in surgery, particularly surgery in the abdominal cavity. However, the development of intracranial surgery was slow because of the paucity of knowledge of cerebral localization.

A few early post-Listerian pioneers of neurological surgery began to exploit the benefits of antiseptic surgery with the limited knowledge of brain function. During the last part of the nineteenth century, neurological surgery was performed by a handful of general surgeons who had become interested in diseases of the nervous system. The first textbook on surgery of the nervous system was written in 1870 by Ernst von Bergmann of Germany. Bergmann, the dominant surgeon in Berlin, instituted an aseptic operative ritual, an advance over the Listerian antiseptic technique.[42]

Pierre Paul Broca, of Paris, was the first surgeon to neurologically localize an occult intracranial lesion (an extradural abscess) in the speech area and to drain it surgically in 1876.[4,39] Sir William Macewen, of Glasgow, neurologically localized an abscess in Broca's lobe in 1876; he advised surgery but was not allowed to proceed. Autopsy proved his diagnosis to be correct. Macewen, utilizing neurological localization and Listerian antiseptic surgical techniques, was the first to successfully remove a tumor (meningioma) of the dura mater in 1879; the patient made a long-term recovery. Macewen localized and removed five additional lesions before 1884. Between 1883 and 1886, he reported five laminectomies performed for paraplegia, in some cases caused by pressure from granulomatous tumors on the spinal cord. He was a surgical pioneer—a remarkable and versatile genius (Fig. 1-5).[2,31,35,36]

Francesco Durante of Rome diagnosed an olfactory groove meningioma and successfully removed it in May 1884.[10,11] Rickman J Godlee, Lister's nephew, in association with A Hughes Bennett of London, was persuaded by David Ferrier, who also had consulted with Hughlings Jackson, to remove a tumor from a patient's right midmotor area. With the collaboration of Jackson and Lister, the glioma was subtotally excised from the right midmotor region. The operation, performed on November 25, 1884, provided further acceptance and impetus for the developing specialty of neurological surgery.[1,21]

Sir Victor Horsley, of London, was prepared to develop surgery of the nervous system by virtue of his training in antiseptic neurosurgery, neuroanatomy, neurophysiology, and neuropathology (Fig. 1-6). He may properly be regarded as the first specialized surgical neurologist. Previous

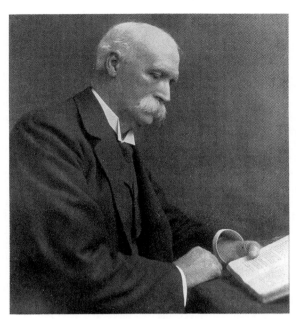

Figure 1-5 Sir William Macewen (1848–1924), pioneer British neurological surgeon. Courtesy of William Hodge and Co., Ltd., London. (From Bowman.[2])

general surgeons had had the courage to operate on the nervous system but lacked the stimulus of colleagues whose attention centered on the brain. Horsley, as a result of his associates at the National Hospital's Institute of Neurology, was encouraged to explore new territory for his surgical talents. Their acceptance of Horsley and his work was a remarkable impetus for neuroscience and neurological sur-

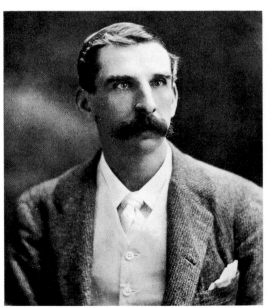

Figure 1-6 Sir Victor Horsley (1857–1916), the first specialized surgical neurologist. Courtesy of the *British Medical Journal*, July 29, 1916.

gery.[24,26–28] Neither he nor Macewen left many personal disciples to posterity. They were individualists.

Contemporaneous with Horsley were a number of leading general surgeons in Europe who made special endeavors in the field of neurological surgery. Fedor Krause of Berlin, founder of German neurological surgery, was one of the first to study the human cerebral cortex in detail. In a lightly anesthetized patient on whom he was operating for a cortical scar, he carefully explored the motor area and other cortical regions with unipolar faradic stimulation while three assistants observed the responses. His findings were recorded in a publication in 1908–1911. He placed the leg area of the homunculus at the vertex of the convexity, instead of in the paracentral area on the medial surface, an error that was not corrected until 1940. His observations on stimulation of the brains of epileptics led him to conclude that "the faradic stimulation of the cerebral cortex in the operating room represents an indispensable method of investigation. It offers the only way to obtain accurate information regarding the central convolution." His works culminated in his remarkable textbook in 1911 on surgery of the brain and spinal cord.[22]

In Paris, Thiery de Martel provided surgery for the French neurologists. He modeled his work on that performed and reported by Horsley. Clovis Vincent, a neurologist, established modern neurological surgery in France. He started as Babinski's assistant in neurology and transformed the neurological wards at the Pitié into neurosurgical ones. Later with the aid of the Rockefeller Foundation, a chair of neurosurgery was established for him at the Faculté de Médicine.

Otfrid Foerster (1873–1941), of Breslau, joined the ranks of young functionally and morphologically oriented investigators who were interested in the new concepts of localization. He was influenced by Wernicke, with whom he published an atlas of the brain in 1903. According to his biographer, Zülch, Jackson and Sherrington were his heroes. His classical investigations through analysis of hundreds of cortical stimulations carried out during operations for epileptogenic scars of World War I head-injured persons, and analysis of the functional results of the excision of those scars, gained moderate success for the patients and considerable knowledge for Foerster. Shortly after electroencephalography was introduced in 1929 by Berger, Foerster and Altenburger were the first to describe electrocorticography. They applied it to brain tumor localization and focal epilepsy in 1935. On the occasion of Jackson's 100th birthday celebration in 1936, Foerster concisely reported on the stimulation and ablation of the precentral complex.[15,22] A detailed account of his experiences with cerebral localization was published in Bumke's *Handbook of Neurology* in 1936.

Shortly before the turn of the century, Vladimir Bechterev, the notable physiological neurologist of Petrograd, attracted Ludwig Puusepp to his team and created the first academic chair accorded to surgical neurology. With it, Puusepp acquired an international reputation, although his career was blighted by wars and political upheavals.

In North America at this time, WW Keen, Jr, in Philadelphia, acquired a considerable reputation in cranial surgery, among his other surgical endeavors (Fig. 1-7).[23] He became America's earliest pioneer neurological surgeon and

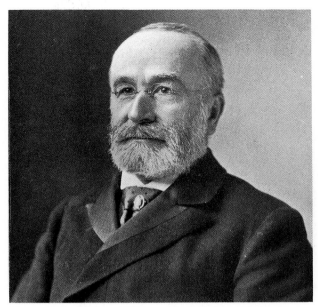

Figure 1-7 William Williams Keen (1837–1932), pioneer American neurological surgeon. Professor of surgery, Thomas Jefferson University College (1889–1907). Courtesy of Historical Section of the National Library of Medicine, Bethesda, Maryland.

contributed to the early development of the specialty. Joseph Lister, who elucidated the antiseptic principles in the practice of surgery in 1867, delivered a stimulating lecture at the International Medical Congress in Philadephia in September 1876. Prior to this time almost no surgeon in America had employed Listerian principles; the concept was also slow in being accepted in Europe. Keen, familiar with Pasteur's work and the great need to control surgical infection, was fully convinced of the practical importance of Lister's contributions. He adopted the antiseptic system on October 1, 1876, the first surgeon in Philadelphia, and one of the first in America, to do so.

Keen was familiar with the contemporary contributions to brain surgery by William Macewen in Glasgow and Victor Horsley in London, both of whom had adopted Listerian antiseptic methods of surgery. In agreement with Horsley and Macewen, Keen recognized the desirability of suturing the dura mater at the completion of the procedure to minimize the chance of cerebrospinal fluid leakage and cerebral herniation. Keen was the first American to successfully remove a large intracranial meningioma in 1888. Such a tumor had been removed only twice previously in Europe (Macewen and Durante). He provided the first recorded case in America of electrical stimulation of the human cortex during a craniotomy for epilepsy.[32]

Harvey Cushing, of Baltimore, decided to specialize in surgical neurology by 1899 (Fig. 1-8). He was fortunate to have WS Halsted as a surgical mentor and William Osler of the new Johns Hopkins School of Medicine at Baltimore as an inspiring medical teacher. Halsted had developed an ideal surgical technique that fully utilized the advantages of anesthesia and asepsis for the first time, and Cushing inherited

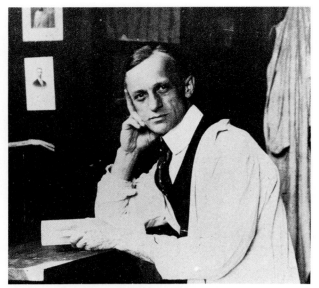

Figure 1-8 Harvey Cushing (1869–1939), founder of the American school of neurological surgery, pictured in 1907 in his laboratory at The Johns Hopkins Hospital. (From Fulton.[17])

this technique. Halsted was also the pioneer of specialization in surgery, encouraging his protégés to specialize in some area of surgery. At first he discouraged Cushing from specializing in neurological surgery on the basis that this speciality was likely to be too unrewarding. He nonetheless provided Cushing with generous opportunities, including a year's travel and study in Europe in 1900–1901. Cushing sternly set himself the task of becoming the best surgical neurologist in the world.

Cushing was the first to map the human cerebral cortex with faradic electrical stimulation in the conscious patient.[8] His results from neurological procedures were so far superior to anything achieved up to that time that they seemed almost incredible. In 1912 he became professor of surgery at

TABLE 1-8 Pioneer Neurological Surgeons[23]

WW Keen, Philadelphia	1837–1932
Francesco Durante, Rome	1844–1934
William Macewen, Glasgow	1848–1924
Rickman J Godlee, London	1849–1925
Fedor Krause, Berlin	1856–1937
Victor Horsley, London	1857–1916
Anthony Chipault, Paris	1866–1920
Harvey Cushing, Boston	1869–1939
Charles H Frazier, Philadelphia	1870–1936
Charles A Elsberg, New York	1871–1948
Thierry de Martel, Paris	1875–1940
Ludvig Puusepp, Tartu, Estonia	1875–1942
NN Burdenko, Moscow	1876–1946
Ernest Sachs, St. Louis	1879–1958
Clovis Vincent, Paris	1879–1947
Walter E Dandy, Baltimore	1886–1946
Makoto Saito, Nagoya	1889–1950
Mizulo Nakata, Nigata	1893–1975

Harvard. His brilliant junior, Walter Dandy, succeeded him at Johns Hopkins. By 1912 Cushing had already achieved international fame as a surgical neurologist and as an expert in pituitary disorders and physiology. He founded the first school of American neurological surgery.[7,17,19,25,37]

More or less contemporaneous with Cushing, and of independent development, were Charles H Frazier, of Philadelphia; Ernest Sachs, of St. Louis; Charles Elsberg, of New York; and Edward Archibald, of Montreal. Frazier had trained with von Bergmann and Virchow in Berlin. Sachs was trained by Horsley in London, Elsberg by von Mikulicz-Radecki in Breslau, and Archibald by Horsley and Gowers in London. Each of these men made distinctive contributions to surgical neurology. Together, they and others founded the Society of Neurological Surgeons in 1920, with Cushing as the first president and Sachs as secretary-treasurer.[9] Eighteen pioneer neurological surgeons are listed in Table 1-8.[23]

References

1. Bennett AH, Godlee RJ. Excision of a tumour from the brain. *Lancet* 1884; 2:1090–1091.
2. Bowman AK. *The Life and Teaching of Sir William Macewen; A Chapter in the History of Surgery.* London: Hodge, 1942.
3. Breasted JH. *The Edwin Smith Surgical Papyrus.* Chicago: The University of Chicago Press, 1930.
4. Broca P. Diagnostic d'un abcès situé au niveau de la region du langage: trépanation de cet abcès. *Rev d'Anthrop* 1876; 5:244-248.
5. Clarke E, Dewhurst K. *An Illustrated History of Brain Function.* Berkeley: Univ California Press, 1972.
6. Clarke E, O'Malley CD. *The Human Brain and Spinal Cord.* Berkeley: Univ California Press, 1968:458–575.
7. Cushing H. Surgery of the head. In: Keen WW (ed.), *Surgery: Its Principles and Practice.* Philadelphia: Saunders, 1908; Vol 3, pp 17–276.
8. Cushing H. A note upon the faradic stimulation of the postcentral gyrus in conscious patients. *Brain* 1909; 32:44–53.
9. Dott N. The history of surgical neurology in the twentieth century. *Proc R Soc Med* 1971; 64:1051–1055.
10. Durante F. Estirpazione di un tumore endocranico. *Arch Soc Chir* 1885; 2:252–255.
11. Durante F. Contribution to endocranial surgery. *Lancet* 1887; 2:654–655.
12. Feindel W (ed.) (Thomas Willis). *The Anatomy of the Brain and Nerves. Tercentenary Edition 1664–1964.* Montreal: McGill Univ Press, 1965.
13. Ferrier D. Experimental researches in cerebral physiology and pathology. *W Riding Lunatic Asylum Med Rep* 1873; 3:30–96.
14. Ferrier D. *The Functions of the Brain.* London: Smith, Elder, 1876.
15. Foerster O. Ueber die Bedeutung und Reichweite des Lokalisationsprinzips im Nervensystem. *Verh Dtsch Ges Inn Med* 1934; 46:117–211.
16. Fritsch G, Hitzig E. Ueber die elektrische Erregbarkeit des Grosshirns. *Arch Anat Physiol* 1870; 37:300–332.
17. Fulton JF. *Harvey Cushing: A Biography.* Springfield, Illinois: Charles C Thomas, 1946.
18. Gall FJ, Spurzheim G. *Anatomie et Physiologie du Système Nerveux en Général, et du Cerveau en Particulier: Avec des Observations sur la Possibilité de Reconnaître Plusiers Dispositions Intellectuelles et Morales de l'Homme et des Animaux par la Configuration*

de Leurs Tetes. Paris: F Schoell, 1810-1819 (Vols I and II by Gall and Spurzheim; Vols III and IV by Gall).

19. Goldring S. The need to trace our roots in difficult times: the 1985 AANS presidential address. *J Neurosurg* 1985; 63: 485–491.

20. Gowers W. *Clinical and Physiological Researches on the Nervous System*. 1: *On the Localization of Movements in the Brain*. London: Churchill, 1875.

21. Green JR. The beginnings of cerebral localization and neurological surgery. *BNI Quart* 1985; 1(1):12–28.

22. Green JR. Cerebral localization during the past century. *BNI Quart* 1985; 1(2):26–40.

23. Green JR. William Williams Keen, Jr.: Pioneer American neurological surgeon. *BNI Quart* 1985; 1(4):15–28.

24. Green JR. Sir Victor Horsley: A centennial recognition of his impact on neuroscience and on neurological surgery. *BNI Quart* 1987; 3(2):2–16.

25. Horrax G. Some of Harvey Cushing's contributions to neurological surgery. *J Neurosurg* 1944; 1:3–22.

26. Horsley V. Brain-surgery. *Br Med J [Clin Res]* 1886; 2: 670–675.

27. Horsley V. Remarks on ten consecutive cases of operations upon the brain and cranial cavity to illustrate the details and safety of the method employed. *Br Med J [Clin Res]* 1887; 1:863–865.

28. Horsley V. The Croonian Lecture: On the mammalian nervous system, its functions and their localization, determined by an electrical method. *Philos Trans R Soc Lond* 1891; 182:267–326.

29. Jackson JH. On the anatomical and physiological localisation of movements in the brain. *Lancet* 1873; 1:84–85, 162–164, 232–234.

30. Jefferson G. The prodromes to cortical localization. In: *Sir Geoffrey Jefferson: Selected Papers*. Springfield, IL: Charles C Thomas, 1960:113–131.

31. Jefferson G. Sir William Macewen's contribution to neurosurgery and its sequels. In: *Sir Geoffrey Jefferson: Selected Papers*. Springfield, IL: Charles C Thomas, 1960:132–149.

32. Keen WW. Three successful cases of cerebral surgery: including (1) the removal of a large intracranial fibroma; (2) exsection of damaged brain tissue; and (3) exsection of the cerebral centre for the left hand; with remarks on the general technique of such operations. *Am J Med Sci* 1888; 96:329–357, 452–465.

33. Lister J. On the antiseptic principle in the practice of surgery. *Lancet* 1867; 2:353–356.

34. Lister J. Illustrations of the antiseptic system of treatment in surgery. *Lancet* 1867; 2:668–669.

35. Macewen W. Tumour of the dura mater: convulsions; removal of the tumour by trephining; recovery. *Glasgow Med J* 1879; 12:210–213.

36. Macewen W. Intra-cranial lesions, illustrating some points in connexion with the localisation of cerebral affections and the advantages of antiseptic trephining. *Lancet* 1881; 2:581–582.

37. Ojemann RG. The tradition of Harvey Cushing commemorated by a stamp in the Great American stamp series. *J Neurosurg* 1987; 67:631–642.

38. Phillips CG, Zeki S, Barlow HB. Localization of function in the cerebral cortex: past, present and future. *Brain* 1984; 107: 327–361.

39. Schiller F. *Paul Broca: Founder of French Anthropology, Explorer of the Brain*. Berkeley: Univ California Press, 1979.

40. Sherrington CS. *The Integrative Action of the Nervous System*. New Haven: Yale Univ Press, 1947.

41. Taylor J. *Selected Writings of John Hughlings Jackson*. London: Hodder and Stoughton, 1931–32; New York: Basic Books, 1958.

42. Walker AE. Introduction to: Horsley V: *The Structure and Functions of the Brain and Spinal Cord*. Philadelphia: Blakiston, 1892; Birmingham, AL: Classics of Neurology & Neurosurgery Library, Gryphon Editions, 1985.

2

Magnetic Resonance Imaging of Supratentorial Neoplasms

Michael T. Modic
Sarah M. Beale

The inherent tissue contrast sensitivity and multiplanar imaging capability of magnetic resonance (MR) positions this modality as the best first test and often most definitive examination in the evaluation of patients with suspected brain lesions. The wide range of tissue contrast available with the utilization of various pulse sequences and paramagnetic contrast agents is the basis of MR's superiority over computed tomography (CT) in detecting tissue changes. This, coupled with the ability to image directly in any plane allows morphological alterations to be better appreciated in a true three-dimensional sense, allowing better localization and characterization.

To appreciate the advantages and disadvantages of the modality, consideration must be given not only to intrinsic tissue characteristics but to technical parameters. Toward that end, it is reasonable to consider MR first from a technical viewpoint. Next, the signal intensity changes produced by pathological tissues, as well as the histological substrate of secondary changes must be integrated with a basic knowledge of the neuropathological categories related to anatomic location. Lastly, it is important to consider nonneoplastic differential considerations in formulating a final impression of the imaging study.

Technical Considerations

As the presenting symptom complex in patients with intracranial neoplasms is rarely specific, the initial technical parameters of an examination should provide the maximum sensitivity to the widest possible spectrum of disease processes. This can be followed by more tailored approaches to improve specificity if necessary. This in practice has led most examinations to be performed with sequences which emphasize T1 and T2 tissue changes.[8] A long time of repetition (TR) sequence (2000 to 3000 ms) with an early and late echo (15 and 90 ms) provides an excellent screen for tissue changes. The axial plane is employed most commonly because of its familiarity, but sagittal images may be best for evaluation of the region of the pineal gland, cerebral aqueduct, and other midline structures. Coronal planes are particularly useful for calvarial, convexity, parasellar, temporal lobe, or skull base lesions. A subsequent T1-weighted spin echo or gradient echo sequence is then employed either in the same or an orthogonal plane for further tissue characterization and anatomic localization. A 5-mm slice thickness with a 256×265 matrix provides a reasonable compromise between voxel size for spatial resolution and signal-to-noise ratio for contrast sensitivity. Thinner slices (such as, 1 to 2 mm) may be necessary for better characterization of smaller lesions. With adequate signal-to-noise ratio (especially at higher fields, 1 to 1.5 tesla) a single excitation for T2-weighted spin echo sequences and two excitations for T1-weighted or gradient echo sequences will usually produce a diagnostic head examination in less than 20 min of scan time. Flow-compensated sequences, special coils, and optimized bandwidths are technical issues which can further improve the diagnostic quality of the exam.

Tissue Contrast and Morphological Considerations

Conventional radiographic methods are almost wholly dependent on differences in electron density. The MR image, on the other hand, is a reflection of a complex interaction of T1 and T2 relaxation times, proton density, and flow. T1 and T2 are intrinsic properties of tissues and are not a function of the instrumentation or pulse sequences used to deduce them. They are tissue specific and are related to the magnetic field strength, the macromolecular constituents of cells, their disposition, and their conformation as sensed by tissue water molecules diffusing throughout the intracellular and extracellular regions of tissue.[21] Simplistically put, alterations in the MR signal intensity are related to changes in tissue water content, especially in the extracellular space. This results in most abnormalities being identified as a decreased signal on T1-weighted images (prolonged T1 relaxation time) and increased signal intensity on T2-weighted images (prolonged T2 relaxation time; Fig. 2-1).[5]

Tissue changes may be noted on T2-weighted sequences before any attenuation alteration or contrast enhancement is noted on CT or on T1-weighted images with gadolinium. The reason for this is that subtle alterations in the blood-brain barrier may allow abnormal water accumulation, but the barrier may still remain relatively resistant to the passage of contrast media, whether iodinated or paramagnetic.[6] The resulting signal intensity is, however, further complicated by the inherent heterogeneity of tissue, which is often compounded by calcification, cysts, hemorrhage, and necrotic areas which can result in a wide range of signal intensities.

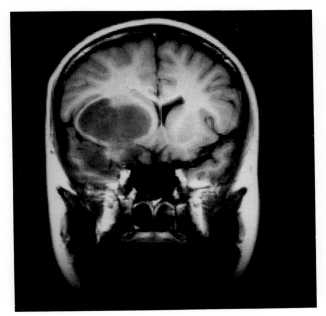

A

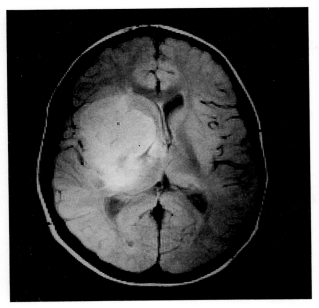

B

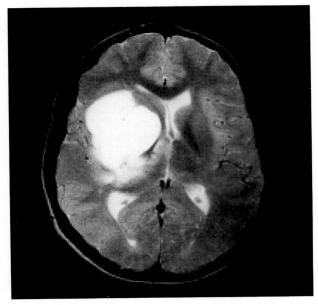

C

Figure 2-1 Astrocytoma. *A*. T1-weighted coronal. *B, C*. Intermediate and T2-weighted axial sequences, respectively. There is a large ovoid mass of decreased signal intensity on the T1-weighted sequences. It has an increased signal intensity on intermediate and T2-weighted sequences. It has irregular margins and a slightly heterogeneous core. There is a small amount of edema noted on the T2-weighted sequences posteriorly and obvious mass effect with subfalcial herniation and effacement of the lateral ventricle.

In addition, in the case of gliomas with areas of different histology, there may be additional differences in signal intensity based on vascularity, oxygenation, etc.

Less commonly, tissue abnormalities will exhibit the opposite signal intensity changes. For instance, increased signal intensity will be noted on T1-weighted sequences (decreased T1 relaxation time) in the presence of fat (Fig. 2-2A), blood (Fig. 2-2B; proton electron dipole-dipole paramagnetic effect, e.g., extracellular methemoglobin or gadolinium diethylenetriamine pentaacetic acid [Gd-DTPA]), or a viscous proteinaceous complex (Fig. 2-2C). Decreased signal intensity on T2-weighted images (decreased T2 relaxation time) suggests flow, some types of calcium (Fig. 2-3A;

reduced mobile proton density), or a magnetic susceptibility effect (Fig. 2-3B; e.g., hemorrhage with intracellular deoxyhemoglobin).

In addition to basic tissue contrast considerations, the appearance of neoplasms will be affected by physiological and morphological alterations such as disruption of the blood-brain barrier and vasogenic edema, hemorrhage, cyst formation, mass effect, herniation, and hydrocephalus, all of which are important in developing a differential diagnosis.

Edema and disruption of the blood-brain barrier are often associated with brain neoplasms. Brain edema may be secondary to alterations of the normal blood-brain barrier resulting in abnormal leakage of water and plasma proteins with a preferential accumulation in the larger extracellular spaces of white matter with respect to those of gray matter. This increased water content usually results in increased signal intensity on T2-weighted and decreased signal intensity on T1-weighted images, producing an increased sensitivity to abnormal interstitial water, a hallmark of MR.[7,30] While this vasogenic edema pattern is sometimes a helpful differentiating factor between ischemic and neoplastic processes, it may mask the nidus of a tumor, a problem not unique to

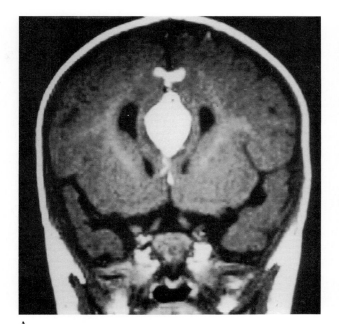

A

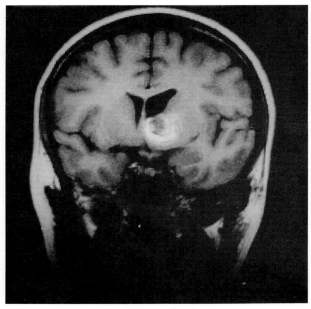

B

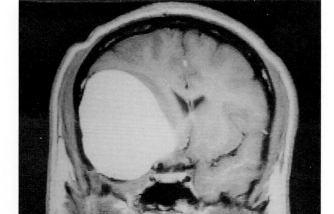

C

Figure 2-2 Increased signal intensity on T1-weighted images. *A*. Coronal T1-weighted spin echo sequences demonstrating a mass with increased signal intensity in the midline which is a lipoma of the corpus callosum. The increased signal intensity is secondary to the short T1 of fat. *B*. Coronal T1-weighted spin echo sequence demonstrating a high signal intensity rim surrounding a lower signal intensity core in the left thalamic region. The high signal intensity rim represents methemoglobin in the periphery of a thalamic hematoma. *C*. Coronal T1-weighted sequence demonstrating a large right-sided extra-axial lesion with marked mass effect and high signal intensity. At surgery this was an epidermoid.

MR but seen with CT as well. Vasogenic edema is less likely to spread across the corpus callosum to the contralateral hemisphere than a neoplasm itself. The vasogenic edema pattern is not specific for a malignant process, as it can be seen with inflammatory or toxic insults.

Cyst formation may be a helpful differential sign and is better characterized on MR than CT. Benign cysts usually demonstrate a well circumscribed, uniformly thin wall and signal intensity characteristics which usually parallel those of cerebrospinal fluid (CSF).[20] The signal intensity characteristics, however, may show wide variability related to the chemistry of the contents as well as from the effects of mo-

tion. Cystic craniopharyngiomas, colloid cysts, Rathke's cleft cysts, and some epidermoid tumors may demonstrate increased signal intensity on T1 related to their chemical contents. Cysts associated with malignant lesions usually demonstrate an irregular wall and intensity characteristics different from those of CSF, especially on T1-weighted or intermediate (long TR/short TE) pulse sequences. In general, the signal intensity on these sequences is higher than that of CSF. A fluid level within the cyst is indicative of a cellular or chemical heterogeneity and results from the different signal intensity characteristics of the contents.[20]

Calcification is appreciated on CT as higher attenuation than adjacent brain parenchyma. Its appearance on MR is more complex and is related to the chemical structure of the calcium itself. In most cases, calcification is less well seen on MR spin echo sequences than on CT.[10] When seen, it is usually of a decreased signal intensity on both T1- and T2-weighted sequences secondary to low mobile proton density. However, calcification may appear hypo-, iso-, or hyperintense. On T1-weighted sequences, calcification has been noted in certain situations to be hyperintense, and this is thought to be due to a paramagnetic effect which has been demonstrated with calcium phosphate[2] or secondary to ossification with marrow formation, resulting in a fat signal as can be seen in the falx. Calcification may also demonstrate a magnetic susceptibility effect which will be more obvious on gradient echo sequences, resulting in a decreased signal intensity.[10]

Obstructive hydrocephalus secondary to tumors is well appreciated on both T1- and T2-weighted images. With more T2-weighted sequences, interstitial edema is well appreciated as a diffuse high signal intensity in the periventricular region. These are usually smooth, symmetrical changes and need to be differentiated from other nonspecific periventricular white matter changes that can occur in patients undergoing chemotherapy or radiation therapy as well as nonneoplastic disorders such as multiple sclerosis. Sagittal images may be particularly useful in patients with hydrocephalus for direct visualization of the aqueduct.

Mass effect is almost always present with supratentorial neoplasms. Subfalcial, uncal, transtentorial, and tonsillar herniations are usually better appreciated than with CT because of the multidimensional imaging capability of MR. Likewise, convexity or base lesions can be better delineated because of the lack of bony artifact or averaging with adjacent brain, resulting in improved depiction of more subtle signs such as buckling of the gray-white junction.

Intracranial hemorrhage resulting from neoplasms is not uncommon; the incidence has been reported to range from 1 to 14 percent. Of the primary intracranial neoplasms, hemorrhage occurs most frequently in relationship to pituitary neoplasms. Other neoplasms that have been reported to bleed include glioblastoma multiforme, low grade gliomas, ependymomas, choroid plexus papillomas, sarcomas, and meningiomas. The incidence of hemorrhage in metastatic neoplasms is highest in melanoma, hypernephroma, bronchogenic carcinoma, and choriocarcinoma. Less commonly, metastases of thyroid and breast neoplasms have been reported to be associated with hemorrhage.[11] The factors involved in determining the signal intensity of an intracranial hemorrhage are complex and are to a certain extent related to location, oxygenation of tissues, age, and clearance. Similar to evolving intraparenchymal hematomas, hemorrhagic neoplasms undergo changes in their appearance that can be categorized into three distinct intensity patterns, or stages. The first, in the acute stage, is characterized as iso- or hypointense on short TR/TE sequences and as hypointense on long TR sequences. The hypointense changes on the long TR/TE images is thought to be secondary to intracellular deoxyhemoglobin. In the subacute stage there is a develop-

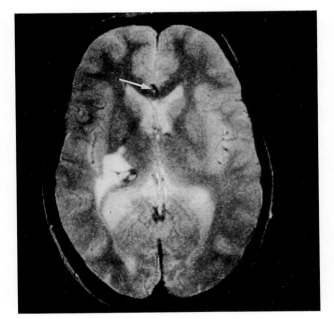

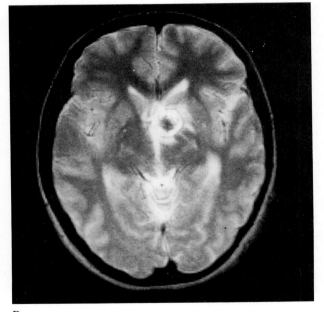

A B

Figure 2-3 Decreased signal intensity on T2-weighted images. *A.* Axial T2-weighted spin echo sequence demonstrating a high signal intensity lesion in the posterior thalamus and internal capsule region on the right. The medial portion of the lesion demonstrates a decreased signal intensity which on CT was heavily calcified. Note the decreased signal intensity in the interhemispheric region anterior to the corpus callosum which represents a flow void within the anterior cerebral arteries (*arrow*). *B.* Axial T2-weighted sequence which demonstrates a high signal intensity rim surrounding a decreased signal intensity core in the left thalamic region. This is the T2-weighted sequence through the same region as depicted in Figure 2-2B. The decreased signal intensity core represents intracellular met- and deoxyhemoglobin in this thalamic hemorrhage.

ing hyperintensity on short TR sequences, with a hypo- or mixed intensity on long TR sequences without evidence of a well-defined hypointense rim. The increased signal intensity in the periphery of the hematoma on the short TR/TE sequences is thought to be secondary to a paramagnetic effect of extracellular methemoglobin that forms secondary to cell lysis. In the more chronic stages there is hyperintensity noted on both short and long TR sequences with a well-defined hypointense rim on long TR sequences. This hypointense rim is secondary to ferritin and hemosiderin in the capsule of the hematoma.[14]

There are certain features that, when present, could be helpful in differentiating a hemorrhagic neoplasm from a primary intraparenchymal hemorrhage. An underlying neoplasm should be suspected in any hemorrhage that evolves slowly, develops central or eccentric hyperintensity as it evolves, or exhibits a mixed signal intensity pattern. While somewhat controversial, the appearance of a hemosiderin rim can be seen with both entities.[1,11]

Paramagnetic Contrast Agents

At this time, gadolinium DTPA is the only contrast agent approved for use with MR. Studies with gadolinium DTPA have shown levels of contrast enhancement equal to or greater than those of iodinated contrast agents with CT. In addition, paramagnetic contrast agents make T1-weighted sequences, with their inherently higher signal-to-noise ratio, more sensitive. It does not cross the intact blood-brain barrier and is excreted unchanged through the kidneys. Its molecular size and behavior with reference to a disrupted blood-brain barrier are similar to those of iodinated contrast media. To date, neither renal toxicity nor hypersensitivity has been documented. The primary effect of the paramagnetic contrast agent is shortening of T1 and T2 relaxation times. This effect is concentration related and, in doses used clinically, usually results in a more obvious shortening of the T1 relaxation time and hence an increased signal intensity on T1-weighted spin echo sequences. With higher concentrations, T2 shortening predominates and results in decreased signal intensity on both T1- and T2-weighted sequences.[13,31]

Paramagnetic contrast agents such as gadolinium DTPA are large molecules that require both intact perfusion and gross active disruption of the blood-brain barrier for their accumulation within the diseased tissue. However, only minimal blood-brain barrier breakdown may be needed for water to leak out into abnormal tissues. Such water accumulation may predate the more severe blood-brain barrier disruption needed for leakage of large proteins across this barrier. This water change is an inherent contrast-enhancing substance for T2-weighted spin echo sequences and is the reason diseased tissue such as demyelinating plaques may be detected on T2-weighted sequences even without active blood-brain barrier breakdown. It is also the reason why unenhanced T2-weighted spin echo sequences are usually as sensitive as gadolinium-enhanced T1-weighted sequences for the detection of intra-axial lesions. It is implausible that gadolinium DTPA would accumulate in a site that did not

also contain abnormal amounts of water. Nevertheless, experience indicates that small metastatic foci may be better seen with gadolinium DTPA on both T1- and T2-weighted sequences, primarily because they are more conspicuous after gadolinium on T1-weighted sequences than on T2-weighted sequences, where they may be hidden by the high signal intensity of adjacent CSF. In addition, the presence of enhancement of gadolinium provides important information regarding perfusion and the status of the blood-brain barrier. As with CT and iodinated contrast, both techniques can mask the presence of underlying hemorrhage if only contrast studies are performed. Separation of tumor and surrounding edema is inaccurate on both CT and MR, even when focal enhancement surrounding the lesion is noted. The changes of enhancement indicate the site of the greatest blood-brain barrier disruption, not the tumor margins. Histological studies have shown that tumor spread can go beyond that of the enhancing ring surrounding the neoplastic lesions.[6]

The utilization of paramagnetic contrast agents in extra-axial lesions is more clear-cut. Their location over the convexities and at the skull base may make them less conspicuous and subject to partial volume averaging. In addition, some lesions (e.g., meningiomas) may possess tissue signal characteristics similar to those of normal brain. Unlike intra-axial lesions, extra-axial lesions lack a blood-brain barrier and therefore are ideal candidates for enhancement with a paramagnetic contrast agent. Meningiomas, acoustic neuromas, and leptomeningeal disease have all been reported to enhance markedly following the administration of paramagnetic contrast agents.[3]

Anatomic Location

With the preceding technical and tissue contrast considerations in mind, it is important to consider the anatomic location of an abnormality in further developing differential considerations. Towards that end, we will now consider some of the common tumor types that we are likely to encounter in the intra-axial, extra-axial, intraventricular, and midline locations.

Intra-axial Lesions

Astrocytomas

Supratentorial astrocytomas are usually solid and infiltrating masses with an appearance that will roughly vary with grade. Although not consistent, low grade tumors typically show less signal intensity change on both T1- and T2-weighted sequences and may be manifested only as a loss of distinction between normal gray and white matter. Vasogenic edema, if present, is usually minimal and hemorrhage is very uncommon (Fig. 2-4). Higher grade lesions, such as anaplastic tumors, usually demonstrate high signal intensity on T2-weighted images which may be heterogeneous depending upon the histology. On T1-weighted sequences these lesions are more conspicuous but demonstrate de-

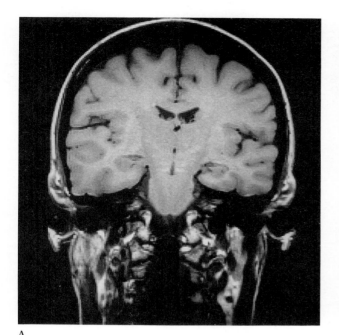

A

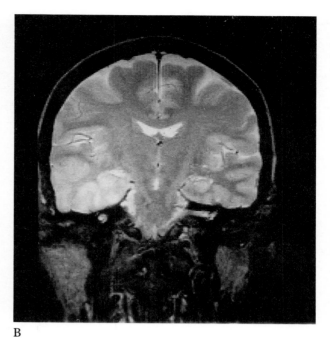

B

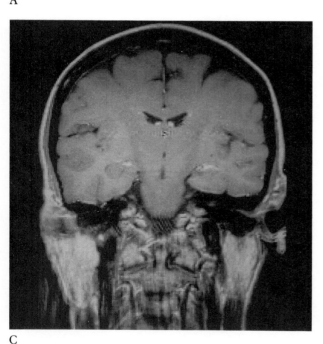

C

Figure 2-4 Low grade astrocytoma. *A.* Coronal T1-weighted sequence through the temporal lobes. The only abnormality is a vague fullness to the temporal lobe on the right as compared to the left as evidenced by some superior displacement of the sylvian fissure. Note also that the gray-white junction is slightly blurred on the right when compared to the left. *B.* Coronal T2-weighted sequence through the same location. Note the subtle increased signal intensity of the inferior aspect of the temporal lobe on the right when compared to the left. *C.* Coronal T1-weighted sequence after the administration of gadolinium DTPA. There is no obvious enhancement. At surgery, a low grade infiltrating astrocytoma was identified. The fact that there is abnormal increased signal intensity on T2 without evidence of enhancement on the gadolinium studies suggests that the disruption of the blood-brain barrier is not gross.

creased signal intensity relative to normal brain parenchyma (Fig. 2-1). Vasogenic edema is usually obvious, but hemorrhage remains uncommon. The highest grade lesion, glioblastoma multiforme, is usually associated with more irregular margins; marked vasogenic edema may extend across the midline through the central white matter structures. Intratumoral hemorrhage is not uncommon and has a variable appearance, as discussed previously. Additional signal heterogeneity may reflect necrosis, cyst formation, or calcification. The central core of the tumor may occasionally be separated from the vasogenic edema by less intense signal changes. Cystic changes do occur but are more frequent in astrocytomas of the posterior fossa, particularly in the pediatric age group. Once cysts are noted, the signal intensity is usually greater than that of CSF on T1-, intermediate, and T2-weighted sequences.

Contrast enhancement, reflecting a disruption of the blood-brain barrier, is usually more obvious in intermediate and higher grade tumors and may be absent in low grade malignancies.[12] While the degree of mass effect and associated edema may vary from none with very low grade astrocytomas to marked with glioblastoma multiforme, it usually remains less than for metastases of similar size.

Oligodendrogliomas

These lesions have a predilection for frontal lobe involvement and appear similar to other low to intermediate grade solid neoplasms with an increased signal intensity on T2-weighted images predominating and less obvious signal changes on T1. Large and extensive calcifications may be relatively inconspicuous on spin echo sequences and are better appreciated by CT and by MR gradient echo sequences. Mass effect and surrounding edema can be minimal.

Ganglioneuromas, Gangliogliomas

These lesions occur most often in children. The most common supratentorial locations are the temporal lobes and the vicinity of the third ventricle. These lesions usually ap-

pear as solid masses with heterogeneous increased signal intensity on T2-weighted sequences and less obvious T1-weighted changes. They can be single or multiple. There is less mass effect and edema than one would expect with the size of these lesions (Fig. 2-5).

Metastatic Disease

Multiplicity, marked vasogenic edema, and mass effect are the hallmarks of this process (Fig. 2-6). The central portion of these tumors is often separated from the high signal intensity of the edema by slight differences in T1 and T2 relaxation times.[5,6,9] The incidence of hemorrhage is highest in melanoma, hypernephroma, choreocarcinoma, and bronchogenic carcinoma. Increased signal intensity changes on T1-weighted images in patients with metastatic melanoma may be secondary to melanin or hemorrhage. Evidence indicates, however, that hemorrhage exerts a stronger influence on the signal characteristic than melanin (Fig. 2-7).[11] Paramagnetic contrast agents may increase the sensitivity of MR to the detection of small foci that may not be appreciated on routine T2-weighted sequences (Figs. 2-6 and 2-7).[6] Likewise, leptomeningeal metastases, most commonly seen with lung cancer, breast cancer, and lymphoma, are best appreciated with paramagnetic contrast agents, which should be employed routinely if these differential considerations are suspected.

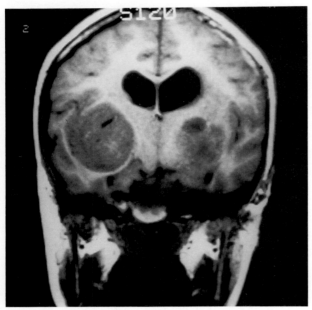

A

Figure 2-5 Ganglioglioma. *A.* Coronal T1-weighted spin echo sequence. *B, C.* Axial intermediate and T2-weighted spin echo sequences. Bilateral, inhomogeneous, lobulated lesions without marked mass effect are noted. These bilateral lesions are histologically proven gangliogliomas.

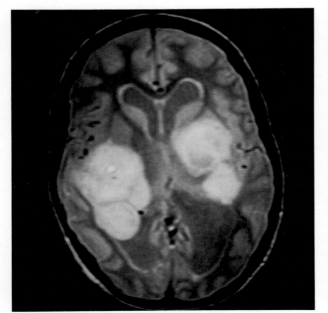

B

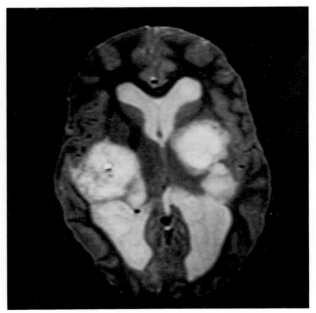

C

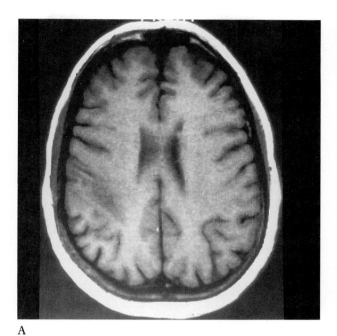

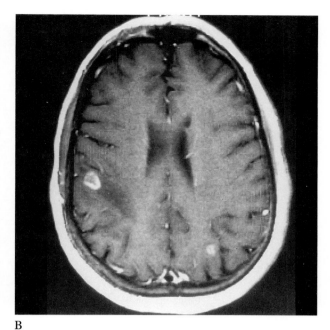

A

B

Figure 2-6 Metastatic breast carcinoma. *A*. Axial T1-weighted spin echo sequence. *B*. Axial T1-weighted spin echo sequence following the administration of gadolinium DTPA. *C*. Axial T2-weighted spin echo sequence. Note that on *A* there is only a subtle decreased signal intensity noted in the parietal lobe on the right. Following the administration of gadolinium DTPA (*B*) there is enhancement noted in the lateral aspect of this region as well as a second lesion in the contralateral hemisphere posteriorly. There is vasogenic edema on the T2-weighted image, surrounding the right hemisphere lesion. There is also increased signal intensity suggestive of vasogenic edema associated with the left hemispheric lesion. It is not as obvious as on the Gd-DTPA study, and it could be mistaken for averaging with adjacent CSF.

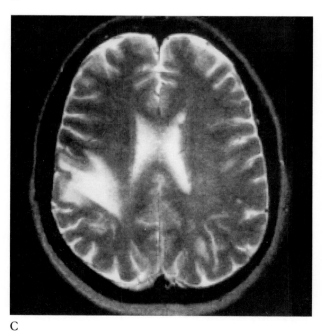

C

Primary central nervous system (CNS) lymphoma is relatively rare, most frequently occurring in the fifth and sixth decades.[17] It can be seen at any age in patients with acquired immunodeficiency syndrome (AIDS) and can be a cause of differential confusion. It most often presents as a lesion(s) greater than 2 cm in diameter, with a ringlike appearance on T2-weighted images due to central T2 shortening.[28] Secondary CNS lymphoma can arise within the brain parenchyma or the meninges and may be multicentric. It has a predilection for the midline or paramedian structures and usually presents as an infiltrating mass with less mass effect and edema than are usually associated with metastatic disease. Its signal intensity characteristics are similar to those of other solid tumors, and on imaging grounds alone, there are no distinguishing features separating the metastatic from primary variety. There is a greater incidence of leptomeningeal involvement in metastatic lymphoma when compared to primary lymphoma of the central nervous system (Fig.

2-8).[10] As mentioned above, the leptomeningeal involvement is better detected by utilizing gadolinium DTPA in conjunction with T1-weighted sequences.

Intraventricular Lesions

Ependymomas

Supratentorial involvement is more common in children than adults. Supratentorial ependymomas usually occur along the ependymal surface of the third or lateral ventricle

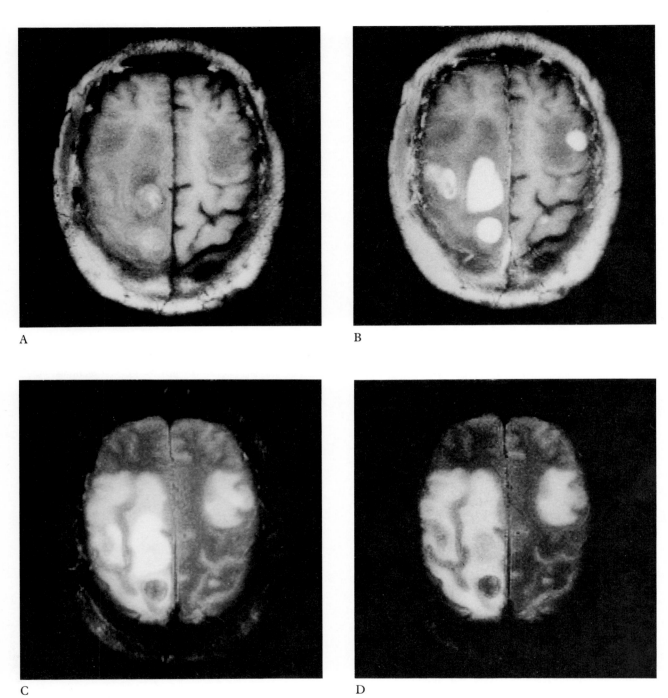

A

B

C

D

Figure 2-7 Metastatic melanoma. *A*. Axial T1-weighted spin echo sequence. *B*. Axial T1-weighted spin echo sequence following gadolinium DTPA. *C*. Axial T2-weighted spin echo sequence. *D*. Axial T2-weighted spin echo sequence following gadolinium DTPA. On the nonenhanced study (*A*) there are areas of edema noted in both hemispheres as well as ovoid lesions of increased signal intensity suggestive of some type of paramagnetic effect, either hemorrhage or melanin. Following the administration of gadolinium DTPA (*B*) multiple focal areas of enhancement indicative of disruption of the blood-brain barrier are noted. At a slightly higher level, the nonenhanced T2-weighted spin echo sequence (*C*) demonstrates multiple areas of vasogenic edema suggestive of disruption of the blood-brain barrier. Following the administration of gadolinium DTPA, the cores of two of these lesions in the right hemisphere show a further decrease in signal intensity which is greater T2 shortening secondary to accumulation of gadolinium DTPA.

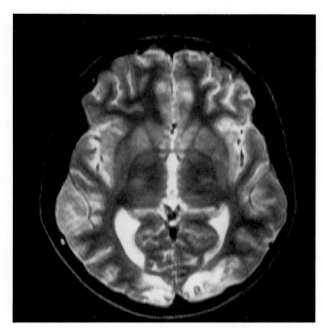

Figure 2-8 Leptomeningeal metastases (lymphoma). Increased signal intensity is noted in the occipital lobes bilaterally on this axial T2-weighted sequence, secondary to leptomeningeal involvement. T1-weighted sequences in this same locale were normal.

but may appear intraparenchymal in the supratentorial region. Signal intensity changes are similar to those of other solid tumors and the differential consideration is usually based on its peri- or intraventricular location. While ependymomas are usually well circumscribed, they can have malignant degeneration and aggressive behavior with spread via CSF seeding. Thus, it is useful to study these patients with gadolinium DTPA, which is more sensitive than nonenhanced examinations for the evaluation for potential CSF seeding which can be masked by the high signal intensity on T2-weighted spin echo sequences.

Choroid Plexus Papillomas

These usually appear as lobulated, somewhat heterogeneous hyperintense lesions on T2-weighted sequences in the region of the choroid plexus. Choroid plexus carcinomas are characterized by invasion of the adjacent brain parenchyma. Both lesions can cause marked ventricular dilation secondary to overproduction of CSF. When small, these lesions may be masked by the high signal intensity of the surrounding CSF on T2-weighted sequences. On T1-weighted sequences, the signal intensity is usually similar to that of adjacent brain parenchyma.[22]

Colloid Cysts

These are most often found in the region of the foramen of Monro. Their signal intensity is variable, but in contradistinction to other types of intraventricular lesions, they may commonly present with a high signal intensity on T1-

weighted sequences and a decreased central core of signal intensity on T2-weighted sequences (Fig. 2-9).[19] The differential in this situation is with much less common intraventricular lesions such as intraventricular craniopharyngiomas and/or Rathke's cleft cysts.

Intraventricular astrocytomas and meningiomas can also occur but are more common in an intra-axial or extra-axial location, respectively. The signal intensity characteristics are similar regardless of the location, although there is certainly less vasogenic edema associated with these lesions when they are intraventricular (Fig. 2-10).

Midline Lesions

Pineal Region Tumors

The differential diagnosis of a solid lesion in this location is usually that of a germ cell–origin tumor (germinoma, teratoma), pineal cell–origin tumor (pineocytoma, pineoblastoma), metastasis to the pineal gland, and an epidermoid or dermoid tumor. The multidimensional imaging capability of MR is extremely useful for precisely localizing lesions in this area (Fig. 2-11).[22]

Pineal germinomas are the most common lesion in this location and are best appreciated on sagittal sections, where any resulting mass effect or hydrocephalus secondary to displacement and compression of the midbrain tectum and aqueduct can be appreciated. They are usually hyperintense on T2-weighted images and frequently heterogeneous, reflecting focal calcification, hemorrhage, and cyst formation.

Tumors of pineal cell origin are more common in young females. Pineocytomas are usually well-defined homogeneous lesions, whereas pineoblastomas are typically more irregular and invasive.

Epidermoids, Dermoids, Teratomas

Epidermoids may occur in the midline or laterally depending upon their time of formation. Early inclusion results in midline lesions, while later inclusions result in increasing laterality. These are usually well-defined cystic structures containing cholesterol and keratinized debris. Their internal architecture is slightly heterogeneous. They are slightly increased on T1 and T2 relative to CSF, but a very high signal intensity on T1 has also been reported (Fig. 2-2C). Dermoids are frequently in the midline. Two-thirds are hyperintense on T1-weighted sequences, suggestive of fat. All are hyperintense on T2-weighted sequences. Teratomas have a more marked heterogeneity on both T1 and T2 sequences, and a variable but usually increased signal intensity. All of these lesions usually demonstrate a smooth margin, mass effect, and little or no associated edema. Calcification may be difficult to see on spin echo sequences.[23,27]

Extra-axial Lesions

Meningiomas

Meningiomas are the prototype of extra-axial lesions. Eighty-five percent of meningiomas are supratentorial, and

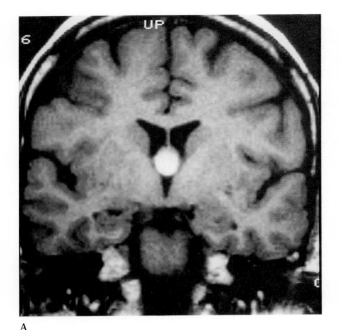

A

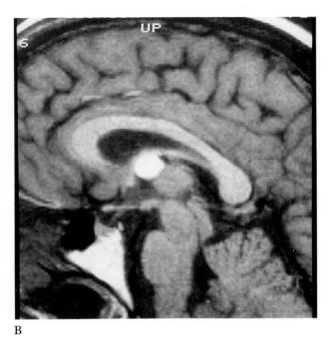

B

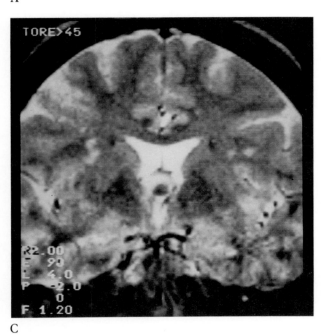

C

Figure 2-9 Colloid cyst. *A.* Coronal T1-weighted spin echo sequence. *B.* Sagittal T1-weighted spin echo sequence. *C.* Coronal T2-weighted spin echo sequence. Note the ovoid mass located at the foramen of Monro on all three images. There is an increased signal intensity on the T1-weighted images and a rim of high signal intensity surrounding a decreased signal intensity core on the T2-weighted images.

the most common locations are parasagittal, over the convexity, and along the sphenoid wing. On nonenhanced MR studies they are sometimes difficult to distinguish on the basis of contrast alone from adjacent brain parenchyma (Fig. 2-12). Mass effect may be the only sign. In approximately 20 percent of cases they demonstrate hypointensity on T1- and hyperintensity on T2-weighted images (Fig. 2-13). They are often separated from the brain by an adjacent low intensity capsule which may be related to dense fibrous tissue or displaced vessels with flow void. The internal matrix typically

has a uniform granular appearance, but focal calcification may alter this appearance.[32]

Nerve Sheath Tumors

Nerve sheath tumors such as schwannomas involve one or more cranial nerves. They are iso- or hypointense on T1-weighted images and typically are hyperintense on T2-weighted images. They are more common in the posterior fossa than supratentorially.

Both nerve sheath tumors and meningiomas demonstrate intense enhancement following the administration of paramagnetic contrast media, which may be important for determining their margins relative to adjacent brain parenchyma or for determining multiplicity (Fig. 2-14).[3] This is particularly important in patients with neurofibromatosis, where multiplicity is more common and lesions of various sizes are often found.

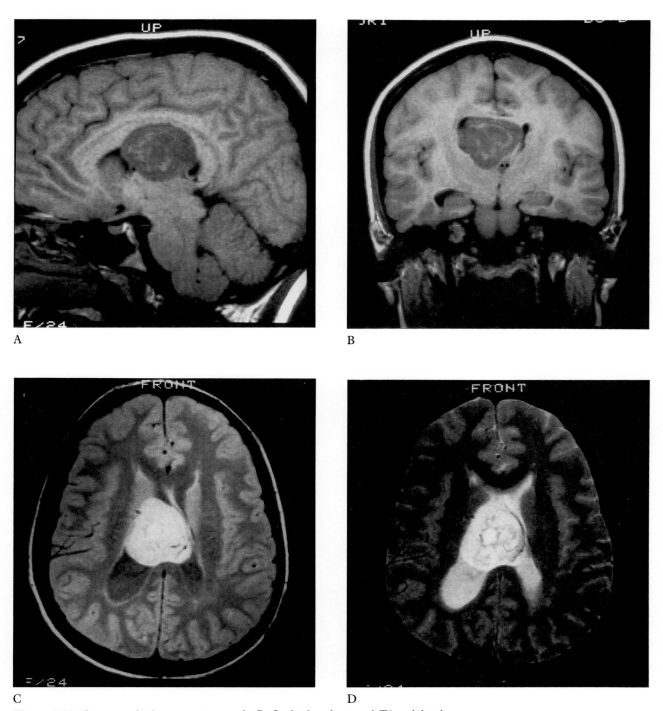

A

B

C

D

Figure 2-10 Intraventricular astrocytoma. *A, B.* Sagittal and coronal T1-weighted spin echo sequences. *C, D.* Axial intermediate and T2-weighted sequences. A large lobulated heterogeneous mass of decreased signal intensity on T1- (relative to brain parenchyma) and increased signal intensity on intermediate and T2-weighted images is noted within the right lateral ventricle.

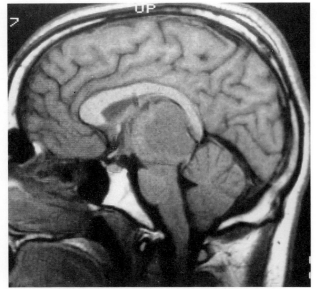

A

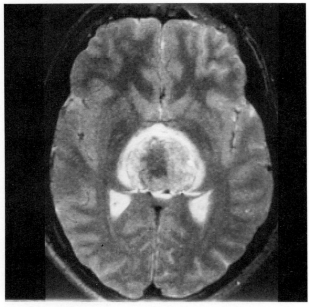

B

Figure 2-11 Pineoblastoma. *A.* Sagittal T1-weighted spin echo sequence. *B.* Axial T2-weighted spin echo sequence. There is a large lobulated mass with a heterogeneous signal intensity on both T1- and T2-weighted images located in the region of the posterior third ventricle. There is marked distortion and invasion of the adjacent midbrain.

Calvarial Lesions

Involvement of the calvarium itself may be manifested by a loss of the normal decreased signal intensity of the cortical

bone and an abnormally high signal intensity on T2-weighted images within the diploic space. Differential considerations include epidermoids, hemangiomas, eosinophilic granulomas, and metastases. The multidimensional imaging capability of MR can be used to present the diploic space and cortical bone in various projections, facilitating identification and localization (Fig. 2-15).

Nonneoplastic Differential Considerations

In general, the lesions which may be considered in the differential diagnosis are demyelinating plaques, infarcts, vascular malformations, aneurysms, and areas of dysplastic brain such as heterotopic gray matter or hamartomas. Lastly, and often impossible to distinguish from malignant disease, are inflammatory changes such as abscesses.

In demyelinating disease, areas of abnormal signal intensity are often noted in the white matter or at the gray-white junction. These can be single or more commonly multiple and are usually associated with some periventricular changes. In general, edema and mass effect are absent even when the lesions are quite large (Fig. 2-16).

An infarct, particularly in its early stages when it is associated with ischemic edema, may be difficult to separate from an infiltrating neoplasm. In general, the mass effect will dissipate anywhere from 4 to 7 days. An infarct typically involves a vascular distribution and involves the gray and white matter equally.

Vascular malformations, when patent, typically demonstrate areas of signal void suggestive of flowing blood. In addition, there are often signal intensity changes in the adjacent parenchyma suggestive of calcification or hemorrhages of various ages. Cavernous angiomas and/or cryptic vascular malformations may present as single focal or multiple lesions with high signal intensity on both T1- and T2-weighted images and a heterogeneous matrix (Fig. 2-17).[15] The signal intensity changes usually reflect hemorrhage of varying age and adjacent tissue changes. Unless recent hemorrhage has occurred, most vascular malformations are conspicuously lacking in vasogenic edema and mass effect. The presence of a hypointense rim on T2-weighted images composed of both hemosiderin and ferritin is also typical of the chronic stage.

Aneurysms, when patent, will demonstrate a flow void within the lumen on both T1- and T2-weighted images. Partially thrombosed aneurysms, however, may present a complex signal intensity picture and may be difficult to separate from a solid mass. A location near a vessel and an ovoid appearance are strongly suggestive. Aneurysms which have recently ruptured present a complex appearance not just of the aneurysm itself but of the adjacent brain parenchyma resulting in mass effect and vasogenic edema. In these cases, the presence of flow void and signal intensity changes suggestive of hemorrhage is an indication that an aneurysm or vascular malformation may be present.

The association of intracranial tumors with neurofibromatosis is well known. In addition, small focal areas of increased signal intensity within the brain parenchyma on T2-weighted sequences have been identified. Although the exact nature of these lesions remains unclear it has been pos-

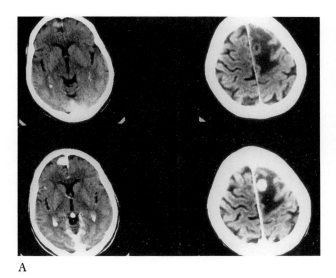

A

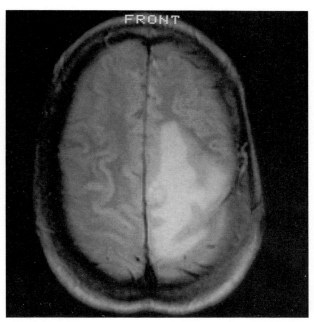

B

Figure 2-12 Meningioma and breast carcinoma metastases. *A.* Nonenhanced (*above*) and enhanced (*below*) contiguous CT images. Note the high signal intensity on the nonenhanced CT in the upper left image adjacent to the falx on the right. This enhances densely following the administration of contrast material (*lower left image*). Vasogenic edema is identified on a slightly higher slice with an enhancing lesion following the administration of contrast media (*right images*). *B, C.* Axial intermediate and T2-weighted sequences, respectively. Note that the meningioma is not discernible from adjacent brain on the intermediate sequence on the right. On the more T2-weighted sequence, the meningioma is of a decreased signal intensity relative to brain parenchyma (*arrows*). The metastatic focus is well seen on both sequences. This case also illustrates that the angulation of the section is often different on CT and MR.

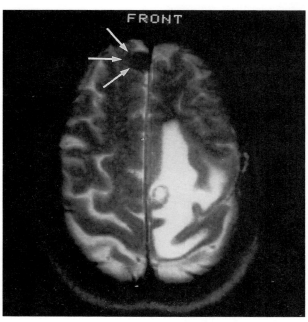

C

tulated that they represent focal areas of heterotopic or possibly dysplastic tissue. They are located primarily in the basal ganglia and internal capsule, with other lesions seen in the midbrain, cerebellum, and subcortical white matter. CT and T1-weighted MR images reveal few or no abnormalities in corresponding locations.[4,16]

Subependymal hamartomas in tuberous sclerosis are often heavily calcified and may produce little alteration of the MR signal intensity. They may be seen best by their extension into the CSF-containing ventricle. Gradient echo sequences appear to be sensitive to these lesions and their typical subependymal location is characteristic. Contrast enhancement is identified in some of these lesions, which may be an indication that there has been a transition to a giant cell astrocytoma.

Abscesses may be difficult to distinguish from metastatic or primary CNS neoplasms. They may be single or multiple and associated with profound vasogenic edema. The problems they may cause are best typified by considering the difficulty in making a specific diagnosis in patients with

AIDS. These patients may demonstrate a variety of signal intensity changes within the brain parenchyma. Most reports have described focal solid lesions as being secondary to toxoplasmosis or primary CNS lymphoma, with the former being the most common. Focal lesions suggest a focal infection or tumor, whereas diffuse white matter changes may be seen secondary to direct infection of the brain with the human immune deficiency virus resulting in a diffuse white matter pattern.[28]

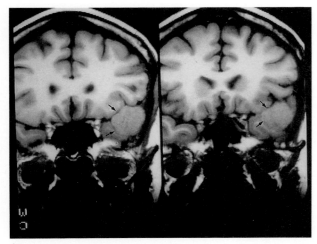

A

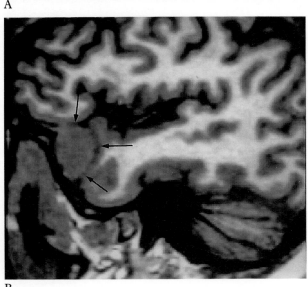

B

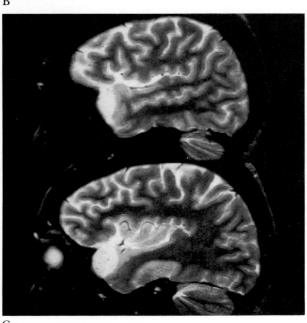

C

Figure 2-13 Sphenoid wing meningioma. *A*. Depicts contiguous coronal T1-weighted sections through the sphenoid wing. *B*. Parasagittal T1-weighted gradient echo sequence through the same region. *C*. Depicts contiguous parasagittal T2-weighted sequences. Notice that on *A* and *B* the meningioma (*arrows*) is identified as an extra-axial mass with a signal intensity similar to adjacent cortical gray matter. There is high signal intensity noted in the same region on the parasagittal T2-weighted sequences.

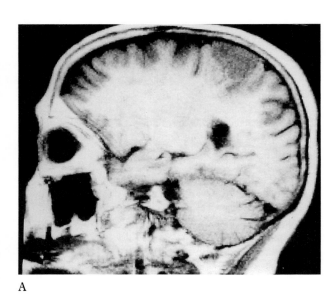

A

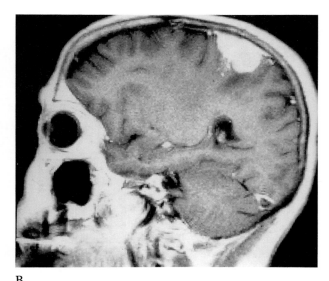

B

Figure 2-14 Convexity meningioma. *A*, *B*. Sagittal T1-weighted spin echo sequences before and after the administration of gadolinium DTPA. Note the dense enhancement of the meningioma following the administration of gadolinium.

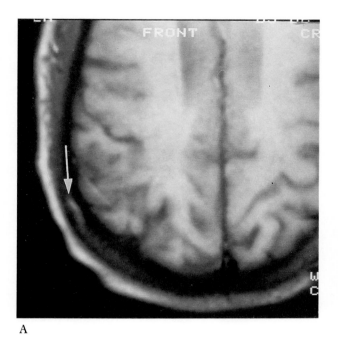

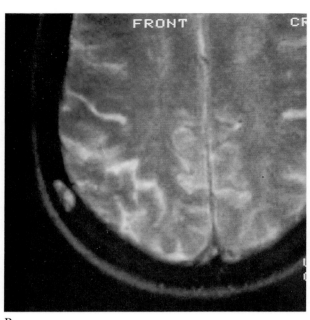

A   B

Figure 2-15 Calvarial hemangioma. *A, B*. Axial T1- and T2-weighted spin echo sequences. There is a vague area of increased signal intensity noted in the diploic space overlying the posterior parietal region on the right on the T1-weighted sequence (*arrow*). On the T2-weighted sequence this region is more obvious as an area of high signal intensity within the diploic space. The high signal intensity surrounding the calvarium on both sequences is the subcutaneous fat.

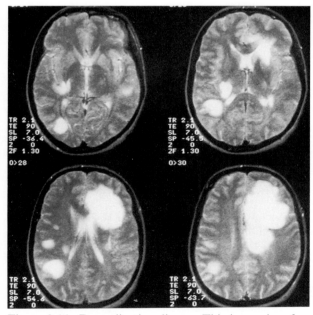

Figure 2-16 Demyelinating disease. This is a series of contiguous T2-weighted axial images through the brain. Note the multiple focal area of high signal intensity bilaterally. Note the relative absence of mass effect for the size of these lesions. Biopsy demonstrated these to be regions of demyelination.

Heterotopic gray matter, a neuronal migration disorder, presents as focal masses with a signal intensity identical to that of cortical gray matter on all sequences.[29] These may present in the central white matter or in a periventricular location. They are often associated with a seizure disorder.

The Future

While more specific and quantitative tissue characterization remains a goal of MR, work to date with measurements of proton relaxation times has been disappointing. While normal brain tissue shows only small interindividual variations, pathological entities have been characterized by wide variations and overlap, precluding reliable diagnosis based on quantitative evaluation of T1, T2, and proton density alone.[18] More recently, phosphorus and proton spectroscopy have shown encouraging results in helping to assess intracranial lesions based on their metabolism and biochemistry. Early indications suggest that these techniques will prove useful not only for the separation of malignant versus benign tissue but also as an aid in following the effects of treatment.

Lastly, despite the superior sensitivity to and improved localization of brain pathology before open surgery,[24] CT has remained the modality most commonly used for stereotactic needle biopsy. This, in part, has been because of technical issues related to the design of magnet-compatible localization devices and surgical equipment and fears regarding

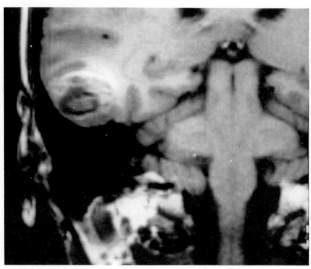

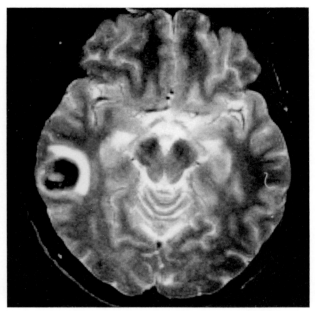

A   B

Figure 2-17 Vascular malformation. *A.* Coronal T1-weighted spin echo sequence. *B.* Axial T2-weighted spin echo sequence. Note in *A* the decreased signal intensity core surrounded by high signal intensity in the temporal lobe on the right. On the T2-weighted sequence this region shows marked decreased signal intensity surrounded by a high signal intensity rim. These changes are consistent with hemorrhage in the subacute stage. The increased signal intensity in the periphery of the lesion on the T1-weighted spin echo sequence is secondary to extracellular methemoglobin. The decreased signal intensity on the T2-weighted sequence in the core is secondary to intracellular deoxyhemoglobin. The high signal intensity rim on the T2-weighted sequences is adjacent parenchymal edema. This lesion demonstrates some mass effect, and at angiography no evidence of a vascular malformation was noted. At surgery and subsequent histological analysis this was found to be a vascular malformation which had recently bled. This case illustrates the differential problem in hemorrhagic lesions.

the ability of MR to detect very acute hemorrhage related to the biopsy itself. While preliminary, these problems have been addressed and appear to be surmountable.[25,26]

References

1. Atlas SW, Grossman RI, Gomori JM, et al. Hemorrhagic intracranial malignant neoplasms: spin-echo MR imaging. *Radiology* 1987; 164:71–77.
2. Atlas SW, Grossman RI, Hackney DB, et al. Calcified intracranial lesions: detection with gradient-echo-acquisition rapid MR imaging. *AJNR* 1988; 9:253–259.
3. Berry I, Brant-Zawadzki M, Osaki L, et al. Gd-DTPA in clinical MR of the brain: 2. Extraaxial lesions and normal structures. *AJNR* 1986; 7:789–793.
4. Bognanno JR, Edwards MK, Lee TA, et al. Cranial MR imaging in neurofibromatosis. *AJNR* 1988; 9:461–468.
5. Brant-Zawadzki M, Badami JP, Mills CM, et al. Primary intracranial tumor imaging: a comparison of magnetic resonance and CT. *Radiology* 1984; 150:435–440.
6. Brant-Zawadzki M, Berry I, Osaki L, et al. Gd-DTPA in clinical MR of the brain: 1. Intraaxial lesions. *AJNR* 1986; 7:781–788.
7. Brant-Zawadzki M, Kelly W. Brain tumors. In: Brant-Zawadzki M, Norman D (eds.), *Magnetic Resonance Imaging of the Central Nervous System*. New York: Raven, 1987:151–185.
8. Brant-Zawadzki M, Norman D, Newton TH, et al. Magnetic resonance of the brain: the optimal screening technique. *Radiology* 1984; 152:71–77.
9. Claussen C, Laniado M, Schörner W, et al. Gadolinium-DTPA in MR imaging of glioblastomas and intracranial metastases. *AJNR* 1985; 6:669–674.
10. Dell LA, Brown MS, Orrison WW, et al. Physiologic intracranial calcification with hyperintensity on MR imaging: case report and experimental model. *AJNR* 1988; 9:1145–1148.
11. Destian S, Sze G, Krol G, et al. MR imaging of hemorrhagic intracranial neoplasms. *AJNR* 9:1115–1122, 1988.
12. Felix R, Schörner W, Laniado M, et al. Brain tumors: MR imaging with gadolinium-DTPA. *Radiology* 1985; 156:681–688.
13. Gadian DG, Payne JA, Bryant DJ, et al. Gadolinium-DTPA as a contrast agent in MR imaging: theoretical projections and practical observations. *J Comput Assist Tomogr* 1985; 9:242–251.
14. Gomori JM, Grossman RI, Goldberg HI, et al. Intracranial hematomas: imaging by high-field MR. *Radiology* 1985; 157:87–93.

15. Gomori JM, Grossman RI, Goldberg HI, et al. Occult cerebrovascular malformations: high-field MR imaging. *Radiology* 1986; 158:707–713.
16. Hurst RW, Newman SA, Cail WS. Multifocal intracranial MR abnormalities in neurofibromatosis. *AJNR* 1988; 9:293–296.
17. Jack CR Jr, Reese DF, Scheithauer BW. Radiographic findings in 32 cases of primary CNS lymphoma. *AJNR* 1985; 6:899–904.
18. Just M, Thelen M. Tissue characterization with T1, T2, and proton density values: results in 160 patients with brain tumors. *Radiology* 1988; 169:779–785.
19. Keller IA, Pinto RS, Sands SF, et al. The MR spectrum of colloid cysts: therapeutic implications. *AJNR* 1987; 8:963 (abstr).
20. Kjos BO, Brant-Zawadzki M, Kucharczyk W, et al. Cystic intracranial lesions: magnetic resonance imaging. *Radiology* 1985; 155:363–369.
21. Koenig SH, Brown RD III. The raw and the cooked, or the importance of the motion of water for MRI revisited. *Invest Radiol* 1988; 23:495–497.
22. Kortman KE, Bradley WG. Supratentorial neoplasms. In: Stark DD, Bradley WG Jr (eds.), *Magnetic Resonance Imaging*. St. Louis: Mosby, 1988:375–424.
23. Kortman KE, Van Dalsem W, Bradley WG. MRI of intracranial epidermoid tumors. *Radiology* 1985; 157:71P.
24. Krol G, Galicich J, Arbit E, et al. Preoperative localization of intracranial lesions on MR. *AJNR* 1988; 9:513–516.
25. Mamourian AC, Rhodes RE, Duda JJ, et al. MR-directed brain biopsy: feasibility study. *AJNR* 1988; 9:510–512.
26. Mueller PR, Stark DD, Simeone JF, et al. MR-guided aspiration biopsy: needle design and clinical trials. *Radiology* 1986; 161:605–609.
27. Newton DR, Lawson TC III, Dillon WP, et al. Magnetic resonance characteristics of cranial epidermoid and teratomatous tumors. *AJNR* 1987; 8:945 (abstr).
28. Olsen WL, Longo FM, Mills CM, et al. White matter disease in AIDS: findings at MR imaging. *Radiology* 1988; 169:445–448.
29. Osborn RE, Byrd SE, Naidich TP, et al. MR imaging of neuronal migrational disorders. *AJNR* 1988; 9:1101–1106.
30. Russell DS, Rubinstein LJ. *Pathology of Tumors of the Nervous System*, 4th ed. Baltimore: Williams and Wilkins, 1977:361–370.
31. Weinmann HJ, Brasch RC, Press WR, et al. Characteristics of gadolinium-DTPA complex: a potential NMR contrast agent. *AJR* 1984; 142:619–624.
32. Zimmerman RD, Fleming CA, Saint-Louis LA, et al. Magnetic resonance imaging of meningiomas. *AJNR* 1985; 6:149–157.

3

Magnetic Resonance Imaging of Posterior Fossa Masses

Victor Waluch
Peter Dyck

One of the earliest recognized advantages of magnetic resonance imaging (MRI) over computed tomography (CT) was in the imaging of the posterior fossa. This region, as opposed to the supratentorial compartment, imposes extreme hardship upon CT. The thick bony walls generate such severe Hounsfield artefacts on CT scans that small lesions, even on contrast-enhanced studies, can be hidden and larger ones obscured. This bony envelope, while playing such havoc with CT, is completely transparent to MRI. MRI is thus able to look into the posterior fossa unencumbered and extract details that heretofore were the province of the surgeon and the pathologist.

The value of any imaging modality is determined by its sensitivity and specificity. Throughout the central nervous system (CNS), MRI has been shown to generally possess more intrinsic tissue contrast than CT and often even more than CT with intravenous contrast. The sensitivity of MRI has been further enhanced now that a contrast agent has been approved for clinical use (Magnevist; Berlex, Parsippany, NJ). The specificity of an imaging modality, which may roughly be thought of as the ability to narrow the differential diagnosis, is dependent on the amount of independent information the modality can extract about the lesion. Even without contrast, MRI can extract most of the information available to CT. With the recent improvements in resolution and slice thickness and its ability to image in any arbitrary plane, MRI can extract much more useful anatomic information as well.

Although it is now nearly incontrovertible that MRI is the imaging modality of choice in the imaging of the posterior fossa, there are some problems unique to MRI. MRI imaging is time-consuming and requires a good deal of cooperation on the part of the patient, not often possible with the acutely ill or demented patient. In addition, naturally occurring motion such as vascular blood flow and CSF pulsations can degrade MRI images, sometimes severely. Claustrophobic patients often cannot undergo the examination. MRI is still relatively contraindicated for pregnant patients and patients with intracranial aneurysm clips, pacemakers, and ferromagnetic fragments near sensitive organs such as the eye.

Techniques

There are literally hundreds of operator-controlled parameters to choose from in setting up an MRI examination. They range from choice of sequence (spin echo, inversion recovery, gradient recalled echo, etc.) to choice of parameters within the sequence [repetition time (TR), echo time (TE), inversion time (TI), etc.]. Furthermore, there are choices of slice thickness, resolution, and projection.

In the CNS, most strategies are two-step: lesion detection and lesion characterization. Most CNS lesions have prolonged relaxation values so that T2-weighted sequences, usually spin echo, with long TRs and long TEs (e.g., TR/TE = 2000 ms/30 to 80 ms), will image them as high-intensity lesions, while normal brain parenchyma appears gray. Unfortunately, most of the internal structure of a lesion will take on a similar high-intensity appearance, making it difficult to characterize the internal structure of the lesion. Surrounding edema also having prolonged relaxation parameters may obscure the boundaries of the lesion. Additional information is then usually obtained by spin echo sequences having short TRs and TEs, the so-called T1-weighted sequences (e.g., TR/TE = 500 ms/20 ms). These sequences are rapid and can be averaged multiple times to give high-resolution, high-quality images to define the anatomy. Because they are so rapid, they can also be run in various projections to further characterize the lesion.

Other approaches also exist. The most interesting of these is direct three-dimensional imaging using gradient-recalled echo techniques, as recently developed by researchers at Siemens (Erlangen, West Germany; Fig. 3-1). In this approach, the brain is imaged isotropically, that is, the imaging voxel is the same size in all dimensions, commonly less than a millimeter on each side. Since the entire head is represented mathematically, the data can be reconstructed to yield a high-resolution slice from any direction desired without the step-off problems common to CT reconstruction. In addition, if appropriate computer hardware is available, surface views and cutaway views may be created so that one may look into the brain while still seeing the surface details. This can be done at varying depths so that the surgeon can, in real time, walk through the different layers of tissue on the way to the lesion, a sort of computer simulation run prior to surgical exploration.

In spite of its sophistication, MRI in most cases cannot distinguish the various tumors of the posterior fossa strictly by their MRI appearance. The more internal structure MR images, the more the tumors resemble each other. Solid medulloblastomas with the appropriate T1 and T2 images frequently appear to have lucencies or cysts. Meningiomas

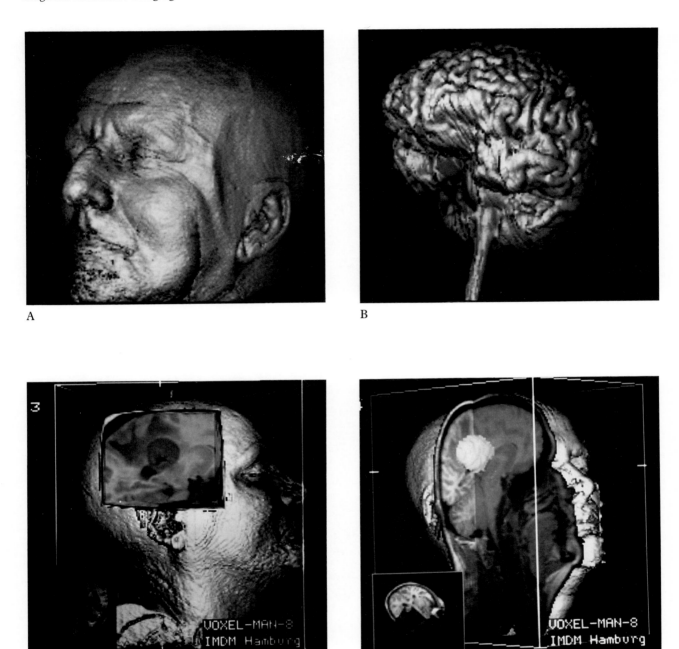

A

B

C

D

Figure 3-1 Three-dimensional imaging. The data set used to generate these images was obtained by means of an isotropic 3-D acquisition with resolution of less than 1 mm in all dimensions. The data can be selected to reconstruct the surface of the head or any internal structure, A and B, or to give a cutaway view, as shown in C and D. (Courtsey of Siemens, Erlangen, West Germany.)

can simulate acoustic neurinomas, and cystic astrocytomas can appear just like hemangioblastomas. Accurate diagnosis still requires a detailed clinical history and neurological examination, as well as a detailed study of the morphology.

Neuroepithelial Tumors

Cerebellar Astrocytomas

Cerebellar astrocytomas can occur at any age. In children, the astrocytoma is one of the most prevalent of the posterior fossa tumors, and the cerebellar astrocytoma is nearly the exclusive property of this age group.[4] These tumors can arise in the vermis or in a hemisphere. They can be solid, monocystic, or mixed. All portions of these tumors tend to have high proton density and long relaxation times. On T2 images they tend to appear as high-intensity masses, with their cystic components, if any, tending to be of very high intensity. Detailed internal structure can best be demonstrated on moderately T1 weighted images, whereupon their cystic or solid nature becomes evident (Fig. 3-2). In the monocystic types, a mural nodule can frequently be identified (Fig. 3-3).

MRI, with its multidimensional capability, is ideally suited for demonstrating morphology. Sagittal and coronal images can define the exact cephalocaudal extent of the tumor. The distortion of the fourth ventricle and its recesses can be well evaluated. Exophytic growth into the ventricle and the cisterns, and invasion of the peduncles can be assessed. In general, the degree of intensity difference between the tumor and the normal parenchyma increases with the grade of the tumor, as does the amount of edema, which can mask the extent of the tumor. The primary disadvantage of MRI in the evaluation of cerebellar astrocytomas is its insensitivity to calcium, which can be demonstrated by CT in some 22 percent of these tumors.[6] Calcifications are rarely present in hemangioblastomas and are infrequent in medulloblastomas.

Brain Stem Gliomas

Although primary brain stem tumors are termed *gliomas*, they are usually astrocytomas. In this location, they are primarily a tumor of childhood with a peak incidence between 3 and 9 years.[5] Their origin is usually the pons, and they may extend into the midbrain, medulla, and cerebral hemispheres. When small they are difficult to detect by CT as they enhance poorly and may not cause pontine enlargement. In the past, cisternography CT was employed to better define the pontine contours and minimize the effect of bone artefacts. Even then, however, clinically evident tumors could go undetected unless the pontine enlargement was prominent or asymmetrical.

On MR images even the low-grade, early tumors are of a detectably higher intensity than the surrounding uninvolved tissue on T2 images (Fig. 3-4). The cystic nature of the tumor can best be determined on T1 images, much in the same way as their cerebellar counterparts (Fig. 3-5). Al-

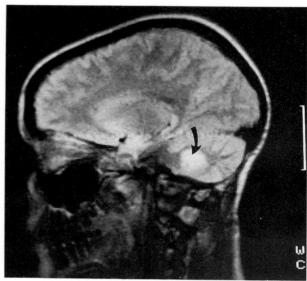

A

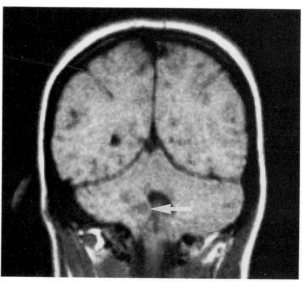

B

Figure 3-2 Cerebellar astrocytoma. On the spin density image in *A*, TR/TE = 2000/35, the spherical lesion (*arrow*) has a uniform high intensity without evidence for internal structure. On the T1 image *B*, TR/TE = 500/35, the tumor exhibits multiple cystic lucencies (*arrow*). The coronal projection is ideal for demonstrating the bulging of the tumor into the fourth ventricle.

though experience with MRI contrast in these tumors is limited, it is not expected that they will be enhanced to any great degree, much as in CT.

Ependymomas

Although ependymomas constitute only some 5 percent of primary intracranial tumors, nearly half of these occur in the

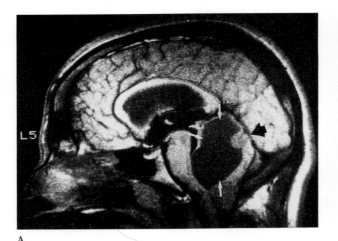

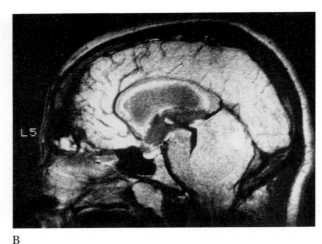

A

B

Figure 3-3 Cystic astrocytoma. Tl image *A*, TR/TE = 500/40, reveals a low-intensity mass within the vermis obliterating the fourth ventricle (*small arrows*). That the mass is not a CSF cyst can be deduced from the moderate T2 image *B*, TR/TE = 1500/40, where the cyst has a much higher intensity than the CSF of the distended ventricles. *Thick arrow* in *A* identifies the mural nodule. (Courtsey of Dr M Solomon, Peninsula Imaging Center, Burlingame, CA.)

first two decades of life. Nearly all ependymomas occur in the midline, usually arising from the ependyma of the floor of the fourth ventricle. Ependymomas grow to fill and obstruct the fourth ventricle while exerting considerable mass effect upon the brain stem and the cerebellum. They may grow through the egresses of the fourth ventricle and spread into the subarachnoid space and the cervical region. Calcifications to a varying degree are present in some 50 percent of

these tumors.[9] They are usually solid but often may contain small cysts or foci of necrosis.

Even on moderately weighted T2 images, ependymomas tend to be of higher intensity than the surrounding structures, with the cystic portions varying from hypointense to slightly more intense than the solid components. On T1 images the cystic portions are hypointense, unless hemorrhage is present (Fig. 3-6). Images in several dimensions are

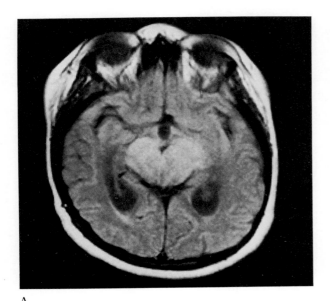

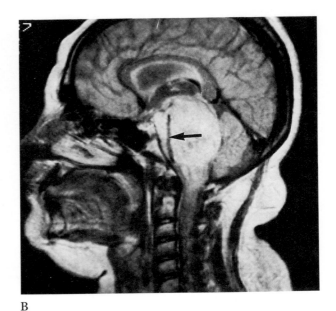

A

B

Figure 3-4 Solid brain stem glioma. T2 images *A* and *B*, both TR/TE = 1800/40, reveal a giant exophytic brain stem glioma extending from the cervicomedullary junction to the midbrain. The basilar artery is encased in the tumor (*arrow in B*). The fourth ventricle is compressed, resulting in moderate hydrocephalus.

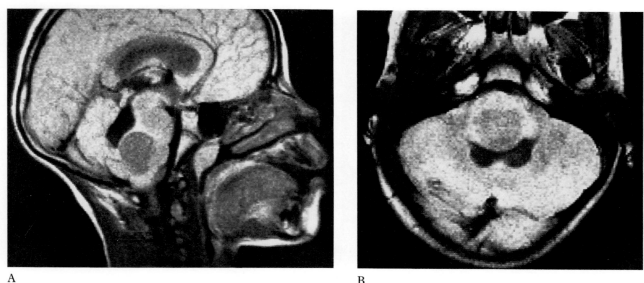

A   B

Figure 3-5 Cystic brain stem glioma. Intermediate-weighted sagittal image *A*,
TR/TE = 1500/35, shows the origin of a cystic tumor in the medulla. There is obstruction of the exit foramina of the fourth ventricle with resulting hydrocephalus.
The axial image *B*, TR/TE = 2100/35, better delineates the lateral extension of the
tumor.

very useful for demonstrating the origin of these tumors,
thus distinguishing them from medulloblastomas (Fig. 3-7).
Edema is only moderate and may aid in the detection of the
tumor boundaries on T2 images. MRI contrast agents

are expected to play a significant role in the detection of sub-
arachnoid extension and seeding, currently a problem for
MRI due to cerebrospinal fluid (CSF) pulsation artefacts
(Fig. 3-8).

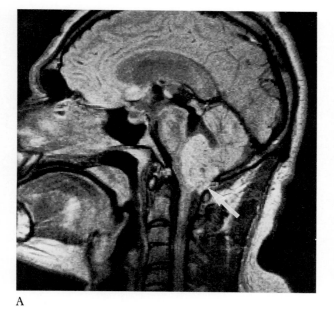

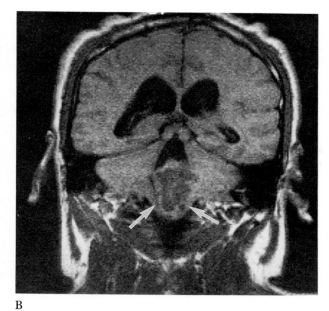

A   B

Figure 3-6 Ependymoma of the fourth ventricle. Spin density image *A*, TR/TE =
1900/35, shows a medium high-intensity, slightly heterogeneous mass arising from
the floor of the fourth ventricle and compressing the medulla. A portion of the mass
extends below the foramen magnum (*arrows* in *A* and *B*). The partially cystic nature
of this tumor is demonstrated to better advantage on the T1 image *B*, TR/TE =
600/34.

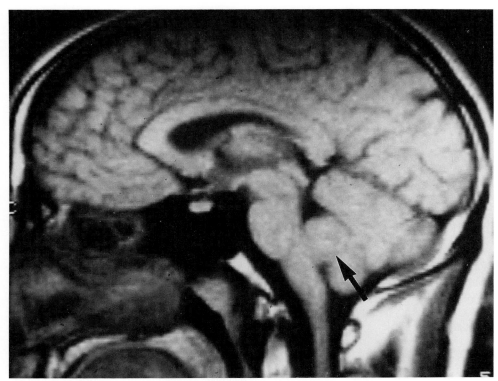

Figure 3-7 Subependymoma of the fourth ventricle. T1 image, TR/TE = 500/28, shows an intraventricular mass arising from the floor of the fourth ventricle (*arrow*). The tumor is isointense to the cerebellum on this T1 image. (Courtesy Dr M Solomon, Peninsula Imaging Center, Burlingame, CA.)

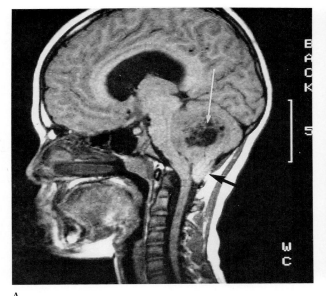

A

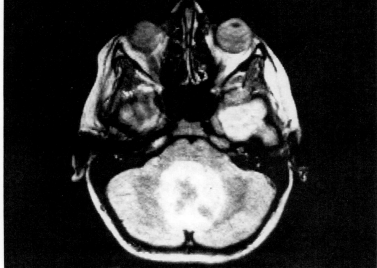

B

Figure 3-8 Ependymoma of the fourth ventricle in an 8-year-old male. T1 sagittal image *A*, TR/TE = 600/17, and axial spin density image *B*, TR/TE = 3000/28. This large tumor is seen to fill the fourth ventricle and invade the cerebellum. Mass effect upon the pons, without invasion, is clearly seen in *A*. The lesion contains multiple small cysts (*long arrow* in *A*) and does not incite edema formation within the cerebellum (*B*). Herniation of the cerebellar tonsils through the foramen magnum is well demonstrated in *A* (*short arrow*). (Courtesy of Dr V Runge, New England Medical Center, Boston, MA.)

Medulloblastomas

Medulloblastomas make up some 4 to 10 percent of all brain tumors but are the second most common posterior fossa tumor in children. They are most frequently found in the fourth venticle arising from the posterior medullary velum. These tumors are rapidly growing and locally invasive and may extend outside the fourth ventricle and present in the cisterns. Seeding of the subarachnoid space is common.[2] Once invasion of the contiguous structures occurs, edema is frequently extensive.

On T2 images, these tumors usually appear as hyperintense masses but may have hypointense foci. The edema surrounding the tumor usually completely obscures the boundaries of the tumor. On T1 images these tumors appear with an intensity that may differ only slightly from brain parenchyma, so that these images may not aid in defining the boundary (Fig. 3-9). Medulloblastomas generally enhance with contrast so that MRI enhancement agents will be quite useful in demarcating the tumor, in accurately defining biopsy sites, and in the detection of subarachnoid seeding.

Nerve Sheath Tumors

Acoustic Neurinomas

Of all the intracranial nerve sheath tumors, the schwannoma of the eighth nerve is the most common. Its origin is predominantly from the Schwann cells of the vestibular division of the eighth cranial nerve, usually at the Schwann cell–glial junction. The location is often within the internal auditory canal (IAC) but it may originate within the cerebellopontine angle (CPA). If their origin is within the IAC, they usually grow toward the brain stem, forming an oval mass in the angle that resembles a scoop of ice cream on a cone.

These tumors enhance brightly with iodinated contrast agents and may be detected within the CPA on enhanced CT studies. Strictly intracanalicular tumors cannot be detected, as they are obscured by bone artefacts generated by the bony walls of the canal, so that a gas cisternography CT study must be employed.

All acoustic neurinomas have a high proton density and prolonged relaxation times and appear as hyperintense, occasionally heterogeneous, rarely cystic masses on T2 images (Fig. 3-10). On T1 images, their intensity can vary from hypointense to slightly hyperintense relative to the pons (Figs. 3-10 and 3-11). When a strictly IAC tumor is extremely bright on T1 images, the possibility of a hemangioma, usually of the seventh nerve, must be considered, as these lesions are invariably markedly hyperintense.

In a double blind study, MRI has been shown to be as accurate as CT and gas cisternography CT in the detection of these lesions.[3] MRI is rapidly becoming the modality of choice in imaging the acoustic complex. Furthermore, MRI also has the advantage of detecting other causes of neurosensory hearing loss not usually detectable by CT, such as multiple sclerosis or a small brain stem glioma. Since acoustic neurinomas enhance brightly with MRI contrast agents, it is hoped that these agents will extend MRI's sensitivity down

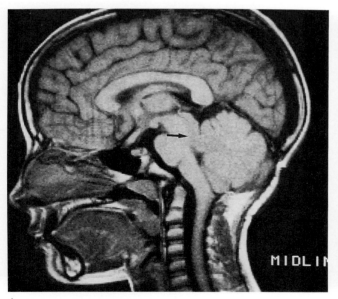

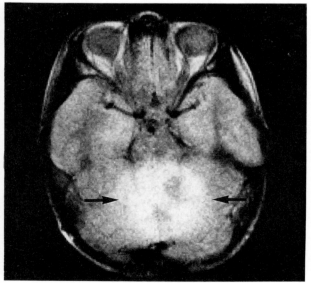

A   B

Figure 3-9 Infiltrating medulloblastoma. Midline sagittal T1 image *A*, TR/TE = 500/34, demonstrates enlargement of the vermis and a bridging mass extending across the fourth ventricle invading the pons (*arrow A*). The tumor is nearly isointense with the cerebellum on this T1-weighted image. Axial image *B*, TR/TE = 1900/35, also fails to delineate the tumor due to the presence of diffuse edema (*arrows*). Perhaps more heavily T1 weighted sequences would have been more useful. Alternatively, a contrast agent would have been useful but was not available.

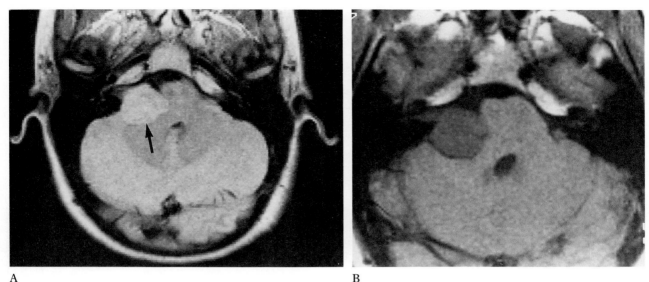

A   B

Figure 3-10 Large acoustic neurinoma. Even moderately T2-weighted sequences usually demonstrate acoustic neurinomas as high-intensity masses (*arrow A*), TR/TE = 1900/35, with the intensity becoming hypointense with respect to the pons on T1 image *B*, TR/TE = 600/30. The interface between the tumor and brain is well demarcated in all cases.

to the millimeter level, thus enabling early detection of these tumors and their removal with a high probability of preserving nerve function (Fig. 3-11*B* and *C*).

Neurinomas of Other Cranial Nerves

With nearly the same accuracy, MRI can detect small neurinomas on other cranial nerves, particularly those of the trigeminal, vagus, and hypoglossal nerves. Their appearance is similar to that of acoustic neurinomas, and the multidimensionality of MRI can be used to follow their extension from the intracranial to the extracranial compartments.

Meningeal Tumors

Some 10 percent of intracranial meningiomas occur in the posterior fossa. They arise from the dura of the tentorium, the cerebellar convexity, the surface of the clivus, the cranial nerves, and the posterior surface of the temporal bone. If they are near the porus acusticus, they may simulate acoustic neurinomas. They are the second most frequent lesion in the CPA.

Meningiomas present a problem for MRI. The relaxation times of meningiomas are extremely variable, so that these tumors can be iso-, hypo-, or hyperintense with respect to brain parenchyma on all imaging sequences (Figs. 3-12 and 3-13). If isointense, they may go undetected unless they are large or are inciting edema in the adjacent brain parenchyma. Their frequent calcification and the hyperostosis of adjacent bone, which aid in their detection by CT, are invisi-

ble by MRI except in those tumors that are extensively calcified, in which case MRI might detect a signal void. Previously, one had to resort to CT scans to reliably detect these tumors. However, it appears that MRI contrast agents enhance these tumors to the same or greater extent than in CT. Thus, enhanced MRI should be at least as sensitive as CT in the detection of these masses (Fig. 3-13*D*).

Blood Vessel Tumors

Hemangioblastoma, the primary characteristic of the von Hippel–Lindau complex, is a nonmalignant tumor that makes up some 10 percent of posterior fossa tumors. It is the most common primary intra-axial posterior fossa tumor in adults. Hemangioblastomas originate in the vermis, the cerebellar hemisphere, the fourth ventricle, and the dorsal aspect of the medulla and pons. These tumors are usually cystic (70 percent), containing proteinaceous fluid, with mural nodules representing the solid component of the tumor. Large vessels surrounding the tumors are frequently seen.

On T1 images, the solid components of the tumor are of similar intensity to the cerebellum. The cystic components are usually hypointense due to their very prolonged relaxation times. On T2 images, the solid components are usually hyperintense with respect to the cerebellum, often of similar intensity to the surrounding edema. The cystic components are often extremely bright on T2 images (Fig. 3-14).

The detection of the mural nodule is aided by the use of multiple projections to minimize partial volume averaging problems. In addition, MRI contrast agents brightly en-

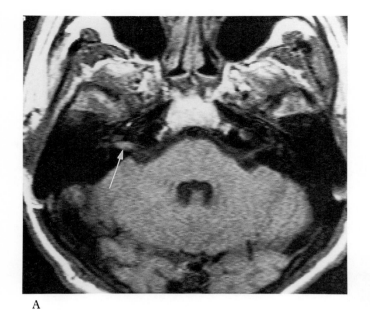

A

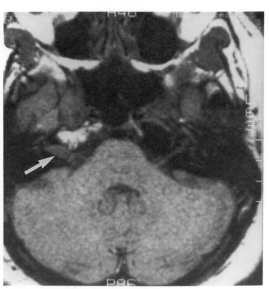

B

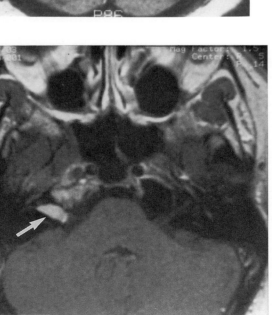

C

Figure 3-11 Acoustic neurinoma in the internal auditory canal. In *A*, a small, moderately hyperintense, strictly intracanalicular acoustic neurinoma is clearly evident within the IAC (*arrow*). When IAC masses are this bright relative to the pons on T1-weighted images, TR/TE = 650/40, the possibility of a facial nerve hemangioma should be raised. In *B*, TR/TE = 800/20, a large hypointense IAC neurinoma is difficult to distinguish from an enlarged canal (*arrow*). The tumor is easily identified after contrast enhancement, *C*, TR/TE = 800/20. (Courtesy of Dr VM Haughton, Medical College of Wisconsin, Milwaukee, WI.)

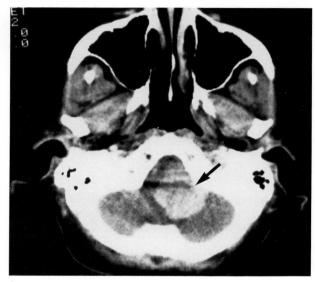

A

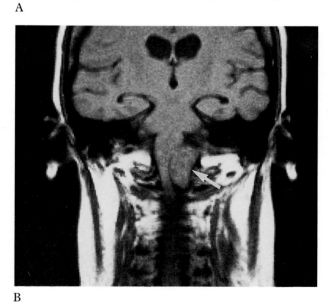

B

Figure 3-12 Foramen magnum meningioma. CT in *A* demonstrates an enhancing lesion in the lower brain stem (*arrow*) originally interpreted as intra-axial. Sagittal and coronal projections *B*, TR/TE = 700/34, helped define the mass as extra-axial (*arrow*), leading to the correct diagnosis and therapy.

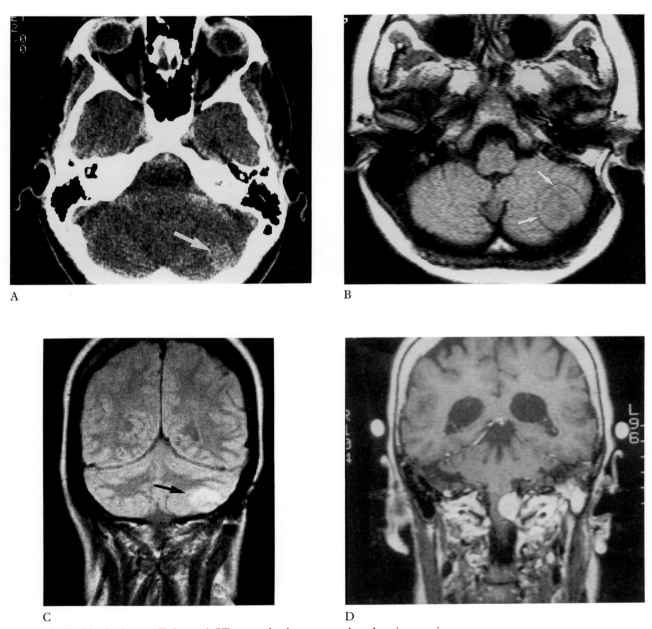

Figure 3-13 Meningiomas. Enhanced CT scan, *A*, shows a poorly enhancing meningioma (*arrow*). On the T1 image *B*, TR/TE = 650/40, the lesion is equally subtle and can only be detected by its mass effect and its thin interface with the cerebellum (*arrows*). On the T2-weighted coronal image *C*, TR/TE = 1900/35, the lesion is identified as a region of increased intensity. There is no edema within the cerebellum, consistent with the clinically quiescent nature of this lesion. *D*, TR/TE = 800/20, shows a brightly enhancing foramen magnum meningioma in another patient. (*D* courtesy of Dr VM Haughton, Medical College of Wisconsin, Milwaukee, WI.)

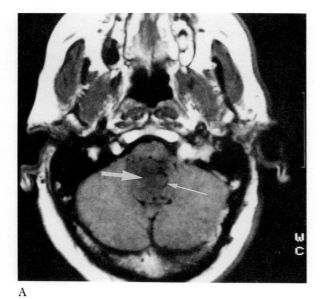

A

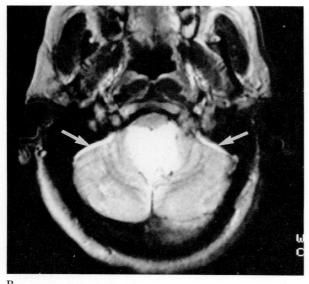

B

Figure 3-14 Hemangioblastoma. A midline cerebellar hemangioblastoma is shown in a patient with von Hippel-Lindau syndrome (*large arrow A*). The lesion is crossed by several serpentine lucencies in *A*, TR/TE = 650/20 (*thin arrow*), which develop some flow enhancement in *B*, TR/TE = 3000/45, and are poorly seen, demonstrating their vascular nature and suggesting the diagnosis. Flow enhancement is also seen in the sigmoid sinuses in *B* (*arrows*). (Courtesy Dr V Runge, New England Medical Center, Boston, MA.)

hance the mural components of these tumors, making even small nodules detectable, perhaps obviating an angiogram.

Other Posterior Fossa Lesions

Chordomas

Posterior fossa chordomas usually arise from the clivus and skull base. When these tumors are small, sagittal and coronal scans may define their origin and distinguish them from meningiomas. When large, these projections define their extent and direction of growth, thus aiding greatly in both surgical and radiation therapy planning.[7] Their soft tissue extent is best defined by spin density and T2 images, on which they are generally hyperintense to muscle but hypointense relative to fat (Fig. 3-15). Detailed evaluation of bone destruction is best left for CT.

Paragangliomas

In our opinion the definitive workup of these tumors includes CT bone studies. The glomus tumors along Jacobson's nerve and in the jugular bulb may permeate the adjacent bone. Although high-resolution MRI may detect some of this permeation, it cannot provide the highly detailed bony landmarks often necessary to plan the surgical excision. MRI's primary role is in the recognition of the presence of these tumors and distinguishing them from other lesions in the same locations.

Glomus jugulare tumors can be identified on MRI images by their "salt and pepper" appearance on T2-weighted images within the jugular bulb and fossa, which distinguishes them from vagus neurinomas and meningiomas, which are usually homogeneous (Fig. 3-16). The high-intensity foci in these tumors may be a result of slowly flowing blood, and the low-intensity foci to solid components and rapidly flowing blood. The presence of these tumors should be distinguished from the complex signals that are frequently present due to slow, turbulent blood flow within the sigmoid sinus and jugular bulb.[10] Additional flow-sensitive sequences can be employed to identify normal flow effects and avoid serious misinterpretation (Fig. 3-14B).

Choroid Plexus Papillomas

These are rare intracranial lesions, representing less than 1 percent of primary brain tumors. They are usually benign and originate from the choroid plexus. Although they are most common in children, their location within the fourth ventricle is usually found in adults.[12]

On MRI images their origin may be determined by imaging in multiple projections. They are hyperintense on T2 images and hypointense on T1 images and have a heterogeneous, lobulated appearance.[8] They readily enhance and their extent within the ventricle and cisterns can be evaluated with MRI contrast agents (Fig. 3-17).

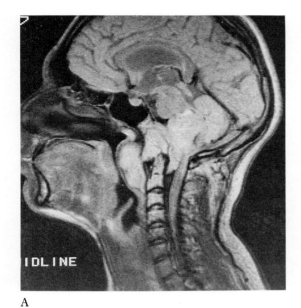

A

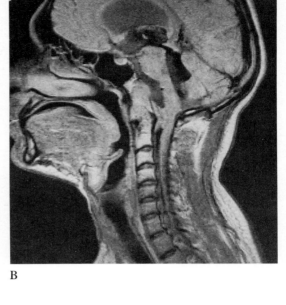

B

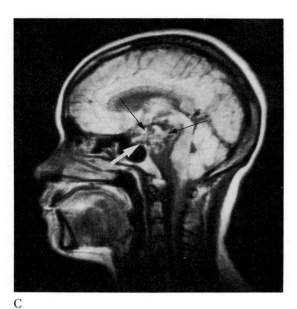

C

Figure 3-15 Chordoma. *A* is a preoperative and *B* a postoperative image, both TR/TE = 1900/35. An unusual chondroid chordoma whose large size obscures its origin. There is invasion of the brain stem, the pharyngeal area, and the condyles and extension into the spinal canal. The information obtained from the multiple projections helped to accurately define the extent of the tumor and permit a staged operative approach. A more typical chordoma containing calcification is demonstrated in *C*, TR/TE = 1000/30 (*arrows*).

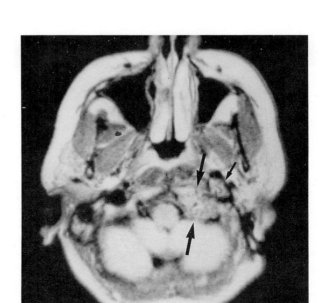

Figure 3-16 Glomus jugulare tumor. A large speckled mass occupies the left jugular fossa and invades the adjacent bone (*arrows*), TR/TE = 2000/35.

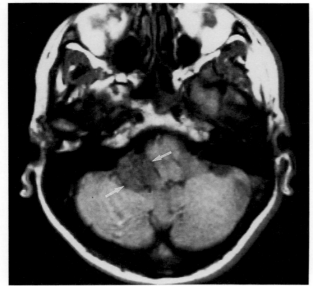

A

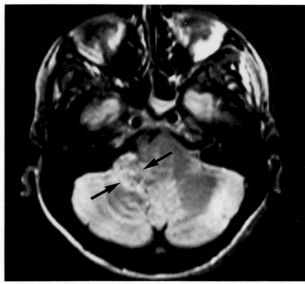

B

Figure 3-17 Choroid plexus papilloma. T1 image *A*, TR/TE = 650/25, and spin density image *B*, TR/TE = 3000/25, demonstrate a large choroidal mass located in the right lateral recess of the fourth ventricle in a 28-year-old woman (*arrows*). The T1 image defines the boundaries of the lesion well. The mass enhances inhomogeneously after MRI contrast administration (*C*). (Courtesy of Dr V Runge, New England Medical Center, Boston, MA.)

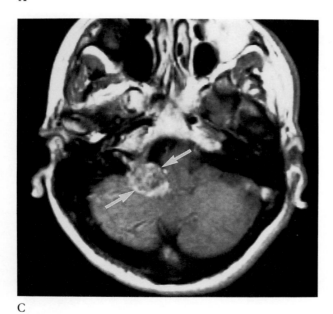

C

plicity of tumors will aid in the diagnosis of metastatic disease. MRI contrast agents should also help in the detection of extra-axial metastases which are notoriously difficult to identify due to the presence of CSF pulsation artifacts (Fig. 3-19).

Metastatic Tumors

The varied primary malignancies yield a variety of MRI appearances for their metastases. Metastases can be cystic, solid, or mixed. When isointense, their detection is aided by the surrounding edema that is generated by the breakdown of the blood-brain barrier. Often, however, this same edema masks the tumor and makes the metastasis indistinguishable from an infarct (Fig. 3-18). The use of MRI contrast agents will become mandatory in such cases, particularly in those cases where a stereotactic biopsy is planned and an exact focus must be identified. In addition, MRI contrast agents will help in distinguishing metastases from primary tumors. These agents have been shown to make visible even the smallest of metastases, so that the identification of a multi-

Cysticercosis

In our southern California practice, with its large Mexican and South American population, we have diagnosed more central nervous cysticercosis than primary brain tumors. The role of MRI and CT in the diagnosis of these lesions is complementary. CT is best in the detection of calcified larvae, which are invisible to MRI. Cysticerci in the subarachnoid and intraventricular regions are best detected by MRI. The cystic forms of these parasites generally contain a fluid that is nearly indistinguishable from CSF. A scolex can nearly always be identified, especially through the use of multiple imaging projections. When intraventricular, the cyst wall can be identified on high-quality MR images. The solid forms are more readily identified since they appear as high-intensity masses on T2 images. They may be free-float-

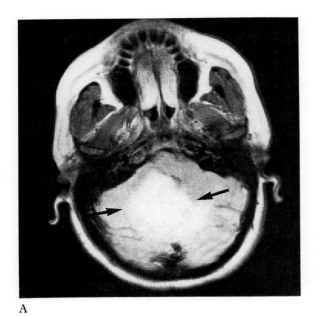
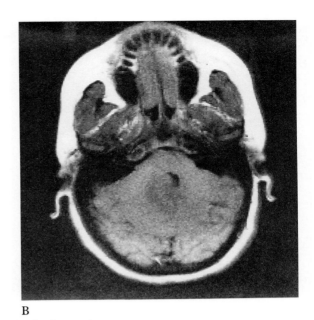

A   B

Figure 3-18 Cerebellar metastasis from breast carcinoma. Spin density image *A*, TR/TE = 1900/35, demonstrates a large area of hyperintense edema involving both hemispheres and the right cerebellar peduncles in a patient with a known breast carcinoma (*arrows*). Although a hypointense region appeared on the T1 image *B*, TR/TE = 500/30, an accurate biopsy site could only be determined by contrast CT, which showed a 5 mm enhancing focus within the central portion of the hypointense area.

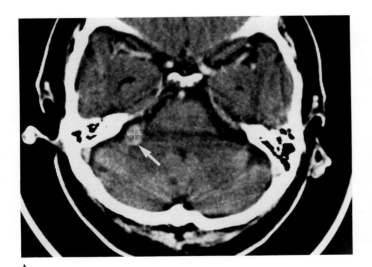
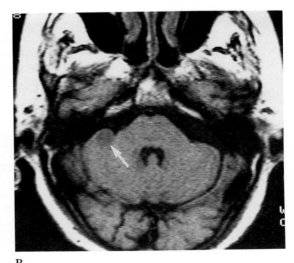

A   B

Figure 3-19 Cerebellar metastasis from lung carcinoma. Enhanced CT shows an enhancing metastatic deposit in the right CPA (*arrow* in *A*). The MRI showed a vague area of increased intensity in this region on the T2-weighted images. The T1 high-resolution image *B*, TR/TE = 650/34, showed a subtle lucency (*arrow*) in the tip of the flocculus, the location of the metastatic deposit. This was appreciated only after perusal of the CT scan. It is in cases like these that MRI contrast agents will play an important role.

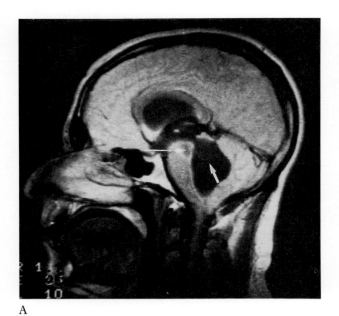
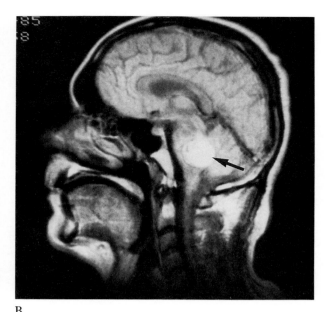

A   B

Figure 3-20 Cysticercosis. Moderate T1 image *A*, TR/TE = 1100/35, shows a subtle cyst projecting through the aqueduct into the fourth ventricle (*short arrow*). A parenchymal cyst is also present in the pons (*long arrow*). A high-intensity, solid cysticercus is located in the fourth ventricle in another patient (*arrow in B*), TR/TE = 2000/35.

ing within the ventricular system or adherent to its walls. In this form they may easily be confused with primary intraventricular tumors (Fig. 3-20). In this case, the greatest aid in their diagnosis is the patient's Spanish surname.

Since MRI can readily detect intraventricular parasites and their locations, a single-stage procedure of parasite removal, fenestration, and ventricular shunting may be performed instead of the multiple-stage procedure usually undertaken.

Dermoids, Epidermoids, Teratomas

The appearance of these masses depends on their composition. The fatty and oily components of dermoids and teratomas are usually hyperintense on both T1 and T2 images, whereas regions containing pieces of solid calcium appear black (Fig. 3-21). The inclusion of hair and pultaceous material can lead to intermediate intensities. Epidermoids contain keratin and frequently appear with CSF intensity on T1 images and moderately hyperintense on T2 images.[11] When located in the CPA, their identification can be aided by the use of heavily T2-weighted images and by their interdigitating conformity to the local spaces. Epidermoids of the temporal bone can be distinguished from cholesterol granulomas, since the latter lesions contain blood products and are hyperintense on T1 images.

Hemorrhage

The appearance of hemorrhage on MR images depends on its age.[1] Acute hemorrhages are nearly isointense with the brain and cannot be identified as such on either T1 or T2 images, although increased water signal may be seen. As the clot ages, the red cells lyse and release their hemoglobin. The hemoglobin undergoes transition from oxyhemoglobin to deoxyhemoglobin to methemoglobin. In this final state, the methemoglobin acts as a strong paramagnetic contrast-enhancing agent. Thus, the intensity of the clot goes from isointense, to slightly more intense, to very hyperintense as the methemoglobin fraction grows. The appearance of these transitions varies with the field strength of the MRI equipment, being apparent slightly earlier on ultralow field strength than at moderate or high field strength systems (0.35 to 1.5 tesla).

The appearance of hemorrhage on MR images complements that of CT. When bright on CT, the lesions are barely detectable on MRI. As the CT density fades, MRI intensity rises. In the chronic phase, the center of the hematoma remains a moderate-intensity focus on T2 images with a low-intensity ring surrounding it created by hemosiderin deposits. Therefore, the choice of modality for imaging depends on the age of the lesion. CT is better in acute events, and MRI is superior after several days.

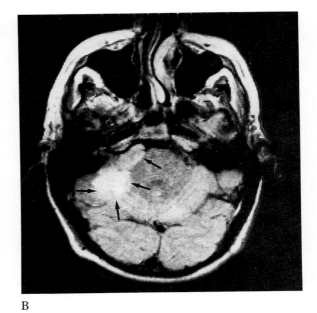

B

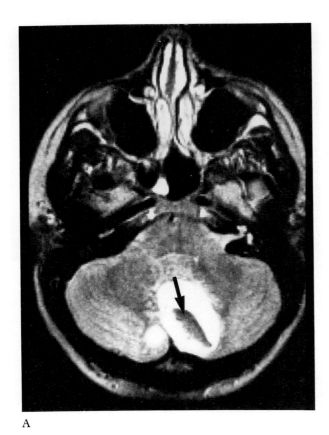

A

Figure 3-21 Teratoma and epidermoid. T2 image *A*,
TR/TE = 2000/80, demonstrates a cerebellar teratoma
having high-intensity areas consisting of fats and oils and
a low-intensity portion corresponding to calcium (*arrow*).
A mixed-intensity epidermoid (*arrows*) in *B*, TR/TE =
1900/35, is seen to insinuate itself into the local folds of
the cerebellum. On the T1 image *C*, TR/TE = 500/30,
the lesion is of low intensity but contains an unusual
high-intensity focus representing either blood products or
fatty materials (*arrow*). (*A* courtesy of Dr M Solomon,
Peninsula Imaging Center, Burlingame, CA.)

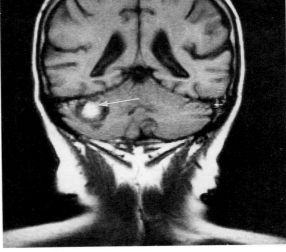

C

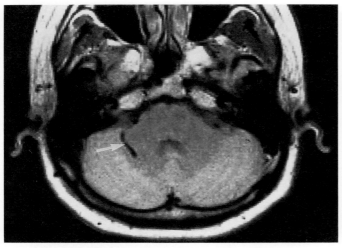
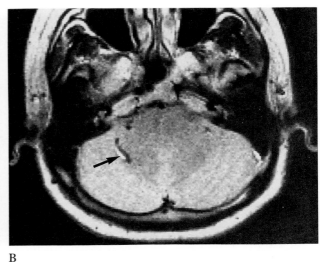

A   B

Figure 3-22 Arteriovenous malformation. First and second echo images *A* and *B* demonstrate a draining vein (*arrow*) from a cryptic vascular malformation. On the second echo *B*, the even echo rephasing phenomenon of slow flow is demonstrated by the bright streak adjacent to the vessel (*arrow in B*). TR/TE = 1900/35 in *A* and 1900/70 in *B*.

Vascular Malformations

Arterial malformations can easily be detected as flow voids in serpentine vessels. Small venous and capillary malformations are difficult to detect due to their size. However, a draining vein can often be discovered and the presence of a lesion inferred (Fig. 3-22). Cavernous hemangiomas usually appear as mottled foci of high intensity, presumably due to stagnant or slow-flowing blood. Often a ring of low-intensity will surround these hemangiomas to give them a characteristic appearance (Fig. 3-23). The low intensity is thought to be

the result of severe T2 shortening induced by residual hemosiderin deposits from previous subclinical hemorrhage.

References

1. Bradley WG Jr. MRI of hemorrhage and iron in the brain. In: Stark DD, Bradley WG Jr (eds.), *Magnetic Resonance Imaging.* St Louis: Mosby, 1988:359–374.
2. Chin HW, Maruyama Y, Young AB. Medulloblastoma: recent advances and directions in diagnosis and management: Part I. *Curr Probl Cancer* 1984; 8:4–54.
3. House JW, Waluch V, Jackler RK. Magnetic resonance imaging in acoustic neuroma diagnosis. *Ann Otol Rhinol Laryngol* 1986; 95:16–20.
4. Koos WT, Miller MH. *Intracranial Tumors of Infants and Children.* St Louis: Mosby, 1971.
5. Lassman LP, Arjona VE. Pontine gliomas of childhood. *Lancet* 1967; 1:913–915.
6. Naidich TP, Lin JP, Leeds NE, et al. Primary tumors and other masses of the cerebellum and fourth ventricle: differential diagnosis by computed tomography. *Neuroradiology* 1977; 14:153–174.
7. Oot RF, Melville GE, New PFJ, et al. The role of MR and CT in evaluating clival chordomas and chondrosarcomas. *AJNR* 1988; 9:715–723.
8. Schellhas KP, Siebert RC, Heithoff KB, et al. Congenital choroid plexus papilloma of the third ventricle: diagnosis with real-time sonography and MR imaging. *AJNR* 1988; 9:797–798.
9. Segall HD, Zee CS, Naidich TP, et al. Computed tomography in neoplasms of the posterior fossa in children. *Radiol Clin North Am* 1982; 20:237–253.
10. Waluch V, Bradley WG Jr. NMR even echo rephasing in slow laminar flow. *J Comput Assist Tomogr* 1984; 8:594–598.
11. Yuh WTC, Barloon TJ, Jacoby CG, et al. MR of fourth-ventricular epidermoid tumors. *AJNR* 1988; 9:794–796.
12. Zimmerman RA, Bilaniuk LT. Computed tomography of choroid plexus lesions. *J Comput Tomogr* 1979; 3:93–103.

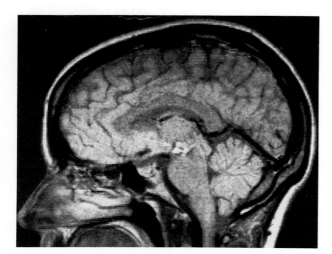

Figure 3-23 Cavernous hemangioma. This moderate T1 image, TR/TE = 1500/35, demonstrates an irregular high-intensity focus in the pons. The rim of hypointensity surrounding the lesion (arrow) is due to deposits of hemosiderin from old subclinical bleeding.

4

Magnetic Resonance Imaging of Craniovertebral Junction Lesions

Russell J. Asleson
Victor M. Haughton

Both spin echo and gradient echo techniques may be needed for imaging the craniovertebral junction (CVJ). T1-weighted images, which show the contours of the cord and brain stem, are efficiently obtained with spin echo techniques. With a short repetition time (TR) and echo time (TE), T1-weighted spin echo images have short acquisition times and little artifact from cerebrospinal fluid (CSF) pulsations. Intra-axial abnormalities are often better demonstrated on T2-weighted images, which can be obtained expeditiously with gradient echo imaging and relatively short acquisition time or with spin echo images obtained with long TR and long TE. Cardiac or peripheral gating or gradient moment nulling are needed to minimize artifacts due to CSF motion in T2-weighted images. Gradient echo techniques are generally faster than spin echo sequences but are more susceptible to artifacts.[1] Bone contours are shown and gray and white matter differentiated better on gradient echo images than with spin echo images. Blood flowing in the major arteries and veins can be demonstrated effectively with gradient echo techniques and gradient moment nulling.

Sagittal plane imaging is most useful for evaluation of the brain stem and cervical spinal cord and their relationship to the bony structures of the CVJ. Axial and, less commonly, coronal images are obtained as needed. The CVJ may be studied with a head coil, especially if the entire brain is to be studied, or with a surface coil, especially when the upper cervical region is to be included.

Magnetic Resonance Anatomy at the Craniovertebral Junction

Osseous structures at the CVJ are identified because of the lack of signal from the cortical margins and the moderately intense signal of fat in bone marrow in a short TR and TE spin echo image. On gradient echo images, the signal intensity of bone marrow and cortical bone is lower than on spin echo sequences. Bone contours are therefore more readily defined with gradient echo sequences than with their spin echo counterparts.[5] The posterior rim of the foramen magnum is usually conspicuous as a low signal region on sagittal images. The thinner anterior rim is less conspicuous; however, its position on most scans can be determined because of the high signal from bone marrow in the clivus (Fig. 4-1). A fat pad normally seen superior to the dens also identifies the inferior extent of the clivus. The cortical margins of C1 and C2 also have very low signal intensity. Marrow in C1 and the body and posterior elements of C2 has high signal intensity in the short TR and TE images. The cancellous bone of the odontoid process often has a lower signal intensity than the rest of C2 (Fig. 4-2).

Synovial joints of the occipitoatlantal and atlantoaxial articulations are seen particularly well on coronal MR images. A thin band of intermediate to high signal intensity, representing articular cartilage, is identified in magnetic resonance (MR) (especially T1-weighted) images between the low signal intensity of the cortical margins of opposing articular surfaces. The synovial joint between the anterior arch of C1 and the odontoid process has a similar signal intensity characteristic but is better seen on sagittal images.

The anterior longitudinal ligament and the atlanto-occipital membrane together are seen on sagittal T1-weighted images as a low-intensity band extending from the anterior aspect of the body of C2 cephalad to the anterior arch of C1 and to the inferior aspect of the occipital bone anterior to the basion. Posterior to the atlanto-occipital membrane and superior to the dens a high signal intensity from a fat pad is normally identified. The apical ligament of the dens is seen as a thin dark band surrounded by fat extending from the superior dens to the basion.

The ligament complex posterior to the dens includes the posterior longitudinal ligament, the superior extension of the tectorial membrane, and the cruciform ligament.[7] On sagittal T1-weighted images a relatively low signal intensity band representing the ligament complex can be seen extending from the posterior aspect of the C2 vertebral body cephalad to the posterior aspect of the basion. When the CSF has low signal intensity, as in T1-weighted images, the posterior ligament complex is difficult to identify. On T2-weighted sequences the CSF has a higher signal intensity than the ligaments so that the ligaments can be distinguished (Fig. 4-3). The synovial joint between the posterior aspect of the dens and the cruciform ligament is difficult to identify with routine MR sequences.

In sagittal T1-weighted images, the pons, medulla, upper cervical spinal cord, cerebellar vermis, fourth ventricle, and cisterna magna are useful landmarks. In the T1-weighted images the fourth ventricle and cisterna magna have a low signal intensity characteristic of CSF. The basilar and vertebral arteries may be seen as structures anterior to the pons and medulla with no signal intensity unless the signal from flowing blood is enhanced by techniques such as gradient moment nulling or gating. In axial and coronal T1-weighted images, the distinctive belly of the pons, the lobulations of the medulla oblongata, the ovoid shape of the upper cervical

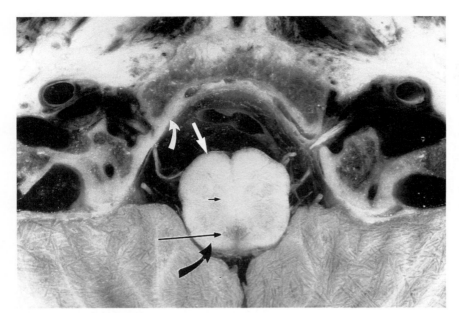

Figure 4-1 Anatomic landmarks in the medulla oblongata illustrated by an (*A*) axial cryomicrotomic section and (*B*) axial proton density weighted MR image at the level of the midmedulla. The pyramidal tract (*white straight arrows*), medial lemniscus (*small arrows*), central gray matter (*long arrows*), nucleus gracilis and nucleus cuneatus (*black curved arrows*), and cortical bone of the anterior margin of the foramen magnum (*white curved arrows*) are labeled.

A

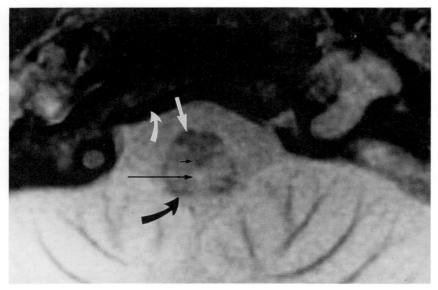

B

cord, and the paramidline location of the cerebellar tonsils are easily recognized. The hypoglossal canals are seen on coronal images as "C" shaped low-signal cortical rims in the occipital bone at the anterolateral aspects of the foramen magnum.

MR images depict in detail the intrinsic anatomy of the upper cervical spinal cord and medulla oblongata (Figs. 4-1 and 4-2).[5,9] Distortions of these normal intrinsic landmarks are important signs of infiltrating processes. Gray and white matter at the CVJ are best differentiated on T2-weighted gradient echo images.[6] Midline sagittal images with this technique show the central gray matter in the upper cervical

spinal cord as a relatively high signal intensity line within the ventral half of the cord (Fig. 4-3). At the CVJ, the central gray matter is located centrally in the cord, posterior to the decussation of the pyramidal tracts. As it nears the obex, the high signal intensity of the gray matter lies closer to the dorsal than the ventral surface of the brain stem. Axial T2-weighted gradient echo images show the high signal intensity of the central gray matter to have a butterfly pattern in the upper cervical cord. In contrast to the gray matter, the pyramidal tracts located anteriorly, the posterior columns (fasciculus gracilis and fasciculus cuneatus), and the other white matter tracts have a lower signal intensity. At the level

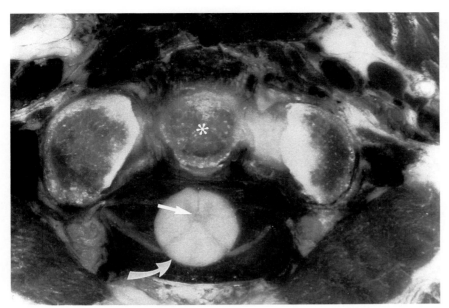

A

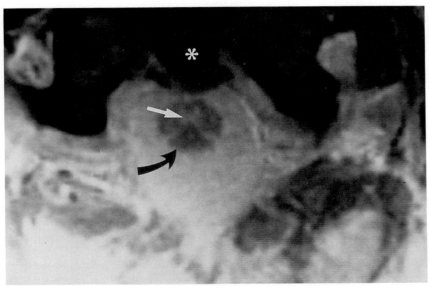

B

Figure 4-2 Anatomic landmarks at the CVJ illustrated by an (*A*) axial cryomicrotomic section and (*B*) proton density weighted MR image. The odontoid process (*asterisk*), central gray matter (*white arrows*), and fasciculus gracilis and fasciculus cuneatus (*curved arrows*) are identified.

of the decussation of the pyramidal tracts, no butterfly pattern is identified. On axial T1-weighted images, the central gray matter of the upper cervical cord has a higher signal than the adjacent white matter tracts (in contrast to the signal intensity relationship in the brain).

Exactly at the CVJ, several intrinsic landmarks can be recognized normally. Axial images show the central gray matter as a triangle-shaped region of high signal intensity. The spinal trigeminal nuclei are visible as high signal intensity regions located posterolaterally in the cord.[9] The supraspinal nuclei are also seen as high signal intensity structures cephalad to the anterior horns.

Above the CVJ proper, axial images show the prominent median fissure of the medulla. The pyramidal tracts, which form the anterior margin of the cord, have a low signal intensity. The central gray matter located dorsal to the middle of the brain stem is a round region of high signal intensity slightly more cephalad in the medulla. Axial T1-weighted images also show the inferior olivary nuclei projecting from the anterolateral margin of the brain stem.

Following the intravenous administration of gadolinium diethylenetriamine pentaacetic acid (Gd-DTPA) in T1-weighted images, the spinal cord and medulla normally show no change in signal intensity ("contrast enhance-

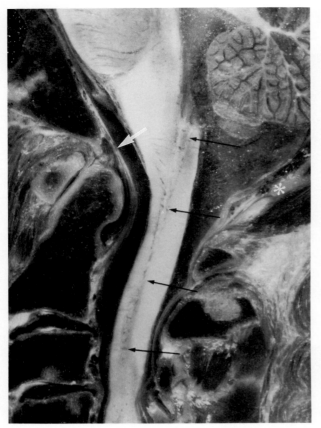

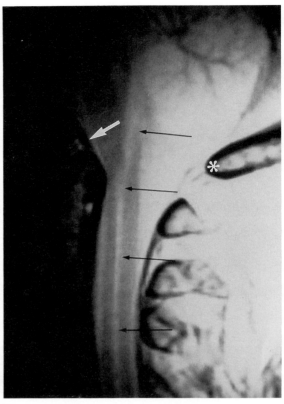

B

A

Figure 4-3 Anatomic landmarks in the upper cervical spinal cord and medulla. In the (*A*) sagittal cryomicrotomic section and (*B*) T2-weighted MR image, the central gray matter (*long arrows*), tectorial membrane, cruciform ligament complex (*white arrow*), and opisthion (*asterisk*) are identified.

ment"), while many extra-axial structures do normally enhance. Enhancement of the brain stem or spinal cord indicates an absence or breakdown of the normal endothelial barrier to the leakage of contrast medium. The C2 nerve roots, some intradural veins, and the venous plexus surrounding the dural sac are enhanced. In larger arteries or veins, enhancement is not usually detected because signal is lost from rapidly flowing blood. Enhancement in dura, medullary bone, and fat can be measured but is usually not perceived on inspection of MR images.

Congenital Abnormalities

The congenital abnormalities of the CVJ that are referred for imaging are the Chiari malformations and osseous abnormalities such as platybasia, basilar impression, etc. The former are indications for MR. The latter are effectively demonstrated by plain roentgenograms.

The position and appearance of the cerebellar tonsils suggest the diagnosis of Chiari malformation. "Peg"-shaped tonsils extending 3 mm or more below the foramen magnum indicate a Chiari malformation. Normally shaped tonsils up to 2 mm below the foramen magnum are within normal limits.[2]

The Chiari I malformation is differentiated by the fourth ventricle in normal position or slightly inferiorly displaced and a normal cerebellar vermis and medulla oblongata. On sagittal images the spinal cord should be examined for central low signal indicative of an intramedullary syrinx, which is seen in over half of the patients with a Chiari I malformation (Fig. 4-4). Hydrocephalus or CVJ osseous abnormalities may be present.

The MR findings in the Chiari II malformation are more complex than in the Chiari I deformity. In sagittal short TR images, caudal displacement of the cerebellar vermis, often to the C2-C3 level, is characteristic (Fig. 4-5). The fourth ventricle and brain stem are also displaced caudally. The fourth ventricle may be small because of compression by the adjacent tonsils and cerebellar vermis in the upper cervical spinal canal, or enlarged due to associated hydrocephalus. The anterior surface of the pons may be flattened against the clivus, which may be abnormally concave. Inferior displacement of the medulla oblongata may produce a characteristic kink in the brain stem. Sagittal images often show the inferior portion of the quadrigeminal plate in a horizontal orientation with a pointed appearance posteriorly because of fusion of the inferior colliculi. The distance between the mamillary bodies and the upper surface of the pons may be longer than the normal 1.2 cm.[8] The normal flow void in the region of the aqueduct may be absent because of aqueductal stenosis. Flow in the aqueduct can be confirmed with special gradient-echo sequences.[1]

MR often demonstrates the abnormalities in the dural partitions and brain in Chiari II malformations. Axial images may show interdigitation of the cerebral hemispheres indicative of falx cerebri hypoplasia or a wide incisura because of hypoplasia of the tentorium.[10] Sagittal images may show the torcular in an abnormally low position. An enlarged massa intermedia is another sign of a Chiari II malformation seen in the sagittal images. Gray matter heterotopia can be identified in some patients with a Chiari II malformation. Hydrocephalus is common. Sagittal images of the spinal cord should be examined for syringomyelia. A meningomyelocele, nearly always present in association with the Chiari II malformation, is detected with sagittal or axial MR images of the lower spine.

In the rare Chiari III malformation, more severe abnormalities of the brain are present. Portions of malformed cerebellum are located in a high cervical or CVJ meningoencephalocele.

Rheumatoid Arthritis

MR imaging accurately depicts the bony and soft tissue changes of the CVJ due to rheumatoid arthritis (RA), and their effect on adjacent neural structures. On sagittal short TR images, inflammatory synovial proliferation ("pannus") is identified because of abnormal soft tissues and erosions of adjacent bone (Fig. 4-6). The erosions characteristically are seen on the anterior, posterior, and superior margins of the odontoid process near synovial joints of the atlas and axis. The erosions are accompanied by a tissue with intermediate signal intensity representing the pannus or thickened ligaments. The normal high signal intensity fat pad seen between the basion and the tip of the odontoid process may be obliterated by the pannus.

In some cases of RA, sagittal MR images demonstrate subluxation of the craniovertebral articulations, especially if the head is flexed. Excessive flexion during the examination must be avoided because of the risk of spinal cord compression. The same measurements of atlantoaxial subluxations which are made in roentgenograms can be used in MR images.[4] In addition, MR images may show pannus interposed between the dens and C1, which prevents reduction of some subluxations.

Compression of the medulla or upper cervical spinal cord in RA is effectively evaluated by MR. Subluxations at the CVJ or retrodental pannus which compress the cord are

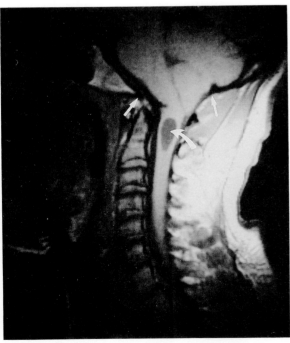

A

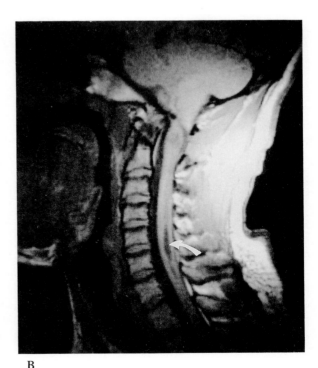

B

Figure 4-4 Chiari I malformation with intramedullary cyst. *A, B.* Sagittal MR images (TR 800, TE 20) show the cerebellar tonsils protruding below the foramen magnum (*straight arrows*). An intramedullary cyst (*curved arrows*) is present in the cervical spinal cord.

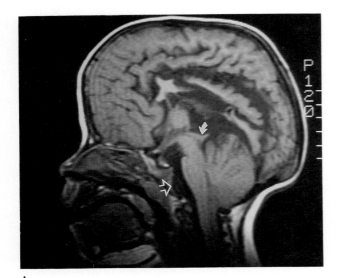

A

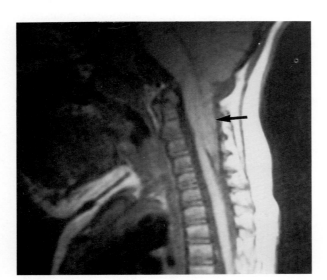

B

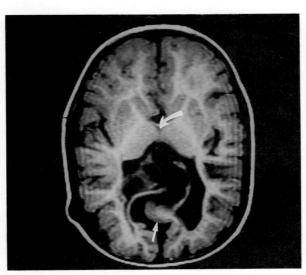

C

Figure 4-5 Chiari II malformation. *A, B.* Sagittal MR images (TR 500, TE 20) show the caudal position of the cerebellar vermis (*black arrow*), concavity of the clivus (*open arrow*), and deformity of the tectum (*small curved arrow*). Dysgenesis of the corpus callosum is also identified. *C.* An axial MR image (TE 500, TE 20) shows interdigitation of the cerebrum (*small arrow*), indicating hypoplasia of the falx. A large massa intermedia (*large curved arrow*) is also present.

demonstrated by sagittal MR images. Vascular compromise can be detected in some cases in axial images by the finding of a narrowing of the signal void normally present in the vertebral and basilar arteries. To demonstrate intrinsic cervical spinal cord abnormalities such as myelomalacia secondary to cord compression, T2-weighted MR images (SE with long TR and TE or gradient echo) are obtained in sagittal or axial planes. In these images, myelomalacia or cord edema appear as high signal intensity regions in the cord. Gradient echo images may also demonstrate some occult fractures of the dens, which occasionally occur in RA. Fractures appear as linear high signal intensity regions through dark bone on T2-weighted gradient echo images.

Neoplasms

The intra-axial and extra-axial primary and secondary tumors that occur at the CVJ are effectively demonstrated by MR. The intramedullary tumors of the CVJ include brain

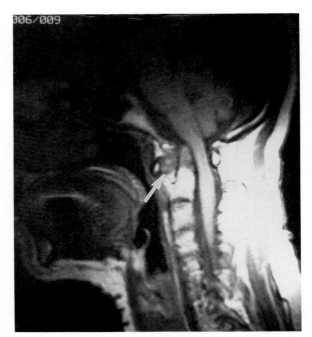

Figure 4-6 Rheumatoid arthritis at the CVJ. Inflammatory tissue (*arrow*) is seen interposed between the anterior arch of C1 and the odontoid process. The spinal canal is narrowed at C1 due to subluxation.

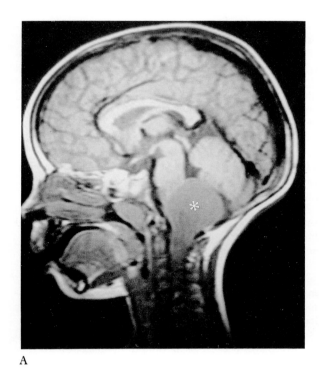

A

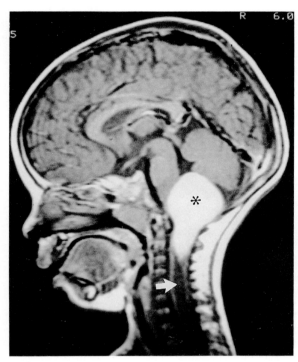

B

Figure 4-7 Astrocytoma at the CVJ. *A.* Sagittal MR image (TR 500, TE 20) shows a large tumor *(asterisk)*. *B.* Image obtained following intravenous Gd-DTPA administration shows marked enhancement of the tumor. An intramedullary cyst *(arrow)* is also present.

stem and upper cervical cord gliomas. The tumors which expand the brain stem are most commonly astrocytomas. Tumors arising near the fourth ventricle, extending caudally to include the CVJ, are commonly ependymomas. Tumors that spread to the CVJ from the upper cervical spinal cord are usually glial tumors.

The short TR images, having the best anatomic detail, show expanding intramedullary tumors effectively. On sagittal short TR images, intra-axial tumors are usually hypointense (Fig. 4-7) or, less commonly, isointense relative to the normal brain stem. In cases of hemorrhage in which some degradation of red cells has occurred, high signal regions may be evident. Vessel displacement and encasement can be recognized by noting the location and caliber of the tubular regions of signal void within and adjacent to the tumor.

Most brain stem glial tumors have high signal intensity on long TR images. The region of abnormality is usually larger on long TR than on short TR images. A rim of high signal intensity characteristic of edema is less common in brain stem tumors than in cerebral glial tumors.

Short TR images following the intravenous administration of Gd-DTPA may be useful in the evaluation of intramedullary tumors because of the enhancement of signal intensity at sites of blood-brain barrier breakdown (Fig. 4-7). Although not all glial tumors enhance, enhancement may be useful to direct a biopsy to the solid portion of the tumor.

Meningioma, the most common extra-axial tumor at the foramen magnum, has a characteristic appearance on MR image. On short TR images, meningiomas are isointense or slightly hypointense with respect to the brain stem. Displacement of the spinal cord by the meningioma is usually demonstrated. On T2-weighted images, meningiomas are usually hypointense; the fibrous meningiomas have a lower signal intensity than the more cellular ones. Meningiomas markedly enhance with intravenous Gd-DTPA (Fig. 4-8), with a 200 to 500 percent increase in signal intensity.[3]

Neurofibromas at the CVJ on short TR images are usually slightly hyperintense with respect to the spinal cord. On T2-weighted images, they are often hypointense. They consistently enhance with intravenous Gd-DTPA. The detection of neurofibromas, especially of the smaller ones, is facilitated with intravenous contrast medium (Fig. 4-9).

Until the availability of MR and Gd-DTPA, leptomeningeal metastases were difficult to detect radiographically. With unenhanced long or short TR images, such metastases are not conspicuous. Short TR images with enhancement show nodular regions of high signal intensity on dural and pial surfaces in cases of leptomeningeal tumor. Melanotic metastases may have high signal intensity without intravenous contrast medium because of the paramagnetic properties of melanin.

Chordomas at the CVJ in short TR images have intermediate to low intensity in contrast to the normal moderately high signal in bone marrow in the clivus. The characteristic finding in chordoma is destruction of the clivus. In short MR images, the high signal intensity of bone marrow in the

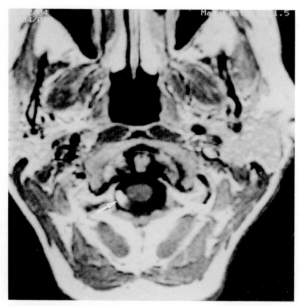

Figure 4-8 Meningioma at C1. An axial MR image (TR 600, TE 20) obtained following intravenous Gd-DTPA administration shows the meningioma (*arrow*). The small unenhanced portion (low signal intensity) of the tumor represents a cyst.

clivus may be replaced with the lower signal intensity of the tumor. Displacement of the brain stem may be seen. Calcifications which may be readily apparent in CT images are in MR inconspicuous or represented as regions of low signal in

the tumor. In gradient echo images, the regions of calcification are accentuated as low signal intensity.

Epidermoid tumors at the CVJ typically have an inhomogeneous low signal intensity on short TR images and high signal intensity on long TR images. Strands or septae of fibrous tissue separating the cystic spaces have a lower signal intensity than the cystic portions of the tumor on short TR images.

Neurenteric cysts at the CVJ are rare (Fig. 4-10). They have low signal intensity on short TR images. A defect in the adjacent vertebrae is a characteristic finding. The spinal cord may be displaced. The cyst may be difficult to distinguish from the adjacent subarachnoid space.

Lipomas have a characteristic high signal intensity on short TR images, and lower signal intensity on T2-weighted images. They are usually isointense with fat elsewhere. They are not common at the CVJ.

Carcinoma has intermediate intensity on short TR images and hyperintensity on long TR images. Carcinomas may spread to the CVJ from the nasopharynx or by hematogenous spread to osseous structures. Multiple myeloma has an appearance similar to that of carcinoma.

Arteriovenous malformations (AVMs) can be identified on MR images because of the abnormal enlarged feeding or draining vessels. On short and long TR images, the vessels are usually tubular structures with absent signal. In some cases, bright signal is seen in the venous structures because of flow-related enhancement. Hemorrhage or thrombosis may also produce high signal intensity on short TR images due to methemoglobin. Areas of low signal on long TR images may signify the presence of hemosiderin or in acute hematomas the presence of deoxyhemoglobin. Gradient echo sequences with specially designed pulses that enhance

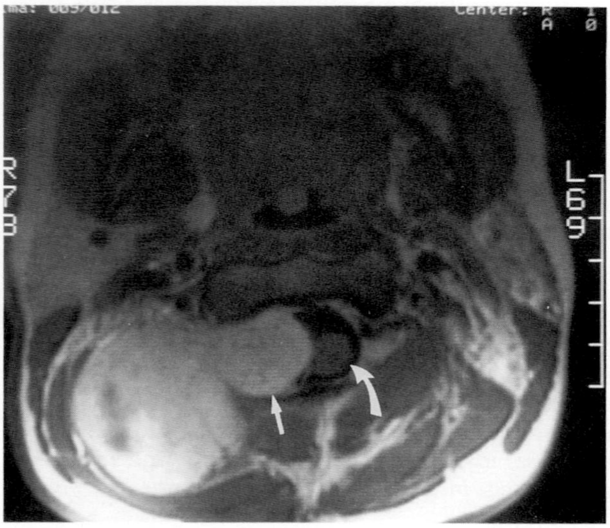

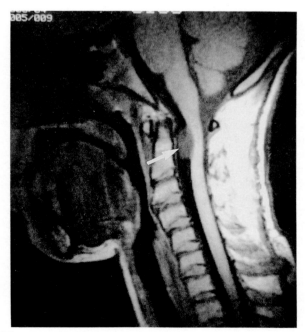

Figure 4-10 Neurenteric cyst. A sagittal MR image (TR 800, TE 20) shows a relatively low intensity mass (*arrow*) displacing the spinal cord posteriorly.

Figure 4-9 Neurofibroma at C2. An axial MR image (TR 800, TE 20) obtained following intravenous Gd-DTPA administration shows that the tumor has both intradural (*arrow*) and extradural components. The spinal cord (*curved arrow*) is displaced.

the signal of flowing blood can be performed to verify AVMs.

Intramedullary Cysts

Syringomyelia and hydromyelia are two conditions in which cysts (syrinxes) are formed within the spinal cord. MR images readily demonstrate such cystic intramedullary processes.[11] Both short and long TR images are useful in the evaluation of intramedullary cysts. The sagittal plane is most useful for screening and for demonstrating the longitudinal extent of the syrinx and the presence of septations within it. Axial images are obtained to confirm or further characterize the intramedullary abnormalities.

The signal characteristics of the fluid within syrinx cavities may be useful diagnostically. In many non-neoplastic intramedullary cysts, the signal intensity of the cyst fluid is the same as that of CSF in all pulse sequences. A higher signal intensity in the cyst than in CSF in T2-weighted images (without cardiac or peripheral gating) suggests less movement of the fluid in the cyst than in the subarachnoid space. In these cases, the cyst may be under high pressure. This sign may be useful in selecting patients for cyst decompression. Blood, which may increase the signal intensity in T1-weighted images, is rarely found in benign intramedullary cysts. When the cyst has a lower signal intensity than CSF in T2-weighted images, a sign that the fluid may contain a high concentration of protein, a neoplastic cyst rather than a non-neoplastic intramedullary cyst should be considered.

In cases of intramedullary cyst, associated abnormalities may provide important diagnostic information. Sagittal images, used to evaluate the position of the cerebellar tonsils and vermis, may permit the diagnosis of a coexisting Chiari malformation (see above). Diastematomyelia is another developmental abnormality that may be associated with a syrinx.

Congenital intramedullary cysts must be distinguished from those resulting from an intramedullary neoplasm or from myelomalacia (Fig. 4-11), which may have similar MR appearances. On long TR images, areas of high signal in the spinal cord without expansion of the cord more likely represent gliosis or myelomalacia than cyst or neoplasm. A neoplasm almost invariably enlarges the cord. Cysts usually have better defined margins than do neoplasms. Enhancement following the administration of Gd-DTPA is seen in many intramedullary tumors, but not usually in myelomalacia and gliosis. Therefore, intravenous contrast enhancement may be used with MR to differentiate neoplastic from non-neoplastic conditions of the cord (Fig. 4-7).

Artifacts may obscure or mimic intramedullary cysts. High contrast interfaces, such as between the spinal cord and CSF, generate truncation artifacts. Truncation artifact in the spinal cord is seen as a linear shadow paralleling the cord and located centrally in the cord. This artifact may simulate enlargement of the central canal. Truncation artifact is minimized by increasing the number of encoding

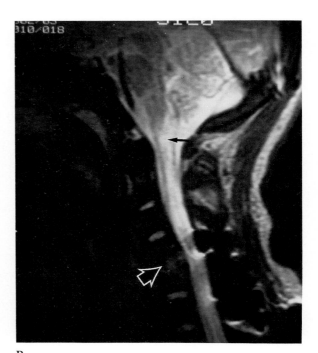

A   B

Figure 4-11   Post-traumatic myelomalacia associated with a fracture-dislocation at C4-5. *A*. A T1-weighted MR image (TR 600, TE 20) shows an ill-defined low signal intensity in the upper cervical cord (*arrow*). *B*. A T2-weighted image (TR 2571, TE 80) shows high signal in the cord (*black arrow*). The disc space at C4-5 (*open arrow*) is obliterated, and slight kyphosis is present. The signal void (*curved arrow*) is an artifact from a metallic clip.

steps, i.e., by increasing the matrix from 128 to 256 or more steps. Motion artifacts, due to CSF pulsations or patient motion, create linear ill-defined "ghosts" which degrade image quality and may obscure syringomyelia or simulate it if it superimposes on the cord silhouette. Peripheral pulse or cardiac gating minimizes pulsation artifacts.

References

1. Atlas SW, Mark AS, Fram EK. Aqueductal stenosis: evaluation with gradient-echo rapid MR imaging. *Radiology* 1988; 169:449–453.
2. Barkovich AJ, Wippold FJ, Sherman JL, et al. Significance of cerebellar tonsillar position on MR. *AJNR* 1986; 7:795–799.
3. Breger RK, Papke RA, Pojunas KW, et al. Benign extra-axial tumors: contrast enhancement with Gd-DTPA. *Radiology* 1987; 163:427–429.
4. Bundschuh C, Modic MT, Kearney F, et al. Rheumatoid arthritis of the cervical spine: surface-coil MR imaging. *AJR* 1988; 151:181–187.
5. Czervionke LF, Daniels DL. Cervical spine anatomy and pathologic processes: applications of new MR imaging techniques. *Radiol Clin North Am* 1988; 26:921–947.
6. Czervionke LF, Daniels DL, Ho PSP, et al. The MR appearance of gray and white matter in the cervical spinal cord. *AJNR* 1988; 9:557–562.
7. Daniels DL, Williams AL, Haughton VM. Computed tomography of the articulations and ligaments at the occipito-atlanto-axial region. *Radiology* 1983; 146:709–716.
8. El Gammal T, Mark EK, Brooks BS. MR imaging of Chiari II malformation. *AJR* 1988; 150:163–170.
9. Ho PSP, Yu S, Czervionke LF, et al. MR appearance of gray and white matter at the cervicomedullary region. *AJNR* 1989; 10:1051–1055.
10. Naidich TP, Pudlowski RM, Naidich JB, et al. Computed tomographic signs of the Chiari II malformation. Part 1: Skull and dural partitions. Radiology 1980; 134:65–71.
11. Sherman JL, Barkovich AJ, Citrin CM. The MR appearance of syringomyelia: new observations. *AJNR* 1986; 7:985–995.

5

Magnetic Resonance Imaging of Sellar and Parasellar Lesions

Walter Kucharczyk
Roger M. L. Smith

The sella turcica and parasellar region are fascinating areas for the radiologist and surgeon alike. The anatomy is intricate, and the pathology is diverse. Many different imaging modalities have been used for the assessment of this area, but for the most part the introduction and widespread use of high-resolution computed tomography (CT) relegated its imaging predecessors, such as plain skull roentgenograms, pluridirectional tomography, and pneumoencephalography, to obsolescence. Magnetic resonance imaging (MRI) is now widely available, and a considerable body of experience has been accumulated in evaluating this region. MRI has much to offer in comparison to CT. Its major advantages are its superior soft tissue contrast and multiplanar imaging. Also, there is no artifact from bone, contrast agents are generally not required, and the patient is not exposed to ionizing radiation. However, MRI is still not universally accepted as a superior imaging test. Many centers that have had considerable experience with both CT and MRI advocate the preferential use of MRI over CT.[7,9] Others are less enthusiastic.[4,10] Regardless of which of these philosophies one believes, it is useful to review the normal anatomy of this area as it appears on MRI and to look at the more common types of pathological entities which occur in this area.

Equipment and Technique

MR images with optimal spatial and contrast resolution and minimal background noise are required. In general, high-field-strength units (1.0 to 2.0 tesla) are best for this purpose. Midfield units operating between 0.3 and 1.0 tesla can produce adequate images, but when the finest detail is re-

quired without unacceptable background noise levels, the high-field unit is generally superior.

Images are obtained in the sagittal, coronal, or axial plane or a combination thereof. Usually, time constraints preclude acquisition in all three planes. It is generally accepted that coronal images are the most useful, particularly when examining the pituitary gland.[4,5,7,9,10] Coronal images allow the gland to be examined for asymmetries, and there is minimal partial volume artifact from the cavernous sinuses and carotid arteries. The sagittal image is useful in demonstrating midline anatomy and the orientation of the sella turcica and pituitary gland relative to the sphenoid sinus. It is particularly useful when tumors extend out of the sella turcica. In cases of extrasellar extension, it is important to demonstrate the direction of extent of the lesion because it may alter the choice of surgical approach. Axial images are of limited usefulness. Generally, only one or two consecutive axial images can be obtained through the pituitary gland, and these may be subject to considerable partial averaging effects from the sphenoid sinus below and the suprasellar cistern above. Axial sections can be useful for evaluating the cavernous sinus and the medial temporal fossa on each side. In practice, images are acquired in only the sagittal and coronal planes. If upon review other views are thought to be potentially useful, they are obtained as individual circumstances dictate.

Detailed spatial resolution is of the utmost importance because many lesions in this area are very small. This requires small pixel size and thin slices. Most current MR images are capable of obtaining images as thin as 2 or 3 mm. In-plane resolution finer than 0.5 mm on side can be obtained. However, the use of very small pixels results in images which are very grainy. Generally, pixel sizes approximately 0.8 mm on side are optimal. These can be achieved with a 20-cm field of view and a 256 × 256 matrix.

There are a wide variety of imaging pulse sequence options. T1-weighted images appear to be the most sensitive and provide the best anatomic detail for extra-axial structures. The pituitary gland and parasellar region are no exception to this general rule. T1-weighted sequences demonstrate the soft tissues of this area very well as intermediate gray structures within the dark surrounding CSF. T1-weighted images can also be obtained in a relatively shorter period of time compared to T2-weighted images. T2-weighted images, which are extremely useful in evaluating the parenchyma of the brain, generally do not display the anatomy of the base of the brain as well as the T1-weighted sequences. They are also susceptible to motion artifacts from pulsating CSF in the cisterns. There are several methods of compensating for this CSF movement such as cardiac gating or specialized gradient pulses. But T2-weighted images take longer to acquire, and it is more difficult to resolve the intrinsic anatomy of the pituitary gland, to visualize the pituitary infundibulum, and to see the optic chiasm. For these reasons, T1-weighted images are the imaging sequence of choice. They may be obtained using either a spin-echo technique or an inversion recovery technique. Spin-echo sequences are favored because they are more widely available, there is a wider body of experience with them, and they provide more slices per unit time than inversion recovery.

TABLE 5-1 Magnetic Resonance Imaging Technique for Examination of the Sella Turcica and Parasellar Region*

Variable	Sequence 1, "T1-Weighted"	Sequence 2, "T1-Weighted"	Sequence 3, "T2-Weighted"†
Type	Spin echo	Spin echo	Spin echo
Plane	Sagittal	Coronal	Coronal
TR (ms)	400–700	400–700	2000–2800
TE (ms)	20	20	35 and 70
Slice (mm)	3	3	5
Matrix	256 × 256	256 × 256	256 × 256
Field of view (cm)	20	20	20
Averages	4	4	1
Exam time (min)	~10	~10	~10

*All sequences performed with a head coil and a multislice mode.
†Supplementary T2-weighted sequence. CSF flow compensating gradients are required.

Finally, because of the requirements of fine spatial detail, signal averaging is required to produce a visually pleasing and diagnostic image. This increases imaging time in a direct linear relationship to the number of signal averages. Therefore, compromise is reached between obtaining good images and still being practical as far as time constraints are concerned. Furthermore, long imaging sequences increase the opportunity for patient motion to degrade all the images. A reasonable balance is to limit the number of signal averages to four.

In summary, the optimum technique consists of using a head coil, sagittal and coronal T1-weighted images, the thinnest possible slices, pixel sizes approximately 0.8 mm per side, and four signal averages. This allows the entire region to be covered in two planes, and examinations are kept to less than 30 min in length. Occasionally, a supplementary T2-weighted sequence is used if the T1-weighted sequences do not demonstrate any abnormality and there is a very compelling reason to believe that a lesion has been overlooked. A T2-weighted sequence is also used if the remainder of the brain needs to be examined (Table 5-1).

Normal Anatomy

The sella turcica is located in a midline depression in the sphenoid bone. It contains the anterior and posterior lobes of the pituitary gland and the distal portion of the pituitary stalk. It is covered by a dural reflection, the diaphragma sellae. Above this lies the suprasellar cistern, which contains the supraclinoid carotid arteries and the optic tract, chiasm, and nerves, and through which travels the pituitary stalk. Lateral to the sella turcica are the cavernous sinuses containing the carotid arteries, cranial nerves III, IV, and VI, and the first two divisions of the fifth cranial nerve. Anteriorly, it is bounded by the tuberculum sellae and anterolaterally by the anterior clinoid processes. Anteroinferiorly, the foramen rotundum conducts the maxillary branch of cranial nerve V. Posteriorly, there are the smaller posterior clinoid processes, the dorsum sellae, and the interpeduncular cistern containing cranial nerves III and IV. Inferiorly, the sella turcica has a thin floor of cortical bone, below which lies the air-containing sphenoid sinus. The sinus is extremely variable in size. Adjacent to the posteroinferior cavernous sinus lies Meckel's cave, containing the gasserian ganglion. Immediately below and lateral to the gasserian ganglion, the third branch of the fifth cranial nerve exits through the foramen ovale.

The midline sagittal section is extremely useful in delineating a great deal of this anatomy (Fig. 5-1A). The pituitary gland is seen within the hemispherical sella turcica. The anterior lobe of the gland is an intermediate gray, very similar to the white matter of the cerebral hemispheres in intensity. The posterior lobe is much smaller and is typically nestled in a small depression in the dorsum (Fig. 5-1A and B). It has a rather unique appearance in that it is extremely bright on the T1-weighted sections. The pituitary stalk is seen to angle anteriorly as it descends from the hypothalamus to the pituitary gland. Normally, the stalk is approximately 1 mm in transverse diameter. The size of the pituitary gland is vari-

Figure 5-1 Normal anatomy. A. Midline sagittal T1-weighted MR image (SE 600/20). This high-resolution MR image demonstrates the anterior and posterior lobes of the pituitary gland, the air-containing sphenoid sinus, the dorsum sellae, the suprasellar cistern, the mamillary bodies, the infundibulum and infundibular recess, and the optic chiasm and chiasmatic recess. B. Axial T1-weighted MR image (SE 600/20). The anterior pituitary lobe occupies most of the sella turcica. It is an intermediate gray intensity, approximately the same as the white matter of the temporal lobe or the brain stem. The posterior lobe is much smaller and is located in a concavity in the dorsum sellae. It is hyperintense. The marrow space of the posterior clinoid processes flank either side of the posterior lobe. C–E. T1-weighted MR images (SE 600/20). Coronal sections through the posterior (C), middle (D), and anterior (E) portions of the sella turcica. The arrows indicate the optic tracts, chiasm, and nerves. Posteriorly, Meckel's cave is lateral to the sella, below which V3 exits from the foramen ovale (C). The midcoronal section shows the pituitary gland, which is bilaterally symmetric about its midline axis (D). It is bounded laterally by the medial cavernous sinus wall (which cannot be resolved as a distinct structure). The carotid arteries are clearly seen in the cavernous sinuses. The lateral wall of the cavernous sinus and the CSF of the medial temporal fossa are of low signal intensity. The suprasellar cistern, of dark gray intensity, contains the infundibulum and the optic chiasm. The anterior section through the sella turcica shows the maxillary branch of the fifth cranial nerve in the foramen rotundum, fat within the superior orbital fissure, and the prominent marrow space of the anterior clinoid processes (E).

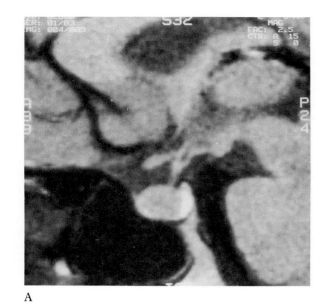

A

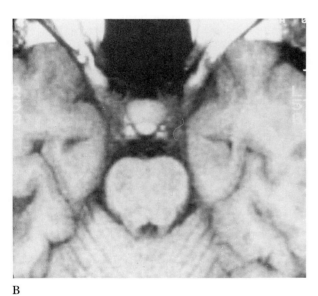

B

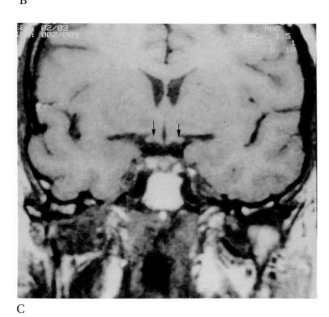

C

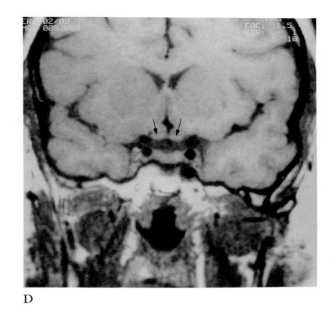

D

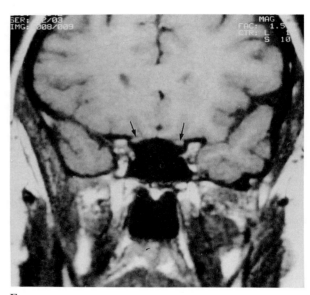

E

Figure 5-1

able. The generally accepted upper limits of normal for diameter is approximately 9 mm. Magnetic resonance and CT measurements correlate very well in this regard.

The optic chiasm is seen immediately anterior to the pituitary stalk in the suprasellar cistern. The CSF in the suprasellar cistern is a dark gray. The third ventricle and its inferior recesses, the optic and infundibular recesses, are well seen immediately above the optic chiasm and infundibulum, respectively. The floor of the sella turcica, formed by thin cortical bone, is difficult to appreciate, particularly if the sphenoid sinus is large. There is no appreciable contrast interface between dark cortical bone and the dark air-containing sinus. Parasagittal sections are of limited usefulness, primarily because parts of these sections contain the cavernous sinus and carotid arteries which loop through this area. This causes troublesome partial volume averaging effects and may lead to misinterpretation of images.

Coronal images are particularly useful for evaluation of the pituitary gland and cavernous sinuses (Fig. 1C through E). The coronal section through the midbody of the pituitary gland generally demonstrates symmetry about the stalk. Its superior surface may be either flat, concave, or convex. Upward convexity is in itself not indicative of an intrapituitary mass because such a convexity is often present at the point where the infundibulum inserts into the gland. Above the gland, the fibrous diaphragma sellae is generally not seen as a distinct structure because immediately above it lies the CSF of the suprasellar cistern. Because both of these tissues are approximately of the same signal intensity (dark gray on T1-weighted images), the thin diaphragma is poorly seen, if it is seen at all. The supraclinoid carotid arteries and their bifurcations are seen as regions of signal void (due to the flowing blood within them) in the suprasellar cistern. The optic chiasm is a biconcave disc in cross-section. It has approximately the same signal intensity as the pituitary gland. Immediately above it is the hypothalamus, which forms the inferior and lateral walls of the third ventricle. Only a thin layer of CSF separates the optic chiasm from the hypothalamus, but they can be distinctly seen as separate structures. The clinoid processes, both anterior and posterior, are variable in size and in the amount of marrow they contain. Typically, the anterior processes are larger. They are of high intensity centrally, surrounded by a dark ring of cortical bone.

Laterally lie the cavernous sinuses. The carotid artery is the most prominent structure in the cavernous sinus. It is circular in coronal cross section and is devoid of signal. The remainder of the sinus is composed of venous channels, septa, and cranial nerves. Cranial nerves III and IV and the ophthalmic branch of V have a consistent anatomical relationship to the carotid artery, being superolateral, directly lateral, and inferolateral to the artery, respectively. They can occasionally be seen on the lateral cavernous sinus wall on MRI.[3] The sixth cranial nerve lies within the sinus itself and is generally too small to be seen consistently. The mandibular branch of the fifth nerve is well visualized as it exits from the gasserian ganglion through the foramen ovale. Similarly, the maxillary branch of the nerve can reliably be seen within the foramen rotundum. The venous channels of the cavernous sinus itself have a rather heterogeneous appearance. Regions of flow void are not consistently seen,

perhaps because the flow is too sluggish or because the channels are too small. The lateral cavernous sinus wall together with the CSF in the medial middle cranial fossa form a low-signal-intensity boundary between the medial temporal lobe and the sinus. The medial cavernous sinus wall is extremely thin and cannot be resolved as a distinct structure between the pituitary gland and the cavernous sinus proper.

Meckel's cave is immediately lateral to the posterior portion of the cavernous sinus. Frequently, the gasserian ganglion can be seen within it.

Pathology

General Considerations

The most common lesions in this region are the pituitary adenoma, craniopharyngioma, meningioma, carotid aneurysm, and optic and hypothalamic gliomas, each of which arises from relatively distinct anatomical sites. Therefore, a concise differential diagnosis can usually be established by localizing the lesion to a particular structure. The excellent anatomical detail on MRI facilitates this process. Analysis of the signal intensity may then further refine the differential diagnosis.

In addition to these common disorders, there are many uncommon neoplastic and infiltrative diseases which affect this area. These include (but are not limited to) germinoma, lymphoma, leukemia, chordoma, metastasis, nasopharyngeal carcinoma, sarcoidosis, and histiocytosis X. Although these rarer entities merit some mention, detailed discussion is reserved for the common lesions.

Pituitary Adenomas

Pituitary adenomas are common, benign, epithelial tumors which arise from the anterior lobe of the pituitary gland. The clinical presentation and classification depends primarily on whether they are functioning (secretory) or nonfunctioning (nonsecretory). From the radiological perspective, it is best to classify adenomas based on their size, those under 1 cm in diameter being considered microadenomas and those greater than 1 cm in diameter being considered macroadenomas.

The role of MRI in the diagnosis of microadenomas is to confirm the clinical diagnosis, to localize the tumor, and to determine the involvement of adjacent structures. Thin-section T1-weighted images are best for this purpose.

The typical microadenoma appears as an area of focal hypointensity within the intermediate intensity of the anterior lobe (Fig. 5-2).[4,7,9,10] It is usually well defined, with a distinct border. Most are laterally situated. They may be associated with superior displacement of the upper gland surface (focal convexity upward) and/or displacement of the pituitary stalk to the opposite side. There may also be focal remodeling of the sella floor beneath the adenoma. These latter three signs are less reliable because quite often the normal gland may display similar features. The most reliable sign is that of the focal hypointensity. Quite often the differ-

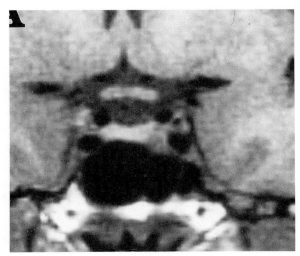

Figure 5-2 Microadenoma of the pituitary gland. T1-weighted MR image (SE 600/20). There is a focal hypointensity, 4 mm in diameter, on the left side of the gland. The gland is otherwise normal. This appearance is typical of a small, laterally situated adenoma.

ence in intensity between the small adenoma and the normal gland is small. This often necessitates photographing the images at narrow windows or carefully reviewing the images on the operator's console.

To date, there have been no reliable means of distinguishing between various types of microadenomas. The prolactin-secreting adenoma appears identical to the ACTH- and growth hormone-secreting adenoma. Their intensity is in no way dependent on the hormone they secrete. Approximately half of all microadenomas are prolactin-secreting, and of the remainder, there is an approximately equal incidence of ACTH- and growth hormone-secreting tumors. A small minority (less than 10 percent) are rarer types (TSH-, FSH-, LH-secreting). The one pattern that is apparent is that the ACTH-secreting adenomas present at a smaller size, almost certainly because they cause significant clinical problems while they are small. This has been well established in the CT and surgical literature and has been the experience with MRI as well.[5,7]

There is general disagreement in the literature as to how accurate MRI is in the detection of microadenomas. Only a few small series have been reported. The reported sensitivity of MR has varied from 55 to 100 percent.[7,9,10] Our own experience has been favorable. We were able to accurately localize 10 of 11 surgically proven microadenomas, the one false-negative being a 5-mm-in-diameter ACTH-secreting adenoma.[7]

It is probable that most false-negative examinations will continue to be with small adenomas, particularly in Cushing's disease. MRI, currently limited to 2 or 3 mm in slice thickness, cannot reliably detect lesions which are smaller than the slice is thick. One recent large surgical series, reporting on the size of ACTH-secreting microadenomas, noted that the median size was 3 mm.[11] Therefore, the problem is quite obvious.

There are two current developments which may further improve the MRI diagnosis of microadenomas. One is the development of volume imaging techniques in which 1-mm or thinner slices can be achieved. These are currently available, although their implementation is somewhat hampered by the long imaging times involved. The concurrent development of fast imaging techniques using gradient echoes in conjunction with volume acquisitions may be the solution required to detect very small lesions in clinically acceptable imaging times. Second is the introduction of MRI contrast agents into clinical practice. Paramagnetic contrast agents have been used on an investigational basis for several years, the most notable of which is gadolinium diethylenetriamine pentaacetic acid (gadolinium-DTPA). This agent behaves in an analogous fashion to iodinated contrast agents used in computed tomography in that it crosses regions that do not have an intact blood-brain barrier. The normal pituitary gland is perfused by such agents. It enhances on T1-weighted sections. Adenomas, interestingly, are not perfused initially to the same degree. Therefore, on immediate postinjection images (0 to 10 min after injection), their relative hypointensity compared to the normal gland is increased. If delayed images are obtained, the contrast agent appears to slowly permeate into the lesion. The adenoma may then be hyperintense to the pituitary gland.[5]

Macroadenomas are well seen on MRI, as they are on CT. MRI is indicated for diagnosis, differential diagnosis, staging, and evaluation of adjacent structures (Fig. 5-3). The advantages of MRI over CT are superior visualization of the carotid arteries and optic chiasm and direct multiplanar display of the tumor in relation to parasellar structures.

Whereas the detection of the larger adenoma is straightforward, the differential diagnosis can be difficult. Occasionally, pituitary adenomas may be indistinguishable from

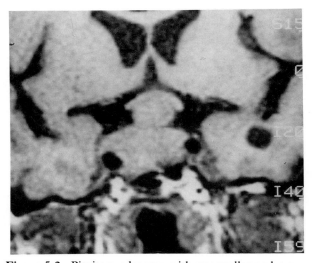

Figure 5-3 Pituitary adenoma with suprasellar and cavernous sinus extension. T1-weighted MR image (SE 600/20). The pituitary adenoma extends laterally, with tumor visible in the cavernous sinus. There is encasement of the carotid artery. The carotid artery lumen is of normal caliber.

meningiomas and even craniopharyngiomas. However, the important clinical distinction between an adenoma and an aneurysm is easily made. The adenoma is, in the majority of cases, an intermediate gray, whereas the aneurysm is either black, due to flowing blood, or very bright if it is thrombosed. Therefore, with MRI it is possible to confidently exclude the presence of a significant vascular abnormality which would preclude trans-sphenoidal surgery.

The ability to obtain images in multiple planes is useful for determining the extrasellar extent and involvement of adjacent structures. This may be a determining factor in choosing transcranial rather than trans-sphenoidal surgery, particularly if the tumor extends far laterally into the middle fossa or anteriorly over the tuberculum.

Superior extension is the most common route of spread outside the sella turcica. Usually a waistlike constriction can be seen around the tumor at the point where it extends above the sella turcica. The relationship of the optic chiasm and supraclinoid carotid arteries to the superior aspect of the tumor is well seen (Fig. 5-3).

Although the superior extent can be precisely delineated, lateral extension is more problematic because of the inability to reliably visualize the medial cavernous sinus wall. Because of this, it is difficult to confidently confirm or exclude the extension of an adenoma into the cavernous sinus, unless such extension is gross, in which case the diagnosis is readily evident. In gross cavernous sinus extension, prominent lateral bowing of the lateral cavernous sinus wall is observed (Fig. 5-3). Contrast agents may aid in the diagnosis of subtle cavernous sinus invasion.

In cavernous sinus extension, the relationship of the carotid artery to the tumor and the effect of the tumor on the vessel lumen is easily seen due to the high contrast provided by the flow void within the carotid artery lumen (Fig. 5-3). Although pituitary adenoma extension into the cavernous sinus is quite common, it is rare to see constriction of the carotid lumen, the more common finding being displacement or encirclement of the vessel without constriction.

Inferior extension of an adenoma causes either remodeling of the floor of the sella turcica or frank erosion through the floor into the sphenoid sinus or sphenoid bone. It may be difficult if not impossible to determine whether the inferiorly extending adenoma is eroding through the bone of the floor or merely remodeling it, because there is no contrast between the cortical bone and the air-containing sinus. Inferior extension is seen as asymmetric downward protrusion of a soft tissue mass from the inferior aspect of the gland.

There is a subgroup of tumors, the invasive adenomas, which preferentially grow through the rigid bony floor or into the cavernous sinus rather than take the path of least resistance into the suprasellar cistern. This type of invasive biologic behavior is well recognized but unexplained. Many of these are microadenomas. They carry a worse prognosis because complete surgical resection is difficult. They do not have any distinguishing imaging features other than their pattern of growth.

Hemorrhage into adenomas is a frequent MRI observation. Whereas previously it was thought that intrapituitary hemorrhage was seen only in the clinical syndrome of pituitary apoplexy, it is apparent that hemorrhage into an adenoma may be clinically occult. Very often portions of adeno-

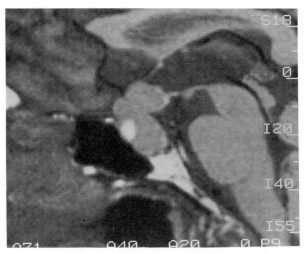

Figure 5-4 Pituitary macroadenoma with suprasellar extension and hemorrhage. T1-weighted MR image (SE 600/20). A large tumor arises from the sella turcica and extends into the suprasellar cistern. The relationship of the tumor to the optic chiasm and stalk is clearly seen. The high intensity in the midportion of the tumor is due to hemorrhage (which was clinically occult).

mas, both large and small, can be seen to have hemorrhagic foci (Fig. 5-4). These were previously unappreciated but are now being detected with increasing frequency due to the high soft-tissue contrast afforded by MRI. In true cases of pituitary apoplexy, a large hemorrhage typically occurs within a relatively large adenoma. The diagnosis is evident both clinically and on the MR scan, which shows an area of high signal intensity representing hemorrhage into the gland. Pituitary apoplexy also is recognized to occur in the postpartum female.

Craniopharyngiomas

Craniopharyngioma is another common benign tumor of the parasellar region. There is a well-known bimodal age distribution. Children are affected most frequently; there is a second later and smaller incidence peak in the fifth and sixth decades of life. These tumors arise from epithelial remnants of Rathke's cleft. Their gross pathology is variable even within the same tumor, where there may be solid tissue, various types of cysts, and calcification. This is reflected in their MRI appearance, where virtually any pattern is possible. The majority are closely related to the pituitary infundibulum, usually on its anterior aspect. Most of these tumors are suprasellar in location, but they may extend down into the sella turcica. A minority may be entirely intrasellar. Rarely they may occur purely within the third ventricle. They may be invasive locally, and it may be impossible to see clean tissue planes between the tumor and adjacent structures such as the optic chiasm, hypothalamus, uncus, and pituitary gland.

Their image intensity is varied as it reflects the tumor constituents. Usually a cyst is seen, but the intensity of the cyst may be high or low on the T1-weighted image. Low intensity indicates the presence of a serous type of fluid or, as reported in one case, keratin.[12] The cyst is more commonly extremely bright. This high signal intensity is found in the "machine oil" cysts. The cause of the high intensity is thought to be due to hemorrhagic products or cholesterol crystals.[12] Solid components of the tumor do not have any particularly unique characteristics to them. If calcification is present and is dense, it will be seen as a region of signal dropout. However, MRI is relatively insensitive to the presence of calcium, and lesser degrees of calcification may be entirely overlooked (Fig. 5-5).[6] In this regard, CT may offer a more specific differential diagnosis by its ability to detect small amounts of calcification.

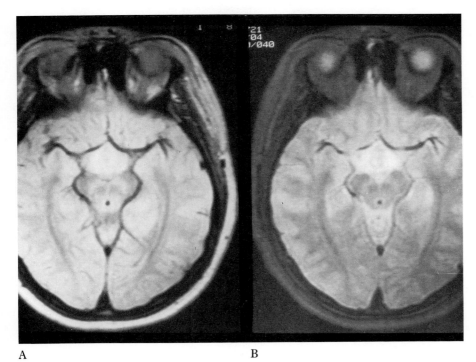

A   B

Figure 5-5 Craniopharyngioma with central calcification. *A* and *B*. T2-weighted MR images (SE 2000/70 and 2000/35). *C*. CT scan. The central calcification visible on the CT scan escapes detection on the MR images.

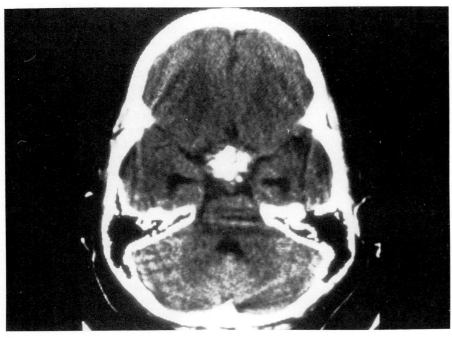

C

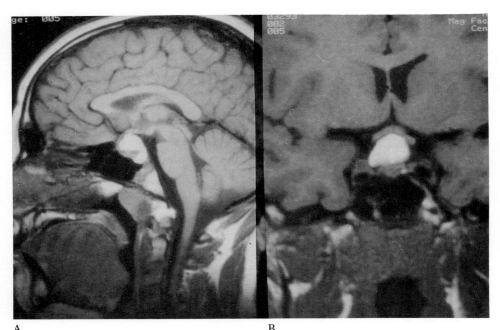

A   B

Figure 5-6 Craniopharyngioma. *A* and *B*. T1-weighted MR images (SE 600/20). A high-intensity suprasellar mass is seen. The high intensity within the tumor is due to old hemorrhagic products. There is a small central area of intermediate gray intensity representing solid tumor tissue.

These tumors may attain a very large size and may extend laterally into the middle fossa, superiorly to invaginate the third ventricle, or posteriorly into the interpeduncular and prepontine cisterns. As a general rule, a large suprasellar mass with a variety of components is most likely to be a craniopharyngioma (Fig. 5-6). The classic case is a suprasellar mass in which a high-intensity cyst is present combined with small amounts of solid tissue and/or calcification. Cases in which there are both suprasellar and intrasellar components and in which no calcification can be seen may be difficult to distinguish from a pituitary macroadenoma.

Rathke's Cleft Cysts

The nomenclature relating to cysts derived from Rathke's cleft is confusing. The simple epithelial cyst, the colloid cyst of the pituitary gland, and the pars intermedia cyst all have very similar histology. These cysts all have an epithelial wall with a single cell layer. For the purposes of this discussion, they may be considered as a signal entity. Small Rathke's cleft cysts are extremely common findings at autopsy but rarely cause clinical problems. However, there can be secretory cells present within the walls of these cysts. They may enlarge as these secretions accumulate, with resultant compression of the surrounding normal pituitary gland, or on rare instances, they may rise out of the sella turcica and compress the optic chiasm (Fig. 5-7). They arise from epithelial remnants of Rathke's cleft and, therefore, their location is quite predictable: the anterior half of the sella turcica or directly in front of the pituitary stalk in the suprasellar cistern. However, the intensity of the cyst contents is variable depending on whether the secreted material is a simple serous fluid or a viscous mucus and also depending on whether it contains cellular debris.[8] If the cellular compo-

nent within the cyst is abundant, the lesion may appear solid and the differential diagnosis between it and a pituitary adenoma or craniopharyngioma may be impossible.

Meningiomas

Meningiomas of the medial sphenoid wing, tuberculum sellae, diaphragma, and dorsum are not rare. Unfortunately, they are problematic lesions for MRI. In most cases, the T1 and T2 relaxation times of meningiomas are very similar to those of gray matter. Furthermore, they often display the *en plaque* type of growth pattern. Therefore, there may be no obvious evidence of a mass, and there may be no perceptible interface or contrast between these two tissues. For that reason, there is a relatively high incidence of false-negative MRI examinations for meningiomas.

However, if the tumor is seen, the differential diagnosis is limited. Their signal intensity and morphology are well characterized. Typically, they have a wide dural attachment, particularly those occurring on the planum or tuberculum sellae (Fig. 5-8). Close scrutiny of the sagittal images through this area may demonstrate separation of the meningioma from the pituitary gland more clearly than is possible on CT.

Currently, CT is preferable to MRI for the evaluation of meningiomas. Enhancement on CT is profuse; therefore, the tumor is easily detected. CT is also more sensitive to the detection of calcification and hyperostosis of underlying bone. Each of these features facilitates CT diagnosis.

MRI intravenous contrast agents will be very beneficial in evaluating meningiomas of the skull base. As noted earlier, these agents are analogous to iodinated agents used in computed tomography. Meningiomas enhance intensely with gadolinium-DTPA, and this greatly improves the de-

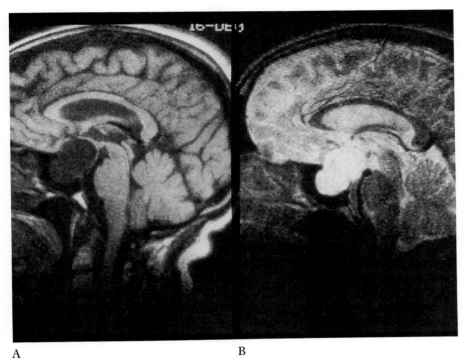

A   B

Figure 5-7 Large Rathke's cleft cyst. *A.* T1-weighted MR image (SE 600/20). *B.* T2-weighted MR image (SE 2000/70). A space-occupying lesion approximately 2 cm in diameter is seen within the anterior sella turcica and anterior to the infundibulum within the suprasellar cistern. The optic chiasm is elevated superiorly. This patient presented with bitemporal hemianopsia secondary to chiasmatic compression. This is a rare presentation of a large Rathke's cleft cyst. The lesion is of identical intensity to the cerebrospinal fluid in the ventricles on both the T1- and T2-weighted sections. At surgery, a simple cyst with CSF-like fluid was found. Most Rathke's cleft cysts are very small and are incidental findings at autopsy. Symptomatic cysts are uncommon.

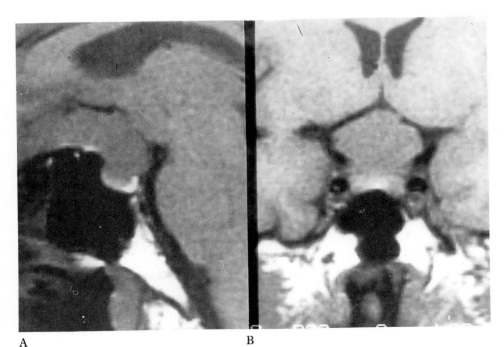

A   B

Figure 5-8 Tuberculum sellae meningioma. *A* and *B.* T1-weighted MR images (SE 600/20). The tumor is very similar to gray matter in intensity. It can clearly be seen to be separate from the pituitary gland. This excludes the diagnostic possibility of pituitary adenoma.

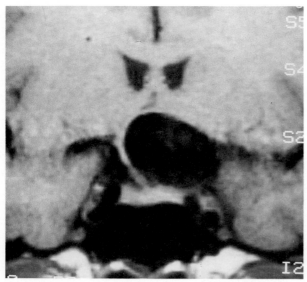

Figure 5-9 Carotid aneurysm. T1-weighted MR image (SE 600/20). There is a well-defined, dark lesion contiguous with the left carotid artery, rising into the suprasellar cistern with displacement of the infundibulum to the right and elevation of the optic chiasm. This appearance is pathognomonic of a nonthrombosed aneurysm.

lineation of the extent of such tumors and their relationship to vessels of the skull base.

Aneurysms

Vessels and vascular abnormalities are extremely well delineated on MRI because of the natural contrast present between the signal void of flowing blood and the higher signal intensities of adjacent tissue. For this reason, vessels, vascular anomalies, and aneurysms have an easily recognizable appearance on magnetic resonance images. The nonthrombosed aneurysm is black, has well-defined margins, and is contiguous to a vessel (Fig. 5-9). Thrombosis within an aneurysm is also quite distinctive in appearance. The thrombus has high signal intensity on the T1-weighted images and usually has a dark rim on the T2-weighted sections. This is thought to be due to hemosiderin in the wall of the aneurysm or in the adjacent brain.

Carotid aneurysms originating within the cavernous sinus itself, at the origin of the ophthalmic artery, or from the supraclinoid carotid artery are equally well seen. However, a normal MR scan does not exclude the presence of an aneurysm. Selective cerebral arteriography remains the definitive diagnostic procedure for these lesions.

Optic Gliomas, Hypothalamic Gliomas

These two lesions may be indistinguishable from one another radiologically and surgically. Optic gliomas may extend superiorly into the hypothalamus and hypothalamic gliomas may extend downward to incorporate the optic chiasm or tract. When lesions are smaller, the optic chiasm and hypothalamus can be separated from one another and the diagnosis is facilitated.

Optic gliomas occur in children and adults. They may involve the intraorbital or intracranial portions of the nerve. In children they are usually seen in patients with neurofibromatosis and are often bilateral. There are often abnormalities in the optic radiations of such patients. In many cases this represents tumor extension along the optic radiations. However, it has become apparent over the past several years that patients with neurofibromatosis often have multiple white matter abnormalities in anatomic areas remote from the optic radiations. The etiology of these findings has not been established, but they are presumed to be either hamartomas or dysplastic white matter. It is therefore difficult to stage the posterior extent of optic gliomas in the neurofibromatosis patient because it is impossible to distinguish what is presumably a hamartoma from an infiltrating glioma. The adult optic glioma tends to have a more aggressive biologic behavior, but the imaging findings are identical to those seen in childhood.

It is particularly important to determine the extent of an optic glioma if excision is being contemplated. The tumor characteristically appears as a thickening of the optic nerve and/or chiasm on T1-weighted sections (Fig. 5-10).[1,2] On T2-weighted sections it is of higher signal intensity than normal nerve. Oblique images directly along the long axis of the optic nerve are extremely beneficial in determining the transition between normal and abnormal optic nerve.

The hypothalamic glioma may be histologically identical to the optic glioma. It too can present as a suprasellar mass, and when it does so, it is difficult to separate it from the optic nerve. Useful differential imaging features are that the optic glioma has a propensity to grow along the optic pathways or posteriorly along the optic radiations. The hypothalamic glioma does neither. Clinically, the hypothalamic tumor presents primarily with hypothalamic dysfunction, the optic glioma with visual loss. This may be the most useful differential point. MRI is useful in delineating the extent of hypothalamic tumors into the brain and suprasellar cistern (Fig. 5-11).

The Empty Sella Turcica

This entity refers to a large sella turcica that is filled with CSF extending downward from the suprasellar cistern. It is due to a larger than normal hiatus in the diaphragma sellae. This exposes the sella turcica to the transmitted pulsations of CSF within the suprasellar cistern. This may cause enlargement of the sella and flattening of the pituitary gland. The findings on MRI, and on CT for that matter, are a large sella turcica occupied by CSF. The pituitary gland is flattened along the floor of the sella turcica, usually in the posterior-inferior portion. The pituitary stalk can be seen to traverse this CSF space from the median eminence of the hypothalamus down to the flattened pituitary gland (Fig. 5-12). This is an important feature to ascertain because it virtually excludes the possibility that the sella turcica is occupied by a space-occupying cyst. Cysts and other space-

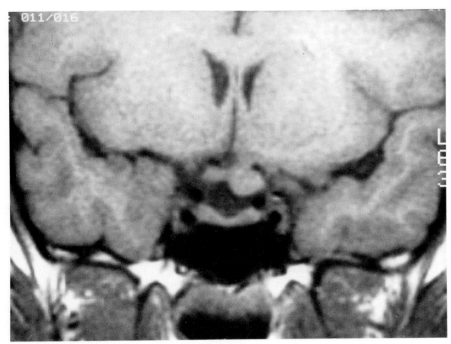

Figure 5-10 Optic glioma. T1-weighted MR image (SE 600/20). There is thickening of the left side of the optic chiasm. This is the typical appearance of a chiasmatic glioma.

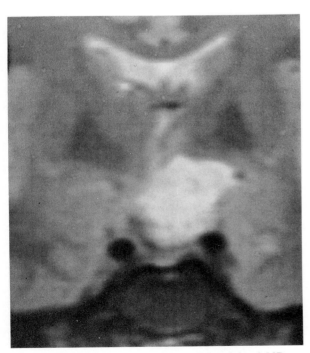

Figure 5-11 Hypothalamic glioma. T2-weighted MR image (SE 2000/70). The tumor is clearly seen as arising from the hypothalamus. The tumor extends down into the suprasellar cistern, displacing the optic chiasm. This T2-weighted image shows the tumor as a high-intensity area within the brain substance.

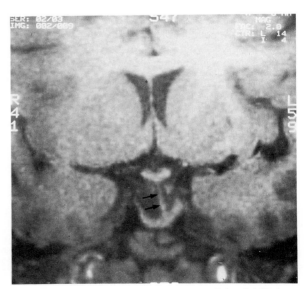

Figure 5-12 Empty sella turcica. T1-weighted MR image (SE 600/20). CSF fills the majority of the sella turcica. The pituitary gland is flattened posteriorly and inferiorly within the enlarged sella turcica. The pituitary stalk maintains its normal course from the median eminence to the pituitary gland (*arrows*).

occupying lesions deviate the stalk away from its normal course.

Other Lesions

The parasellar region is involved with a wide variety of other abnormalities, although most are rare, as mentioned in the introduction to this chapter.

Many disorders can infiltrate the pituitary stalk, basal meninges, and inferior aspect of the brain. Most notable of these are sarcoidosis, histiocytosis X, germinoma, lymphoma, and leukemia. Each of these can cause thickening of the pituitary stalk, a suprasellar mass, or focal lesions in the inferior aspect of the brain. The stalk thickening is best seen on the T1-weighted sagittal or coronal images, whereas the focal lesions in the brain often require T2-weighted sections for optimal visualization.

Optic neuritis can simulate an optic nerve tumor. Both cause nerve enlargement. The two entities can be distinguished by interval follow-up. The untreated glioma will continue to grow, albeit usually slowly. In neuritis, the nerve will return to normal in size and may actually become atrophic. Examination of the entire brain is particularly useful in this setting. The finding of multiple white matter lesions may establish the diagnosis of multiple sclerosis.

A variety of tumors occur in the sphenoid bone and clivus. The most common of these are chordoma, metastasis, and nasopharyngeal carcinoma. The intensities of these lesions are not sufficiently distinct to permit confident differentiation. The most useful diagnostic features are the location of the tumor and the associated findings.

The chordoma is almost always in the midline of the clivus. It usually expands the bone but commonly breaks through the cortex and has large excrescences posteriorly into the prepontine cistern or anteriorly into the nasopharyngeal soft tissues. Nasopharyngeal carcinoma extends upward into the bones of the skull base. Usually the primary lesion can be seen within the nasopharynx, and for this reason the nasopharynx must be closely scrutinized when abnormalities are seen within the sphenoid bone and clivus. Metastases may affect any bone within the skull base. Identification of a clival lesion which does not fit the typical pattern of chordoma or nasopharyngeal carcinoma should arouse suspicion of a metastasis and a search for a primary lesion should be instituted. The primary tumors most often associated with skull base metastases are carcinomas of the lung, breast, and kidney. All tumors which affect the skull base have common imaging features in terms of signal intensity: they replace the high signal intensity of marrow fat normally seen on the T1-weighted sections. On T2-weighted sections, they are usually hyperintense to marrow, although the degree of hyperintensity is variable.

References

1. Albert A, Lee BCP, Saint-Louis L, et al. MRI of optic chiasm and optic pathways. *AJNR* 1986; 7:255–258.
2. Azar-Kia B, Naheedy MH, Elias DA, et al. Optic nerve tumors: role of magnetic resonance imaging and computed tomography. *Radiol Clin North Am* 1987; 25:561–581.
3. Daniels DL, Pech P, Mark L, et al. Magnetic resonance imaging of the cavernous sinus. *AJNR* 1985; 6:187–192.
4. Davis PC, Hoffman JC, Spencer T, et al. MR imaging of pituitary adenoma: CT, clinical, and surgical correlation. *AJNR* 1987; 8:107–112.
5. Dwyer AJ, Frank JA, Doppman JL, et al. Pituitary adenomas in patients with Cushing disease: initial experience with Gd-DTPA-enhanced MR imaging. *Radiology* 1987; 163:421–426.
6. Holland BA, Kucharczyk W, Brant-Zawadzki M, et al. MR imaging of calcified intracranial lesions. *Radiology* 1985; 157:353–356.
7. Kucharczyk W, Davis DO, Kelly WM, et al. Pituitary adenomas: high-resolution MR imaging at 1.5 T. *Radiology* 1986; 161:761–765.
8. Kucharczyk W, Peck WW, Kelly WM, et al. Rathke cleft cysts: CT, MR imaging, and pathologic features. *Radiology* 1987; 165:491–495.
9. Kulkarni MV, Lee KF, McArdle CB, et al. 1.5-T MR imaging of pituitary microadenomas: technical considerations and CT correlation. *AJNR* 1988; 9:5–11.
10. Marcovitz S, Wee R, Chan J, et al. The diagnostic accuracy of preoperative CT scanning in the evaluation of pituitary ACTH-secreting adenomas. *AJNR* 1987; 8:641–644.
11. Pojunas KW, Daniels DL, Williams AL, et al. MR imaging of prolactin-secreting microadenomas. *AJNR* 1986; 7:209–213.
12. Pusey E, Kortman KE, Flannigan BD, et al. MR of craniopharyngiomas: tumor delineation and characterization. *AJNR* 1987; 8:439–444.

6
Magnetic Resonance Imaging of Cerebrovascular Diseases

Linda Gray
Russell A. Blinder
William T. Djang

Magnetic resonance imaging (MRI) is an ideal modality for the evaluation of vascular disorders of the central nervous system (CNS). MRI provides high resolution images of the brain in multiple planes, allowing lesions to be localized accurately. It is also very sensitive in detecting pathologic alterations in tissue composition and edema. Many imaging sequences provide high contrast between flowing blood and tissue. This allows blood vessels to be imaged without intravenous contrast administration. Extravascular blood has characteristic signal changes over time that allow accurate diagnosis of hemorrhage and hematoma. Unlike computed tomography (CT), MR images of the posterior and temporal fossae are not degraded by surrounding bone. Newer techniques allow for projectional angiography of the major intracranial vessels.

Strategies of Imaging

Standard MRI is based on nuclear properties of hydrogen. MR images reflect the different relaxation times of protons within different tissue components. The differences in relaxation times are responsible for the contrast in MR images. Image contrast is manipulated by the choice of specific pulse sequences. The principal pulse sequences are spin echo (SE), gradient refocused echo (GRA), and inversion recovery (IR). Spin echo imaging is the pulse sequence primarily utilized in brain imaging and consists of a 90-degree pulse followed by a 180-degree pulse. This is followed by an echo delay time (TE) after which a signal is sampled. TR represents the total time between 90-degree repetitive pulses.

Images may be either T1-weighted (short TR and TE) or T2-weighted (long TR and TE). Any abnormal signal intensity generally reflects a change in tissue water composition. T1-weighted images generally demonstrate more anatomic detail and show decreased intensity with increased amounts of free water. T2-weighted images show increased intensity with increased amounts of free water, a condition which is generally associated with pathologic processes. The effects seen may be nonspecific; that is, infarcts, tumors, and other pathologic processes may all demonstrate increased signal on T2-weighted images. However, increased specificity can often be achieved with gadolinium enhancement.

Gradient refocused echo images are obtained using radiofrequency pulses which generally create flip angles of less than 90 degrees. They allow shorter acquisition times and also may be T1- or T2-weighted. An additional feature is increased sensitivity to "magnetic susceptibility" (T2*) which occurs in the presence of blood products and iron deposition.

Two topics relevant for vascular disease imaging deserve special attention. Blood flow effects are complex and are pulse sequence dependent. On a simplified model, high velocity flow appears on spin echo images as an area of signal void or signal loss related to so-called time of flight effects and phase dispersion caused by turbulence. Thus, arterial channels are usually well displayed. Slow flow, however, may appear as areas of brighter signal intensity, predominantly related to entry slice phenomena. These effects are best seen in cortical veins. With gradient refocused techniques, parameters may be manipulated to cause marked increased signal intensity in vascular channels. Thus a near angiographic effect is produced which may be helpful in characterizing vascular lesions. Newer techniques include three-dimensional volume imaging and postprocessing techniques which allow three-dimensional projection angiograms of the vasculature of the head and neck. Loss of flow enhancement characteristics can be used as presumptive evidence of vessel thrombosis, such as with sagittal sinus thrombosis.

Intracerebral hemorrhage also has a characteristic MR appearance. The age and evolutionary features of hemorrhagic lesions and the presence of underlying cerebral abnormalities can thus be well documented by MRI. The MR appearance is predominantly governed by the state of blood breakdown products. Deoxyhemoglobin, the predominant component of acute hematomas, appears isointense to hypointense on T1-weighted images and markedly hypointense on T2-weighted images. Methemoglobin, the major component of subacute hematomas, initially appears bright on T1-weighted images and has a low signal on T2-weighted images. With cell lysis, subacute hematomas become bright on T1- and T2-weighted images. Hemosiderin present within chronic hematomas and located generally around the periphery of hematomas is iso- to hypointense on T1-weighted images and markedly hypointense on T2-weighted images.

One limitation of MR is relatively poor sensitivity in detecting calcifications. CT may be needed to document the presence of calcium. However, the greater sensitivity of MR in detecting tissue abnormalities, in documenting blood flow, and in detecting and characterizing cerebral hemorrhage means that MR will be generally superior to CT in evaluating cerebral vascular diseases.

In the evaluation of cerebral ischemia and infarction, axial SE imaging represents the first line of evaluation. T1- and T2-weighted images should be obtained. T1-weighted images can demonstrate the high signal intensity of subacute hemorrhagic components which may be present within an infarction. T2-weighted images will demonstrate the high signal intensity of cytotoxic and vasogenic edema. Use of the sagittal or coronal plane can aid in demonstrating infarcts within the brain stem or cerebellum. Coronal images will improve the detection of infarcts near the vertex. Use of gradient refocused acquisition, which is sensitive to changes in magnetic susceptibility because of the absence of the 180-degree refocusing pulse, can improve the detection of hemorrhagic components within infarcts. Most lesions of the CNS (i.e., infarction, ischemia, neoplasms, infection, trauma, demyelinating processes, and gliosis) have prolonged T1 and T2 values, but the administration of gadolinium diethylenetriamine pentaacetic acid (Gd-DTPA) may add specificity in distinguishing among these abnormalities.

In the evaluation of aneurysms, the detection of acute subarachnoid hemorrhage is best evaluated with CT scanning. Angiography is still indicated for the detection of aneurysms, as MRI can miss small aneurysms. MRI may be helpful for detecting completely thrombosed aneurysms not seen by angiography. Clot at different stages of degradation will be identifiable within the lumen of the aneurysm. Any flow within the aneurysm will be detected as a flow void on SE sequences. The best plane for evaluation may need to be determined at the time of evaluation.

Axial SE images will distinguish the types of hemorrhagic components present within a brain hematoma. Gradient refocused acquisition will detect subtle areas of deoxyhemoglobin and hemosiderin. Different planes of imaging will help in characterizing the size and location of the hematoma. If a hemorrhagic neoplasm is suspected, Gd-DTPA administration may be helpful for demonstrating an enhancing tumor nodule.

Arteriovenous malformations can be demonstrated on SE images. Large feeding vessels and draining veins appear as signal voids because of rapid dephasing of protons due to rapidly flowing blood. Areas of slow flow or venous flow may demonstrate increased signal intensity. Thrombus within vessels also may demonstrate increased signal intensity on both T1- and T2-weighted images, representing stages of blood degradation. Gradient refocused acquisitions which are more heavily T1-weighted (i.e., an approximately 60-degree flip angle) will demonstrate increased signal intensity in vessels with flowing blood. MR angiography is a new technique utilizing T1-weighted gradient refocused acquisition in a three-dimensional mode. Bright signal intensity emanating from both arteries and veins is present at the same time; therefore, the degree of arteriovenous (AV) shunting cannot be determined by this technique. Cryptic vascular malformations that are not visible on angiography may demonstrate old blood products, thus suggesting the diagnosis. A hypointense rim around the lesion may represent evidence of old hemorrhage and hemosiderin within the lysosomes of macrophages. CT is more sensitive in detecting small calcified lesions; however, MR is more sensitive for detecting subacute and chronic blood products related to small vascular malformations.

Both T1- and T2-weighted SE images in coronal and axial planes should be obtained for the evaluation of venous sinus thrombosis. If the signal intensity emanating from the superior sagittal sinus is isointense or hypointense on T1-weighted images and hypointense on T2-weighted images, gradient refocused acquisition (GRA) can be helpful in demonstrating absence of flow within the sinus. Normal flow within the superior sagittal sinus would be demonstrated on GRA images as bright in signal intensity; absence of this bright signal would be consistent with absent flow. If the signal intensity within the superior sagittal sinus is bright on both T1- and T2-weighted SE images, suggesting methemoglobin formation, GRA imaging will not add information (the signal intensity emanating from the sinus will be hyperintense).

Cerebral Ischemia and Infarction

MRI is more sensitive than CT to most cerebral pathology because of the better inherent contrast between normal and pathologic tissues. One of the major reasons for different signal intensities between tissues is the amount of free water within the tissues. Cerebral ischemia, as well as other pathologic processes, increases the free water content of tissue.[11]

In two studies (20 and 55 patients), MRI was found to be more sensitive than CT in imaging cerebral infarction.[15,56] Patients with multiple infarct dementia secondary to subcortical atherosclerotic encephalopathy (SAE or Binswanger's disease) were found to show foci of edema or demyelination that was not visualized by CT.[15] Due to the lack of artifact from bone, MRI is superior to CT for the evaluation of infarction in the brain stem and cerebellum.[15,20]

Experimenters using animal models found that MRI can often accurately show ischemia as early as 30 min after occlusion of a major cerebral vessel.[14,15,18,22,46,55,57] The characteristic changes of infarction are prolongation of T1 and T2 relaxation times in areas corresponding to the vascular distribution. These areas show decreased intensity on T1-weighted images and increased intensity on T2-weighted images (Fig. 6-1).[17,23] A distinction between acute and chronic infarction can generally be made. Both acute and nonacute infarcts demonstrate prolonged T1 and T2 values. However, chronic infarcts are associated with overlying cortical atrophy. In the case of hemorrhagic infarcts, there can be difficulty differentiating acute hemorrhagic infarcts from nonhemorrhagic infarcts within the first 2 days of onset. A few days must elapse before blood products undergo a decrease in T1 causing high signal on T1-weighted images. MRI may also be able to image areas of reversible ischemia (Fig. 6-2). MRI is unable to distinguish between infarction, ischemia, and edema because all have areas of prolonged T1 and T2 relaxation times.[35,38,56]

Lacunar infarcts appear as focal areas of decreased signal intensity on T1-weighted images and increased signal intensity on T2-weighted images. The acute lacunar infarcts, those studied within 1 week of onset, are seen only on T2-weighted images. Chronic lesions, those more than 1 week

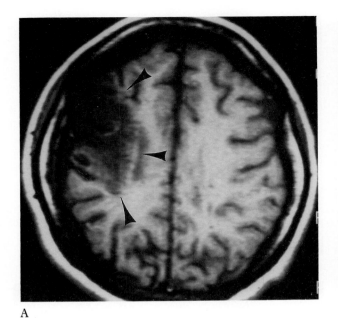

A

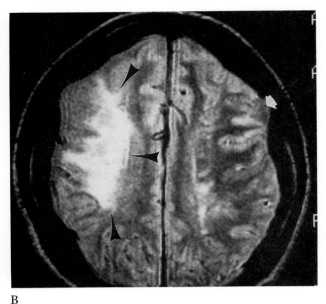

B

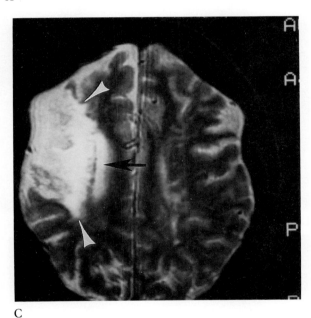

C

Figure 6-1 Old right parietal infarct. *A.* A T1-weighted image (TR 500, TE 20) showing decreased intensity of the right parietal cortex and white matter *(arrowheads).* *B.* A mildly T2-weighted image (TR 2000, TE 30). The intensity of the infarct *(black arrowheads)* is greater than that of CSF *(white arrow).* *C.* A T2-weighted image (TR 2000, TE 80) shows that the infarct *(arrowheads)* is isointense to the CSF in right lateral ventricle *(arrow).*

of age, are seen on both T1- and T2-weighted images.[37] Among 21 patients imaged by both CT and MR, MR identified lesions in 19, whereas CT showed lesions in only 11. The sensitivity of MR during the acute phase of ischemia is most likely due to its ability to detect small changes in tissue water content by T2-weighted images.[16]

Gd-DTPA is an intravenous contrast agent currently used in MRI. Gd-DTPA shortens T1 relaxation time through enhanced proton relaxation, thus causing a bright signal on T1-weighted images. Cerebral infarcts often "enhance" with gadolinium administration. The degree of enhancement depends upon the extent of breakdown of the blood-brain barrier, the amount of collateral circulation

present, and the degree of compression of the capillary bed due to vasogenic edema. These phenomena also affect the iodinated contrast enhancement of infarcts studied by CT, but MRI using gadolinium may be more sensitive to the effects of vasogenic edema and the degree of collateral circulation. Also, gadolinium enhancement of infarcts may be greater than iodinated contrast enhancement due to the superior contrast resolution of MR when compared with CT.[36] With CT, maximal contrast enhancement of infarcts is usually seen between 4 and 18 days after infarction.[60] In patients, the earliest gadolinium enhancement of infarcts is at 6 days after the event, but in cats such enhancement may be detected as early as 16 h after the experimental occlusion of the middle cerebral artery.

The pattern and character of enhancement on MR images closely correlate with those on CT scans. MR enhancement occurs within the first 3 min after injection and continues to increase by 30 min. By 55 min, enhancement in medium-aged infarcts continues but begins to decline in late infarcts. Enhancement of periventricular lesions or chronic asymptomatic lacunar-type infarcts does not occur, whereas symptomatic lacunar infarcts do enhance.[60]

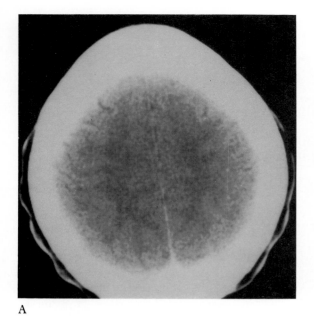

A

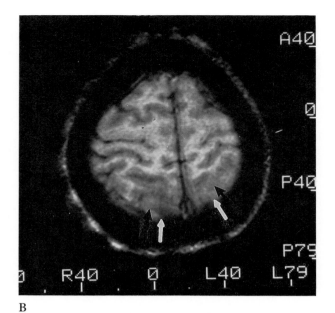

B

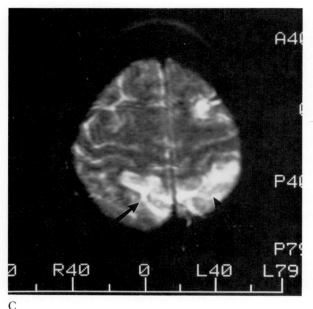

C

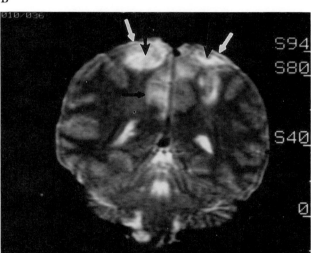

D

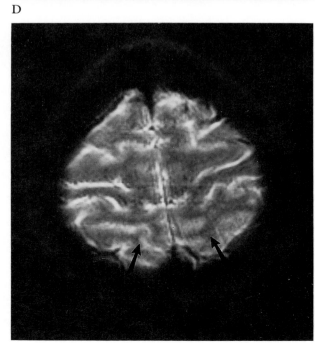

E

Figure 6-2 Reversible ischemia in a patient with porphyria. *A.* A noncontrasted CT scan was normal. *B.* A T1-weighted image (TR 500, TE 20) shows hypointensity of the posterior parietal regions bilaterally *(arrows)* with loss of sulcal and gyral definition. *C, D.* T2-weighted images (TR 2000, TE 80) demonstrate hyperdensity in the areas of ischemia on axial *(C)* and coronal *(D)* images *(arrows).* *E.* A T2-weighted (TR 2000, TE 80) MR scan 2 weeks later shows that the areas of signal abnormality have reverted to normal *(arrows)*, demonstrating reversible ischemia.

Deep White Matter Lesions

Areas of hyperintensity on T2-weighted images within the periventricular region or deep white matter have several different etiologies. Analysis of pathologic specimens has demonstrated such lesions to be areas of infarction, demyelination, or gliosis, ventricular diverticuli, or prominent Virchow-Robin spaces. These different types of lesions can generally be distinguished by location, morphologic appearance, and intensity on long TR, short TE images.[12,13,39,40,48]

Lacunar infarcts are generally less than 1 cm in greatest diameter and are hyperintense relative to brain parenchyma on long TR, short TE sequences. They may be slit-like, round, or ovoid. They are produced by an occlusion of a penetrating vessel secondary to atheromata, fibrinoid necrosis, or embolization.[12]

Virchow-Robin spaces are isointense relative to CSF on all pulse sequences. They are perivascular spaces that result from an invagination of the subarachnoid space surrounding a vessel wall as it penetrates into the brain parenchyma. They surround arteries, veins, and venules but not capillaries. Prominent Virchow-Robin spaces are found in the basal ganglia or white matter, and there is generally no alteration of the adjacent brain tissue. They tend to be round or linear in appearance. They can often be seen on successive axial sections beginning above the level of the bifurcation of the internal carotid artery and may persist through the variable thickness of the putamen.[12]

Infarction, gliosis, or periventricular atrophic demyelination cannot be distinguished by MR. They appear hyperintense relative to brain parenchyma on long TR, short TE sequences. Perivascular atrophic demyelination consists of atrophy and shrinkage of axons and myelin with gliosis surrounding thickened tortuous vessels in the white matter. Such lesions can be distinguished from multiple sclerosis plaques by their subcortical location; multiple sclerosis plaques usually occur in the periventricular white matter and may involve the corpus callosum and brachium pontis.[39] Although similar in appearance to prominent Virchow-Robin spaces, perivascular atrophic demyelination may result from chronic low-grade vascular insufficiency.[12,40] Low-grade vascular insufficiency appears to produce atrophy of tissue rather than acute tissue necrosis as ordinarily caused by ischemic or occlusive vascular disease.[40]

Intracranial Hemorrhage

The MR appearance of a hematoma is dependent upon the degradation products of hemoglobin, which is a paramagnetic substance.[26,34] Many factors affect the breakdown products of a hematoma and thus its MR appearance. Some of the contributing factors include pH, oxygen tension, integrity of intact red cell membranes, and an increase in hematocrit caused by clot retraction. Theoretical explanations for the different signal intensities observed include proton relaxation enhancement, preferential T2 proton relaxation enhancement, and changes in magnetic susceptibility.

Proton relaxation enhancement describes the interaction between electrons of a paramagnetic substance and the protons of water. It results in shortening of T1 and T2 relaxation times. Proton relaxation enhancement is exhibited primarily by methemoglobin. Preferential T2 proton relaxation enhancement is a result of proton spin dephasing, which is primarily a T2 effect. No significant effect on T1 is produced. Paramagnetic substances which are insoluble or intracellular create local magnetic fields (changes in magnetic susceptibility) resulting in preferential T2 proton relaxation enhancement. This means that phase coherence is more readily lost, thus T2 is shortened. This effect is exhibited by intracellular deoxyhemoglobin and methemoglobin and insoluble hemosiderin. With lysis of the cells, preferential T2 proton relaxation enhancement is lost.

SE imaging is designed to eliminate field inhomogeneities with a 180 degree refocusing pulse which improves the appearance of the images by improving the signal-to-noise ratio. The consequence in blood imaging is to decrease those effects of field inhomogeneity that are caused by magnetic susceptibility. Gradient refocused acquisitions eliminate the 180 degree refocusing echo and consequently are sensitive to field inhomogeneities and therefore areas of magnetic susceptibility. Increasing field strength increases the effect of magnetic susceptibility and preferential T2 proton relaxation enhancement on signal intensity.

The evolution of a hematoma can be artificially divided into stages: hyperacute (within the first few hours), acute (0 to 7 days), subacute (7 to 21 days), and chronic (21 days or greater) (Table 6-1).[21,24,25,28] The hyperacute hematoma is hypointense on T1-weighted images and hyperintense on T2-weighted images (prolongation of T1 and T2 relaxation times) because the blood remains in solution at this time and behaves similarly to water. At this time, the signal intensities are indistinguishable from those of other intracranial masses.[25] Hyperacute hemorrhage consists of intact red blood cells with oxygenated hemoglobin. There is no paramagnetic effect and no relaxation enhancement.

Within a short period of time, reduction of hemoglobin occurs, causing the formation of deoxyhemoglobin. The MR appearance of an acute hematoma is isointense to slightly hypointense (in comparison to gray matter) on T1-weighted images; there is a central hypointensity on T2-weighted im-

TABLE 6-1 Magnetic Resonance Imaging Characteristics of Hematomas

Hematoma Degradation Product	Location	Time Course	Signal Intensity	
			T1-Weighted Images	T2-Weighted Images
Deoxyhemoglobin	Center	1–7 days	Isointense, hypointense	Hypointense
Intracellular methemoglobin	Periphery	7–21 days	Hyperintense	Hypointense
Extracellular methemoglobin	Periphery	7–21 days	Hyperintense	Hyperintense
Hemosiderin	Periphery	>21 days	Isointense, hypointense	Hypointense

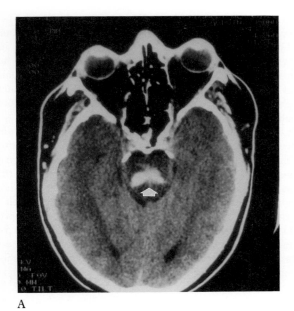

A

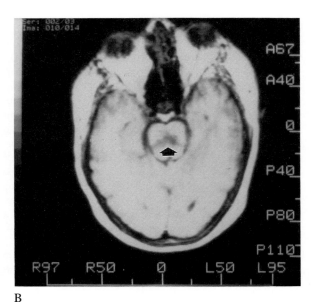

B

C

Figure 6-3 Acute pontine hemorrhage. *A*. A noncontrast CT scan shows the increased attenuation of hemorrhage within the pons (*arrow*). *B*. A T1-weighted image (TR 500, TE 20) demonstrates that the area of hemorrhage is isointense to slightly hypointense with respect to gray matter (*arrow*). *C*. A T2-weighted image (TR 2000, TE 80) shows the area of hemorrhage to be hypointense (*arrow*) with respect to gray matter.

ages (Fig. 6-3). The absence of T1 shortening (bright signal) is related to the insolubility of intracellular deoxyhemoglobin and thus the lack of dipole-dipole interactions between the protons of the water molecules, preventing proton relaxation enhancement. The low signal intensity on T2-weighted images is related to the magnetic susceptibility effects of intracellular deoxyhemoglobin which is paramagnetic. This appearance is accentuated at high field strength. Parenchymal edema adjacent to the hematoma appears after 24 h and is isointense or mildly hypointense on T1-weighted images and hyperintense on T2-weighted images. The edema subsequently resolves over several weeks.[7,28,29,32,62]

Subacute hematomas initially demonstrate peripheral hyperintensity on T1-weighted images which later shows increased signal on T2-weighted images (Fig. 6-4). The hyperintensity seen on T1-weighted images begins along the periphery to subsequently fill in the hematoma in the chronic phase. Hyperintensity on T1-weighted images along the margins of the hematoma corresponds to the development of methemoglobin, resulting from the oxidation of deoxyhemoglobin. Methemoglobin is able to interact with water molecules. The bright signal intensity observed on T1-weighted images is attributed to T1 shortening caused by proton electron dipole-dipole interaction between water molecules and methemoglobin. Other factors may also con-

tribute to the high signal intensity such as high spin density and increased hemoglobin concentration.[32] Initially, T2-weighted images of subacute hematomas show a low signal intensity which is the result of selective T2 proton relaxation enhancement of intracellular methemoglobin. Therefore, pure intracellular methemoglobin is hyperintense to gray matter on T1- and hypointense on T2-weighted images. Eventually, as cell lysis occurs and the methemoglobin becomes extracellular, the effect disappears. The low signal intensity is replaced by high signal intensity on T2-weighted images, primarily a consequence of the long T2 of a dilute solution. Within 2 to 3 weeks the hematoma is hyperintense on both short and long SE sequences. Surrounding edema causes hypointensity on T1-weighted images and hyperintensity on T2-weighted images in the adjacent white matter. A hypointense rim surrounding the intracerebral hematoma,

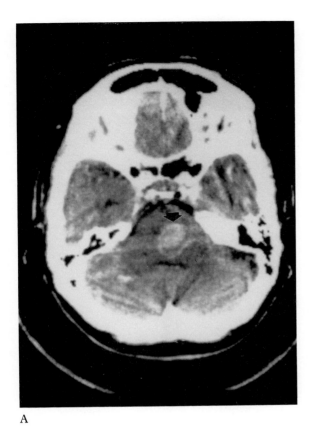

A

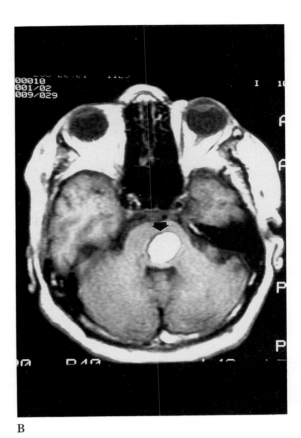

B

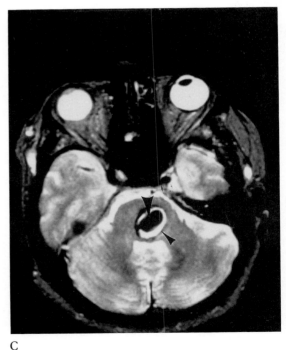

C

Figure 6-4 Subacute pontine hemorrhage. *A.* A noncontrast CT scan shows the increased attenuation of a hemorrhage in the pons *(arrow)*. *B.* A T1-weighted image (TR 500, TE 20) demonstrates the increased intensity of the hemorrhage consistent with methemoglobin *(arrow)*. *C.* A T2-weighted image (TR 2000, TE 20) shows the increased intensity of a peripheral rim which represents extracellular methemoglobin *(small arrowhead)*. The low intensity center represents intracellular methemoglobin *(large arrowhead.)*

best seen on T2-weighted images, represents hemosiderin within macrophages. It has also been suggested that this represents a ring of gliosis and/or granulation tissue because it may correspond to the ring blush seen around a hematoma on contrasted CT images.[28,41] It is possible that the thickness and magnitude of the hypointense rim may be indicative of the total amount of hemoglobin resorbed from an old hematoma. Due to the short T1 relaxation time, certain regions of a subacute hematoma may be difficult to distinguish from a melanotic melanoma or from fat.[29]

The resolution of a hematoma becomes apparent at 3 weeks. At this time, chronic hematomas demonstrate a slowly decreasing intensity in the cavity on T1-weighted images. Over time the lesions become almost isointense with CSF. There is greater hypointensity around the periphery on T2-weighted images which is mainly due to the distribu-

tion of superparamagnetic hemosiderin through the granules in the lysosomes of macrophages (Fig. 6-5).[30] Chronic hematomas lack the surrounding edema. They may be centrally hyperintense with a peripheral rim of hypointensity

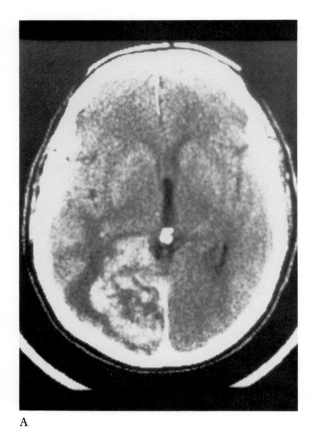

A

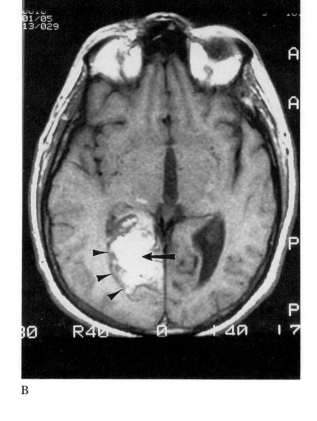

B

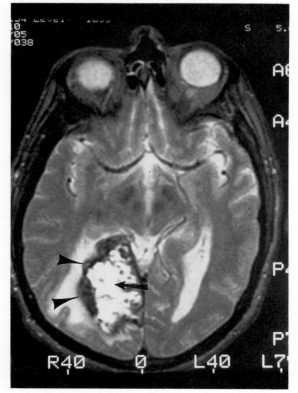

C

Figure 6-5 Three-week-old hemorrhagic infarct. *A.* A noncontrast CT scan depicts the high attenuation of hemorrhage with surrounding edema in the right occipital lobe. *B.* On a T1-weighted image (TR 500, TE 20), the hyperintense center represents methemoglobin *(arrow)* and the hypointense to isointense rim represents hemosiderin *(arrowheads).* *C.* On a T2-weighted image (TR 2000, TE 80), the hyperintense center represents extracellular methemoglobin *(arrow)* and the irregular, thick hypointense rim represents hemosiderin *(arrowheads).*

representing hemosiderin or the central portion may become CSF-like in intensity with the hemosiderin rim on T2-weighted images. Eventually, the center may become completely resorbed and only the presence of a hemosiderin scar may suggest a previous hemorrhagic lesion (Fig. 6-6).[27]

MR is useful for depicting intracranial hemorrhage but cannot always distinguish non-neoplastic from neoplastic causes of hemorrhage. Yet a distinction between non-neoplastic and neoplastic hemorrhage may often be made. Findings on SE images that might indicate a neoplastic cause of hemorrhage are signal heterogeneity, the presence of nonhemorrhagic tumor tissue, a decreased or absent he-

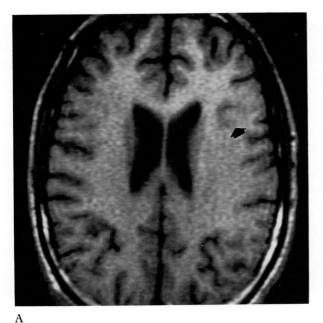

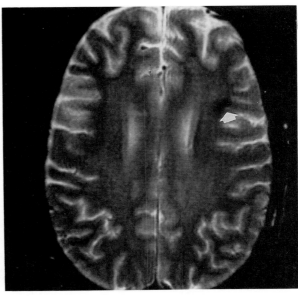

A

B

Figure 6-6 Left frontal brain contusion. *A.* A T1-weighted image (TR 500, TE 20) from an MR scan obtained 1 year after injury shows an isointense lesion in the area of a prior contusion, which represents hemosiderin (*arrow*). *B.* A T2-weighted image (TR 2000, TE 80) shows a hypointense lesion, again representing hemosiderin (*arrow*).

mosiderin ring, delayed evolution of the hematoma, and persistent surrounding edema.

There is an overall heterogeneity and more complex appearance to neoplastic hematomas. The temporal evolution of hemorrhage secondary to a neoplasm is delayed. Signal changes associated with deoxyhemoglobin may persist for weeks and changes consistent with methemoglobin may persist for months. The delay in evolution of the hemorrhage is thought to be related to intratumoral hypoxia delaying the chemical evolution of the hematoma. The rim of hypointensity indicating hemosiderin is irregular, diminished, or absent in neoplastic hemorrhages. This may be related to breakdown in the blood-brain barrier leading to more efficient removal of hemosiderin-laden macrophages. Persistent perilesional edema, even when the hemorrhage is in the subacute or chronic phase, may be another finding suggesting a hemorrhagic neoplasm. Finally, focal abnormal tissue that does not have the signal intensity pattern of a hematoma suggests a tumor.[4,7]

GRA has been useful in demonstrating evidence of old hemorrhage. This is attributed to its sensitivity to the magnetic susceptibility arising from paramagnetic blood breakdown products which shorten the T2*. Areas of hemorrhage may be missed with SE techniques. This is because SE techniques, which have a 180-degree refocusing pulse, rephase losses due to field inhomogeneities, removing the effect of T2*. In 30 of 61 cases reported by Atlas et al., GRA imaging demonstrated more hemorrhagic lesions than SE images.[5]

GRA imaging may have an adjunctive role in the evaluation of intracranial hemorrhage at high field strength.

Aneurysms

Aneurysms may be caused by congenital defects of the media, vestigial remnants of embryonic vessels, arteriosclerotic vascular disease, trauma, or infection.[19,49] Saccular aneurysms with a diameter of 5 mm or less do not rupture as frequently as those with a diameter of over 1 cm. The cardinal diagnostic sign of a ruptured aneurysm is acute, severe headache. CT remains the modality of choice for noninvasively detecting the presence of subarachnoid blood because MRI does not adequately visualize fresh subarachnoid blood within the CSF.[2] Currently MRI cannot definitively exclude the presence of an aneurysm. However, MRI can permit the diagnosis of an aneurysm based on the identification of a mass showing blood flow signal in a characteristic location, contiguous to a parent vessel. On SE imaging sequences, nonthrombosed aneurysms show a signal void due to the rapid flow of blood.[10,61] Often the site of bleeding can be pinpointed by MRI. When multiple aneurysms are present in a patient with subarachnoid hemorrhage and CT is inconclusive as to the source of bleeding, MRI may occasionally show a subacute clot adjacent to the ruptured aneurysm (Fig. 6-7).[33] Angiography remains the definitive procedure for the diagnosis of small aneurysms but only demonstrates the interior of the lesion in continuity with the circulation. In completely thrombosed aneurysms, MR is often better able to demonstrate the extent of the lesion than angiography or CT.

MRI clearly delineates the size, residual lumen, and extra-axial location of giant aneurysms. Large aneurysms usually have an inhomogeneous signal due to the presence of slow-flow regions within the aneurysm and laminated thrombus in various stages of organization (Fig. 6-8).[2,3,53] Perianeurysmal hemorrhage can cause hyperintensity on T1 images and either hypo- or hyperintensity on T2-weighted images depending on the age of the hemorrhage. Giant aneurysms can occasionally be difficult to differentiate from enhancing extra-axial tumors (meningiomas, pituitary adenomas, craniopharyngiomas) on CT examination.[9] Olsen et al. were able to diagnose a giant aneurysm in 12 of 15 cases using MRI because of the presence of blood flow phenomena.[53] Calcification is better demonstrated by CT than by MRI. Occasionally calcification can be seen as areas of hypodensity on all MRI sequences. Clipping a calcified giant aneurysm is technically more difficult and may carry greater risk than clipping a noncalcified aneurysm. If calcification is not imaged on MR, it may still be present. CT is then needed to further search for the presence of calcium.[2]

Arteriovenous Malformations

Traditionally, cerebral angiography has been the mainstay for establishing the diagnosis of an intracranial arteriovenous malformation (AVM). However, MR has virtually replaced CT and to some extent angiography as the modality of choice for screening patients with potential vascular malformations. In addition, gradient refocused acquisitions improve the detection and definition of these lesions.[2]

AVMs are clinically the most dangerous of all vascular malformations. They may hemorrhage and can be associated with brain atrophy secondary to a steal phenomenon.[49] AVMs are masses of arteries, arterialized veins, and veins. The arteries are of smaller caliber and are distinguishable from the draining veins, which are larger.[44] The component vessels may be compact or relatively loose. The interposed parenchyma is gliotic and hemosiderin-laden. Calcification can be present in vessel walls. Arterial saccular aneurysms can be found concurrently with AVMs.

CT scanning after intravenous contrast administration will demonstrate vascular enhancement and, in some cases, enlarged vessels. The pattern of vascular enhancement can suggest the diagnosis of vascular malformation; occasionally, however, a vascular tumor or enhancement within an

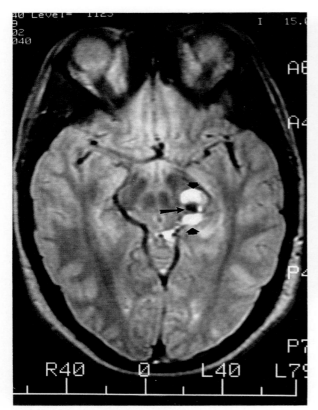

A

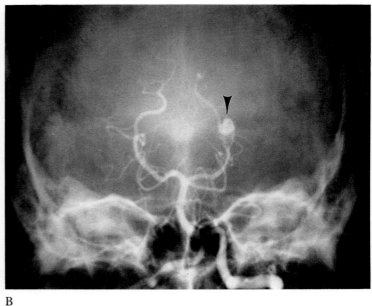

B

Figure 6-7 Left posterior cerebral artery aneurysm. *A.* An MR image (TR 2000, TE 30) demonstrating a circular region of low signal intensity that represents a flow void in the lumen of the aneurysm (*long arrow*). The perianeurysmal hyperintensity represents an adjacent clot (*short arrows*). *B.* An arteriogram verifies the aneurysm (*arrowhead*).

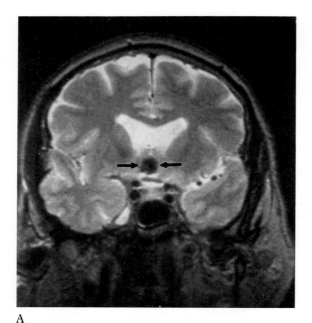

A

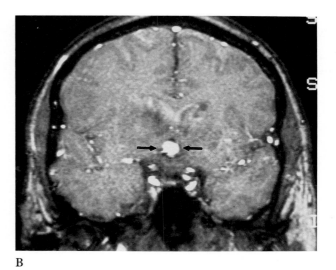

B

Figure 6-8 Giant anterior communicating artery aneurysm. *A*. A T2-weighted image (TR 2000, TE 80) shows a signal void in the suprasellar cistern, representing the aneurysm (*arrows*). *B*. On gradient refocused acquisition, flowing blood appears hyperintense in vessels and in the aneurysm (*arrows*). *C*. An arteriogram depicts the aneurysm (*curved arrow*) that separates the anterior cerebral arteries (*arrowheads*).

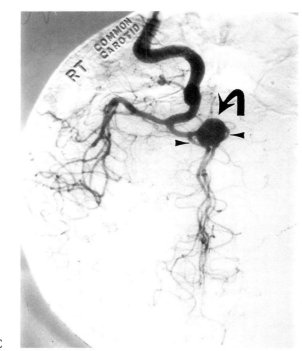

C

area of infarction can have a similar appearance.[43] If hemorrhage is present, enhancement will be nonspecific and fail to indicate the vascular nature of the lesion.[44]

MRI can achieve a definitive diagnosis without the use of ionizing radiation or intravenous contrast material. The typical MR appearance consists of a honeycomb vascular pattern with a signal void in the center. Tubular areas of signal void representing arteries and veins emanate from the center of the lesion (Fig. 6-9). Differentiating regions of signal void on SE images as regions of blood flow rather than calcification or hemorrhage can be obtained by using GRA. GRA imaging can be particularly useful in delineating vascular structures adjacent to the inner table of the skull. The presence of hemosiderin may limit the GRA imaging technique. Marked signal dropout due to the sensitivity to magnetic susceptibility effects can occur. The limitations of GRA imaging require that it be used complementary to standard SE imaging in defining vascular lesions.[2,50]

MRI and angiography are also complementary. MRI correctly assesses the extent of involvement and can localize the nidus.[52,58] If the lesion is considered unresectable, an angiogram may not be needed. Angiography is superior to MR and CT for showing the details of the distal distribution of the vessels, including any external carotid supply,[58] and for

showing the dynamics of the blood flow to, through, and away from the malformation.

Occult Vascular Malformations

MR cannot distinguish among intraparenchymal cavernous hemangiomas, capillary telangiectasias, and small thrombosed AVMs. Such lesions ordinarily are not visualized angiographically and are therefore called occult vascular malformations. Cavernous angiomas are characterized histopathologically by sinusoidal vascular channels with an absence of intervening brain tissue.[49] They may be calcified or ossified and have surrounding gliosis and hemorrhage. Capillary telangiectasias are formed by small vessels dispersed in

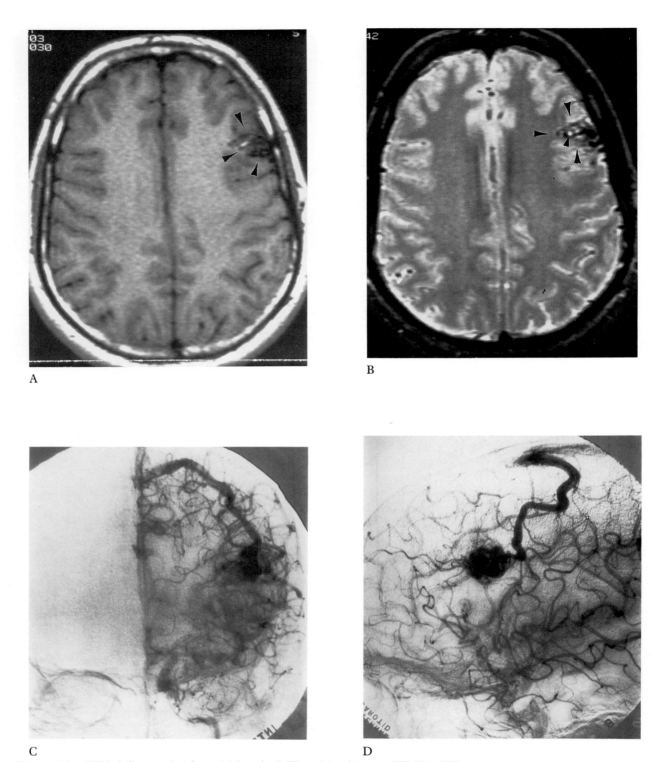

Figure 6-9 AVM, left posterior frontal lobe. *A.* A T1-weighted image (TR 500, TE 20) demonstrates serpentine areas of hypointensity which represent flow in the vessels of the AVM *(arrowheads);* the single area of hyperintensity represents a small subacute hematoma. *B.* A T2-weighted image (TR 2000, TE 30) shows serpentine areas of hypointensity representing blood flow *(arrowheads).* Again, the single area of hyperintensity represents a small subacute blood collection *(small arrowhead). C, D.* Anteroposterior and lateral views of an arteriogram show the tangle of vessels and a large early draining vein extending to the superior sagittal sinus.

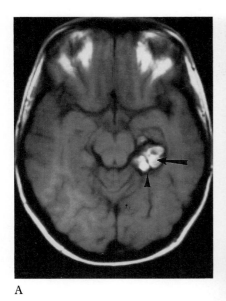

A

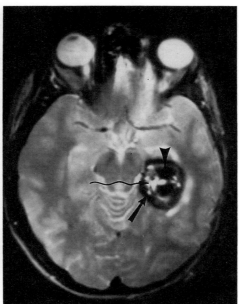

B

Figure 6-10 Thrombosed AVM. *A.* On a T1-weighted image (TR 500, TE 20), the hyperintense center represents intracellular methemoglobin (*arrow*); the peripheral hypointense ring represents hemosiderin (*arrowhead*). *B.* On a T2-weighted image (TR 2000, TE 80), the hypointense center represents intracellular methemoglobin (*arrowhead*). Areas of hyperintensity correspond to extracellular methemoglobin (*wavy arrow*). The hypointense rim is due to hemosiderin (*arrow*).

brain tissue, especially in the pons; the involved area of the brain may contain gliotic cells stained with hemosiderin.[19] Hemosiderin-laden macrophages may surround the angioma or telangiectasia, and iron deposition within glial cells of the adjacent white matter may be present.

Patients with occult vascular malformations may present clinically with a seizure disorder or with an acute neurologic deficit secondary to hemorrhage. Often these lesions are found incidentally.[42,49] Cavernous angiomas are usually single lesions; however, studies have been reported where 50 percent of cases had multiple lesions.[49,59]

The typical MR appearance of an occult vascular malformation on a T2-weighted image is a central focus of high signal intensity consistent with subacute or chronic hemorrhage. This is surrounded by a peripheral zone of low intensity attributed to hemosiderin deposition (Figs. 6-10 and 6-11).[31,51,54] The distinction between a cavernous hemangioma and a hemorrhagic neoplasm may be difficult. Occult vascular malformations will generally have an absence of both associated edema and nonhemorrhagic tissue consistent with tumor. They will have a hemosiderin ring and display the temporal evolution of a hematoma.[2,45] They are often single, so the presence of multiple lesions suggests the possibility of metastases. CT may be helpful in defining calcification, which is fairly unusual in untreated cerebral metastases.[59] Primary and secondary hemorrhagic neoplasms can

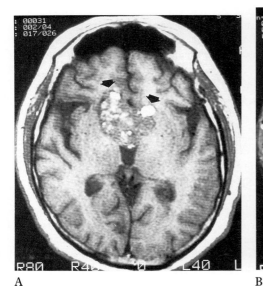

A

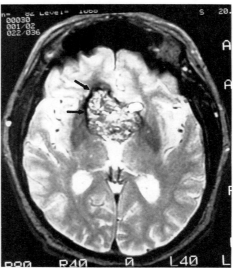

B

Figure 6-11 Cavernous hemangioma. *A.* A T1-weighted image shows a suprasellar mass of mixed signal intensity within the brain parenchyma. Areas of hyperintensity represent subacute hemorrhage (methemoglobin) (*arrows*). *B.* On a T2-weighted image, areas of hyperintense signal represent subacute blood deposits. There is a peripheral rim of hemosiderin (*arrows*).

appear identical to occult vascular malformations and in questionable cases a follow-up examination should be obtained.[59]

Venous Angiomas

The characteristic features of a venous angioma on MRI are a curvilinear streak of very low signal strength on T2-weighted images corresponding to the transcerebral draining vein. The curvilinear vascular channel may appear to receive drainage from a spoked-wheel-like collection of small tapering medullary veins, sometimes in a radial pattern. The large draining vein empties into a larger cortical vein, dural sinus, or subependymal ventricular vein. A region of increased signal on T2-weighted images, corresponding to the venous angioma body, is often visible. This area of increased signal has been attributed to an increased blood pool within the body of the venous angioma.[6] T2-weighted images depict the lesion better than CT or T1-weighted images.[54] Gradient refocused acquisition MRI will confirm the presence of flowing blood within incidentally discovered venous malformations.[2]

Venous Sinus Thrombosis and Venous Infarction

Venous sinus thrombosis is often difficult to diagnose clinically. MRI offers advantages over angiography and digital subtraction angiography in that it is noninvasive and may be more reliable than CT.[8]

MR experience indicates that there is an orderly evolution of MR signal intensity associated with venous thrombosis. This is a process similar to that which occurs in intraparenchymal hemorrhage. In the initial acute stage, the normal flow void in the sagittal sinus is not seen in any plane or imaging sequence. Fresh thrombosis is isointense on T1-weighted images and hypointense on T2-weighted images. In the subacute phase, the thrombus becomes hyperintense initially on T1-weighted images and then also on T2-weighted images. Later changes, seen approximately 2 weeks after presentation, reveal the beginning of recanalization with resumption of a flow void in the previously thrombosed vessel.[47]

Gradient refocused acquisitions can be helpful to confirm the diagnosis of superior sagittal sinus thrombosis. Normally, the superior sagittal sinus will demonstrate high signal with GRA imaging. In the early stages of sagittal sinus thrombosis when SE techniques demonstrate low signal on T1- and T2-weighted images, the high signal intensity of flow will be absent in the superior sagittal sinus. In the subacute phase, when SE images demonstrate high signal on both T1 and T2 images, the GRA images will also demonstrate high signal intensity related to shortened T1 and lengthened T2 in the clot. In the subacute phase, when GRA

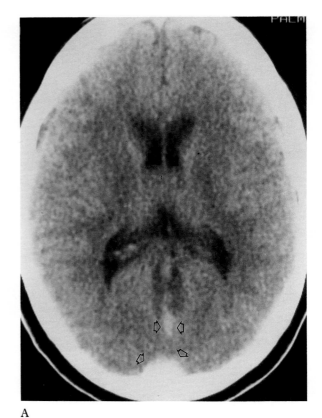

A

Figure 6-12 Early sagittal sinus thrombosis. *A.* A noncontrast CT scan shows a high attenuation thrombus in the straight and superior sagittal sinuses (*open arrows*). *B,* *C.* T1-weighted images demonstrate an isointense to hypointense thrombus in the transverse and superior sagittal sinuses; the intensity represents the deoxyhemoglobin of the acute thrombus (*arrows*). *D.* A T1-weighted image in a midline sagittal plane shows a hypointense to isointense acute thrombus in the superior sagittal and straight sinuses (*arrows*). *E.* On a T2-weighted image, the superior sagittal sinus appears markedly hypointense (*arrowheads*), corresponding to the deoxyhemoglobin of the acute thrombus. *F.* Gradient refocused acquisition shows that flow within the basilar artery is present (*long arrows*). The absence of a bright signal in the superior sagittal and straight sinuses represents absence of flow (*short arrows*).

imaging could be confusing, the diagnosis can be made on the basis of SE images (Figs. 6-12 and 6-13).[47]

Venous infarcts appear as areas of increased signal on T2-weighted images. They typically involve the subcortical white matter of the cerebral or cerebellar hemispheres. If these areas are bright on T1- and T2-weighted images, hemorrhagic infarction, which is frequently associated with dural sinus thrombosis, is present (Fig. 6-14).[1]

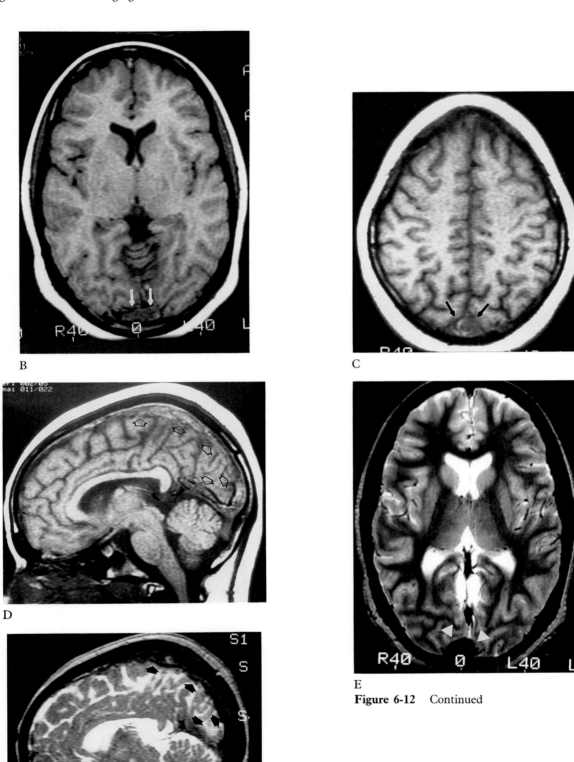

B

C

D

E

Figure 6-12   Continued

F

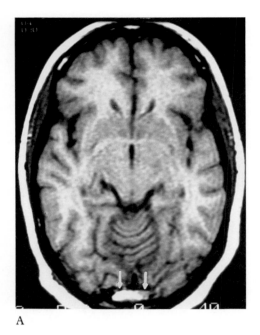

A

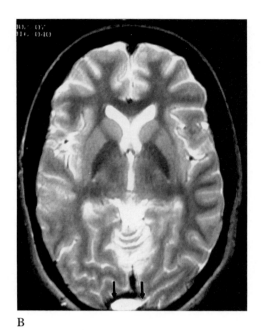

B

Figure 6-13 Late sagittal sinus thrombosis. *A*. On a T1-weighted image, the hyperintense signal in the superior sagittal sinus represents a subacute thrombus (methemoglobin) *(arrows)*. *B*. On a T2-weighted image, the hyperintense signal in the superior sagittal sinus represents extracellular methemoglobin in a subacute thrombus *(arrows)*. *C*. On GRA, the hyperintense signal from the superior sagittal sinus corresponds to subacute blood, which is bright due to the short T1 and long T2 effect of GRA *(arrowhead)*. Partial recanalization is also present *(arrow)*.

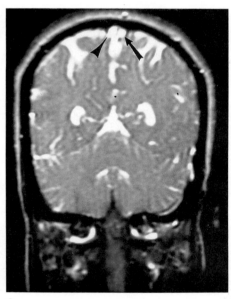

C

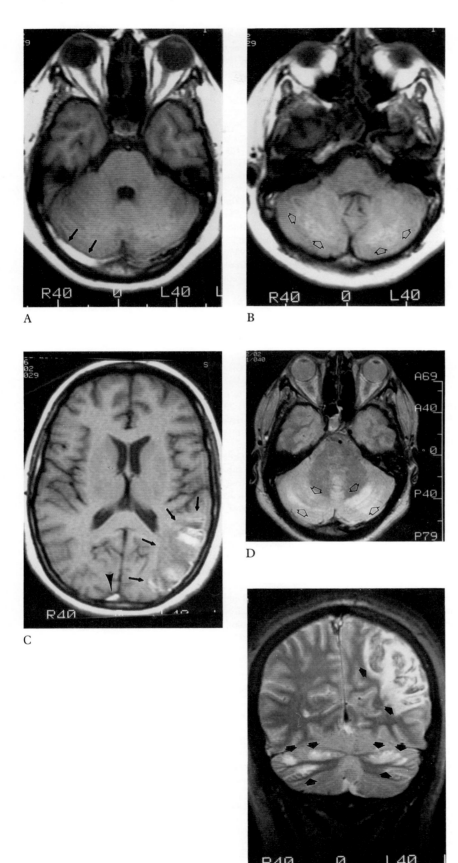

Figure 6-14 Sagittal sinus thrombosis and deep venous infarcts. *A.* On a T1-weighted image, hyperintensity in a transverse sinus represents a subacute thrombus *(arrows)*. *B.* On a T1-weighted image there is hyperintensity within the cerebellar hemispheres, corresponding to subacute hemorrhage within venous infarcts *(open arrows)*. *C.* On this T1-weighted image, hyperintensity in the superior sagittal sinus corresponds to subacute thrombosis (methemoglobin) *(arrowhead)*. Hyperintensity in the left posterior parietal region represents subacute hemorrhage in a venous infarct *(arrows)*. *D.* A T2-weighted image shows increased signal in the cerebellar hemispheres bilaterally, corresponding to venous infarcts *(open arrows)*. *E.* A coronal T2-weighted image demonstrates both left parietal and bilateral cerebellar hemispheric infarcts *(arrows)*.

A

B

C

D

E

Summary

MRI is often the diagnostic modality of first choice in diagnosing vascular lesions of the brain. CT is superior in detecting calcification within aneurysms and cavernous angiomas and detecting the presence of acute subarachnoid hemorrhage or hemorrhage within an acute infarct. Otherwise, in general, MR currently equals or surpasses CT in evaluating cerebrovascular disorders. Newer techniques in instrumentation will allow for better resolution and shorter scan times. Techniques are currently being developed that will allow angiograms to be produced on MR images, that will measure the perfusion rates of tissues, and that will evaluate the adequacy of perfusion by measuring the high energy phosphates present by spectroscopy. MRI is a relatively young field, and its usefulness will continue to grow over the years.

References

1. Anderson SC, Shah CP, Murtagh FR. Congested deep subcortical veins as a sign of dural venous thrombosis: MR and CT correlations. *J Comput Assist Tomogr* 1987; 11:1059–1061.
2. Atlas SW. Intracranial vascular malformations and aneurysms: current imaging applications. *Radiol Clin North Am* 1988; 26:821–837.
3. Atlas SW, Grossman RI, Goldberg HI, et al. Partially thrombosed giant intracranial aneurysms: correlation of MR and pathologic findings. *Radiology* 1987; 162:111–114.
4. Atlas SW, Grossman RI, Gomori JM, et al. Hemorrhagic intracranial malignant neoplasms: spin-echo MR imaging. *Radiology* 1987; 164:71–77.
5. Atlas SW, Mark AS, Grossman RI, et al. Intracranial hemorrhage: gradient-echo MR imaging at 1.5 T: comparison with spin-echo imaging and clinical applications. *Radiology* 1988; 168:803–807.
6. Augustyn GT, Scott JA, Olson E, et al. Cerebral venous angiomas: MR imaging. *Radiology* 1985; 156:391–395.
7. Barkovich AJ, Atlas SW. Magnetic resonance imaging of intracranial hemorrhage. *Radiol Clin North Am* 1988; 26:801–820.
8. Bauer WM, Einhäupl K, Heywang SH, et al. MR of venous sinus thrombosis: a case report. *AJNR* 1987; 8:713–715.
9. Belec L, Cesaro P, Brugieres P, et al. Tumor-simulating giant serpentine aneurysm of the posterior cerebral artery. *Surg Neurol* 1988; 29:210–215.
10. Biondi A, Scialfa G, Scotti G. Intracranial aneurysms: MR imaging. *Neuroradiology* 1988; 30:214–218.
11. Bradley WG Jr. Magnetic resonance imaging of the central nervous system. *Neurol Res* 1984; 6:91–106.
12. Braffman BH, Zimmerman RA, Trojanowski JQ, et al. Brain MR: pathologic correlation with gross and histopathology. 1. Lacunar infarction and Virchow-Robin spaces. *AJNR* 1988; 9:621–628.
13. Braffman BH, Zimmerman RA, Trojanowski JQ, et al. Brain MR: pathologic correlation with gross and histopathology. 2. Hyperintense white-matter foci in the elderly. *AJNR* 1988; 9:629–636.
14. Brant-Zawadzki M, Pereira B, Weinstein P, et al. MR imaging of acute experimental ischemia in cats. *AJNR* 1986; 7:7–11.
15. Brant-Zawadzki M, Solomon M, Newton TH, et al. Basic principles of magnetic resonance imaging in cerebral ischemia and initial clinical experience. *Neuroradiology* 1985; 27:517–520.
16. Brown JJ, Hesselink JR, Rothrock JF. MR and CT of lacunar infarcts. *AJR* 1988; 151:367–372.
17. Bryan RN, Willcott MR, Schneiders NJ, et al. NMR evaluation of stroke in the rat. *AJNR* 1983; 4:242–244.
18. Buonanno FS, Pykett IL, Brady TJ, et al. Proton NMR imaging in experimental ischemic infarction. *Stroke* 1983; 14:178–184.
19. Burger PC, Vogel FS. *Surgical Pathology of the Nervous System and Its Coverings.* New York: Wiley, 1976:331–336.
20. Bydder GM, Steiner RE, Thomas DJ, et al. Nuclear magnetic resonance imaging of the posterior fossa: 50 cases. *Clin Radiol* 1983; 34:173–188.
21. De La Paz RL, New PFJ, Buonanno FS, et al. NMR imaging of intracranial hemorrhage. *J Comput Assist Tomogr* 1984; 8:599–607.
22. DeWitt LD. Clinical use of nuclear magnetic resonance imaging in stroke. *Stroke* 1986; 17:328–331.
23. DeWitt LD, Buonanno FS, Kistler JP, et al. Nuclear magnetic resonance imaging in evaluation of clinical stroke syndromes. *Ann Neurol* 1984; 16:535–545.
24. Di Chiro G, Brooks RA, Girton ME, et al. Sequential MR studies of intracerebral hematomas in monkeys. *AJNR* 1986; 7:193–199.
25. Dooms GC, Uske A, Brant-Zawadzki M, et al. Spin-echo MR imaging of intracranial hemorrhage. *Neuroradiology* 1986; 28:132–138.
26. Edelman RR, Johnson K, Buxton R, et al. MR of hemorrhage: a new approach. *AJNR* 1986; 7:751–756.
27. Gomori JM, Grossman RL, Goldberg HI, et al. High-field spin-echo MR imaging of superficial and subependymal siderosis secondary to neonatal intraventricular hemorrhage. *Neuroradiology* 1987; 29:339–342.
28. Gomori JM, Grossman RI, Goldberg HI, et al. Intracranial hematomas: imaging by high-field MR. *Radiology* 1985; 157:87–93.
29. Gomori JM, Grossman RI, Hackney DB, et al. Variable appearances of subacute intracranial hematomas on high-field spin-echo MR. *AJR* 1988; 150:171–178.
30. Gomori JM, Grossman RI, Steiner I. High-field magnetic resonance imaging of intracranial hematomas. *Isr J Med Sci* 1988; 24:218–223.
31. Griffin C, De La Paz R, Enzmann D. Magnetic resonance appearance of slow flow vascular malformations of the brainstem. *Neuroradiology* 1987; 29:506–511.
32. Hackney DB, Atlas SW, Grossman RI, et al. Subacute intracranial hemorrhage: contribution of spin density to appearance on spin-echo MR images. *Radiology* 1987; 165:199–202.
33. Hackney DB, Lesnick JE, Zimmerman RA, et al. MR identification of bleeding site in subarachnoid hemorrhage with multiple intracranial aneurysms. *J Comput Assist Tomogr* 1986; 10:878–880.
34. Hayman LA, Ford JJ, Taber KH, et al. T2 effect of hemoglobin concentration: assessment with in vitro MR spectroscopy. *Radiology* 1988; 168:489–491.
35. Hecht-Leavitt C, Gomori JM, Grossman RI, et al. High-field MRI of hemorrhagic cortical infarction. *AJNR* 1986; 7:581–585.
36. Imakita S, Nishimura T, Naito H, et al. Magnetic resonance imaging of human cerebral infarction: enhancement with Gd-DTPA. *Neuroradiology* 1987; 29:422–429.
37. Kapelle LJ, van Gijn J. Lacunar infarcts. *Clin Neurol Neurosurg* 1986; 88:3–17.
38. Kertesz A, Black SE, Nicholson L. The sensitivity and specificity of MRI in stroke. *Neurology* 1987; 37:1580–1585.
39. Kertesz A, Black SE, Tokar G, et al. Periventricular and subcortical hyperintensities on magnetic resonance imaging: "rims, caps, and unidentified bright objects." *Arch Neurol* 1988; 45:404–408.
40. Kirkpatrick JB, Hayman LA. White-matter lesions in MR im-

aging of clinically healthy brains of elderly subjects: possible pathologic basis. *Radiology* 1987; 162:509–511.

41. Komiyama M, Baba M, Hakuba A, et al. MR imaging of brainstem hemorrhage. *AJNR* 1988; 9:261–268.

42. Kucharczyk W, Lemme-Pleghos L, Uske A, et al. Intracranial vascular malformations: MR and CT imaging. *Radiology* 1985; 156:383–389.

43. Leblanc R, Levesque M, Comair Y, et al. Magnetic resonance imaging of cerebral arteriovenous malformations. *Neurosurgery* 1987; 21:15–20.

44. Lee BCP, Herzberg L, Zimmerman RD, et al. MR imaging of cerebral vascular malformations. *AJNR* 1985; 6:863–870.

45. Lemme-Plaghos L, Kucharczyk W, Brant-Zawadzki M, et al. MRI of angiographically occult vascular malformations. *AJR* 1986; 146:1223–1228.

46. Levy RM, Mano I, Brito A, et al. NMR imaging of acute experimental cerebral ischemia: time course and pharmacologic manipulations. *AJNR* 1983; 4:238–241.

47. Macchi PJ, Grossman RI, Gomori JM, et al. High field MR imaging of cerebral venous thrombosis. *J Comput Assist Tomogr* 1986; 10:10–15.

48. Marshall VG, Bradley WG Jr, Marshall CE, et al. Deep white matter infarction: correlation of MR imaging and histopathologic findings. *Radiology* 1988; 167:517–522.

49. McCormick WF. Vascular diseases. In: Rosenberg RN (ed.), *The Clinical Neurosciences*. New York: Churchill Livingstone, 1983; 3:35–83.

50. Needell WM, Maravilla KR. MR flow imaging in vascular malformations using gradient recalled acquisition. *AJNR* 1988; 9:637–642.

51. New PFJ, Ojemann RG, Davis KR, et al. MR and CT of occult vascular malformations of the brain. *AJR* 1986; 147:985–993.

52. Noorbehesht B, Fabrikant JI, Enzmann DR. Size determination of supratentorial arteriovenous malformations by MR, CT and angio. *Neuroradiology* 1987; 29:512–518.

53. Olsen WL, Brant-Zawadzki M, Hodes J, et al. Giant intracranial aneurysms: MR imaging. *Radiology* 1987; 163:431–435.

54. Rigamonti D, Drayer BP, Johnson PC, et al. The MRI appearance of cavernous malformations (angiomas). *J Neurosurg* 1987; 67:518–524.

55. Salgado ED, Weinstein M, Furlan AJ, et al. Proton magnetic resonance imaging in ischemic cerebrovascular disease. *Ann Neurol* 1986; 20:502–507.

56. Sipponen JT. Visualization of brain infarction with nuclear magnetic resonance imaging. *Neuroradiology* 1984; 26:387–391.

57. Sipponen JT, Kaste M, Ketonen L, et al. Serial nuclear magnetic resonance (NMR) imaging in patients with cerebral infarction. *J Comput Assist Tomogr* 1983; 7:585–589.

58. Smith HJ, Strother CM, Kikuchi Y, et al. MR imaging in the management of supratentorial intracranial AVMs. *AJR* 1988; 150:1143–1153.

59. Sze G, Krol G, Olsen WL, et al. Hemorrhagic neoplasms: MR mimics of occult vascular malformations. *AJR* 1987; 149:1223–1230.

60. Virapongse C, Mancuso A, Quisling R. Human brain infarcts: Gd-DTPA-enhanced MR imaging. *Radiology* 1986; 161:785–794.

61. Worthington BS, Kean DM, Hawkes RC, et al. NMR imaging in the recognition of giant intracranial aneurysms. *AJNR* 1983; 4:835–836.

62. Zimmerman RD, Heier LA, Snow RB, et al. Acute intracranial hemorrhage: intensity changes on sequential MR scans at 0.5 T. *AJR* 1988; 150:651–661.

7

Magnetic Resonance Imaging of Intracranial Infections

Robert A. Zimmerman

At present the limitations of magnetic resonance (MR) in examining patients with infectious diseases of the central nervous system (CNS) are several: (1) long data acquisition times, on the order of minutes, may permit motion during a portion of that scan time that results in a degraded or uninterpretable set of images; (2) support equipment, such as intubation devices, respirators, intravenous pumps, electrocardiographic recording instruments, and other devices must be made so that they are not ferromagnetic (and therefore will not be pulled into the magnet at untoward speed) and so that they will not produce inhomogeneity of the magnetic field or give rise to unwanted radiofrequency (RF) signals (degrading the image); and (3) the support equipment must operate normally in this setting [e.g., to produce an interpretable readout despite the potential interference and deflection of the readout device (electron gun) within such an instrument due to the magnetic field generated by the MR unit].[20]

Despite the inherent difficulties in performing MR, especially on very ill patients, the benefits from the information obtained from the MR images often outweighs the difficulties encountered in performing the study. MR allows direct imaging in any plane, including the axial, coronal, and sagittal. The sagittal and coronal planes are particularly useful in planning surgical approaches because of the correlation to the superficial gyral anatomy that can be made relative to deeper lesions.

In most situations, patient motion can be controlled through cooperation, sedation, or general anesthesia. Not routinely available at present but currently undergoing experimentation are rapid imaging techniques known as ultrafast imaging. These imaging sequences produce images with a data acquisition per image on the order of 20 to 60 ms.[16] Thus there is a future potential for much more rapid scanning.

In addition to multiple direct planes of imaging, MR's contribution to the imaging of CNS infectious diseases stems from the following[20]:

1. Proton density–weighted (PDW) and T2-weighted images (T2WI) show great sensitivity to minimal increases in the local water concentration at the site of pathological processes, such as occurs in areas of inflammation as well as in a variety of noninfectious diseases.
2. MR is highly sensitive in the detection of blood products in the form of deoxyhemoglobin, methemoglobin, and hemosiderin.[3] Such blood products occur at the site of cerebritis, abscess formation, and in association with many hematogenously borne infectious diseases and as part of the spectrum of viral infections.[20]
3. MR clearly shows both the normal and pathologic anatomy of the sulci, fissures, cerebral aqueduct, foramina, and ventricular system. Furthermore, the flow of cerebrospinal fluid (CSF) through the CSF pathways can be shown, especially with cine–MR imaging sequences, which show the motion of CSF to the point that the rate of movement (millimeters per second) can be calculated.[13]
4. With the use of the newly approved (by the Food and Drug Administration) paramagnetic contrast agent, gadolinium-DTPA (Magnavist; Berlex Laboratories, Cedar Knolls, NJ), abnormalities of the blood-brain barrier (BBB) can be demonstrated, such as those that occur at the site of abscesses, cerebritis, and ventriculitis.[14,20] Loculations of pyogenic material with reactive membranes in the extracerebral spaces (subdural and epidural empyemas) can be delineated.

Despite the advantages of MR enumerated above, computed tomography (CT) may be the initial study of choice in selected instances, or the follow-up study of choice when the clinical condition of the patient is rapidly changing or is so unstable that time or the necessity of certain supporting and monitoring equipment does not permit the steps necessary to ensure a safe MR examination. When speed is essential, CT will suffice to show the size of a lesion, such as an abscess, as well as the displacement of the brain and the size of the ventricles.[21] CT has one distinct advantage over MR, and that is its ability to demonstrate with great specificity the presence or absence of gross calcification. With MR, the calcification cannot be visualized with any sensitivity on routine (spin echo) pulse sequences.[7] With pulse sequences designed to show calcification, the specificity is not present because other abnormalities cause similar susceptibility effects that can mimic the MR appearance of calcification.[2] With both CT and MR, the pertinent clinical information is vital to the intelligent interpretation of the imaging findings.

Bacterial Infections

Cerebritis

Cerebritis consists pathologically of an ill-defined area of infected brain characterized by edema, softening, petechial hemorrhages, and vascular congestion.[6] MR shows such an

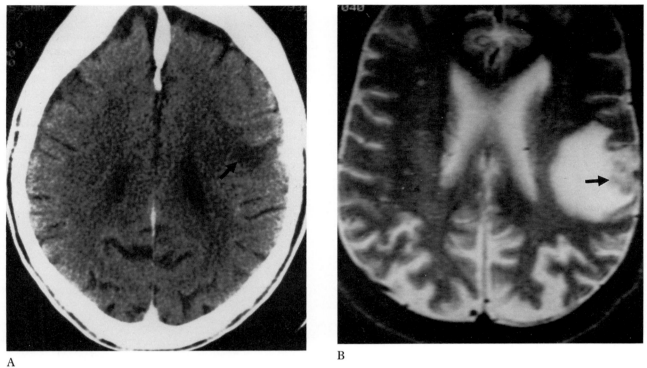

A   B

Figure 7-1 Cerebritis. Male, 51 years old, with a left lower lobe pulmonary infiltrate presenting with the new onset of seizures. *A.* Axial nonenhanced CT shows slight hypodensity in the left frontoparietal region *(arrow)*. *B.* Axial T2WI shows a zone of subcortical white-matter hyperintensity in the left frontoparietal region with a more superficial area of lower signal intensity consistent with a hemorrhagic component *(arrow)*.

area of cerebritis as a region of high signal intensity on PDWI and T2WI because of the increased water content within the edema (Figs. 7-1*B* and 7-2).[20] Other findings that suggest cerebritis are the presence of mass effect and a localization of the process to the corticomedullary juncture when the source is hematogenous. On T2WI the presence of less

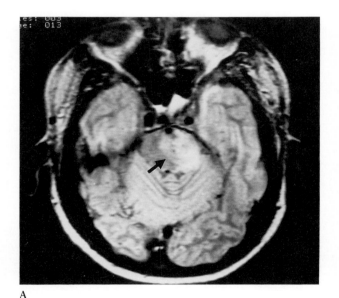

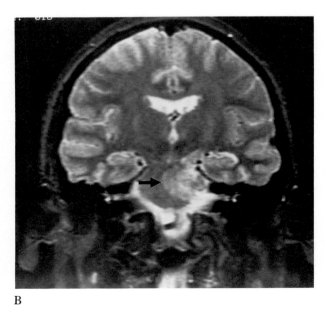

A   B

Figure 7-2 Cerebritis. Young adult with new onset of cranial nerve palsies. *A.* Axial PDW MR image shows high signal intensity in the left pons *(arrow)*. *B.* Coronal T2W MR image shows high signal intensity in the left side of the pons *(arrow)*.

intense foci within the edematous zone suggests areas of pe-techial hemorrhages consisting of intracellular deoxy- or methemoglobin (Fig. 7-1B).[20] T2-weighted and PDW MR images show abnormalities suspicious for cerebritis in a more apparent fashion than CT (Fig. 7-1). Despite the sensitivity of MR in detecting areas of cerebritis, the MR findings lack specificity. Correct interpretation requires correlation to the clinical situation. MR is a good method for follow-up during treatment of clinical cerebritis in order to show resolution or progression to abscess formation.

Brain Abscess

The host response to the cerebritis focus occurs in the form of an attempt to contain the infection (the abscess capsule). Formation of the collagen wall of the abscess capsule is by fibroblasts that arise from superficial blood vessels. There are three layers to the wall: an inner granulation layer, a middle collagen layer, and an outer reactive glial layer. The middle collagen layer, formed by the migrating fibroblasts, gives strength to the capsule, which allows its surgical extirpation. The medial aspect of the capsule, that portion facing the deep white matter and ventricular system, requires the

longest migrational path for the fibroblasts. Thus the inner margin of the capsule tends to be the weakest, and it is from that site that daughter abscesses extend more medially.

CT has proved useful in the identification of abscesses as contrast-enhancing ring lesions that are often surrounded by extensive vasogenic edema (Fig. 7-2A).[5,21] Contrast enhancement occurs in the wall of the abscess capsule because of the abnormality in the BBB associated with the ingrowth of new blood vessels.[6] T1WI show the abscess capsule to have a signal intensity that varies from iso- to hyperintense. Often it is a bright ring, a T1 shortening effect, most likely due to the presence of methemoglobin (Figs. 7-3B and 7-4B).[17,20] The likely etiology for this finding is probably

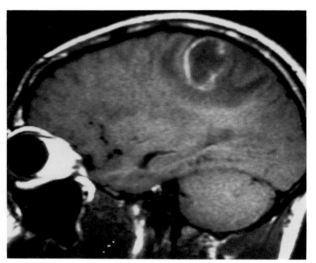

B

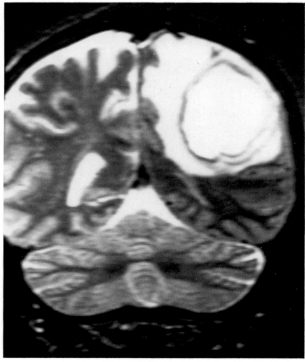

A

Figure 7-3 Brain abscess. Male, 28 years old, with focal seizures and weakness. *A*. Contrast-enhanced axial CT shows a thin rim abscess with marginal enhancement (*arrows*). Surrounding edema is present. *B*. Sagittal T1W MR image shows a margin of high signal intensity consistent with methemoglobin in the wall of the abscess capsule. Surrounding hypointensity is consistent with vasogenic edema. *C*. Coronal T2WI shows the abscess capsule to be hypointense, consistent with intracellular methemoglobin and/or collagen tissue. Surrounding hyperintensity is consistent with vasogenic edema. Note that with this pulse sequence, differentiation cannot be made among the high signal intensity within the abscess, that of CSF, and that of the edematous brain.

C

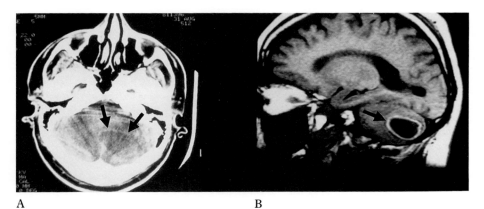

Figure 7-4 Posterior fossa brain abscess. Male, 70 years old, with ataxia. *A*. Contrast-enhanced CT shows a faint, thin rim *(arrows)* of enhancement, partially obscured by artifact. *B*. Sagittal T1WI shows high signal intensity abscess wall *(arrow)*.

A   B

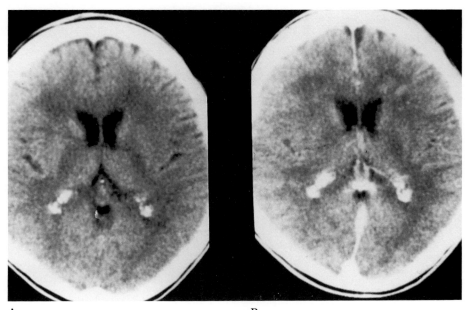

Figure 7-5 Multiple brain abscesses. Demented female, 30 years old. *A*. Axial CT without contrast shows normal brain structure. *B*. Axial CT following contrast administration shows no definite abnormality. *C*. Axial T1WI shows no abnormality. *D*. Axial T1WI following the intravenous injection of Magnevist shows multiple brain abscesses *(arrows)*.

A   B

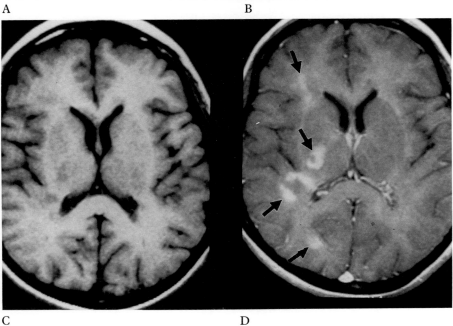

C   D

the incorporation of petechial hemorrhages from cerebritis, or the continued leakage of red blood cells into the forming capsule from the ingrowth of new blood vessels. Depending upon the state of the hemoglobin, if it is intracellular deoxy- or methemoglobin, it will be shown as a focal rim of hypointensity (Fig. 7-3C) on PDWI and T2WI. The fibrous nature of the collagen layer can also contribute to the hypointensity of the abscess capsule on these pulse sequences. An alternative explanation for the signal intensity changes has been raised by Sze and Zimmerman.[17] They postulate that macrophage phagocytosis produces intracellular free radicals which have a paramagnetic effect because of unpaired electrons. Vasogenic edema surrounding the abscess capsule is shown on the PDWI or T2WI as high signal intensity (Fig. 7-3C). Mass effect is well shown on both the T1WI and T2WI. MR demonstrates brain abscesses with a greater sensitivity than CT. Gadolinium-enhanced MR is likely to be the best diagnostic imaging method for diagnosis and follow-up of brain abscesses (Fig. 7-5).

Tuberculosis

Intracranial tuberculomas arise most often from the hematogenous spread of *Mycobacterium tuberculosis* from a primary focus in the lungs. Tuberculous abscesses in the brain are usually shown as multiple small discrete corticomedullary lesions, often containing blood products, that depending upon the pulse sequence, may be either hyper- or hypointense (Fig. 7-6).[18,20] Commonly these are surrounded by small zones of vasogenic edema. The MR appearance of multiple tuberculomas is not specific, as metastasis or multiple occult vascular malformations may produce similar MR appearances.

Figure 7-6 Multiple tuberculomas. Indian male, 55 years old, who presented with seizures. No prior history of tuberculosis. *A.* Axial T2WI shows a zone of high signal intensity edema in the left parieto-occipital region. Centrally within the zone of edema there is a ringlike area of hypointensity (*arrow*) at the site of the tuberculoma. *B.* Coronal PDWI shows a similar finding in the left temporal lobe (*arrow*).

Tuberculous meningitis, a complication of the rupture of a tuberculoma into the subarachnoid space, can be demonstrated on enhanced CT as a thick bright filling-in of the basilar cisterns. On T1WI and T2WI the subarachnoid

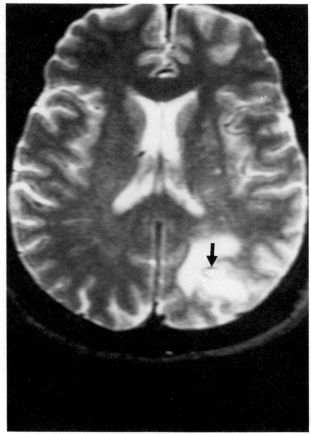

A

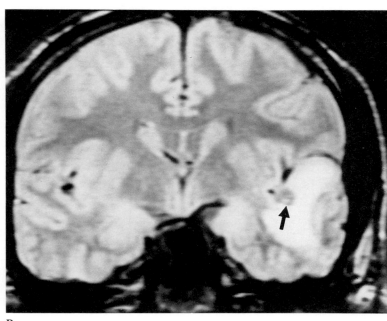

B

changes of tuberculous meningitis are poorly seen. Magnevist-enhanced T1WI hold the best potential for demonstrating MR evidence of tuberculous meningitis.

Bacterial Meningitis

In acute suppurative leptomeningitis, such as is seen with *Haemophilus influenzae* in childhood, pathologically there is an outpouring of polymorphonuclear neutrophils (PMNs), with congestion and hyperemia of the pia and arachnoidal membranes and distention of the subarachnoid space by the infectious exudate.[10] MR shows these findings as a distention of the subarachnoid space and sulci (Fig. 7-7). Blood vessels involved in the inflammatory exudate may become involved in an obliterative infectious process, leading to thrombosis. This leads to infarction of subpial tissues (Figs. 7-8 and 7-9). Depending on the age of the patient and the pulse sequence utilized, infarction will be either hypo- or hyperintense. In the very young infant, under the age of 6 months, the use of T1WI effectively shows the infarction as a hypointensity (Fig. 7-7). This pulse sequence is used in the infant because of the high water content in the unmyelinated white matter[9] (both normal and infarcted tissues are bright). This makes it difficult to distinguish infarcted from normal brain with the T2WI. In the older child, following myelination, the infarcted brain is shown on the PDWI or T2WI as a cortical and subcortical area of high signal intensity (Fig. 7-9). Hydrocephalus can occur as a complication of meningitis due to blockage of the CSF pathways by inflammatory exudate and resultant adhesions (Fig. 7-10*A*). MR is useful in showing the site of blockage and the resultant distention of the proximal CSF pathway. Involvement of the spinal

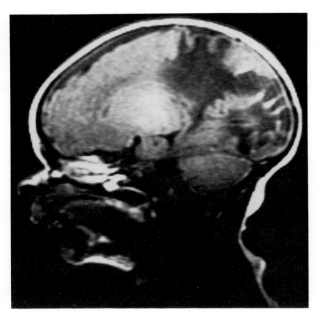

Figure 7-8 Neonatal meningitis due to *Escherichia coli* infection. Sagittal T1WI shows areas of hypointensity within the parieto-occipital white matter consistent with infarction.

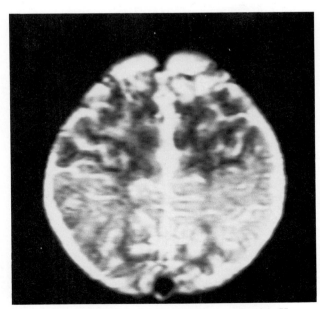

Figure 7-7 Meningitis. Male, 6 months old, with *Haemophilus influenzae* meningitis. Axial T2WI shows marked distention of the subarachnoid space by high-signal-intensity fluid representing the infectious exudate.

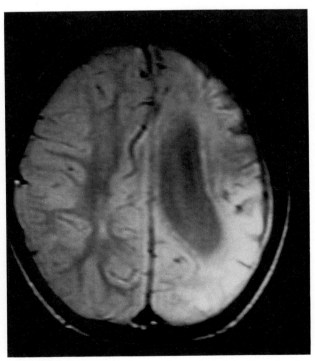

Figure 7-9 Infarction from prior meningitis. Female, 4 years old, with a history of prior beta streptococcus meningitis. Axial PDWI shows dilatation of the left lateral ventricle, with high signal intensity involving the cortex and underlying white matter at the site of infarction.

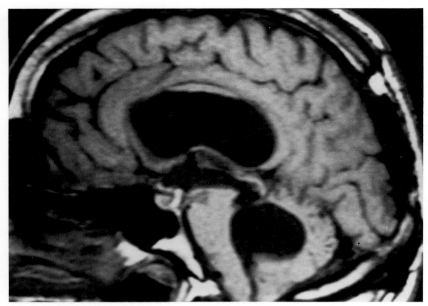

A

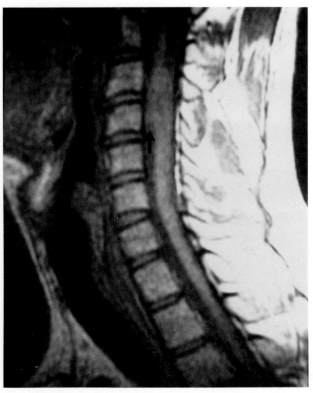

B

Figure 7-10 Postmeningitic hydrocephalus due to adhesions. Cervical spinal cord arachnoiditis. Male, 25 years old, several years after head injury complicated by meningitis with recent development of neck pain. *A.* Sagittal T1WI shows marked dilatation of the lateral ventricle, third ventricle, aqueduct, and fourth ventricle. Cerebellar tonsil is herniated into the foramen magnum. Corpus callosum and cerebellum are stretched over the dilated ventricular system. *B.* Sagittal T1W cervical spine study shows tissue isointense with the spinal cord filling in the anterior subarachnoid space *(arrows)* at the C3-4 level. The finding is consistent with arachnoiditis.

can be formed if this necrosis occurs before treatment has been effective (Fig. 7-11). MR is particularly effective in demonstrating extracerebral fluid collections because of both coronal imaging and the demonstration of fluid as high signal intensity (PDWI and T2WI) in stark contrast to the lower signal intensities of the cortex and calvarium (Fig. 7-11).

Complications of Paranasal Sinus Infections

The intracranial spread of infection from the paranasal sinuses occurs by two methods. The first is direct spread through the wall of the paranasal sinus as a result of osteomyelitis or through foramina leading to contiguous involvement.[15] The second is a spread along the venous connecting pathways via septic phlebitis.[19] Retrograde transmission along the venous channels is possible because they are not protected (by valves) in the facial region. MR is effective in showing opacification of the paranasal sinus on both T1WI

subarachnoid space as a result of meningitis can lead to focal arachnoiditis (Fig. 7-10*B*). Necrosis of the arachnoid can lead to subdural fluid collections. If this occurs after the infectious process has been successfully treated, then the collection is likely to be sterile; however, subdural empyema

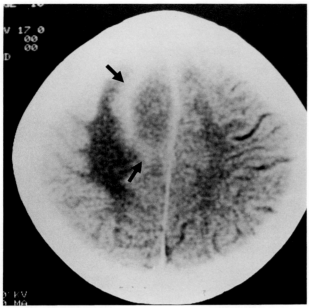

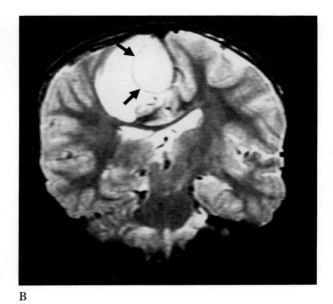

B

A

Figure 7-11 Subdural empyema. Female, 13 years old, presenting with seizures and hemiparesis. *A*. Axial contrast CT shows a focal collection in the right frontal region with a contrast enhancing wall *(arrows)* adjacent to the falx cerebri. There is vasogenic edema in the white matter of the contiguous right cerebral hemisphere. *B*. Coronal T2WI shows a thin hypointense margin outlining the parafalcine subdural empyema *(arrows)*. The falx is displaced to the left. Surrounding vasogenic edema involves the adjacent cortex and subcortical white matter within the right frontal lobe. The corpus callosum is compressed, as is the body of the lateral ventricle.

and T2WI. High signal intensity is found in the infected sinus mucosa with either the PDWI or T2WI (Fig. 7-12). Spread of the infectious process out of the sphenoid sinus into the cavernous sinus and on into the suprasellar cistern is shown as distention of the cavernous sinus, and by obliteration of the normal CSF pathway with the presence of a focal area of high signal intensity (abscess) on the PDWI (Fig. 7-12B, C, and D). Posttraumatic infected hematomas may be well demonstrated by MR, but the signal intensity will not differentiate whether or not infection is present (Fig. 7-13). Retrograde venous extension of septic thrombophlebitis from the infected paranasal sinuses back through the superior ophthalmic vein is shown as enlargement of the vein and lack of the normal flow void because of clotting (deoxyhemoglobin) within the vein (Fig. 7-14A). With retrograde extension of the septic thrombophlebitis through the diploic veins onto the surface of the brain, cortical venous thrombosis occurs and is shown well on either PDWI or T2WI (Fig. 7-14B). High signal intensity edema present surrounding the area of cortical vein thrombosis may be the result of venous infarction and/or cerebritis (Fig. 7-14B). Bacterial infection of the external auditory canal or mastoid air cells such as occurs in childhood or in old age in association with diabetes (malignant external otitis) can lead to involvement of the sigmoid or jugular venous sinus with thrombosis. Compromise of cerebral venous drainage may lead to increased intracranial pressure, hydrocephalus, or papilledema. Computed tomography shows the bone involvement best (Fig. 7-15A), while CT and MR show the mastoid inflammation with air cell opacification. MR shows thrombosis of the involved dural venous sinus best (Fig. 7-15B).

Viral Infections

A wide spectrum of parenchymal changes occur as a result of viral infection. Pathologically the findings may be completely within normal limits or may appear as extensive necrosis, hemorrhage, and edema.[8] In the typical response to the viral infection, PMNs are found in tissue surrounding vessels. Subsequently, the cell reaction changes to mononuclear and lymphoid cells. Vascular congestion and conglomerates of inflammatory cells are then superimposed. A more destructive or thrombotic process producing edema and tissue loss may supervene. The histologic picture depends both on the infective agent and the host response that is mounted.

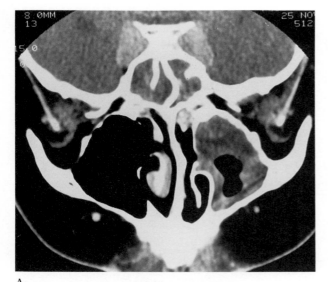

A

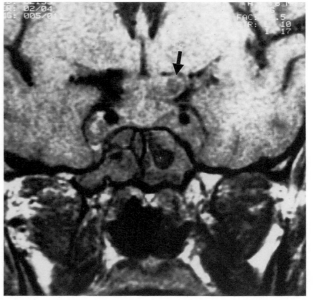

B

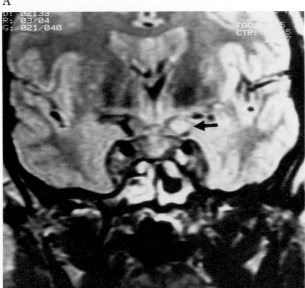

C

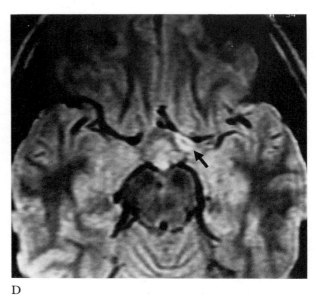

D

Figure 7-12

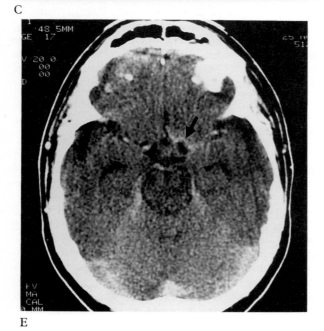

E

96

Figure 7-12 *(opposite)* Sphenoid sinus infection with bilateral cavernous sinus involvement with thrombosis and suprasellar abscess formation. Young male with complicated sinus infection. *A.* Coronal CT following contrast enhancement shows opacification in part of the left maxillary sinus and of both sphenoid sinuses. Cavernous sinuses appear enlarged so that their outward margins bulge laterally. *B.* Coronal T1WI shows opacification of both sphenoid air cells, convex outward bowing of the sinus dura with focal area of high signal intensity consistent with clot or slow flow in the right cavernous sinus. The left side of the optic chiasm is thickened by a soft tissue mass in the suprasellar cistern (arrow). *C.* Coronal PDWI shows high signal intensity inflammatory change within the sphenoid air cells. The cavernous sinuses are distended. A high signal intensity mass is present in the left suprasellar cistern, consistent with an abscess *(arrow).* *D.* Axial PDWI through the chiasmatic cistern shows the high signal intensity abscess on the left *(arrow).* Note the focal thinning of the anterior cerebral artery contiguous with the abscess. *E.* Axial contrast-enhanced CT shows the thin margin of enhancement of the left suprasellar abscess *(arrow).*

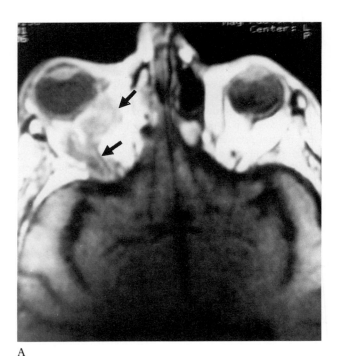

A

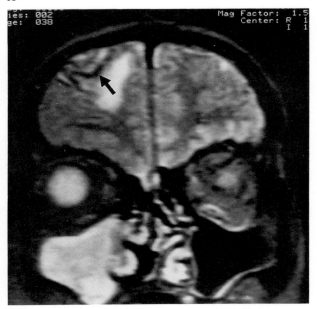

B

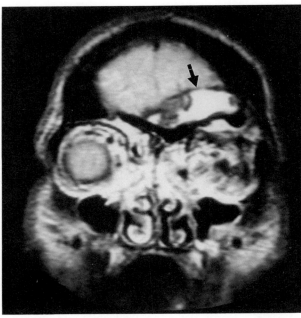

Figure 7-13 Epidural abscess, posttraumatic. Male, 30 years old, with posttraumatic loss of left globe and with fever, chills, and headaches. Coronal T2WI shows high signal intensity changes involving the ethmoid air cells and frontal sinus on the right. These findings are consistent with either blood or inflammatory change. A high signal intensity collection *(arrow)* is also present in the epidural space beneath the left frontal lobe. The collection has a margin of low signal intensity. This finding is consistent with either hematoma or infection. Surgery showed an infected hematoma.

Figure 7-14 Septic thrombophlebitis of the superior ophthalmic vein, sinusitis, cerebral venous infarction. Male, 60 years old, with complicated paranasal sinus infection with new onset of proptosis. *A.* Axial T1WI shows dilatation of the superior ophthalmic vein *(arrows).* There is no flow void within the vein, indicating thrombosis. *B.* Coronal T2WI shows high signal intensity opacification of the right maxillary sinus consistent with sinus inflammatory disease. High signal intensity is seen in the frontal lobe white matter on the right with overlying serpentine hypointensity at the site of a cortical vessel. The hypointensity corresponds to thrombosis of a cortical vein *(arrow),* the hyperintensity to cerebritis and/or infarction or vasogenic edema.

The medical imaging picture depends on the sensitivity of the imaging technique to demonstrating the pathologic processes. Specificity of the imaging information relates to anatomic localization of the findings and correlation of the images to the clinical and laboratory findings.

Intrauterine infection by the cytomegalovirus (CMV) produces a destructive process involving the white matter, leading to gliosis, migrational abnormalities, microcephaly, and mental retardation (Fig. 7-16).[8]

Herpes simplex type 1 (HSV-1) is a ubiquitous virus associated with cold sores that occur around the mouth.

HSV-1 is a common agent involved in the production of encephalitis in both children and adults. In this form it occurs as a reaction to a latent infection. Seizures, personality and behavior changes, with progression to coma are some of the likely clinical manifestations. Pathologically, the infection produces a hemorrhagic, necrotizing involvement of one or both frontal and/or temporal lobes (Fig. 7-17).[8] MR is sensitive in demonstrating the areas of involvement as high signal intensity on T2WI. This is because of the increased fluid content in the involved tissues. HSV-1 infection of the brain is characterized by the sites of involvement, that is, the medial temporal lobes extending into the insular cortex, the multiplicity of sites of involvement, and in the acute stages, the mass effect associated with the disease.[8] The presence of hemorrhagic foci within the area of involvement further supports the diagnosis of herpes simplex infection. In patients surviving the infection, MR is successful in demonstrating the concomitant necrosis and atrophy that occurs (Fig. 7-18).

Acute disseminated encephalomyelitis (ADEM) is not a direct infection of the brain by a virus but a reaction to the virus, most likely of an autoimmune nature, in which a delayed hypersensitivity to myelin basic protein develops, leading to areas of demyelination.[1,4] This typically follows by several weeks a viral infection or occurs in a delayed fashion after a vaccination. Pathologically, there are multiple perivenule zones of demyelination and inflammatory infiltrates in a perivascular distribution. These areas are demonstrated on PDWI and T2WI as focal areas of white-matter high signal intensity, findings consistent with ADEM. These areas are commonly found in the supratentorial white matter (Fig. 7-19) and in the basal ganglia and brain stem.

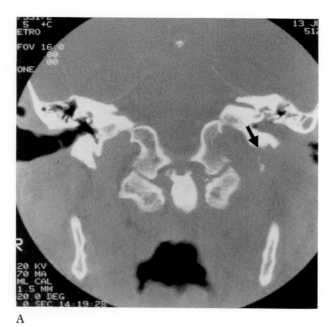

A

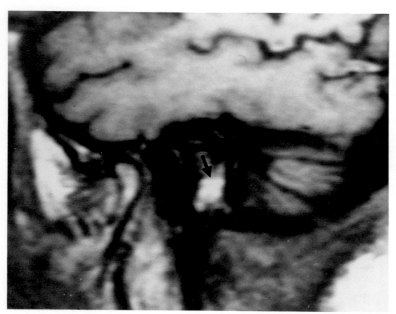

B

Figure 7-15 Malignant external otitis. Diabetic male, 68 years old, with purulent drainage from the left ear. *A.* Coronal contrast-enhanced CT with bone window settings shows opacification of the external auditory canal and partial opacification of the middle ear. Region of the hypotympanum shows bone erosion (*arrow*). This lies adjacent to the jugular fossa, which is more medial. *B.* Sagittal T1WI through the mandibular condyle and jugular canal shows high signal intensity clot within the jugular vein (*arrow*).

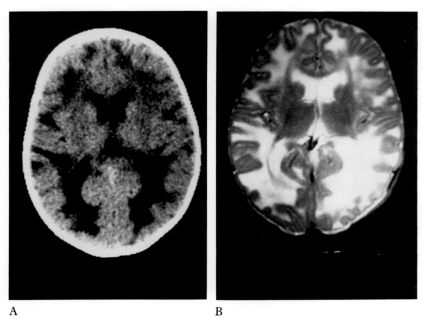

Figure 7-16 Cytomegalic virus disease. Infant, 8 months old, with failure to thrive and a developmental quotient reflecting severe retardation. *A*. Axial CT shows hypodense changes throughout the frontal and temporoparieto-occipital white matter. *B*. Axial T2W image shows marked hyperintensity of the affected white matter. Overall head size was microcephalic.

A   B

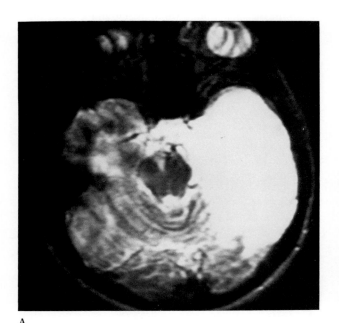

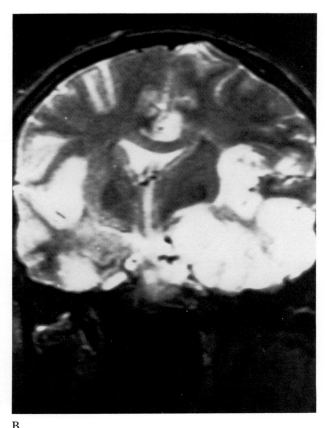

A   B

Figure 7-17 Herpes simplex encephalitis. Female, 30 years old, with coma and seizures. *A*. Axial T2W image shows the left temporal lobe to be high in signal intensity with swelling and mass effect displacing the left cerebral peduncle. *B*. Coronal T2W MRI shows high signal intensity involvement of the left temporal lobe and sylvian cortex, as well as contralateral involvement of the right temporal lobe and sylvian and frontal lobe cortex. Mass effect is present with displacement of the third ventricle and lateral ventricles from left to right with some subfalcine shift.

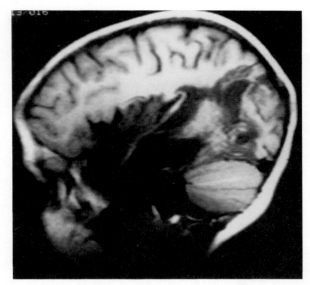

Figure 7-18 Previous herpes simplex encephalitis. Female, 2 years old, examined many months following herpes simplex infection. Sagittal T1WI shows hypointense areas within the temporal lobe consistent with necrotic brain. There is a lack of mass effect.

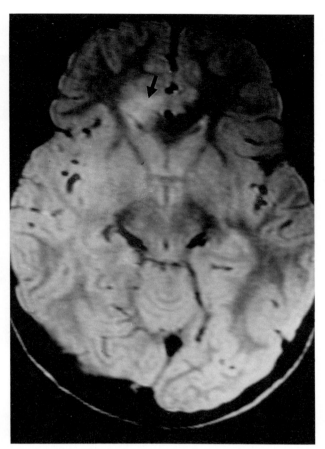

Figure 7-19 Acute disseminated encephalomyelitis. Female, 17 years old, with subtle neurological signs after viral infection. Axial PDWI shows high signal intensity (*arrow*) in the right frontal white matter and genu of the corpus callosum.

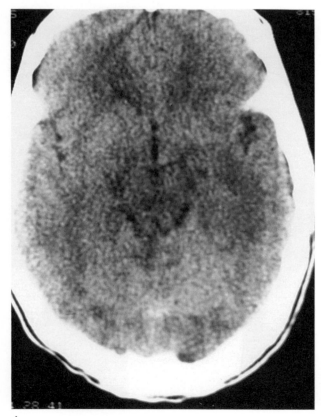

A

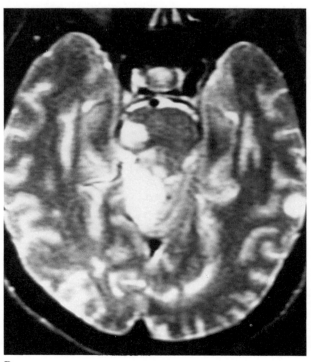

B

Figure 7-20 AIDS. Male, 33 years old, with confusion and cranial nerve palsies. *A.* Axial CT without contrast enhancement shows no focal abnormality. *B.* Axial T2WI shows abnormal high signal intensity involving the right side of the pons and vermis as well as the left temporal lobe.

100

Acquired Immunodeficiency Syndrome (AIDS)

The HTLV-III virus produces a dysfunction of the cell-mediated immune system characterized by inversion of the normal T-helper/T-suppressor cell ratios. Humoral immunity appears to be preserved. Neurological manifestations of various infectious agents occurring in patients with AIDS are highly variable. They depend on the agent, the location, the number, and the rate of progression of the disease. *Toxoplasma gondii*, *Cryptococcus neoformans*, and CMV are among the agents involved.[11,12] The toxoplasma incites a focal inflammatory reaction with perivascular infiltrates of inflammatory cells, areas of vasculitis, and peripheral astrocytosis. *T. gondii* infection in the AIDS patient leads to brain abscesses which are often multiple, with a predilection for the basal ganglia (Figs. 7-20 and 7-21). The MR manifestations of the abscesses are variable but appear most often as areas of high signal intensity of varying size. However, these also often contain areas of mixed signal intensity or of low signal intensity depending on how hemorrhagic the process is (Fig. 7-21). Contrast-enhanced MR with Magne-vist is sensitive in the detection of small areas of early abscess formation (Fig. 7-22). Patients with AIDS are subject to other diseases, including immunodeficiency lymphomas of the brain. At present, neither MR nor CT is satisfactory in differentiating lymphoma from toxoplasma infection. Their differentiation depends on serologic testing for toxoplasmosis, biopsy, or the response of the brain lesions to treatment (e.g., therapy aimed at the toxoplasma organism).

Subacute encephalitis is another important complication of AIDS infection. Atrophy, perivascular parenchymal collections of macrophages and multinucleated giant cells, diffuse astrocytosis, and perivascular lymphocytic infiltrates are found in the white matter. Present evidence indicates that this is due to a direct infection by the HTLV-III virus of the white matter parenchyma. Both CT and MR show, as the initial finding, minimal atrophy with slight sulcal enlargement and ventriculomegaly. MR may also show the white matter to have a high signal intensity on PDWI and T2WI (Fig. 7-23). MR shows this abnormality where CT usually fails.

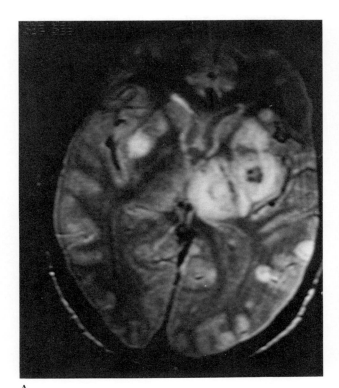

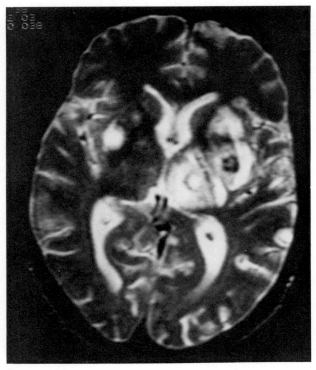

A   B

Figure 7-21   AIDS. Male, 57 years old, with right hemiparesis and seizures. *A*. Axial PDWI shows multiple high signal intensity lesions within the basal ganglia and subcortical white matter (predominantly on the left). Note focal hypointensity within the lesions in the left putamen and thalamus. *B*. Axial T2WI at the same slice location as that shown in *A* shows further hypointensity with the longer time to echo, a finding consistent with deoxyhemoglobin or intracellular methemoglobin. Other high signal intensity lesions are seen, as before. Biopsy-proven toxoplasmosis complicating AIDS.

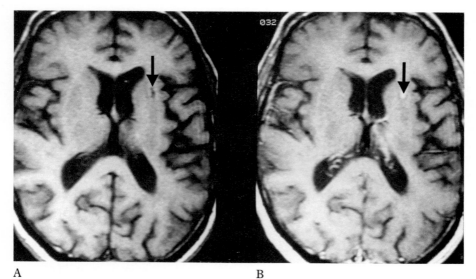

Figure 7-22 AIDS with toxoplasma abscess. Adult male with biopsy-proven toxoplasma abscesses. *A.* T1WI without contrast shows a small hypointensity in the basal ganglia. *B.* Following contrast administration, T1WI shows enhancement at site of toxoplasma abscess.

A   B

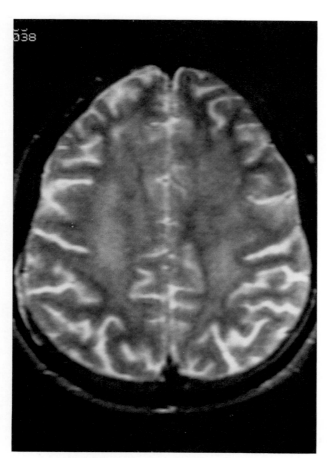

Figure 7-23 AIDS. Demented male, 32 years old, with known AIDS. Axial T2WI shows a diffuse increase in signal intensity throughout the white matter of the centrum semiovale.

Summary

Routine MRI increases the sensitivity of diagnostic imaging in the detection of CNS infections. The use of paramagnetic contrast agents improves this sensitivity in both parenchymal and extracerebral (leptomeningeal) infectious diseases. However, the increased sensitivity is not accompanied by a similar increase in specificity. The imaging findings in many disease states, including those that are infectious and those that are not, may overlap or be identical. Unfortunately, despite the increased sensitivity, at present long scan times and difficulty in monitoring and supporting the patient in the MR environment limit the application of this technology.

References

1. Atlas SW, Grossman RI, Goldberg HI, et al. MR diagnosis of acute disseminated encephalomyelitis. *J Comput Assist Tomogr* 1986; 10:798–801.
2. Atlas SW, Grossman RI, Hackney DB, et al. Calcified intracranial lesions: detection with gradient-echo-acquisition rapid MR imaging. *AJNR* 1988; 9:253–259.
3. Barkovich AJ, Atlas SW. Magnetic resonance imaging of intracranial hemorrhage. *Radiol Clin North Am* 1988; 26:801–820.
4. Dunn V, Bale JF Jr, Zimmerman RA. MRI in children with postinfectious disseminated encephalomyelitis. *Magn Reson Imaging* 1986; 4:25–32.
5. Enzmann DR. *Imaging of Infections and Inflammations of the Central Nervous System: Computed Tomography, Ultrasound, and Nuclear Magnetic Resonance.* New York: Raven Press, 1984:27–79.
6. Enzmann DR, Britt RH, Placone R. Staging of human brain abscess by computed tomography. *Radiology* 1983; 146:703–708.
7. Holland BA, Kucharczyk W, Brant-Zawadzki M, et al. MR imaging of calcified intracranial lesions. *Radiology* 1985; 157:353–356.

8. Leetsma JE. Viral infections of the nervous system. In: Davis RL, Robertson DM (eds.), *Textbook of Neuropathology*. Baltimore: Williams & Wilkins, 1985:704–787.

9. Nowell MA, Hackney DB, Zimmerman RA, et al. Immature brain: spin-echo pulse sequence parameters for high-contrast MR imaging. *Radiology* 1987; 162:272–273.

10. Parker JC Jr, Dyer ML. Neurologic infections due to bacteria, fungi, and parasites. In: Davis RL, Robertson DM (eds.), *Textbook of Neuropathology*. Baltimore: Williams & Wilkins, 1985:632–703.

11. Post MJD, Chan JC, Hensley GT, et al. Toxoplasma encephalitis in Haitian adults with aquired immuno-deficiency syndrome: a clinical-pathologic-CT correlation. *AJNR* 1983; 4:155–162.

12. Post MJD, Hensley GT, Moskowitz LB, et al. Cytomegalic inclusion virus encephalitis in patients with AIDS: CT, clinical and pathologic correlation. *AJNR* 1986; 7:275–280.

13. Ridgway JP, Turnbull LW, Smith MA. Demonstration of pulsatile cerebrospinal-fluid flow using magnetic resonance phase imaging. *Br J Radiol* 1987; 60:423–427.

14. Runge VM, Schoerner W, Niendorf HP, et al. Initial clinical evaluation of gadolinium DTPA for contrast-enhanced magnetic resonance imaging. *Magn Reson Imaging* 1985; 3:27–35.

15. Smith HP, Hendrick EB. Subdural empyema and epidural abscess in children. *J Neurosurg* 1983; 58:392–397.

16. Stehling MJ, Howseman AM, Ordidge RJ, et al. Whole-body echo-planar MR imaging at 0.5T. *Radiology* 1989; 170:257–263.

17. Sze G, Zimmerman RA. The magnetic resonance imaging of infections and inflammatory diseases. *Radiol Clin North Am* 1988; 26:839–859.

18. Whelan MA, Stern J. Intracranial tuberculoma. *Radiology* 1981; 138:75–81.

19. Zimmerman RA, Bilaniuk LT. CT of orbital infection and its cerebral complications. *AJR* 1980; 134:45–50.

20. Zimmerman RA, Bilaniuk LT, Sze G. Intracranial infection. In: Brant-Zawadzki M, Norman D (eds.), *Magnetic Resonance Imaging of the Central Nervous System*. New York: Raven Press, 1987:235–257.

21. Zimmerman RA, Patel S, Bilaniuk LT. Demonstration of purulent bacterial intracranial infections by computed tomography. *AJR* 1976; 127:155–165.

8

Magnetic Resonance Imaging of the Vertebral Column and Spinal Cord

Kenneth D. Miller, Jr.

In recent years, magnetic resonance imaging (MRI) has emerged as a powerful new tool for the diagnostic evaluation of the spine. Imaging in sagittal, coronal, and transverse (axial) planes is easily obtained while the patient lies quietly in a supine position. Whereas CT requires exposure to ionizing radiation and is based on a singular parameter, electron density, MRI is based on several parameters (T1, T2, and proton density) that may be portrayed as different images, providing more information. This chapter studies MRI as applied to imaging of the vertebral column and spinal cord. A variety of pathological entities affecting the spine and spinal cord will be discussed to provide an overview of the current technology.

Surface coils are used for spine imaging, providing superior image quality to examinations obtained by body coil imaging. In our institution we use a marker in the spine surface coil, a test tube containing castor oil, to localize the center of the coil in the sagittal plane. A rapid sagittal localizing scout sequence is obtained using the body coil, patient centering along the spine surface coil thereby noted, and surface coil imaging of the spinal region of interest subsequently begun.

Sagittal imaging sequences are the primary plane of evaluation with magnetic resonance imaging of the spine in contradistinction to computed tomography (CT) with its direct axial images only. Axial MR images of specific levels are obtained to supplement the sagittal images, usually as T1-weighted images. Coronal images are less frequently utilized. It is preferable to obtain oblique axial images that are angled to provide optimal imaging through the intervertebral discs. MR does not have the gantry angulation limitations of CT. A slice thickness of 4 or 5 mm is typically used for spine examinations, although under some circumstances

3-mm slices may be obtained. Commonly, spin echo T1-weighted [short repetition time (TR)/short echo time (TE)] and dual echo T2-weighted sagittal images are obtained for spine imaging. The long TR/short TE first echo images of the dual echo T2-weighted sequence are variably referred to as the spin density, proton density, or balanced images. The long TR/long TE second echo images are referred to as the T2-weighted images (Fig. 8-1).

The higher-field-strength magnet systems such as 1.5 tesla may utilize gradient echo imaging in addition to the conventional spin echo imaging. Gradient echo images may be obtained in much less imaging time than conventional spin echo imaging sequences. Gradient echo images display greater edge enhancement than spin echo images, which may improve spur and disc margin delineation thus providing additional information. Because of bone edge enhancement and white CSF signal, low flip-angle (10 to 15 degrees) oblique axial images are being used to supplement standard spin echo T1-weighted oblique axial images. They may also be used in sagittal sequences at times. It is also possible to generate gradient echo images at other flip angles. Those gradient echo images obtained with angles approaching 90 degrees have a more T1-type image appearance, whereas images obtained with angle flips of 50 to 60 degrees resemble the spin density images. The images obtained with flip-angles of 50 to 60 degrees delineate the lumbar facet joints well and may be used in assessing spinal stenosis. Each type of gradient echo image has some applicability in spine imaging under certain circumstances. Gradient echo images are more motion sensitive and result in greater artifact when metal is present than spin echo images.

Primary and Metastatic Neoplasms of the Vertebral Column

CT examination well demonstrates bone destruction and paraspinal extension of tumor and will show tumoral calcification or ossification. But imaging is limited to relatively short segments of spinal evaluation, with the highest resolution images available only in the axial plane. Reconstructed sagittal or coronal images suffer a significant decrease in image quality. On the other hand, MRI may be utilized in any plane with equally good resolution and no need for reconstructed images of lesser resolution. While cortical bone is seen as a signal void with a black appearance, loss of the dark signal may be utilized for determination of bone involvement by tumor. The marrow within the spinal elements is well imaged by MR and has a characteristic normal appearance. Marrow replacement may be thus utilized to evaluate for tumor involvement of the spine and may be appreciated sooner than on CT. MR images may easily demonstrate tumor extension beyond the osseous confines and may demonstrate paraspinal abnormalities, as well as give information about the status of the spinal cord, spinal canal, and intervertebral discs.

T1-weighted images (short TR/short TE) are most useful in spine evaluation for the presence of tumor. Marrow re-

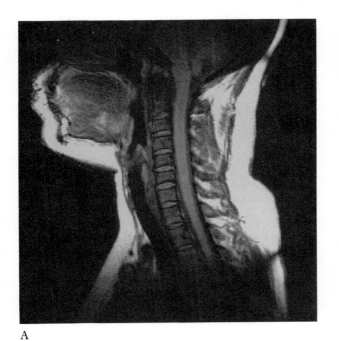

A

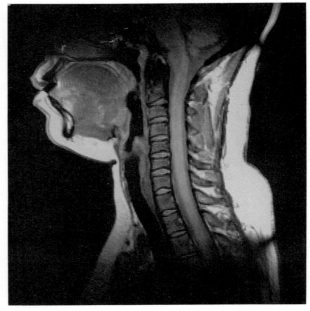

B

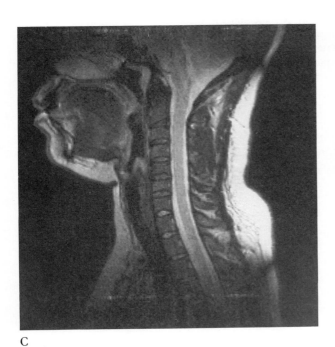

C

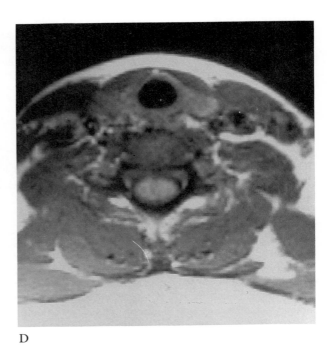

D

Figure 8-1 Normal spin echo MRI examination. *A.* Sagittal T1-weighted image (SE TR 600/TE 25). *B.* Spin density image (SE TR 1600/TE 25). *C.* T2-weighted image (SE TR 1600/TE 90). *D.* Axial T1-weighted image (SE TR 600/TE 25). CSF appears dark on the T1-weighted image, and differentiation between cortical bone and CSF may be difficult. The spin density (proton density, balanced) image allows better delineation between vertebral cortical bone and CSF. The T2-weighted image provides a "myelogram" effect with white, high-signal CSF.

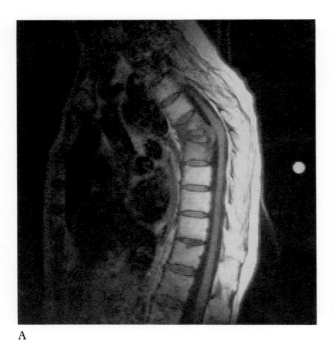

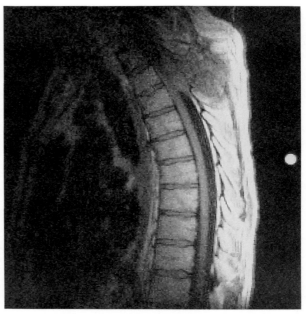

A   B

Figure 8-2 A primary or metastatic tumor involving the spine typically exhibits marrow replacement, which may be seen as an area of decreased signal on T1-weighted images. *A.* Metastatic disease from carcinoma of the breast, with vertebral marrow replacement, compression fractures, and canal impingement (SE TR 500/TE 17). Metastatic involvement of three contiguous vertebral segments can be appreciated. *B.* Upper thoracic primary chondrosarcoma of the posterior elements, with bone involvement, a soft tissue mass, and extension into the spinal canal with spinal cord compression (SE TR 500/TE 25).

placement by tumor, whether primary or metastatic, is typically seen as a decrease in the signal from normal marrow (Fig. 8-2). The T2-weighted images are more variable and may or may not add additional information—the signal from the tumor may increase enough to be dramatically bright, or the signal may increase just enough to become isointense with normal marrow and thus be invisible (Fig. 8-3). For this reason, T1-weighted imaging must always be done. Typically, this is accomplished first in the sagittal plane resulting in the greatest coverage for the single scan sequence. Additionally, the T1-weighted images usually provide the best anatomic detail. Sagittal T2-weighted images are also routinely obtained, even if there are limitations as noted above with some tumors, since we are evaluating symptomatic patients who may or may not have a tumor as the etiology of their symptoms.

Magnetic resonance imaging utilizes multiple image sequences, i.e., spin echo T1-weighted images, spin density (proton density, balanced) images, and T2-weighted images, as well as at times gradient echo images, either low flip-angle T2-type images, larger flip-angle images, or both. Through this compilation of different types of images and different planes of section, the information is gathered. It is from the comparison of such information with normal tissue responses, known patterns of abnormal tissue responses, and altered anatomy that diagnoses begin to evolve.

It has been appreciated that MRI is not very sensitive to the presence of calcium in a lesion, contrary to CT, which is quite sensitive to the presence of calcium. A lesion may contain calcium, and that fact may be completely undetectable with MRI. At other times, a large enough collection of calcification or ossification may be seen as a signal void (black or dark). When seen as a signal void, the darkness of the signal from calcium does not change significantly from the first to the second echo of the dual echo T2 sequence, i.e., it looks about the same on the spin density (proton density, balanced) image as on the T2-weighted image. This is in contrast to the response of hemosiderin deposition within tissue, most commonly seen as a result of remote hemorrhage. Hemosiderin behaves as a paramagnetic substance and becomes much darker in appearance on the T2-weighted image, the second echo image of the T2 sequence (Fig. 8-4). This "blackening" effect with hemosiderin is more dramatic the higher the field strength of the magnet; hence, it is much more readily apparent at 1.5 tesla than at 0.35 or 0.5 tesla.

Another significant advantage of magnetic resonance imaging over CT is the ability to evaluate long segments of the spine on each sagittal sequence. Typically, cervical spine surface coil imaging will include the lower portion of the brain, the base of the skull, the cervical spine with the anterior soft tissues of the neck, and the upper thoracic spine. Thoracic spine imaging will include the conus region and the paraspinal soft tissue. Lumbar spine imaging will extend from the lower thoracic region and conus down through most of the sacrum and will include the prespinal, presacral, and other paraspinal soft tissues. The axial or oblique axial images are used to supplement the sagittal images, as may coronal images. Thus, with sagittal imaging, evaluation of long segments of the spine, even evaluation of the entire spine, becomes feasible, surpassing the limited length of sectional imaging possible with CT. CT, with its ability to show the architectural detail of bone, and with its sensitivity for calcification or ossification, may be utilized supplementally in a specific region where abnormalities have been noted by MR scanning, to help the radiologist to make a more accurate diagnosis.

Metastatic tumors will constitute the largest group of spinal osseous tumors encountered in the ordinary practice. Regardless of tissue type, the lesions tend to be manifested on MRI scans as areas of decreased signal on T1-weighted images due to the replacement of the normal marrow signal. The T2 signal tends to be isointense with, or very little different from, normal marrow. Osteoblastic or calcifying lesions may show decreased signal on both T1- and T2-weighted imaging, but not invariably, because of the intrinsic relative insensitivity of MRI for the presence of calcium. "Wet" tumors having a relatively higher water content may have a brighter T2 signal than normal tissue. This phenome-

non remains true whether the tumor is metastatic or primary.

It has been observed that there is a greater probability of seeing an increased signal on T2 imaging in primary tumors, but the difference in signal characteristics between primary and metastatic lesions is so variable as to not be absolutely reliable for differentiation. The old radiological observation of multiplicity of lesions as indicative of metastatic disease is still more helpful in MRI. Although multiple myeloma and plasmacytoma may show a decreased signal on T1-weighted images and an increased signal on T2-weighted images, we have encountered one case with a signal that was isointense with normal marrow on T1-weighted, spin density, and T2-weighted images.

MRI seems much more sensitive than conventional roentgenograms for the presence of metastatic disease, allows more extensive assessment of the spine with sagittal imaging than axial CT, and provides more anatomic information than radionuclide studies. The presence or absence of multiple segment involvement or contiguous structure extension and the relationship of the tumor to neural structures are easily determined with MRI scanning. MRI may easily delineate the superior and inferior extent of an impinging lesion much easier and quicker and with much less patient discomfort than myelography. The T1-weighted images may demonstrate spinal cord compression, whereas

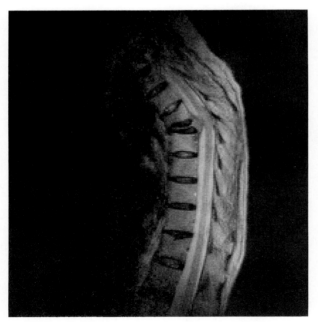
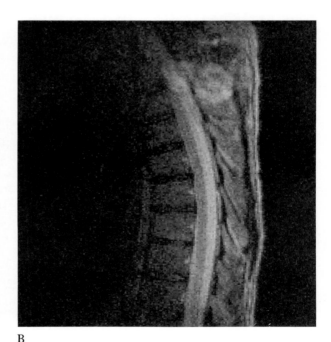

A　　　　　　　　　　　　　　　　　　　　　　　　B

Figure 8-3 T2-weighted imaging of the cases shown in Fig. 8-2. *A.* This demonstrates the potential difficulty a metastatic lesion with an isointense signal on T2-weighted imaging may present (SE TR 1600/TE 120). In the absence of compressive change and mass effect, the lesions could easily be missed because the signal is so similar to that of normal marrow. Even though two abnormal segments with compression are evident, one might consider these compressive changes to be on an osteopenic basis since the marrow signal is so near normal. It is unlikely that the third segment would be considered abnormal when seen only on the T2-weighted image. *B.* An increased signal from the chondrosarcoma is shown (SE TR 1600/TE 120).

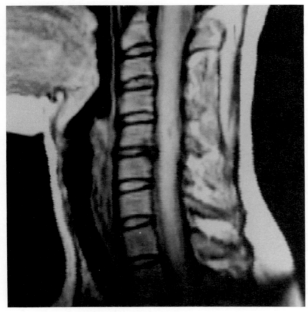

A

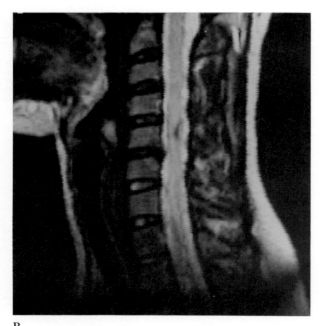

B

Figure 8-4 Cavernous hemangioma of the spinal cord, demonstrating the MRI appearance of hemosiderin deposition as a result of prior hemorrhage. *A*. A lesion within the spinal cord (SE TR 1600/TE 25). Compare the lesion appearance with that in *B* (SE TR 1600/TE 90) and notice the "blackening" effect typical of hemosiderin deposition in the latter image. The patient has hemangiomas in the pons, cervical spinal cord, and thoracic spinal cord.

T2-weighted images best show subarachnoid impingement in the absence of cord impingement.[25]

The cost of an MRI scan compares favorably with myelography followed by CT, especially if the MRI examination is performed on an outpatient basis and myelography followed by CT is done in a hospital setting.[3,25] Furthermore MRI scanning can usually be performed in less time with a definite decrease in patient discomfort compared with the combined myelogram-myelographic CT examinations.[25]

The main disadvantages of MR imaging in tumor patients, as with all patients, include claustrophobia, the inability to bring life support equipment into the scanner room, the incompatability of MRI with the presence of pacemakers or ferromagnetic intracranial aneurysm clips, and patient motion.

Intradural Extramedullary Neoplasms

The ability of MRI to delineate vertebral segments, the spinal canal, the spinal cord, neural foramina and adjacent nerves, and the paraspinal soft tissues has allowed the evaluation of patients for intradural extramedullary neoplasms with ease and precision heretofore unknown. Not only may lesions be delineated anatomically, but the multiparameter imaging (T1, spin density, T2 images) allows a greater degree of tissue typing, thus facilitating the diagnosis of probable tumor type.

Our experience coincides with other reports[5] that neurofibromas and schwannomas typically exhibit an increased signal intensity on T2-weighted images, whether intraspinal, paraspinal, or peripheral in location. On T1-weighted images, they show a signal intensity similar to that of the normal spinal cord.

Meningiomas in the spinal canal show signal characteristics like those of intracranial meningiomas; namely, they are essentially isointense with brain and spinal cord on T1-weighted and T2-weighted imaging and slightly increased in signal intensity on the long TR/short TE spin density images. It is the unusual meningioma that shows increased signal on T2-weighted images. The typical meningioma exhibits no increased signal on T2-weighted images in contradistinction to the typical neurofibroma (Fig. 8-5).

Small lesions such as small drop metastases may not be seen with conventional MR imaging, but investigative work with gadolinium diethylenetriamine pentaacetic acid (gadolinium-DTPA) has been encouraging. Lesions of 2 or 3 mm in diameter have been reported as being apparent with imaging utilizing gadolinium-DTPA when they were not seen on initial imaging, their enhancement occurring as a result of this intravenous MRI contrast agent.[26]

Intrinsic Neoplasms of the Spinal Cord

MRI allows evaluation of the spinal cord for intrinsic lesions, including primary tumors such as ependymomas and astrocytomas, as well as metastatic lesions. It allows differ-

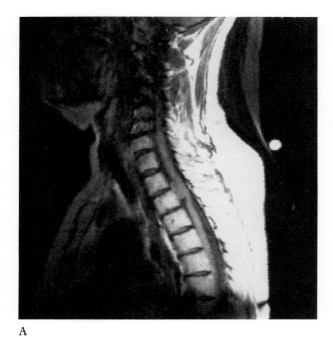

A

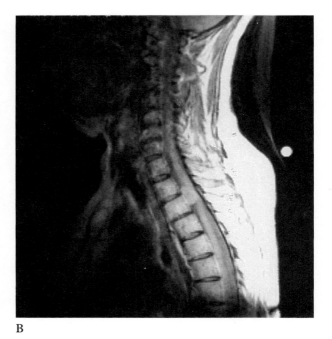

B

Figure 8-5 Thoracic meningioma. The three images demonstrate an upper thoracic intradural extramedullary mass. *A*. The mass is shown to be almost isointense with the spinal cord (SE TR 600/TE 25). In *B* (SE TR 1600/TE 25) the mass shows an increased signal, whereas in *C* (SE TR 1600/TE 90) the lesion appears isointense with the spinal cord. This pattern of tumor response (isointense on T1-weighted imaging, increased signal on spin density imaging, and isointense on T2-weighted imaging) is the common pattern of meningiomas. An increased signal on T2-weighted imaging (long TR/long TE) is uncommon with meningiomas and would favor some other type of tumor.

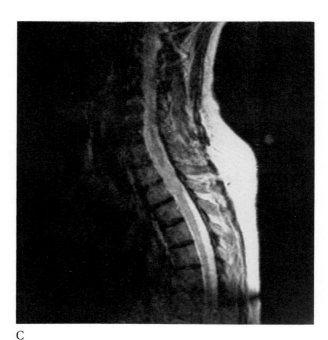

C

entiation of intrinsic tumors from cysts, syringomyelia, or hydromyelia. Intramedullary tumors ordinarily cannot be differentiated from one another as to cell type[6] but are seen as lesions with poorly defined margins, signal inhomogeneity, and lack of isointensity with CSF. This appearance is contrasted with that of syringomyelia and hydromyelia, which tend to exhibit distinct margins, uniform signal intensity, and isointensity with CSF (Fig. 8-6).[27] In difficult cases and to aid in determination of an optimal biopsy site, investigative work with gadolinium-DTPA has shown this MR contrast agent to be of considerable benefit. The tumor will enhance following the intravenous administration of the gadolinium-DTPA, whereas syringomyelia or hydromyelia will not. Additionally, the tumor associated with a syrinx or cyst may be more easily defined utilizing this contrast agent.[24]

Disc Disease, Spondylosis, and Spinal Stenosis

Magnetic resonance imaging with surface coil technology demonstrates the structural anatomy of the spine and pathologic changes unlike any other available imaging modality. The intervertebral discs are easily evaluated for internal de-

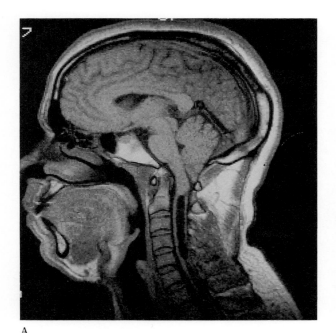

A

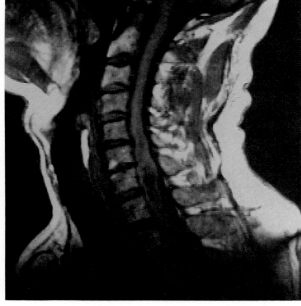

B

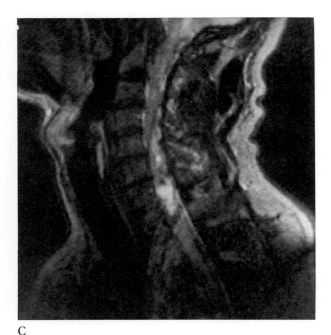

C

Figure 8-6 Comparison of a spinal cord tumor with a syrinx. *A.* A cervical syrinx with an associated Arnold-Chiari malformation (SE TR 500/TE17). The lesion within the spinal cord is well demarcated, homogeneous, and isointense with CSF. Compare this with *B* (SE TR 600/TE 25) and *C* (SE TR 1600/TE 120), which demonstrate a spinal cord tumor which is less distinctly delineated, inhomogeneous, and not isointense with CSF.

generative changes noninvasively with T2-weighted images. Disc contour changes may be assessed easily in various planes with no loss of resolution. Neural structures and soft tissue structures are well delineated in detail that is superior to that of other imaging modalities without the need for contrast material, and osseous structures are depicted in a manner different from that of previously existing imaging techniques. Because of these observations, MRI has proved helpful in the evaluation of intervertebral disc disease, spondylosis, and spinal stenosis. Additionally, MRI provides a

noninvasive tool for the evaluation of the postoperative patient with continued or recurrent symptoms.

T2-weighted imaging (long TR/long TE) results in a bright signal intensity from the central portion of the normal intervertebral disc, whereas the periphery shows a lower signal intensity (Fig. 8-1). Work by Pech and Haughton correlating MR images and anatomic specimens showed the area of increased signal to represent a combination of the nucleus pulposus and the inner portion of the anulus fibrosus, whereas the area of peripheral lower signal coincided with the more collagenous portion of the anulus containing Sharpey's fibers.[20] Usually a thin, low signal linear structure paralleling the vertebral end plates is evident centrally within the higher signal central portion of the disc, but no precisely correlating structure is revealed in anatomic sections.[20] This line has been referred to as the intranuclear cleft.[18] Since it is commonly seen, it apparently represents an MR-sensitive structural variation within the nucleus or an artifact.

The increased signal from the central portion of the disc is a result of higher water content. With aging and degeneration, the water content of the nucleus decreases and it changes to a dessicated fibrous mass, the water loss accompanied by an altered collagen and noncollagenous protein content.[18] The ratio of keratin sulfate to chondroitin sulfate increases, extractability increases, aggregation decreases, and the proteoglycan content decreases.[13,14] During the normal aging process and in specimens of disc herniations (which consistently show biochemical and physiologic changes compatible with premature aging) there is an alteration of the matrix due to the loss of the gelatinous component of the nucleus which is manifested as a progressive change of the disc to fibrocartilage with a loss in the distinction between the anulus and the nucleus as well as a decrease in water content.[18] This results in a loss of signal within the central portion of the disc on T2-weighted imaging.

In addition to allowing the detection of disc degeneration, MRI allows the determination of disc herniation. In herniation with a normal nucleus pulposus, the high signal material of the nucleus may be seen extending peripherally beyond its normal confines as well as producing a focal bulging of the disc margin contour. The degenerative disc with decreased signal from the nucleus may correspondingly exhibit a less intense T2 signal from the protruding component. The herniating nuclear material is seen to be connected to the parent nucleus by a variably thick pedicle of nuclear material (Fig. 8-7). Sequestered (free-fragment) herniations have been described as showing a somewhat higher signal intensity than the degenerated parent nucleus as well as extending superiorly or inferiorly in their posterior or posterolateral extension from the disc space. The sequestered herniation has no pedicle contiguous with the nucleus of the parent intervertebral disc (Fig. 8-8).[16]

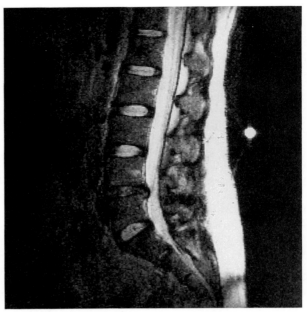

Figure 8-7 Lumbar disc herniation. This image (SE TR 1600/TE 90) demonstrates a decreased signal from the central portion of the L4-5 intervertebral disc, indicating degeneration. There is nuclear herniation with localized disc material extension beyond the vertebral margins. The herniating disc material is continuous with the parent nucleus.

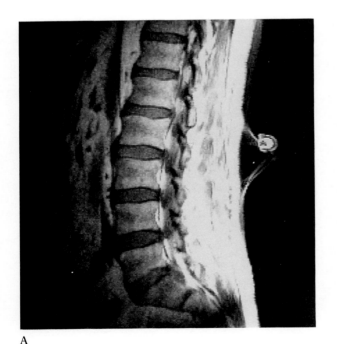

A

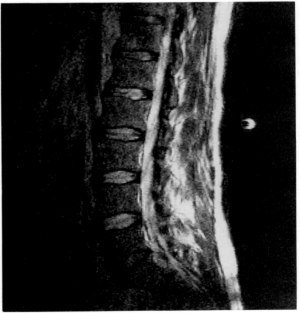

B

Figure 8-8 Sequestered disc herniation. *A*. The herniated disc material at L5-S1 is shown extending downward below the level of the intervertebral disc, behind the S1 vertebral body (SE TR 600/TE 25). *B*. This image (SE TR 1600/TE 90) demonstrates the increased signal of the herniated material. There is no apparent continuity between the herniated nuclear material and the parent nucleus.

Degenerative disc disease may also result in changes in the vertebral bodies. In addition to marginal osteophytic spur formation, MR signal changes have been observed adjacent to the vertebral end plates and are of two types.[19] Type 1 changes show decreased signal intensity on T1-weighted spin echo images and increased signal intensity on T2-weighted images. Histopathologic sections show disruption and fissuring of the end plates and vascularized fibrous tissue. Type 2 changes show increased signal intensity on T1-weighted images and isointense or slightly increased signal intensity on T2-weighted images. These changes are seen to represent yellow (fatty) marrow replacement on histopathologic sections.

Conventional spinal MRI evaluation utilizes a spine surface coil and imaging in the sagittal plane with axial or oblique axial images at appropriate levels. Coronal imaging is often utilized for scout localization images but is not routinely used in imaging. Typically, spin echo sagittal T1-weighted and dual echo T2-weighted (long TR with both short TE and long TE images) scanning sequences are obtained, extending from the parasagittal region beyond the facet joints on one side to the same region on the opposite side. T1-weighted images are commonly utilized for axial imaging. The differentiation of bony spur and disc material may be aided by the additional use of gradient echo images.[10] Gradient echo sequences provide some edge enhancement and show bone as a low signal (dark), which aids in the delineation of bone margins including osteophytic spurs. Disc material exhibits a high signal (bright) with gradient echo imaging, whether it is a normal or degenerated disc. This gradient echo phenomenon of bright disc material and distinct dark spurs may be utilized for the evaluation of whether herniated disc material extends beyond the vertebral body marginal spurs, which seems to be particularly helpful in the cervical region (Fig. 8-9).

The excellent soft tissue contrast associated with MRI allows delineation of paraspinal soft tissues, identification of nerve roots in the foramina and their proximity to adjacent vertebral spurs as well as disc bulges or herniations, delineation of the ligamentum flavum and midline posterior epidural fat, and demonstration of the spinal cord and CSF compartment. With the use of various scanning techniques, the relationship of bone spurs and disc bulges or herniations to the spinal cord, thecal sac, and nerve roots may be evaluated. Cervical spondylosis with canal and foraminal encroachment may be easily demonstrated with sagittal and axial MRI. Not only are bone changes and relationships shown but their relationships to neural elements and associated changes in soft tissue structures are depicted (Fig. 8-10). Likewise, lumbar spinal stenosis may be evaluated with MRI without the ionizing radiation and multiple axial images required for reconstructed sagittal CT images; there is no loss of resolution in the sagittal plane nor is intrathecal contrast material needed.

CT demonstrates bone detail in one way and MRI examinations demonstrate bone detail in another. Cortical bone is seen as a black structure, but marrow shows a signal and MRI allows the recognition of changes in the bone marrow associated with degenerative change. MRI may also be used to advantage in recognizing changes in the facet joints including the articular cartilage and changes in the surround-

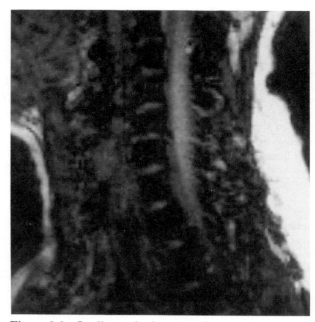

Figure 8-9 Gradient echo imaging of a vertebral spur. The patient exhibited a radiculopathy in the right C6 nerve root distribution. At C5-6 no disc herniation is delineated, but a large lateral osteophytic spur with associated bulging disc material is seen on this sagittal 90-degree flip-angle T1 gradient echo image (FLASH TR 600/TE 37). There is no evidence of disc herniation beyond the spur. The spur is seen to have a black bone effect, whereas the disc material shows a higher signal and may be differentiated from bone, CSF, and other soft tissue.

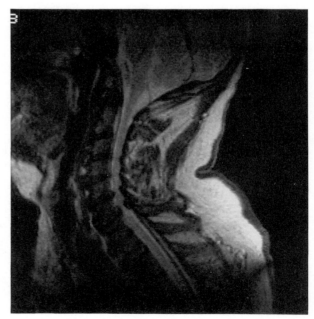

Figure 8-10 Cervical spondylosis. A sagittal image (SE TR 1600/TE 90) shows bone and soft tissue proliferation at C5-6 and C6-7, significantly narrowing the spinal canal and impinging upon the spinal cord.

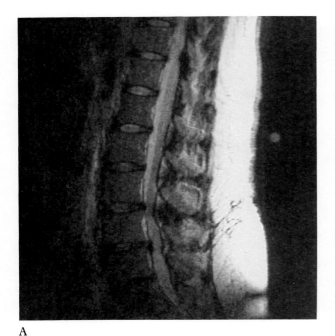

A

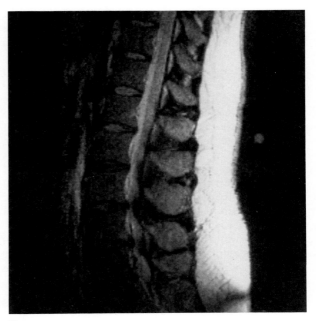

B

Figure 8-11 Lumbar spinal stenosis. Midline (*A*) and parasagittal (*B*) images (SE TR 1600/TE 90) demonstrate posterior and posterolateral spinal canal impingement by bone and soft tissue proliferation with a lesser degree of anterior element degenerative change. *C*. This image (SE TR 700/TE 25) shows the triangular-shaped narrowed spinal canal configuration with hypertrophy of the articular facets and ligamentum flavum.

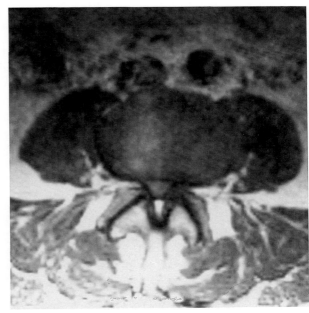

C

ing soft tissues, particularly the ligamentum flavum and displacement of the posterior epidural fat as seen with facet joint and ligamentum flavum hypertrophy. The more T2-weighted images aid in the assessment of the effect of central stenosis on the thecal sac, the CSF being imaged as white without the need for intrathecal contrast material. Sagittal images aid in depiction of the level or levels of posterior abnormalities, measurement of the sagittal diameter of the spinal canal, and evaluation of foraminal stenosis. Axial images allow more precise analysis of the facet joints for osteophyte formation and changes in the articular cartilage, measurement of ligamentum flavum thickening, and measurement of the transverse diameter of the spinal canal (Fig. 8-11).[8]

Recent articles have evaluated the use of magnetic resonance imaging in the postoperative patient. Patients who have undergone anterior discectomy and fusion or corpectomy of the cervical spine may develop canal stenosis or additional disc herniations above or below the fused level.[21] The extensive soft tissue changes seen in the first 10 days after surgery limit the usefulness of MRI in the early evaluation of persistent or new symptoms, with the exception of detecting hemorrhage, which has distinctive signal characteristics.[22]

Arachnoiditis may be detected by MRI and has been described as showing three patterns. Group 1 shows conglomerations of adherent nerve roots residing centrally within the thecal sac; group 2 demonstrates nerve roots adherent to the meninges peripherally, giving the appearance of an empty thecal sac; and group 3 exhibits a soft tissue mass replacing the subarachnoid space.[23]

In evaluating the patient with epidural fibrosis from prior disc surgery who presents with persistent or recurrent symptoms, several observations may be made.[4] Anterior and lateral recess scars appear hypo- or isointense with the anulus intensity on T1-weighted sequences and hyperintense on more T2-weighted sequences. Free fragments demonstrate a slightly hyperintense signal intensity on T1-weighted images relative to epidural fibrosis but have a hyperintense signal intensity on T2-weighted imaging similar to epidural fibrosis. Herniated discs are hypo- or isointense relative to the anulus on all imaging sequences.

Sagittal images may be of help in the differentiation of scar tissue alone from a combination of nuclear herniation and scar tissue in the postoperative patient. Scar tissue is more difficult to identify on sagittal images than on axial images. Also, scar tissue margins are less distinct on sagittal imaging than is recurrent disc herniation. Herniated disc material typically shows contiguity with the parent nucleus and is outlined by a dark margin (Fig. 8-12).

Research with gadolinium-DTPA has indicated its usefulness in the differentiation of scar tissue alone and disc herniation within an area of scar formation. Scar tissue shows heterogeneous enhancement on T1-weighted images, whereas herniated disc material shows no enhancement. Imaging must be performed promptly after injection, preferably within 10 minutes, because disc material may show variable degrees of enhancement on delayed images done 30 minutes or more after injection.[11]

Magnetic resonance imaging of the spine appears to be an effective diagnostic tool for the evaluation of disc disease, spondylosis, and spinal stenosis. It seems to be a practical alternative to myelography and postmyelographic CT scanning, providing more information than nonenhanced CT scanning and more or at least comparable information to myelography and postmyelographic CT scanning. Certainly, it provides anatomic and pathologic information in a much less interventional manner with greater patient comfort than myelography and postmyelographic CT scanning, usually in less time and at a competitive price. MRI is emerging as the procedure of choice for the initial evaluation of the spine after conventional radiography.

Disc Space Infection, Vertebral Osteomyelitis, and Spinal Epidural Sepsis

MRI of the spine with surface coil technique provides a sensitive and accurate diagnostic tool for the evaluation of disc space infection, vertebral osteomyelitis, and spinal epidural sepsis. Vertebral osteomyelitis with disc space infection has a characteristic MRI appearance. T1-weighted images (short TR/short TE) show decreased signal intensity from the vertebral body marrow and intervertebral disc space, with indistinct vertebral end plates on either side of the involved disc. T2-weighted images (long TR/long TE) demonstrate increased signal intensity from the same marrow regions and from the intervertebral disc space. The area of increased signal within the disc space may extend beyond the posterior disc margin (Fig. 8-13).

The signal intensity changes of the marrow and disc space are due to an increase in water content as a result of

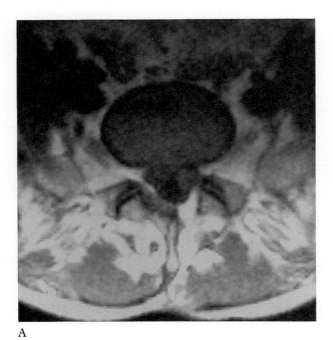

A

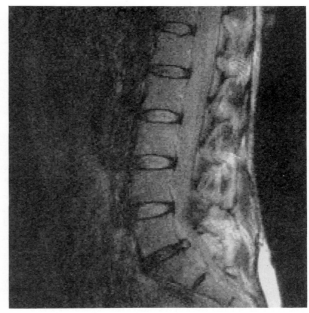

B

Figure 8-12 Recurrent disc herniation. *A.* This axial image (SE TR 240/TE 25) shows bilateral anterior rounded masses of intermediate signal within the spinal canal, with a laminectomy defect posteriorly on the left. *B.* Sagittal imaging (SE TR 900/TE 90) delineates a lesion that is contiguous with the parent disc and exhibits a dark peripheral margin. This represents a recurrent disc herniation.

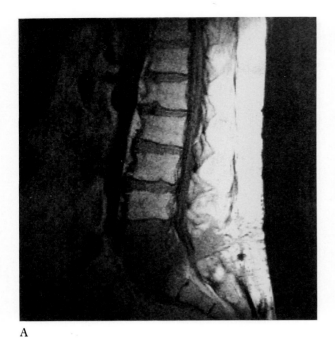
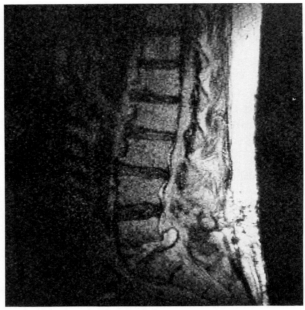

A   B

Figure 8-13 Lumbar discitis. *A.* This sagittal image (SE TR 500/TE 17) shows a decreased marrow signal of the L4 and L5 vertebral bodies with indistinct vertebral end plates and surrounding soft tissue changes. *B.* This image (SE TR 1600/TE 120) shows and increased signal from the L5-S1 intervertebral disc space that extends into the spinal canal.

the inflammatory response associated with the infection. An exudate containing polymorphonuclear leukocytes and fibrin as well as local vascular ischemia with associated edema occur within the marrow. The intramedullary pressure may increase and, combined with the ischemia, bacterial products and enzymes discharged from disintegrating leukocytes may result in bone destruction. Changes in the vertebral end plate and spread of the infection occur.[12,17]

The changes of vertebral osteomyelitis are apparent with MRI at about the same time that radionuclide scans become positive, appearing earlier than changes on conventional roentgenograms.[17] MRI provides more specific anatomic information regarding the level of involvement, the relationship of the osteomyelitis to the thecal sac and neural elements, and the existence of epidural or paraspinal extension of the infectious process. Differentiation between infection with vertebral body and disc space involvement and degenerative disease or neoplastic disease is more easily made with MRI than with radionuclide scans or conventional roentgenograms. The decreased signal intensity on T1-weighted images and increased signal intensity on T2-weighted images of the intervertebral disc space and adjacent vertebral body marrow with more indistinct vertebral end plates appears to be specific for osteomyelitis with disc space infection. Disc space involvement with an abnormal increased signal is not associated with a neoplasm or degenerative disease; a degenerated disc shows a decreased signal on T2-weighted imaging, and a neoplasm tends to spare the disc.

Epidural space infection may occur as a result of extension from adjacent osteomyelitis or discitis; following spinal puncture, a penetrating injury, surgery, or chemonucleolysis; or as a result of hematogenous spread from a remote septic focus in the skin or urinary tract, dental and periodontal disease, intravenous drug abuse, or septicemia. MRI allows demonstration of the infection and the extent and degree of epidural involvement as well as the compressive effect on the adjacent dural sac and underlying spinal cord. T2-weighted images may differentiate the various components of the inflammatory process. An abcess cavity may be seen as a discrete area of markedly increased signal intensity, whereas surrounding inflammatory edema and granulation tissue are depicted as nondiscrete areas of mildly increased signal intensity.[2]

Imaging is typically performed in sagittal and axial planes, with occasional coronal imaging. As noted elsewhere in the chapter, MRI in the sagittal plane with various scanning parameters may provide information about the nature and extent of lesions that is equal to or greater than the information provided by CT scanning. It does not require the instillation of intrathecal contrast material, gives better resolution than sagittal reconstructed CT, utilizes no ionizing radiation, and is competitive costwise to combined myelography and CT scanning. As regards epidural abcesses, Angtuaco et al. noted MR findings were conclusive enough to obviate myelography.[2] Modic et al. found MRI to have a sensitivity of 96 percent, specificity of 92 percent, and accuracy of 94 percent for vertebral osteomyelitis with discitis.[17]

Magnetic resonance imaging provides a superior imaging modality for the diagnosis and anatomic localization of infections involving the spine and their differentiation from other processes. The information may be obtained relatively quickly and at one session in a noninvasive manner.

Tethered Cord Syndrome, Lipomeningocele, Myelomeningocele, and Diastematomyelia

In the evaluation of the individual, usually a child, with suspected spinal dysraphism, prior to the availability of MRI, conventional roentgenograms were followed by myelography and postmyelographic CT scanning. Intrathecal contrast must be instilled and ionizing radiation utilized for both myelography and CT scanning. CT requires the acquisition of multiple axial images and suffers from image resolution degradation when coronal or sagittal reconstruction images are produced. As noted earlier in the chapter, MRI has none of the limitations of resolution degradation in non-axial planes, requires no contrast, involves no discomfort, utilizes no ionizing radiation, and is cost competitive with combined myelography and postmyelographic CT scanning.

MRI has been advocated as the procedure of choice for evaluating children with suspected spinal dysraphism.[1] Thin section (3- to 4-mm) T1-weighted images may be obtained fairly quickly in sagittal, coronal, and axial planes. T2-weighted images or gradient echo T2-type images may also be obtained, usually in the sagittal plane. In our institution, the children are sedated and small children are usually examined using the head coil. Larger individuals may be examined using the spine coil (Fig. 8-14). Because of the possibility of an associated Arnold-Chiari malformation, imaging of the foramen magnum region should be considered, usually by means of a sagittal T1-weighted sequence.

Magnetic resonance imaging has the ability to differentiate fat from other tissues, making it easy to identify intrathecal lipomas that may be associated with the tethered cord syndrome and just as easy to exclude with certainty that there is no associated lipoma. The determination of the presence or absence of tethering may be made with a high confidence level. Likewise, when evaluating meningocele, myelomeningocele, and lipomeningocele, the superior soft tissue contrast and resulting detail are very helpful. Meningocele and myelomeningocele may be differentiated by assessment of the fluid and solid components and correlation with the other components that are delineated. A suspected lipomeningocele may be easily confirmed by MRI; fat has a characteristic appearance and response set on the various imaging parameters that allows its identification with certainty and the determination of its absence as a significant component with equal confidence. The tissue discrimination and detail combined with multiplanar imaging capability make MRI a very useful imaging modality for evaluating the individual with spinal dysraphism. Bone, neural elements, CSF, fat, muscle, fibrous tissue, vascular structures, proteinaceous fluid, and any hemorrhagic blood products may

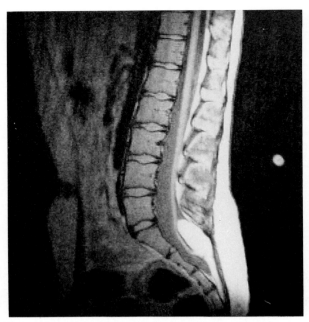

Figure 8-14 Tethered spinal cord with associated intra-spinal lipoma. This sagittal image (SE TR 1600/TE 35) delineates the tethering of the spinal cord and confirms the presence of an associated lipoma within the spinal canal.

be demonstrated and discriminated by MRI. Associated anomalies such as syringomyelia, hydromyelia, and the Arnold-Chiari malformation are easily identified.

In the case of diastematomyelia, magnetic resonance imaging in the coronal plane may easily demonstrate the divided cord, delineating the level and extent of the division consistently on a few images as compared with the numerous axial sections needed with postmyelographic CT scanning (Fig. 8-15).[9] Differentiation between a small bony spicule, a fibrocartilaginous septum, and normal extramedullary structures may prove difficult or impossible with MRI unless the bony septum is large enough to contain fatty marrow centrally.[9] As noted before, associated anomalies may be easily delineated by MRI.

Although myelography may prove necessary in some cases when vulnerable nerve roots are in the proposed surgical field, MRI provides an easy, reliable, informative examination for evaluation of the patient with known spinal dysraphism and for screening of the patient with suspected spinal dysraphism and may provide all the needed imaging information. The procedure may be accomplished in a single session on an outpatient basis, utilizing sedation rather than general anesthesia as is commonly used with myelography and postmyelographic CT scanning. The facts that this is an outpatient procedure without the costs of hospitalization, that no intervention, ionizing radiation, or contrast material are involved, that general anesthesia is not required, and that high resolution multiplanar imaging is possible, make MRI very cost-effective and very appealing as the modern procedure of choice for the evaluation of spinal dysraphism.

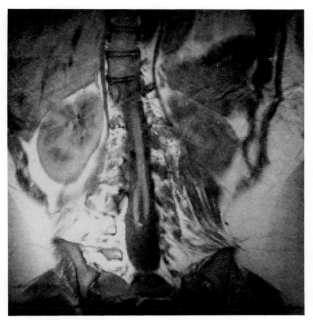

Figure 8-15 Diastematomyelia. This coronal image (SE TR 600/TE 25) shows the split in the low-lying terminal spinal cord.

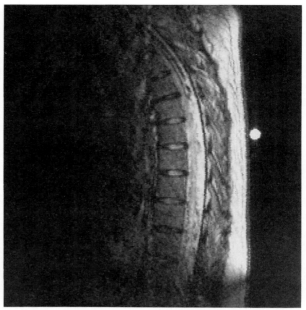

Figure 8-16 Radiculomeningeal spinal vascular malformation. This sagittal image (SE TR 1600/TE 90) shows dark flow voids of vascular structures within the spinal canal about the spinal cord.

Vascular Malformations of the Spine

The ability of MRI to image vascular structures (as flow voids), subacute and chronic blood collections, and hemosiderin deposition in tissue makes the application of MR imaging to the investigation of vascular malformations involving the spine a worthwhile utilization of the diagnostic modality. MRI has demonstrated its superior ability to detect vascular malformations in the brain. Spinal vascular malformations are usually seen as either radiculomeningeal malformations or cavernous hemangiomas of the spinal cord.

Radiculomeningeal-type spinal vascular malformations are now believed to be the most common form of spinal vascular malformation. They are seen best on T2-weighted imaging, presenting as serpentine flow void areas of vascular low signal around the cord (Fig. 8-16).[15] Cavernous hemangiomas of the spinal cord are seen as mixed signal focal lesions, the mixed high (bright) and low (dark) signal intensity indicating the presence of subacute and chronic hemorrhage and a hemosiderin effect with progresseve blackening from first to second echo images of the T2 sequence as noted earlier in the chapter (darker on the long TR/long TE T2-weighted image than on the long TR/short TE spin density image) (Fig. 8-14). Furthermore, cavernous hemangiomas tend not to enlarge the spinal cord, in contradistinction to spinal intramedullary tumors, and tumors usually lack the mixed hemorrhagic signal.[7]

More extensive spinal vascular malformations may also be easily studied by MRI. The vessels may be seen as low signal flow voids. Extensive lesions may show abnormal vessels in the paraspinal soft tissues as well as within the spinal canal. Magnetic resonance imaging may also be used to follow the larger vascular lesions, which may be particularly helpful following therapy.

Magnetic resonance imaging seems well suited for evaluating the patient with a suspected vascular malformation of the spine and may be relied upon to be a sensitive screening tool. Although MRI does not replace spinal arteriography for the determination of the specific supplying arteries of a vascular malformation within the canal, it should be more sensitive than arteriography for the cavernous hemangiomas within the cord, as has been noted to be the case with cavernous hemangiomas in the brain.

References

1. Altman NR, Altman DH. MR imaging of spinal dysraphism. *AJNR* 1987; 8:533–538.
2. Angtuaco EJC, McConnell JR, Chadduck WM, et al. MR imaging of spinal epidural sepsis. *AJR* 1987; 149:1249–1253.
3. Beltran J, Noto AM, Chakeres DW, et al. Tumors of the osseous spine: staging with MR imaging versus CT. *Radiology* 1987; 162:565–569.
4. Bundschuh CV, Modic MT, Ross JS, et al. Epidural fibrosis and recurrent disc herniation in the lumbar spine: MR imaging assessment. *AJR* 1988; 150:923–932.

5. Burk DL Jr, Brunberg JA, Kanal E, et al. Spinal and paraspinal neurofibromatosis: surface coil MR imaging at 1.5T. *Radiology* 1987; 162:797–801.

6. Di Chiro G, Doppman JL, Dwyer AJ, et al. Tumors and arteriovenous malformations of the spinal cord: assessment using MR. *Radiology* 1985; 156:689–697.

7. Fontaine S, Melanson D, Cosgrove R, et al. Cavernous hemangiomas of the spinal cord: MR imaging. *Radiology* 1988; 166:839–841.

8. Grenier N, Kressel HY, Schiebler ML, et al. Normal and degenerative posterior spinal structures: MR imaging. *Radiology* 1987; 165:517–525.

9. Han JS, Benson JE, Kaufman B, et al. Demonstration of diastematomyelia and associated abnormalities with MR imaging. *AJNR* 1985; 6:215–219.

10. Hedberg MC, Drayer BP, Flom RA, et al. Gradient echo (GRASS) MR imaging in cervical radiculopathy. *AJR* 1988; 150:683–689.

11. Hueftle MG, Modic MT, Ross JS, et al. Lumbar spine: postoperative MR imaging with Gd-DTPA. *Radiology* 1988; 167:817–824.

12. Kahn DS, Pritzker KPH. The pathophysiology of bone infection. *Clin Orthop* 1973; 96:12–19.

13. Lipson SJ, Muir H. Experimental intervertebral disc degeneration: morphologic and proteoglycan changes over time. *Arthritis Rheum* 1981; 24:12–21.

14. Lipson SJ, Muir H. Proteoglycans in experimental intervertebral disc degeneration. *Spine* 1981; 6:194–210.

15. Masaryk TJ, Ross JS, Modic MT, et al. Radiculomeningeal vascular malformations of the spine: MR imaging. *Radiology* 1987; 164:845–849.

16. Masaryk TJ, Ross JS, Modic MT, et al. High-resolution MR imaging of sequestered lumbar intervertebral disks. *AJR* 1988; 150:1155–1162.

17. Modic MT, Feiglin DH, Piraino DW. Vertebral osteomyelitis: assessment using MR. *Radiology* 1985; 157:157–166.

18. Modic MT, Pavlicek W, Weinstein MA, et al. Magnetic resonance imaging of intervertebral disk disease. *Radiology* 1984; 152:103–111.

19. Modic MT, Steinberg PM, Ross JS, et al. Degenerative disk disease; assessment of changes in vertebral body marrow with MR imaging. *Radiology* 1988; 166:193–199.

20. Pech P, Haughton VM. Lumbar intervertebral disk: correlative MR and anatomic study. *Radiology* 1985; 156:699–701.

21. Ross JS, Masaryk TJ, Modic MT. Postoperative cervical spine: MR assessment. *J Comput Assist Tomogr* 1987; 11:955–962.

22. Ross JS, Masaryk TJ, Modic MT, et al. Lumbar spine: postoperative assessment with surface-coil MR imaging. *Radiology* 1987; 164:851–860.

23. Ross JS, Masaryk TJ, Modic MT, et al. MR imaging of lumbar arachnoiditis. *AJR* 1987; 149:1025–1032.

24. Slasky BS, Bydder GM, Niendorf HP, et al. MR imaging with gadolinium-DTPA in the differentiation of tumor, syrinx, and cyst of the spinal cord. *J Comput Assist Tomogr* 1987; 11:845–850.

25. Smoker WRK, Godersky JC, Knutzon RK, et al. The role of MR imaging in evaluating metastatic spinal disease. *AJR* 1987; 149:1241–1248.

26. Sze G, Abramson A, Krol G, et al. Gadolinium-DTPA in the evaluation of intradural extramedullary spinal disease. *AJR* 1988; 150:911–921.

27. Williams AL, Haughton VM, Pojuntas KW, et al. Differentiation of intramedullary neoplasms and cysts by MR. *AJR* 1987; 149:159–164.

9

Transcranial Doppler Ultrasonography

David W. Newell
Rune Aaslid
H. Richard Winn

History

In 1959, Satomura first reported the use of Doppler ultrasound to measure flowing blood, initially investigating the peripheral vessels.[25] Since that time, the technology has undergone significant development and refinement. Presently Doppler ultrasonography is extensively used in the evaluation of extracranial vascular disease in combination with echo imaging (duplex scanning).

In 1982, Aaslid et al. reported the ability to record flow velocities in the basal cerebral arteries using Doppler ultrasound and introduced transcranial Doppler (TCD) ultrasonography.[5] This was made possible by utilizing an optimized 2-MHz pulsed range-gated system. With the ability to record flow velocities directly from the intracranial arteries, a new dimension was added to the abilities of Doppler ultrasonography. These developments have made possible the noninvasive evaluation of intracranial stenosis due to atherosclerosis and vasospasm and have also allowed the detection of hemodynamic changes due to a variety of disorders such as extracranial occlusive disease, head injury, intracranial hemorrhage, and conditions causing increased intracranial pressure.

Principles and Equipment

Christian Doppler, an Austrian physicist, described the Doppler effect in 1843 to explain certain astronomical observations. Briefly stated, the Doppler effect describes a shift in the frequency of a wave when either the transmitter of the wave or the receiver of the wave is moving with respect to the wave-propagating medium. Therefore, sound emanating from or reflected by an object moving toward the observer will have a higher frequency in proportion to the speed of the moving object. Conversely, sound emanating from an object moving away from an observer will have a lower frequency in proportion to the speed of the moving object. When using ultrasound to measure the velocity of flowing blood, the ultrasound is emitted by a probe, reflected off the moving blood cells, and the signal is received by the same probe. The shift in the frequency of the reflected ultrasound will be proportional to the velocity of the flowing blood, thus, blood flowing toward or away from the probe will reflect the ultrasound at a higher or lower frequency, respectively.

Doppler ultrasound is well established as a clinical tool to examine the extracranial arteries. Methods have been established using both continuous-wave Doppler and pulsed Doppler employing ultrasonic frequencies between 3 and 10 MHz. Continuous-wave Doppler constantly transmits an ultrasonic beam from a crystal source and simultaneously receives the reflected ultrasound. The receiver records the changes in frequency of the reflected ultrasound produced by moving blood throughout the path of the ultrasonic beam. Pulsed Doppler sends bursts of ultrasound at a regular interval, which is called a pulse repetition frequency. The receiver employs an electronic gate to sample the reflected pulses at certain intervals. Specifically, the gate opens at the time interval required for the ultrasound to be transmitted to and reflected back from a preselected depth. In this way pulsed Doppler is able to record from a specific sample volume at preselected targets.

Transcranial Doppler employs this pulsed range-gated design, which enables sampling of flow velocities at specific sites in and around the circle of Willis, where there is a high concentration of vessels. A 2-MHz ultrasonic frequency is used because this allows penetration through the thin portions of the temporal bone (Fig. 9-1). Studies on ultrasound transmission through the human skull have shown that transmission of up to 35 percent of the power can be achieved through the temporal bone. The diploe has a pro-

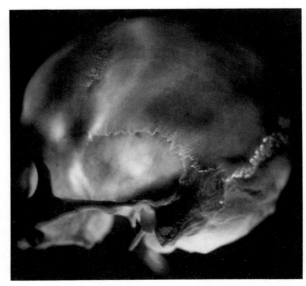

Figure 9-1 Transillumination of the skull illustrates the thin portions of the temporal bone where ultrasound can penetrate.

119

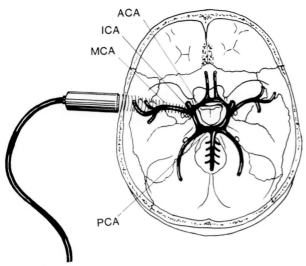

Figure 9-2 Recording from the middle cerebral artery through the transtemporal route. Signals can also be obtained from the ICA, ACA, and proximal PCA through this route.

found effect in scattering the ultrasound due to the bone spicules present. In the thin areas of the temporal bone, the inner and outer layers fuse with no diploe present, thus minimizing the absorption of ultrasound energy.

Three examination routes are available for obtaining signals from the intracranial vessels using TCD ultrasonography: the transtemporal, transorbital, and transoccipital. Through the transtemporal route, signals are obtainable from the middle cerebral artery (MCA), anterior cerebral artery (ACA), intracranial internal carotid artery (ICA), and proximal posterior cerebral artery (PCA) (Fig. 9-2). The transorbital route can be used to examine the ophthalmic artery and ICA. Using the transoccipital approach, signals

can be obtained from the vertebral arteries (VAs) and basilar artery (BA).

Recording of flow velocities from the intracranial arteries has many important implications in the study of cerebral vascular disease. The recorded dimension, velocity, is not a direct measurement of flow, but proportionality does exist between velocity and flow when the arterial diameter remains constant. Lindegaard et al. have demonstrated this relationship by comparing MCA velocity to flow measurements obtained by an electromagnetic flow meter on the carotid artery during carotid surgery.[18] Bishop et al. have compared TCD velocities to cerebral blood flow (CBF) measurements obtained in human subjects using xenon 133.[8] They demonstrated that although resting MCA velocity did not correlate very well with CBF, CBF changes induced by varying the Pa_{CO_2} did correlate well with the change in MCA velocity. Thus when the diameter of the cerebral basal arteries remain constant, changes in the velocities can accurately reflect changes in flow.

The angle of insonation (angle between the ultrasound beam and the vessel being recorded from) also needs to be considered when measuring true velocity. The true flow velocity and the observed velocity will be equal when this angle equals zero degrees. The observed velocity will decrease relative to the true velocity as the angle of insonation increases. The correction will be very small at small insonation angles and will be a product of the cosine of the angle and the true velocity.[1] Thus if the angle between the ultrasound beam and the flow vector is 15 degrees, 97 percent of the true velocity would be observed. If the insonation angle is 60 degrees, then 50 percent of the true velocity is observed (Fig. 9-3). This angle becomes significant when examining the extracranial carotid arteries using ultrasound. The insonation angle used in transcranial applications is small for most of the arteries examined because of their anatomic positions. The change in angles between different observations is also small because of the restrictions of recording sites in the temporal region.

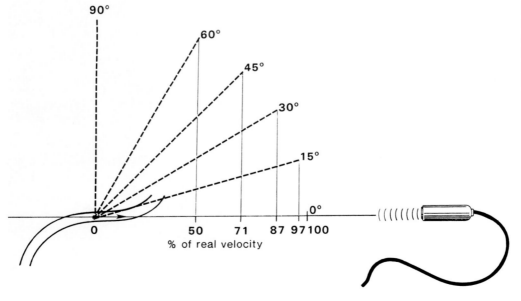

Figure 9-3 The relationship between the angle of insonation and the percentage of the true velocity which will be observed by the recording device.

Stenosis produced by atherosclerosis, vasospasm, or other mechanisms will be reflected by an increase in velocity through the stenotic segment in proportion to the reduction of the cross-sectional area when the same flow is preserved. Thus, for example, if the diameter is reduced to half of the original value by vasospasm, velocity increases to 400 percent of normal.

The frequency changes that are produced by the flowing blood are converted to velocity in centimeters per second (cm/s). Increased frequency shifts indicating blood flowing toward the probe will register as velocity above the zero line on the display screen. Any decreased frequency indicating blood flowing away from the probe will register as a negative deflection on the screen. This directionality is useful in identifying specific arteries and branch points around the circle of Willis.

Technique

As mentioned earlier, the three routes or "windows" for examination of the intracranial vessels are the transtemporal, transorbital, and transoccipital. To focus the probe on a particular artery and obtain a signal is referred to as insonation. In order for one to accurately identify vessels, knowledge of the anatomic position and direction of flow of the various intracranial arteries in normal and pathologic states is essential. The steps in identifying any particular artery are (1) Determine the direction of flow, (2) follow the signal to various depths and determine the spatial relationship of the signal to other known arteries, and (3) determine the response to compression or vibration maneuvers.

Examination through the transtemporal route provides access to the MCA, ACA, ICA, and PCA. Ultrasound transmitting gel is applied to an area just above the zygoma and slightly anterior to the ear. The depth can initially be set at 45 to 50 mm by adjusting the range gate. Generally the strongest signal in this region is the middle cerebral artery. The depth is increased progressively, and one finds a bifurcation usually at 65 mm. A bidirectional signal indicating simultaneous flow toward and away from the probe confirms the position on the ICA termination. The ACA signal can then be followed from this point to a depth of 70 to 75 mm. Aiming the probe inferiorly from the ICA termination will locate the ICA, and aiming it posteriorly will locate the PCA.

The access to the transoccipital "window" is obtained by flexing the patient's head forward and placing the probe just below the cervico-occipital junction. By setting the depth to 45 mm and directing the probe slightly laterally, one can usually find the vertebral artery, and under normal conditions, it will display a signal indicating blood flowing away from the probe. The depth is progressively increased to 80 to 85 mm while following the vertebral artery signal, and at this point the basilar artery is located in the midline. Signals directed toward the probe often are found at 50 to 65 mm, which represent the posterior inferior cerebellar artery.

Through the transorbital route, one can find the ophthalmic artery and also the carotid siphon. The patient's eyes are closed, and the probe is applied to the upper lid. The ophthalmic artery is located at a depth of approximately 40 to 45 mm, and it can be followed to its origin at the carotid artery.

Subarachnoid Hemorrhage and Vasospasm

Perhaps the most promising clinical use of transcranial Doppler ultrasonography is the capacity to noninvasively determine the degree of vasospasm after subarachnoid hemorrhage (SAH). The most significant changes in vessel diameter induced by vasospasm usually occur in the basal arteries. As vasospasm progresses and the vessels narrow, blood flow velocities through the stenotic segments increase and velocities can exceed normal resting values by five to six times. Correlations between residual lumen diameter of the ACA and MCA on angiogram and the changes in velocity on TCD ultrasonography have been observed.[3] The resistance across a stenotic segment is related not only to the degree of stenosis but also to the length of the stenosis. Thus the effect of basal artery narrowing on CBF reduction after subarachnoid hemorrhage will depend on the degree and extent of vessel narrowing, the arterial blood pressure, and the ability of the cerebral circulation to autoregulate and compensate for the vasospasm. In addition, the adequacy of the collateral circulation plays a role. When vasospasm becomes severe enough to reduce CBF to critical levels, neurologic deficits will ensue, frequently in a precipitous manner. The usefulness of TCD ultrasonography is that it can alert the clinician to the degree and extent of vasospasm and can allow institution of proper therapy before neurologic deficit or cerebral infarction takes place. Another potential use of TCD ultrasonography is to aid in the decision about the timing of aneurysm surgery; it may help to avoid untimely operations in asymptomatic patients who are undergoing a rapid but silent progression of vasospasm.

The middle cerebral arteries are the most ideally suited for TCD recordings in vasospasm. They are end arteries with limited leptomeningeal collaterals under normal conditions, so there is a close correlation between the amount of spasm and the increase in velocity seen with TCD ultrasonography. The other intracranial arteries from which recordings are usually made—proximal ACA, PCA, ICA, and the vertebrobasilar system—generally have collateral branches, and depending on the degree of collateralization, the relationship between spasm and increased velocity may not be as close. If an artery with extensive distal collateral vessels narrows in vasospasm, velocity may only increase moderately because collateral channels can provide some of the blood flow demands.

Under normal conditions, blood flow velocities in the middle cerebral artery range from 33 to 90 cm/s with an average value of 62 cm/s.[5] Velocities in excess of 120 cm/s correlate with vasospasm seen by angiography.[3] The divisions are arbitrary after this point, but mean velocities greater than 200 cm/s appear to correlate with severe spasm seen on angiography and are frequently associated with clinical episodes of ischemia and infarction.[29] Seiler et al. found in a group of 39 patients with SAH followed with TCD ultrasonography that if the blood flow velocities did not exceed 140 cm/s, no patient developed a cerebral infarct.[29] Blood flow velocities greater than 200 cm/s were associated with ischemia and infarction, but some patients remained asymptomatic. As a secondary effect of vasospasm, between the 4th and 20th day after SAH, musical tones can sometimes be heard from the loudspeaker of the TCD recording device.[6] The maximum amplitude of these sounds is heard near the carotid termination. The cause of these murmurs is most likely due to the creation of pure-tone frequencies by the vibrations of the arterial walls caused by the periodic shedding of vortices in the transition between laminar flow and turbulent flow. The frequency of the tones appears to correlate with the velocity and therefore the degree of vasospasm.

Time Course of Vasospasm

Since the original description of arterial spasm, several studies have documented the time course of vasospasm using angiography. Allcock and Drake reported that spasm was present in 45 percent of patients less than 3 days after SAH, 41 percent at 3 to 10 days, and 25 percent at more than 10 days.[7] A very detailed study was performed by Weir et al., who took careful measurements from 627 sets of angiograms from 293 patients with aneurysms.[31] These investigators found that vasospasm appeared initially on day 3 after subarachnoid hemorrhage, was maximal at days 6 to 8, and was gone by day 12. These studies, however, provide noncontinuous information in contrast to TCD ultrasonography, which has the advantage of being a noninvasive test which can be performed daily to follow the changes that occur.

Several studies using TCD ultrasonography have looked at the time course of vasospasm.[13,29] In a group of 39 patients with SAH, of whom most were operated on late, vasospasm indicated by an increase in flow velocities on TCD ultrasonography was maximal between days 7 and 12.[29] If the group was broken into subgroups based on the severity of vasospasm, the patients with less severe vasospasm tended to have their maximal increase in velocities later than 7 days. In contrast, a subgroup of patients who died from cerebral infarction had large increases in velocity on days 2 and 3 and high velocities, indicating severe vasospasm, by day 5 after SAH. Harders and Gilsbach reported a series of 50 patients operated on within 72 h after SAH and treated with nimodipine.[13] They found that maximum velocities were reached between the 11th and 20th days after SAH. Figure 9-4 illustrates the time course of the TCD ultrasound velocity changes in a patient who had surgery on day 1 after SAH, received no calcium channel blocker, and did not develop any delayed neurologic deficits.

Correlation of SAH on CT with Velocity

Several reports have pointed out a strong correlation between the amount of blood detected in the basal cisterns on CT scan after SAH and the subsequent development of vasospasm detected by angiography. Fisher et al. studied a group of patients who had CT scans done within 5 days of their SAH and defined four groups based on the amount of blood seen: Group 1, no blood detected; Group 2, diffuse deposition or thin layers with all vertical layers of blood less than 1 mm thick; Group 3, localized clots and/or vertical layers of blood 1 mm or greater in thickness; Group 4, diffuse or no subarachnoid blood but intracerebral or intraventricular clots.[9] Angiograms then done between 7 and 17 days after the subarachnoid hemorrhage showed severe vasospasm in 2 of 11 cases in Group 1, 0 of 14 cases in Groups 2 and 4, and 23 of 24 cases in Group 3. The results indicated that thick clots in the basal cisterns predispose patients to a very high incidence of severe vasospasm. Subsequently, other investigators have confirmed these findings.

Seiler et al. performed a similar study using TCD ultrasonography instead of angiography to assess vasospasm in patients after SAH.[29] In 39 patients, CT scans were done within 5 days after SAH and assessed for the amount of blood in the basal cisterns. The patients were broken into three groups according to the criteria of Fisher et al. The velocities in both MCAs were recorded daily, and the maximum velocities reached were noted. There was a strong correlation between the amount of blood in the basal cisterns and the maximum velocity reached. Eight of nine patients with no blood on the CT scan had maximum velocities below 140 cm/s. In CT Group 3, with thick cisternal clots, 13 of 15 patients had maximum velocities during their hospital course of 140 cm/s or greater, and 9 of 15 had maximum velocities greater than 200 cm/s.

Cerebral Blood Flow and Blood Flow Velocity in Vasospasm

Ischemic deficits from vasospasm occur when the basal vessel diameter becomes reduced to the point of reducing blood flow below levels critical to maintenence of cerebral function. The velocity of blood flowing through the vessel will increase with progressive narrowing until a critical narrowing occurs, diminishing flow. This leads to a nonlinear relationship between velocity and arterial narrowing in severe vasospasm. To correct this effect, a simultaneous index of flow would be helpful. Seiler and Aaslid reported a decreased velocity in the extracranial carotid artery recorded from the neck in SAH patients with intracranial velocities exceeding 200 cm/s.[28] This presumably was due to a reduction in volume flow secondary to the increase in vascular resistance caused by the vasospasm. Lindegaard et al. have applied the concept of the velocity ratio of the MCA/ICA (V_{mca}/V_{ica}) to compensate for changes in CBF.[16] A V_{mca}/V_{ica} ratio greater than 3 was found to correspond to vasospasm seen on angiography. It was also found that the V_{mca} was lower when the spasm was widespread. The V_{mca}/V_{ica} ratio was useful in this setting because it partially corrected for reduced velocities in the MCA caused by a decrease in flow. This ratio may prove to be useful for detecting vasospasm after head injuries because the hyperemia which often occurs may also increase flow velocities beyond the normal range.

Sekhar et al. followed a series of 21 patients with SAH from aneurysm rupture using TCD and CBF measurements performed with stable xenon CT-CBF studies and [133]Xe

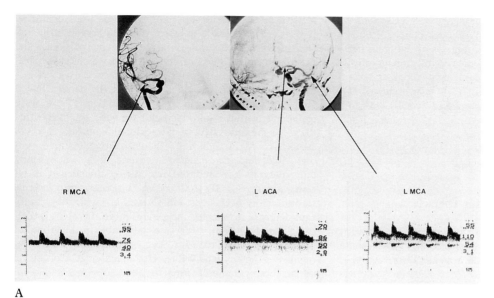

A

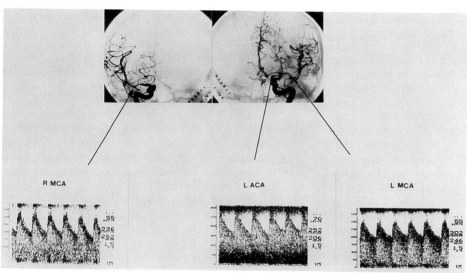

B

Figure 9-4 TCD recordings from a patient with a Grade I SAH from an anterior communicating artery aneurysm. This patient remained asymptomatic despite angiographic vasospasm and increased velocity on TCD ultrasonography. *A*. Angiogram and velocity recordings on day 1 following SAH. *B*. Angiogram and velocity recordings on day 11 following SAH showing vasospasm and increased TCD velocities. *C*. Graph of daily TCD velocity recordings in the same patient following SAH.

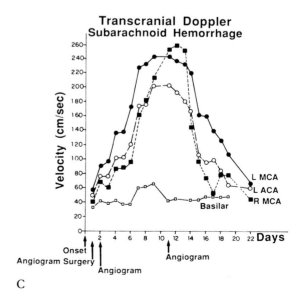

C

washout studies.[30] It was found that increases in TCD velocities preceded the onset of delayed ischemic deficits. In addition, CBF values were decreased in areas of the brain fed by vessels that had high velocities on TCD ultrasonography. It appears that some method of measuring or indexing cerebral blood flow in combination with TCD measurements of velocity may offer the most sensitive and specific way to diagnose critical vasospasm.

Occlusive Vascular Disease

Intracranial Occlusive Vascular Disease

Intracranial stenosis due to atherosclerosis appears less frequently than similar lesions of the extracranial vessels but can be a source of transient ischemic attacks (TIAs). Arteriography has until now been the only way to diagnose these lesions. In patients presenting with TIAs who have normal extracranial noninvasive findings, TCD ultrasonography may be a valuable adjunct to identify those patients with intracranial stenotic lesions. In a study of 11 patients with intracranial occlusive disease, Lindegaard et al. found a clear-cut inverse relationship between the residual lumen diameter of the intracranial stenosis and velocity readings on TCD ultrasonography.[15] It was also noted that with severe stenosis of the proximal middle cerebral artery, recordings distal to the stenosis revealed an abnormally low velocity with a dampened pulse wave indicating flow reduction.

MCA occlusions due to thrombosis or embolism can also be detected by TCD ultrasonography, which can reveal low velocities proximal to the occlusion and absence of a signal distal to the occlusion. The ability to detect MCA occlusions rapidly and noninvasively may have a role in identifying candidates for thrombolytic therapy or in following the time course of occlusion and recanalization and possibly to estimate the prognosis of acute stroke. Halsey recorded MCA blood flow velocities in the hemisphere opposite to the symptoms using TCD ultrasonography in 15 patients presenting with complete hemiplegia of less than 12 hours' duration.[11] The mean velocities were greater than 30 cm/s in seven patients, five of whom made a complete or partial recovery. Velocities of less than 30 cm/s were recorded in the remaining patients. One patient recovered completely and the other seven patients were left with a total paralysis of the hand and arm.

Extracranial Occlusive Vascular Disease

Transient ischemic attacks and stroke can be caused by a variety of mechanisms. Emboli from and hemodynamic effects of extracranial carotid lesions can both play a role. In evaluating patients with carotid bifurcation disease, it can often be difficult to tell which of these mechanisms is responsible. Doppler ultrasonography has achieved a high degree of accuracy in diagnosing extracranial stenosis and identifying hemodynamically significant lesions in the extracranial carotid arteries. The addition of TCD ultrasonography has the advantage of obtaining velocity recordings directly from the arteries supplying the major brain territories. It is therefore possible to assess the final hemodynamic effect due to the extent of extracranial occlusive disease and the adequacy of the collateral network which is variable.

When extracranial occlusion or stenosis causes a hemodynamic change in the MCA, generally the pattern that is seen is a decrease in velocity and a dampened pulse wave ipsilateral to the lesion. Studies have thus far shown that there is a variable effect of extracranial carotid occlusion or stenosis on MCA signals.[24,27] Some patients maintain normal MCA velocities distal to a carotid occlusion, whereas other patients have reduced velocities. Schneider et al. recently reported TCD findings in 39 patients with internal carotid artery occlusions and showed a statistically significant decrease in velocity and pulsatility in the MCA ipsilateral to the occlusion.[27] It was also possible in this group of patients to evaluate the sources of collateral flow from other regions of the circle of Willis. The effects of ICA occlusion on cerebral vasomotor reactivity have also been studied. Ringelstein et al. performed a study of CO_2-induced vasomotor reactivity by recording the changes in MCA velocity induced by Pa_{CO_2} changes using TCD ultrasonography.[24] The study looked at 40 normal subjects and 40 patients with unilateral, and 15 patients with bilateral, ICA occlusions. The results showed that in patients with unilateral ICA lesions, vasomotor reactivity was significantly reduced in both hemispheres but to a greater degree ipsilateral to the occlusion. In the bilateral occlusion group there was also a significant reduction in vasomotor reactivity in both hemispheres compared to normal. There was a significant decrease in vasomotor reactivity in symptomatic compared to asymptomatic patients with unilateral carotid occlusions. These studies suggest that using TCD ultrasonography in combination with physiologic testing may prove useful in identifying patients with cerebrovascular hemodynamic insufficiency.

Head Injury

Although TCD ultrasonography measures velocity and not flow directly, changes in flow can be detected and CBF changes under various conditions can be assessed. For example, Markwalder et al. found that changes in the middle cerebral artery velocity correlated well with changes in the levels of arterial P_{CO_2} in normal human subjects.[20] The V_{mca} changed with expected changes in cerebral blood flow evoked by changes in Pa_{CO_2}. With alterations in Pa_{CO_2}, the distal cerebral vasculature responds by constricting or dilating, thereby changing CBF. Assuming that the diameter of the basal arteries does not change with Pa_{CO_2} changes, a change in velocity readings obtained will directly reflect changes in CBF. A study by Aaslid has demonstrated rapid changes in velocity in the posterior cerebral artery reflecting changes in CBF induced by light and dark stimuli on the retina.[2] These changes occur with 2.3 s of the stimulus and reflect blood flow changes to evoked cortical activity. Autoregulation has also been studied using TCD ultrasonography to record velocity changes induced by rapid changes in blood pressure. One advantage over other CBF measurement methods is that rapid and subtle changes can be detected in humans, allowing the study of phenomena not easily studied otherwise. To use TCD ultrasonography to measure absolute blood flow in human arteries, the cross-sectional area of the artery and the angle of insonation must be known. With further technical developments, this may be possible in the future.

In severe head injury, several pathophysiologic conditions exist that may be evaluated by TCD ultrasonography such as alterations in cerebral blood flow, changes in autoregulation, vasospasm, and increases in intracranial pressure (ICP). There have been only a few reports to date on the use of TCD ultrasonography in head-injured patients, but preliminary findings suggest that it will be a useful diagnostic tool.[26] Obrist et al. and others have demonstrated changes in CBF which occur after severe head injury using xenon washout studies.[22] Decreases in cerebral metabolic rate and CBF paralleled the severity of coma in general, but there was a large group of patients in whom a delayed increase in CBF was found. These increases were out of proportion to the metabolic demands of the brain tissue determined by arteriovenous oxygen differences and CBF. This condition has been termed cerebral hyperemia. There was a positive correlation between the occurrence of cerebral hyperemia and increased ICP.

Vasospasm has also been reported after head injury and can in some cases lead to clinical deterioration. Because either vasospasm or increased CBF can cause an increase in velocity, these two conditions must be differentiated. Distinctions between the two conditions can be made by the following: (1) With cerebral hyperemia, all vessels insonated tend to have high velocities in contrast to vasospasm, which tends to have a more focal nature. (2) If CBF studies are done simultaneously, CBF increases will parallel increases in velocity on TCD ultrasonography with cerebral hyperemia in contrast to significant vasospasm, where CBF will decrease. (3) V_{mca}/V_{ica} ratios will be higher in vasospasm than in cerebral hyperemia. Grolimund et al. found that two groups exist with high velocities after head injury, one group with increased V_{mca}/V_{ica} ratios and another with lower V_{mca}/V_{ica} ratios.[10] It is likely that these two groups represent on the one hand, patients with mild vasospasm, and on the other hand, patients with cerebral hyperemia.

Although ICP levels cannot be determined directly from TCD ultrasonography, Aaslid et al. have shown that in a group of patients undergoing ventricular infusion tests for hydrocephalus, decreased cerebral perfusion pressure could be detected by analysis of the TCD wave forms.[4] Kety et al.[14] were among the first to demonstrate that CBF decreases at high ICP levels, by using quantitative measurements of CBF and ICP. Several investigators using TCD ultrasonography to record from the intracranial vessels have reported a progressive decrease in the diastolic wave form with compromised cerebral perfusion pressure due to increased ICP, progressing to a reverberating pattern that occurs with cerebral circulatory arrest. This pattern occurs when flow is obstructed at the microcirculatory level and the conducting vessel absorbs the arterial pulse wave, distending in systole and contracting in diastole (Fig. 9-5). The detection of a reverberating pattern documenting the arrest of the cerebral circulation may prove to be a useful confirmatory test in determining brain death.[21]

Surgical Monitoring of CBF Changes

TCD ultrasonography has been used to monitor MCA velocities both during carotid endarterectomy (CEA) and cardiopulmonary bypass.[19,23] Using a headband and a movable probe, it is possible to obtain a continuous velocity signal from the middle cerebral artery and thus a measurement of the changes in blood flow during various manipulations such as alteration in blood pressure, onset of cardiopulmonary bypass, or carotid cross-clamping.

During carotid endarterectomy, several methods of assessing the adequacy of the cerebral blood flow during cross-clamping have been used. These methods have included assessment of cerebral activity, using EEG or functional testing during surgery under local anesthesia. Blood flow has also been assessed more directly using stump pressure measurement or regional CBF studies. The results of TCD monitoring during endarterectomy have been reported by several groups. Halsey et al. compared regional CBF using ^{133}Xe to TCD recordings of MCA velocity while simultaneously recording EEG in eight patients undergoing CEA.[12] It

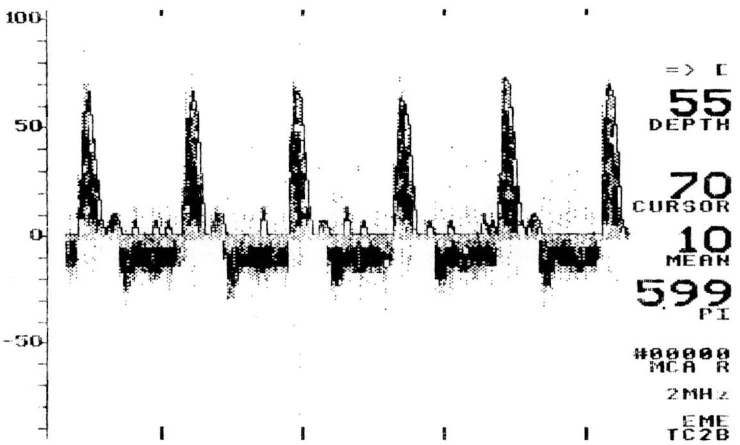

Figure 9-5 The "to and fro" pattern seen in the middle cerebral artery following cerebral circulatory arrest.

was found that there was a considerable variability in the relationship between the mean velocities and the CBF. The systolic/diastolic ratio was more sensitive in detecting changes due to cross-clamping than the mean velocity. It was concluded that while CBF measurements are reflecting cortical blood flow, the TCD tracings may be more indicative of the flow in the basal vessels reflecting blood supply to the deeper perforating vessels. It remains to be determined if TCD ultrasonography will be a reliable monitoring method during carotid endarterectomy and will be able to predict the need for intraoperative shunt placement.

Arteriovenous Malformations

Initial experience using TCD ultrasonography to evaluate patients with arteriovenous malformations (AVMs) has revealed several findings.[17] Feeding arteries to a large AVM show high flow velocities and a low pulse pressure on TCD ultrasonography due to their conduction of high blood flow to a low-resistance vascular bed. Altered CO_2 responsiveness has been demonstrated when comparing in the same patient AVM feeding vessels to other arteries feeding areas of normal brain. The utility of TCD ultrasonography in the management of AVMs is yet to be established, but possible uses include noninvasive detection, serial follow-up in patients undergoing radiation treatment, and possible use in staged obliteration.

Summary

Transcranial Doppler ultrasonography provides a new avenue to study the human cerebral circulation and appears to be very useful in the evaluation of a variety of clinical conditions. It provides for the first time a noninvasive way to assess the degree and extent of vasospasm occurring after SAH. In this way it may be useful in identifying patients at high risk for developing ischemic defects. It also has applications in the evaluation of occlusive cerebrovascular disease such as the diagnosis of intracranial stenosis and occlusion, as well as the assessment of the hemodynamic effects of extracranial disease. TCD ultrasonography also appears useful in monitoring changes in CBF, which occur under a variety of clinical conditions including closed-head injury and other conditions which lead to increases in intracranial pressure.

References

1. Aaslid R. The Doppler principle applied to measurement of blood flow velocity in cerebral arteries. In: Aaslid R (ed.), *Transcranial Doppler Sonography*. New York: Springer-Verlag, 1986:22–38.
2. Aaslid R. Visually evoked dynamic blood flow response of the human cerebral circulation. *Stroke* 1987; 18:771–775.
3. Aaslid R, Huber P, Nornes H. Evaluation of cerebrovascular spasm with transcranial Doppler ultrasound. *J Neurosurg* 1984; 60:37–41.
4. Aaslid R, Lindar T, Lindegaard F, et al. Estimation of cerebral perfusion pressure from arterial blood pressure and transcranial Doppler recordings. In: Miller JD, Teasdale GM, Rowan JO, et al. (eds.), *Intracranial Pressure VI*. Berlin: Springer-Verlag, 1986:226–229.
5. Aaslid R, Markwalder TM, Nornes H. Noninvasive transcranial Doppler ultrasound recording of flow velocity in basal cerebral arteries. *J Neurosurg* 1982; 57:769–774.
6. Aaslid R, Nornes H. Musical murmurs in human cerebral arteries after subarachnoid hemorrhage. *J Neurosurg* 1984; 60:32–36.
7. Allcock JM, Drake CG. Ruptured intracranial aneurysms: the role of arterial spasm. *J Neurosurg* 1965; 22:21–29.
8. Bishop CCR, Powell S, Rutt D, et al. Transcranial Doppler measurement of middle cerebral artery blood flow velocity: a validation study. *Stroke* 1986; 17:913–915.
9. Fisher CM, Kistler JP, Davis JM. Relation of cerebral vasospasm to subarachnoid hemorrhage visualized by computerized tomographic scanning. *Neurosurgery* 1980; 6:1–9.
10. Grolimund P, Weber M, Seiler RW, et al. Time course of cerebral vasospasm after severe head injury. *Lancet* 1988; 1:1173.
11. Halsey JH. Prognosis of acute hemiplegia estimated by transcranial Doppler ultrasonography. *Stroke* 1988; 19:648–649.
12. Halsey JH, McDowell HA, Gelman S. Transcranial Doppler and rCBF compared in carotid endarterectomy. *Stroke* 1986; 17:1206–1208.
13. Harders AG, Gilsbach JM. Time course of blood velocity changes related to vasospasm in the circle of Willis measured by transcranial Doppler ultrasound. *J Neurosurg* 1987; 66:718–728.
14. Kety SS, Shenkin HA, Schmidt CF. The effects of increased intracranial pressure on cerebral circulatory functions in man. *J Clin Invest* 1948; 27:493–499.
15. Lindegaard KF, Bakke SJ, Aaslid R, et al. Doppler diagnosis of intracranial artery occlusive disorders. *J Neurol Neurosurg Psychiatry* 1986; 49:510–518.
16. Lindegaard KF, Bakke SJ, Sorteberg W, et al. A non-invasive Doppler ultrasound method for the evaluation of patients with subarachnoid hemorrhage. *Acta Radiol* (Suppl) 1986; 369:96–98.
17. Lindegaard KF, Grolimund P, Aaslid R, et al. Evaluation of cerebral AVM's using transcranial Doppler ultrasound. *J Neurosurg* 1986; 65:335–344.
18. Lindegaard KF, Lundar T, Wiberg J, et al. Variations in middle cerebral artery blood flow investigated with non-invasive transcranial blood velocity measurements. *Stroke* 1987; 18:1025–1030.
19. Lundar T, Lindegaard KF, Froysaker T, et al. Cerebral perfusion during nonpulsatile cardiopulmonary bypass. *Ann Thorac Surg* 1985; 40:144–150.
20. Markwalder TM, Grolimund P, Seiler RW, et al. Dependency of blood flow velocity in the middle cerebral artery on end-tidal carbon dioxide partial pressure: a transcranial ultrasound Doppler study. *J Cereb Blood Flow Metab* 1984; 4:368–372.
21. Newell DW, Grady MS, Sirotta P, et al. Evaluation of brain death using transcranial Doppler. *Neurosurgery* 1989; 24:509–513.
22. Obrist WD, Langfitt TW, Jaggi JL, et al. Cerebral blood flow and metabolism in comatose patients with acute head injury: relationship to intracranial hypertension. *J Neurosurg* 1984; 61:241–253.
23. Padyachee TS, Gosling RG, Bishop CC, et al. Monitoring middle cerebral artery blood velocity during carotid endarterectomy. *Br J Surg* 1986; 73:98–100.
24. Ringelstein EB, Sievers C, Ecker S, et al. Noninvasive assessment of CO_2 induced cerebral vasomotor response in normal

individuals and patients with internal carotid artery occlusions. *Stroke* 1988; 19:963–969.

25. Satomura S. Study of flow patterns in peripheral arteries by ultrasonics. *J Acoust Soc Jpn* 1959; 15:151–158.

26. Saunders FW, Cledgett P. Intracranial blood velocity in head injury: a transcranial ultrasound Doppler study. *Surg Neurol* 1988; 29:401–409.

27. Schneider PA, Rossman ME, Bernstein EF, et al. Effect of internal carotid artery occlusion on intracranial hemodynamics: transcranial Doppler evaluation and clinical correlation. *Stroke* 1988; 19:589–593.

28. Seiler RW, Aaslid R. Transcranial Doppler for evaluation of

cerebral vasospasm. In: Aaslid R (ed.), *Transcranial Doppler Sonography*. New York: Springer-Verlag, 1986:118–131.

29. Seiler RW, Grolimund P, Aaslid R, et al. Cerebral vasospasm evaluated by transcranial ultrasound correlated with clinical grade and CT-visualized subarachnoid hemorrhage. *J Neurosurg* 1986; 64:594–600.

30. Sekhar LN, Wechsler LR, Yonas H, et al. Value of transcranial Doppler examination in the diagnosis of cerebral vasospasm after subarachnoid hemorrhage. *Neurosurgery* 1988; 22:813–821.

31. Weir B, Grace M, Hansen J, et al. Time course of vasospasm in man. *J Neurosurg* 1978; 48:173–178.

10

The Computer in Neurosurgical Practice

Andrew B. Kaufman

The complexity of accounts receivable management in current neurosurgery practice combined with the availability of cost-effective computerized medical office management systems has led most offices of a single neurosurgeon, and nearly all multiphysician practices, to consider purchase of such a system. Although systems are most commonly purchased for business management, their power, their ease of use, and the availability of inexpensive application software often leads to a desire for additional uses of the computer.

There has been much disappointment felt by those who have purchased a computer system that was inadequate for their needs, too expensive, unable to accommodate even a normal volume of operations much less allow for growth, or too disruptive of customary operational procedures. These problems are predictable in even the most expensive and well-designed computer systems. Numerous stories are available of those who have sustained substantial financial loss and disruption of normal practice by the purchase of well-intentioned but inappropriately designed systems. Even independent consultants, in spite of appropriate qualifications and experience, are prone to error in system selection if the special needs and functions of the neurosurgical practice are not carefully considered. A computer system will not correct disorganization, misfiled information, or neglected paperwork. Most computer systems will reduce the amount of manual paperwork required in the processing of insurance and accounts receivable in a neurosurgery office. Nevertheless, before making any decision to purchase a computer system one should take a close look at the current system for handling those functions for which a computer is proposed, with special attention to current problems in information management and processing. The computer is a general purpose device. Just because it is capable of doing nearly anything with information does not mean it will function satisfactorily in any given implementation. It is more important whether the system will actually improve the efficiency and effectiveness of those functions for which it is to be considered.

Perhaps the most confusing issue for a neurosurgeon contemplating purchase of an office system is the constantly changing nature of the capabilities of hardware and software. It is tempting to defer a decision pending reports of the success of the latest hardware innovations or while awaiting a price reduction, a common occurrence in the natural history of nearly all computer hardware. Nevertheless, at the present time, it would likely be more prudent to determine one's functional requirements for a computer system, consider further desirable but not essential features, and then attempt to determine the availability of systems that will best fulfill these needs. Form should follow function in the choice of an office computer system.[6,11,14]

It is not generally advisable to consider computer automation of a single-physician practice. This is particularly true for a neurosurgical practice, where the volume of transactions is likely to be much less than in many other medical specialties. Existing manual accounting systems supplemented as needed by a computer dedicated to word processing will usually be the most efficient and cost-effective solution for even a busy office of a single neurosurgeon.

How then can a neurosurgeon hope to benefit from this technology and actually enhance and facilitate his or her practice? This guide is provided to aid in the process of making a decision whether to purchase a computer system and to permit the neurosurgeon to ask the right questions and seek appropriate answers so as to enhance the likelihood of a good outcome. A brief review of hardware and available or possible applications software is presented.

Hardware

The hardware or equipment of a computer system is more or less fixed in configuration. Although some additions or modifications can be made to existing hardware, and expansion may be possible, such changes tend to be at the mercy of the specific expertise of the vendor and tend to be expensive. For this reason, and because of the imprecise methods available for predicting actual hardware requirements for a given software application (and particularly in the situation of very large databases such as are the rule in medical office management systems), it is generally wise to consider excess capacity for most capacity-related hardware components. To consider cost, it generally is no more than 20 percent more than the original cost of a hard disk to double the capacity of a drive at the time of original purchase. The physical attributes of the hardware (speed, size, durability, and appearance) will generally be the primary determinants in the selection.

There are four main hardware components in most systems: (1) the central processing unit (CPU); (2) memory; (3) mass storage devices; and (4) input/output (I/O) devices.

Central Processing Unit

This is an electronic device, generally contained within a single or several silicon chips. It is symbolically at the center of all that happens with a system to the extent that all information from any of the four hardware components must pass through the CPU before being directed to its destination for subsequent processing or output. For example, information entered at a keyboard to direct the computer to print a report will first pass through the CPU, where the request will be interpreted and processed, supplementary information will be summoned, directions will be sent out to a mass storage device, and finally the printer will be activated and information for output will be delivered to it. Arithmetic operations generally take place within the CPU. The CPU is one of the least important components of a system with respect to overall system speed in a medical office business application. For certain auxiliary applications mentioned later, such as a spreadsheet, CPU speed may be a relevant consideration. It is the most reliable component of most systems.

Main Memory

When the system is in operation, the main memory is a reservoir for storage of those software components most likely to be needed at any given time. Although main memory is very fast in processing speed, it is also very expensive and consumes large amounts of physical space compared to mass storage devices. Therefore, most applications are designed so that small packets of software are shuttled in and out of memory from hard disks as they are needed for processing by the CPU. Memory is also generally volatile, so that in the event of power failure or other system malfunction, information in memory is readily lost. The software brought into memory is a copy of that already existing elsewhere on a hard disk.

When a system is first started, or booted, it is the *operating system* (discussed below) that is first loaded into memory. This is a copy of information already existing (permanently) on the hard disk. Parts of the *operating system* may be shuttled in and out of memory as needed by the CPU. User instructions indicate to the CPU what *application* software components are to be brought into memory as they are needed. Finally, small amounts of *data* are brought into memory when they need to be modified, analyzed, subjected to mathematical processing, or otherwise processed.

In general, additional memory may be useful only up to a certain point because most software is designed to be swapped in and out of memory. Some systems are designed to create *virtual* memory whereby frequently used batches of software are stored on a hard disk in a physical or logical arrangement such that they may be available for transfer into memory more rapidly than would otherwise be possible. Although this arrangement may be useful, it does not approach main memory in speed.

Mass Storage

This most commonly refers to hard disk devices. The hard disk holds large amounts of data and instructions that are not immediately available to the processor. This is a hardware component where speed and capacity are important in influencing system efficiency and cost. The cost of excess capacity is generally small and worthwhile. The speed of operation of a given application is strongly influenced by the speed with which data and application software modules can be transferred from hard disk to memory and back again. The speed of the hard disk is substantially more important in this respect than the speed of the CPU. Although this hardware component can physically reside outside of the main computer, it is better protected and more efficient if located inside the main system enclosure.

Input/Output Devices

These devices provide the means by which information is put into the system and retrieved from it. A cathode-ray tube (CRT) with an associated keyboard is generally the input device. The system's capacity to accommodate additional CRTs is an important consideration in determining expansion capability. It is a common experience that every clerical and management employee in a medical office will find the computer system essential in their daily work, although sharing of a terminal may sometimes be practical. System capacity is often rated at multiples of four terminals. Simultaneous use of I/O devices may dramatically degrade the performance or response time of a system. Generally, a response time of less than 4 s is desirable. A frequent user of a system who must wait more than 10 s to obtain visual information will likely find the system a hindrance. The physical feel of the keyboard, height of the keyboard, glare from the CRT, and other ergonomic features may be important to a frequent user.

Printers are the next most common I/O devices. Speed, print quality, noise produced, durability, and reliability are important considerations in the selection of a printer. The printer is the most likely component in a system to malfunction and require repair. When printer or printers are selected, it is wise to consider the possible requirement for substituting one printer for another in the event of temporary failure. It is not uncommon for commercial quality printers to generate noise in excess of 62 dB, a generally unacceptable level of noise for an intimate office environment. Internal and external baffling, noise-reducing enclosure, and placement of the printer in a remote location may be helpful if this is a problem. Although a nine-pin dot matrix printer may be adequate and even desirable for generating office reports, even the most expensive 24-pin dot matrix printers may not be acceptable for letters to referring physicians. Daisy wheel, thermal, and laser printers each have advantages and disadvantages if more appealing print quality is preferred.

Printers must have an electronic interface to the computer. A serial interface is a means of transmitting data one bit at a time in sequence. It has the advantage of maintaining a constant speed of transmission even over long distances. A parallel interface may transmit information more rapidly by transmitting multiple bits simultaneously, but the nature of the electronic interface severely limits the distance of the printing device from the computer to no more than 7 ft.

A modem is a device that permits transfer of data over the telephone lines to other computer systems. It is most commonly used in medical office systems for remote electronic submission of insurance claims. An evolving use of these devices is for remote diagnosis and repair of software problems by the systems supplier. Other possible applications would be in utilizing remote databases (e.g., MEDLINE or CompuServe), for the electronic exchange of manuscripts or other alphabetic information, or to gain access to computer bulletin boards.

Backup Hardware

One or more hardware (or software) components of a computer system will periodically, randomly, and unpredictably fail to function normally. This may result in a catastrophic loss of data if appropriate precautions are not taken to anticipate this event. Data loss cannot be reliably prevented, and hence most backup procedures are directed toward restoring data in the event of loss or mechanical breakdown.

Backup battery power supplies are commonly used as a means of dealing with the variations in quality of electrical supply that may exist in some areas or in some commercial buildings. Generally, these devices are designed to sense a voltage fluctuation that would be capable of causing acute failure of a hard disk or other system component. Within milliseconds, this reserve power supply will take over as a source of electricity until the line supply stabilizes. In the event of actual blackout, this power may be utilized for a time interval unique to the unit (generally 5 to 15 min) to permit an orderly shutdown of the computer system.

One of the most common and inexpensive devices for backup is the floppy disk drive included in almost all microcomputer systems. This drive is most commonly used for the purpose of initially transferring software from its usually supplied source on floppy disks onto the system hard disk. However, in systems with a hard disk, the floppy disk drive is often used for daily or monthly backup procedures. Depending upon the nature of the software system and size of the data base, this may be all the backup that is necessary and the cost is nominal. If a daily backup by this procedure takes more than 15 min, then a more rapid device, described below, may be considered.

Some form of serial magnetic tape backup provides the most cost-effective means of ensuring system recoverability. Specifications for such systems often provide the capability of a backup (or restore) rate of 5 Mbyte/min. However, it is important to recognize that the hardware specification for speed of such a device may be a minor consideration if the software backup system is efficiently designed, and may be irrelevant in a poorly designed system where actual performance could be far less than the hardware capability.

A number of different floppy disk–type media and drives are available that have speed capabilities approaching that of a hard disk. These replaceable media may be used as backup devices. They tend to be substantially more expensive than a serial magnetic tape device and may require more operator intervention.

Hardware Installation

Although the CPU, memory, mass storage devices, modem, and backup devices are often contained within the computer console or in immediate proximity to it, the I/O devices may be remote. A direct physical connection by wire or cable, often fragile, is required between the device and the computer console. It is wise and inexpensive to incorporate conduit and appropriate outlets within walls when planning a new medical office, much in the same way that telephone outlets and wiring may be planned. If that has not been done, appropriate planning will be needed to conceal and protect the computer cables. Desk and counter space may be necessary for terminals, stands for printers, proper air circulation for terminals and the computer console, and noise-insulation devices for dot matrix or daisy wheel printers. Keyboards will need to be at the proper height for comfortable typing. Lighting must be such as to prevent distracting glare on terminals.

Hardware Expansion

At some point after successful implementation of a computer system, and often within the first year, there is a desire for system expansion. Planning for this at the time of initial purchase is essential if one is to preserve this valuable capability. Any of the hardware components of a system are capable of restricting the possibility of future expansion. Proper planning can facilitate expansion and markedly reduce the cost of it at a future date. It is very important to go beyond the promises of the vendor and attempt to obtain personal anecdotal experiences of knowledgeable users if one desires to avoid the enormous cost and inconvenience of a premature requirement for replacement of an initially inadequate system.

The hard disk and the input devices (CRT) are the most likely to require expansion. The initial purchase of a hard disk with double the capacity required for full system operation is likely to be a worthwhile and cost-effective system enhancement. A given hardware configuration may have a fixed and absolute maximum capacity for CRTs, or a given software system may rapidly lose performance if too many input devices are in use, even though the hardware may ostensibly permit such a configuration. There is no substitute for information regarding the prior personal experience of other users of a comparable system in determining the limitations of a proposed system with regard to the capability for expansion.

Hardware Maintenance

All hardware will fail at some time. The interfacing of individual hardware components is an exceedingly complex issue usually compounded by the use of devices supplied by different manufacturers or vendors. The most reliable arrangement for hardware maintenance will be one in which a single company has experience with all of the components of a given system and is willing to contract for personal servicing of all components. The annual cost for hardware maintenance will generally be in the range of 7 to 15 percent of the original purchase price of the hardware.

Software

The design and function of the software is usually the most important consideration in any computer system. A poorly written program on a fast machine will run much slower than concise and efficient software running on a slow or older-generation machine. The software of a given system can usually be modified more readily than the hardware.

Operating System

There are three different but related software components in any integrated system. If one is to view the system software in a hierarchical configuration, the operating system would be at the top. This is a part of the software generally supplied by the hardware manufacturer and to some extent specific to the hardware. A UNIX operating system or MS-DOS on a given machine may *function* identically on another machine, even though the actual software code may be quite different. Operating system software may be transferable from one machine to another, but this is not generally assumed to be possible. The operating system is that part of the software that acts as the interface between the specific application software and the hardware. It is responsible for finding a batch of instructions or data on a hard disk and transferring it into memory. It may manipulate, sort, or otherwise process data in memory; it interfaces with the various I/O devices. The operating system is generally cryptic in its syntax and hence is ideally transparent to the user.

An operating system may restrict usage to a single user, be capable of multiuser and/or multitasking operation, or permit a network type of architecture. UNIX is the most widely used multiuser, multitasking operating system in medical office computer systems. This type of operating system is usually much more complex than single-user software because of the complex issues involved in the simultaneous access to a single copy of data.

Because of the wide availability of single-user application software and the relative ease of authoring it, systems suppliers have long sought to share a given body of data using single-user software. The technology of networking of microcomputers has evolved over the last 4 years in an attempt to implement this strategy. It usually involves interfacing several personal computer systems with each other and with some peripheral devices, most commonly a large hard disk and one or more printers. Both hardware and software are required to establish such a *network* and the network software supercedes or supervises the operating system software. These systems generally function somewhat slower than a multiuser software operating system for any given application, assuming comparable skill of the software authors.

The issue of a network architecture versus a multiuser operating system is a common and difficult problem in the choice of a computer system for a neurosurgical practice. The overall functionality of a system for a particular use is the more important determining factor in selection of the best system, irrespective of the particular system architecture.

Software Languages

An office computer system will present to the user application software in understandable syntax. This software, however, must itself be written in a computer language, of which there are many. BASIC, PASCAL, COBOL, and C are some of the languages most commonly used in authoring application software. Programs written in these languages must then be translated into assembly language by some component of the operating system before it can be understood and processed by the system hardware.

Languages may be divided into those that are compiled and those that are interpreted. Simply stated, a compiled language is one in which the original application software is processed by a component of the operating system prior to its use in the system. This operating system translating module is called a compiler, and it translates the software language into a more cryptic language that is directly understandable to the hardware. Individually translated software modules may then be linked together into a coherent, integrated, and efficient body of software that can be used repeatedly by the computer and processed efficiently and rapidly. This translation process must occur only once, and thereafter the code created may be used over and over again until such time as a change is made in the original application software.

An interpreted language is one in which the translation into a machine-readable version occurs each time the application is run. This is a time-consuming process, and hence such software will run more slowly than comparable compiled software.

A language is an essential tool for using and programming a computer. PASCAL, COBOL, and BASIC are examples of high-level languages that are reasonably easy to learn and use. However, by virtue of their being more like the English language and less like native computer code, their translation is more complex and time-consuming. Conversely, assembly language and C are much more difficult to learn and program but are much closer in design to the code required by the hardware and hence more rapid in operation.

Application Software and Pseudolanguages

The software included in an integrated neurosurgical office business system is a type of application software. There are thousands of commercially available applications, written in some high- or low-level computer language. Many of these are general types of software that may be adapted for an array of uses. Examples of this would be commercially available spreadsheets, word processing software, small business accounting packages, and telecommunications software. There are numerous sophisticated packages of database software such as MDBS, Informix, Unify, dBase, and Paradox, to mention a few. Some of these packages have incorporated into them "programming languages," which are not true general purpose programming languages but rather pseudolanguages that permit certain key words to be used to form commands that may then be interpreted by the database software to actually perform the equivalent of several manual database operations in an automated or programmed fashion. This programming capability within the database software has led to the development of some medical office systems run entirely within one of these database packages.

In order for most application software to be processed, each command utilized in the application must be parsed and then translated into a series of appropriate commands of the computer language in which the application was originally written. These commands must in turn be either compiled or interpreted into appropriate assembly or machine language so as to be finally intelligible to the hardware and permit execution of the command. The use of a database programming language or pseudolanguage to develop software as complex as that required for a medical office business system introduces yet another parsing and translating step further removed from the native computer language. This is a time- and memory-consuming process that can only impede performance. Hence, it is not likely that a medical office business system written in one of these general database packages can be efficiently implemented.

Software Maintenance

Software inherently contains errors or "bugs" in spite of the best efforts of producers to test applications prior to their wide circulation. Furthermore, modifications are made to existing software at indeterminate intervals. Changes required to accommodate these situations may be simple or may require a complete and lengthy reinstallation of the software. Finally, operator errors may be made that confound even the most well-planned software. For this reason, software servicing (i.e., maintenance) is as essential as hardware maintenance. Often, software maintenance can be done remotely by modem. The annual charge for software maintenance may be as much as 25 percent of the original cost of the software.

Summary of Software Considerations

The selection of specific application software is the most important decision to be made in implementing a medical office computer system. The functionality of this software should prevail over nearly all other considerations. Nevertheless, important differences in competing software packages may suggest inherent advantages or disadvantages of a given software package. Relevant considerations include (1) whether the software is multiuser, multitasking, or network based; (2) the operating system being used; and (3) the higher-level language in which the application is ac-

tually written. However, all of the above considerations will be irrelevant if the chosen software system is not properly matched to the hardware and if expert and experienced help is not available when needed.

Medical Office Business System

The essence of a system for the management of the business of the medical office is the establishment and maintenance of a database augmented by a mechanism for control of accounts receivable. The database will include demographic information relating to each patient, guarantor (the person responsible for payment of the patient account) information, employment and insurance information, and any codes that indicate circumstances that require special processing. Each time a patient encounter occurs, information will be entered regarding the date of the encounter, a code for the diagnosis, a code for the procedure performed or nature of the encounter, and appropriate financial or medical information. This database will then be utilized to generate bills, produce completed insurance forms or transfer the insurance information electronically, generate data to facilitate follow-up on outstanding balances, generate appropriate business reports, track delinquent insurance claims, etc. Following is a discussion of specific issues that will need to be considered in the control of some of the more common functions relating to this database.

Posting of Accounts Receivable

This operation is the equivalent of manually posting a charge to a patient ledger or making an entry into a single-entry pegboard accounting system. A well-conceived computer-based system permits many of the manual functions to be automated and properly provides a third-party payer with all of the relevant information that may be required by each individual payer. Most computer systems will permit maintenance of multiple fee schedules so that whether a patient is covered by Medicare, a private insurer, or a health maintenance organization (HMO) to whom a discount is extended, the proper charge will be entered automatically at the time of posting of a procedure code. A well-designed system should include security measures to ensure that there is an appropriate audit trail of any changes made to originally billed charges. There should be a facility for specifying those instances in which bills should not be submitted pending the patient's discharge from the hospital, pending receipt of payments from a primary insurer (before a second insurer is billed for the balance), or other special circumstances that commonly arise in contemporary medical economics.

Insurance Processing

Provisions should exist for specifying more than one insurer and distinguishing between third parties that will make payment irrespective of the patient's other available coverage as compared to balance billing in which a secondary insurer is only responsible for the payment of charges not covered by a primary insurer. A given third-party payer may have many different offices throughout the country to which insurance forms should be sent, depending upon the patient's employer. A well-designed system should be able to deal with these problems without user involvement.

Insurance forms should be generated only when desired and should not be computer generated until all required information is included. There must be a mechanism to identify those patients for whom proper and required information has not been entered and hence for whom proper forms will not be generated when otherwise expected.

Electronic claims submission is now available to a varying degree in many localities. Where available, this may result in improved speed of claim processing, less paperwork, and markedly reduced employee time for each claim.

There should be an automated system for tracking those forms submitted for which payment has not been received. An ideal system might supply a monthly report, by insurer, indicating the status of unpaid claims and suggesting that further follow-up is required or generating a letter of inquiry to the appropriate third-party payer.

Billing

The most efficient and inexpensive billing mechanism when a computer system is used is one in which a multipart statement is generated that includes a copy for retention in the office, a peel-open bill for the patient, and a return envelope. The only personnel requirement for processing that remains is for separating or bursting the individual bills, and this can be automated if the volume warrants it. Some systems permit bills to be printed in order of zip code. This sorting may then qualify mailing for discount bulk mail postage depending upon the volume involved.

Collections

A computer system should offer the advantage of being able to customize the reports required to facilitate normal office collection procedures. Collection of delinquent accounts can be processed most effectively when similar categories of accounts can be dealt with at the same time. A computer should permit retrieval of questionable accounts by amount due, third-party payer (or individual patient), zip code, age of account, or any other characteristic that may facilitate the collection process. In many systems, such lists generated may then be linked to a word processing facility for generating personalized form collection letters tailored to the individual requirements of a specified retrieval characteristic.

Census of Hospitalized Patients

Most systems include some mechanism for generating this list. However, unless it is completely integrated with the discharge information in the database, and unless discharge information is promptly entered into the system, the lists generated will not be accurate. Many of the software modules attempting to accomplish this task are in essence a mini-database separate from the integrated system, with a single output report. This report can usually be prepared most efficiently in manual fashion outside the computer system.

Report Generation

All systems include a facility for the generation of numerous kinds of reports relating to the quality, demographic characteristics, financial results, patient diagnostic mix, or volume of a practice. Although there is a tendency to meticulously compare the attributes of one system to another in this regard, it is most likely that very few reports are necessary on any regular basis. Certain end-of-day, end-of-month, and end-of-year reports will be necessary both for hard-copy backup of the computer system and for monitoring of practice performance. Considerable thought should be given to the types of reports desired for this purpose so as to minimize the accumulation of unnecessary space-occupying printed matter.

Ad hoc reports may be extremely useful and provide a capability that is impossible without an automated system. Some examples would be (1) analysis of practice by zip code, (2) a summary of specific procedures of a given type, (3) a listing of all patients on a given drug (in the event of drug recall), (4) listing of all patients with a given diagnosis (in the event of availability of a new medication or procedure), or (5) listing of all referring doctors with numbers of referrals by each. The limiting factor in the capability for a system to be useful in this regard is that the data desired must be contained in the database; furthermore, the system must have the capability for specifying retrieval of a report with the specifications desired. A desirable capability in a practice system would be a simple report-generation language such that the operator could custom design certain reports not previously contemplated.

It is desirable for all reports to be generated on standard letter-size perforated computer paper. Nearly all printers have the capability of generating compressed and regular print of multiple font size so that otherwise wide reports can fit on $8\frac{1}{2}$-in.-wide paper. If this is desired, the software must be capable of specifying appropriate font changes to manage wide reports.

Appointment Scheduling

This is one of the most controversial uses of an office system. One reason is that it is difficult to improve upon many standard practice appointment books readily available at low cost. Nevertheless, with the evolving trend of a marked increase in outpatient diagnostic evaluation, more and more information must be accumulated and be readily available to front-desk office personnel to properly manage time allocated to individual patients and to anticipate reports, x-ray studies, etc., that will need to be available when a patient is seen.

Well-designed software for this task can permit initial entry and updating or modification of this information prior to a patient's arrival so as to minimize delay in the handling of a patient within the office. A well-conceived system will require the entry of minimal information on an established patient, so that entry required by the operator can be quickly accomplished. There should be no need to reenter the patient telephone number, diagnosis, or other already captured information each time a patient schedules an appointment. Automatic generation of a daily appointment listing with necessary notes can eliminate otherwise boring clerical tasks. Many appointment software modules include a facility for tracking patients who fail to report for their appointment.

It is essential that those who will be using this software module personally test it prior to purchase or implementation. Many of the programs offered for this purpose fail to properly utilize graphic and other necessary interfaces that are essential if scheduling by computer is truly to be an improvement over a manual system.

Payroll and Accounts Payable

These items are discussed together because the same principles apply. Unless there are more than 15 employees, or there are unusual volumes of checks issued, these office procedures are most efficiently managed by a manual system. Neither of these office functions utilizes the database required for all of the previously discussed functions. An additional requirement for these functions would be either a dedicated printer for processing of checks or the requirement to manually change from paper to printed checks whenever a check is to be generated.

Correspondence and Word Processing

If the correspondence in the neurosurgical office is confined to letters to referring doctors and comparable correspondence, computer-based word processing will have limited advantage. It will provide for automated correction of common spelling and grammatical errors, a consistent letter format, and the time-saving feature of storage of names and addresses of frequent or occasional correspondents. Because most such letters are rarely edited, the primary advantage of word processing is not applicable.

If manuscripts, edited letters of substantial length, and other edited typewritten output are regularly produced, then the editing capabilities of word processors may prove to be an efficient tool in the office. Word processors can be utilized effectively to create patient-specific educational materials, the personal nature of which could enhance its effectiveness. A word processor integrated with an office management system could automatically prepare personal patient records for forwarding to referral sources, summaries of active and past diagnoses, drug history, allergies, and other useful personal medical information that could be readily stored independent of a more cumbersome complete patient medical record.

Many medical office systems may include a word processing module. Most such software is substantially inferior in quality and capability to that available very inexpensively in dedicated word processor software. If the office application software cannot directly accommodate available word processing software it may be desirable to purchase an inexpensive separate computer system solely for word processing with the capability of also including other readily available and useful software not logically integrated with the office system. An alternative is to adopt a hybrid configuration in which a dedicated MS-DOS (or other) computer may be attached, by software emulation, to the office computer system as a standard terminal for the system. Such a system could also be used *off line* as a stand-alone independent computer system for its word processing, spreadsheet, or other nonintegrated functions. Not to be ignored in considering the advantages of computer-based word processing in all functions for which it is applicable are the extreme legibility, absence of spelling errors, and other mundane advantages offered by this technology.

Computerized Patient Medical Record

Weed first introduced the concept of the problem-oriented medical record. The natural evolution of this concept was an attempt to structure these objectively recorded data to make the information amenable to computer storage and retrieval.[16] Numerous systems have since been developed in an attempt to computerize the medical record.[7] Although many office computer systems offer a medical record software module, most such systems do not accomplish this in a cost-effective, efficient, or useful manner. There is much discussion that the automated medical record is a necessity for the future, but evidence for this is lacking. The obstacles to this at present include the enormous data storage requirements, unacceptably rigid input requirements (if retrieved information is to be presented in a meaningful way), and the human factor of variation in physician training and work habits.

The current trend of substantial national regulatory pressure for quality assurance is a difficult issue with which all hospital medical staffs are currently grappling. When appropriate principles for this process are defined, it is not difficult to imagine that pressure will rapidly develop for a similar process in the practicing physician's office. In such an environment, some form of computerized medical record will be inevitable if only to permit automated generation of required audit data.[9]

There have been many programs developed that permit the patient to input information or respond to questions posed by a computer for the purpose of health-risk appraisal or to acquire a patient profile or history. Although such programs can be very useful to the physician, patient response to such systems has not been consistently favorable. The problem is not patient opposition to such a system of information acquisition. Rather, the time and effort to instruct a patient in use of the input device, mechanical problems with the device, and other similar difficulties have impeded broad acceptance. Physicians have also been reluctant to accept information generated in this fashion and have attempted to verbally verify the computer-generated history so that much of the potential efficiency of such a system is obviated.

In the absence of a complex formal patient medical record system, many office business systems offer the capability to maintain a mini medical record to include active and past diagnoses, social and family history, a summary of services rendered and procedures performed, immunization and drug history, and linear graphic analyses of relevant past laboratory data.

Auxiliary Neurosurgical Practice Applications

Telecommunication Access to Remote Databases

One of the most professionally useful applications for a computer is its ability via telecommunications to gain access to nationally available databases.[2,12] In recent years, most physicians desiring a literature search have learned the efficacy of a computer search of MEDLINE as compared to manually researching the same information through the *Index Medicus*. Until recently, such searches were generally performed through a medical librarian. A private individual can subscribe to MEDLINE and gain similar access. The lexicon required to communicate directly with this bibliographic database can be difficult to learn, and hence several other companies and institutions have developed a simpler language interface so that physicians and other users can communicate with a program that accepts commands in a more familiar jargon and then translates the request into MEDLINE-acceptable commands.[3] Two recent commercial ventures, BRS COLLEAGUE (Saunders) and MEDIS (Mead Data Central), have taken this a step further and make available by computer access a detailed outline or the full text of journal articles.

Utilizing telecommunications software, an office or personal computer at home can now be used to access additional databases for medical and other applications. The AMA has established the AMA Network (AMANET), which offers access to a variety of pharmaceutical, drug interaction, bibliographic, and other databases. The National Cancer Institute maintains a program providing information on currently active chemotherapy and other cancer treatment protocols. A neurosurgery bulletin board (NeuroSIG), distributed on the Compuserve information service network, has been recently established as a neurosurgical forum for the exchange of ideas, posting of information, and the acquisition of public domain software.

Access to many of the above services requires payment of a fee, often quite nominal for the service provided. The only hardware and software required to permit telecommunications access are a modem and appropriate widely available telecommunications software.

At least one company has recently introduced a service for the transmission of MRI and CT images to a central office for neuroradiology consultation. Whether this proves to be a useful service, it serves to illustrate a currently available technology that could be used to permit exchange of information between interested parties, seek quick consultation from colleagues or remote experts, and even to transmit images for remote conferences or submission of manuscripts. A potential competing system exists in rapidly evolving facsimile technology that may permit similar information to be sent with greater resolution.

Some hospitals are making available a database of laboratory and radiology reports so that the neurosurgery office may have direct access to patient data without the current delays inherent in existing personal telephone communication. There are even a few hospitals experimenting with scheduling for the operating room directly from the neurosurgeon's office via computer-to-computer communications. Given the capabilities demonstrated thus far in computer-to-computer telecommunications, it is not difficult to imagine the future utility inherent in this technology.

Continuing Education and Self-Assessment

Numerous research projects and commercial offerings have sought to offer the medium of the personal computer as a medical educational device and personal information system.[5] Typically, a format comparable to that offered in print media but with increased use of a question-and-answer format has been utilized. Often there are rudiments of artificial intelligence techniques incorporated to permit branching to one of multiple areas of further interest depending upon a given response. The nearly exclusive use of text has limited the educational potential, and in instances where information on the computer screen has been supplemented by accompanying graphic images, the advantage over a comparable printed medium is arguable. Nevertheless, the effectiveness of computer-assisted learning has been demonstrated.[4] The most effective programs to date have been simulations of clinical encounters. Well-designed simulations can be stimulating, challenging, and informative.[1]

A recent advance in computer storage capacity, the laser CD-ROM (compact disk–read-only memory), permits storage of up to 106,000 pages of text or very high quality graphic images on a compact disk comparable to that used for audio reproduction.[17,18] Authoring systems are being developed that permit extremely rapid random access to the stored images and that can integrate text and images on a single screen (Heilbrun MP. Personal communication, 1988). The quality of reproduction on currently available equipment is exceptional, permitting accurate interpretation of such items as pathology slides or radiographic [including computed tomographic (CT) and magnetic resonance (MR)] images. Several companies are offering MEDLINE on CD-ROM.

An interactive video-based intelligent tutoring system may be a useful adjunct to residency and other clinically based medical curricula.[10] Such a system would offer the capability of presenting didactic information in uniform fashion to sequential groups of students or residents and also offer an efficient means of introducing new information and deleting that which is obsolete. A good demonstration of such a system is not presently available.

This technology also offers the possibility of storage of vast amounts of reference material in a very small area. The volumes of this textbook would occupy less than 10 percent of a single CD-ROM. Large amounts of reference material with extremely sophisticated indexing capabilities could be stored on a single CD-ROM.

The use of an office or personal computer for continuing self-examination, such that SESAP or SANS could be self-administered via this medium, offers many possibilities for enhancement of the learning experience. The substantial instant analytical capabilities inherent in a computer-administered examination, combined with the graphic capabilities, raises the possibility that written certifying examinations could be administered by this medium. The National Board of Medical Examiners has been working on just such a project for the past 20 years, and that effort is soon to become reality.[8]

Medical Diagnosis

For at least the past 25 years, researchers have attempted to implement a computer-based medical diagnostic system.[13] There is an extensive literature in this regard that nevertheless to date fails to justify this application. A related endeavor has been that of attempting to accurately assess statistical probabilities relating to prognosis in various disease states.[15] Most such work has been an attempt to determine the quantitative risk of assorted variables and then by differential equations to arrive at an overall assessment of statistical probability of a specific disease state or complication thereof. It seems that an attempt to properly index the vast medical literature in any given area with respect to the specific statistical studies available from the accumulated medical literature could serve as a much more accurate source of statistical information frequently sought by patients and lacking in accurate recall by physicians. Such a compendium would lend itself to computer indexing and storage and could be a valuable source of accurate clinical information to supplement text more conveniently obtained in standard book form.

Cost of Medical Office Computer Systems

There is wide variation in the cost of computer systems, only some of which is related to the quality of the hardware and software provided. There are now significant competitive pressures as a result of a substantial number of national vendors offering comparable systems, in addition to unknown numbers of small regional and local computer firms that have developed their own systems. In an attempt to offer some guidelines regarding the cost of a system the following assumptions are made: (1) the system is designed to accommodate more than one user working simultaneously; (2) the system may be configured for as little as a single operator on a single terminal, or for up to a combination of 16 I/O devices; (3) the specific computer and microprocessor used as well as the size of main memory and bulk storage and type of backup device will be configured for the number of physicians in the office; (4) specifications are for a neurosurgical office (i.e., a smaller number of individual transactions as compared to a primary care office); (5) hardware installation (including cables, conduit, etc.) and initial software configu-

ration are included; and (6) the cost of the initial training of all users is included but not the cost of consumable supplies such as paper, statements, etc. The assumptions regarding software are that a basic medical office accounts receivable package includes insurance processing and billing but does not include electronic claims submission. Appointment scheduling is assumed to be included for any system of more than one physician. Medical records modules, word processing, and other auxiliary software discussed earlier are not included. The cost of such a system for one physician should be less than $16,000. For two or three physicians, the cost is likely to be $10,000 per physician, and for each additional physician (up to a total of six), $5000 to $7000 should be added. Electronic claims capability or computerized medical records will add $1500 to $2500 for each module. Word processing, terminal emulation, spreadsheet, and other commercially available software will be in a range of $200 to $700 for each module. Annual hardware and software maintenance is likely to range from 10 to 20 percent of the purchase price. The cost of consumables (paper, insurance forms, statements, binders) will be related to the size of the practice. The largest expenses in this category will be multipart billing statements, which may run $0.12 to $0.40 each, and this expense will be significant in a large practice. The remaining consumable expense should be nominal.

If the system requires any software customization or if there are other charges not covered by hardware and software maintenance agreements, these expenses can be substantial and unpredictable.

Summary

One of the most important decisions to be made in considering an office computer system as an adjunct to neurosurgical practice is whether it is truly worthwhile. A computer will not correct any inherent deficiencies in the patterns of processing office business information. In a well-run office with more than one physician, it will expedite many mundane and repetitious functions and provide an improved method of handling others. If the current system for handling proposed computer functions is working but it would be faster or more convenient to do this by computer, then a good foundation has been established for successful implementation of a computer system. A system is not likely to impose stricter adherence to necessary but poorly or irregularly enforced office routines. It is not likely that there will be economy of office personnel by implementing a computer system, but individual productivity, efficiency, and accuracy may be enhanced.

In assessing the utility of a system, it is useful to categorize proposed office functions as essential, as contrasted to those that are desirable. It is best not to attempt total automation all at once but rather to establish priorities for automation and to implement one system at a time. The emphasis on the evaluation of a proposed system is best placed on the evaluation of function and usefulness of the software, and then on the attempt to select the best hardware options to implement those functions. The single most useful item in the selection of a system is the personal detailed experience of an existing user with a similar system purchased from and serviced by the proposed vendor.

There are many tempting applications available for a doctor's office computer system that tease the imagination of a scientific mind. All, however, require personal involvement of the physician or a well-trained and similarly interested employee if they are to be useful. Most of these applications are of special purpose interest, and unless there is a firm and ongoing commitment to the particular activity involved, the use of the computer for that application will likely fall into disuse and the user of the software will likely forget how to use it. The use of the office computer for mundane business functions is by far the most likely and reasonable justification for purchase of an office computer system, and other applications are best thought of as utility functions of potential value.

Evolving desktop hardware with powerful graphic capability and inexpensive massive storage capability, combined with evolving software technology, provides the capability for use of the office or personal computer as a personal learning center.

The cost of a system, including installation and training but not maintenance, is in the range of $10,000 per physician for two to six physicians (somewhat more at the low end and less as the number of physicians increases). The most consistent cost justification is a lessening in accounts receivable through more consistent and accurate billing and insurance processing, and a more thorough follow-up on delinquent accounts. However, all of the advantages of a computer system may be neutralized by ineffective office procedures and personnel.

References

1. Barnett GO, Hoffer EP, Famiglietti KT. Computers in medical education: present and future. In: Dayhoff RE (ed.), *Proceedings of the Seventh Annual Symposium on Computer Applications in Medical Care*. Silver Spring, MD, IEEE Computer Society Press, 1983: 11–13.
2. Haynes RB, McKibbon KA, Fitzgerald D, et al. How to keep up with the medical literature: V. Access by personal computer to the medical literature. *Ann Intern Med* 1986; 105:810–816.
3. Horowitz GL, Bleich HL. Paperchase: a computer program to search the medical literature. *N Engl J Med* 1981; 305:924–930.
4. Jamison D, Suppes P, Wells S. The effectiveness of alternative instructional media: a survey. *Rev Educ Res* 1974; 44:1–15.
5. Johnson DC, Barnett GO. MEDINFO: a medical information system. *Comput Programs Biomed* 1977; 7:191–201.
6. Mayo GE, Ball MJ. How to select a computerized medical office practice system. *Dis Mon* 1988; 34:4–51.
7. McDonald CJ, Tierney WM. Computer-stored medical records: their future role in medical practice. *JAMA* 1988; 259:3433–3440.
8. Melnick DE. Patient simulation: the computer based examination. In: Ackerman MJ (ed.), *Proceedings of the Ninth Annual Symposium on Computer Applications in Medical Care*. Washington, IEEE Computer Society Press, 1985: 603.
9. Miller PL, Berry TJ. Use of computers in studying quality of care. *QRB* 1980; 6:25–29.
10. Piemme TE. Computer-assisted learning and evaluation in medicine. *JAMA* 1988; 260:367–372.
11. Preece J. *The Use of Computers in General Practice*. New York, Churchill Livingstone, 1983.
12. Scheidt SS, Goldstein H, Blackburn LS. Application of the office or home computer to searching the medical literature. *J Am Coll Cardiol* 1986; 8:1211–1217.
13. Schwartz WB. Medicine and the computer: the promise and problems of change. *N Engl J Med* 1970; 283:1257–1264.
14. Sellars D. *Computerizing Your Medical Office: A Guide for Physicians and Their Staffs*. Oradell, NJ, Medical Economics Books, 1983.
15. Siegel JH, Williams JB. A computer based index for the prediction of operative survival in patients with cirrhosis and portal hypertension. *Ann Surg* 1969; 169:191–201.
16. Weed LL. New premises and new tools for medical education. *Mobius* 1982; 2:24–33.
17. Wertz RK. CD-ROM: a new advance in medical information retrieval. *JAMA* 1986; 256:3376–3378.
18. Wigton RS. The new knowledge bases: CD-ROM and medicine. *MD Comput* 1987; 4:34–38.

11

Treatment of Hemifacial Spasm and Essential Blepharospasm with Botulinum Toxin

Jonathan J. Dutton

Essential blepharospasm is a variably progressive, bilateral, involuntary focal dyskinesia involving the orbicularis oculi muscles. The etiology remains unknown.[9] It is characterized by repetitive, spasmodic, involuntary closure of the eyelids which may vary from increased frequency of blinking to forceful, sustained contraction resulting in functional blindness. Essential blepharospasm is often associated with, and may progress to, Meige's syndrome, a form of craniocervical dystonia involving abnormal eyelid, facial, and oromandibular movements.[6] Although a number of medical and surgical treatments are available for the control of symptoms, there is no known cure for the disease, and no therapy has proved to be consistently effective or long-lasting.

Hemifacial spasm is characterized by unilateral hyperkinetic tonic spasms of muscles innervated by the seventh cranial nerve. In contrast with essential blepharospasm, in hemifacial spasm an anatomic cause appears to be responsible in many cases.[13] Although neurosurgical microvascular decompression at the seventh nerve root exit zone is highly successful in alleviating symptoms, most patients are still treated medically.

Botulinum Toxin

Since 1976, botulinum A toxin has been used in the management of strabismus by weakening opposing extraocular muscles.[18] In 1983, this drug became available for the treatment of facial dystonias on a cooperative prospective clinical research protocol. To date, the results have been consistently impressive, and this drug has become the initial treatment of choice for patients with essential blepharospasm and Meige's syndrome.

Botulinum toxin is a potent inhibitor of transmission at the neuromuscular junction, where it binds irreversibly to presynaptic receptors. Here it interferes with calcium ion metabolism, preventing the release of acetylcholine.[10] Recovery of function occurs slowly over several months as new nerve terminals form on the postsynaptic motor end plate.

So far, purified lyophylized botulinum A toxin (Oculinum) is available only as part of a multicenter research protocol. It is diluted in saline immediately before injection. Patients are treated with 5.0 units (0.002 μg) of toxin in each of two sites per eyelid. The central upper lid is avoided in an attempt to prevent weakening of the levator muscle. An additional 5.0-unit dose is frequently given into the medial brow (procerus muscle) for control of brow spasms. A total dose of 20 to 25 units is typical for each eye, although some patients may require many times this dose for effect. Each injection is delivered in a 0.1-ml volume and is administered subcutaneously or intramuscularly.

Results of Treatment

Nineteen published series have reported on the results of botulinum toxin in the treatment of blepharospasm, with over 2500 injections in nearly 800 patients (Table 11-1).[1–5,7,8,11,12,14,15,17,19–21] In most published accounts, only 0 to 10 percent of patients fail to respond to botulinum chemical denervation. In general, 95 to 98 percent of patients will show measurable reduction in the intensity of orbicularis spasm. The onset of beneficial effect begins 2 to 5 days after toxin injection (Fig. 11-1). The overall mean duration of effect is about 13 weeks (range of means, 6.1 to 17.3 weeks) for each treatment. Although several studies report an increased duration of effect with increasing toxin dose,[7,19] this tendency has not been confirmed in larger series.[3] Patients who have had previous neurectomy or neuromyectomy also show no difference in duration of response. In most studies, hemifacial spasm patients obtain a significantly longer duration of effect (by 2 to 4 weeks) than those with essential blepharospasm,[3,7,20] although the reason for this remains elusive. Patients with Meige's syndrome obtain a significantly shorter response (by 1 to 2 weeks) than do those with essential blepharospasm.[3] Several studies report a decreasing duration of response with increasing treatment number.[5,7,21] However, Dutton and Buckley could show no significant change in duration for 8 successive treatments in 50 patients over a 2-year period, and for 12 repeated treatments in 20 patients over a 3-year period.[3]

About two-thirds of patients treated with botulinum toxin experience at least 75 percent reduction in their spasm intensity. Only 2 to 5 percent fail to show any response at all. The degree of response is similar in all diagnostic groups, and in most reports is not significantly altered with manipulation of toxin dose. Also, as with duration of effect, the degree of response does not seem to decline with increasing treatment number. Previous neurectomy or neuromyec-

138

TABLE 11-1 Summary of Previous Reports on Botulinum Toxin for the Treatment of Blepharospasm and Hemifacial Spasm*

Authors	Patients (No.)	Treatments (No.)	Diagnosis† EB	HS	MS	Sex (F:M)	Age Mean	Range	Response (%)	Mean Duration (wks)	Spasm Intensity‡ Before Treatment	After Treatment
Lingua 1985[12]	13	29	10	3	0	33:10	—	—	100	12	—	—
Scott et al. 1985[19]	39	124	36	0	3	—	—	—	—	9.9	—	—
Shorr et al. 1985[21]	22	57	8	5	9	14:8	—	32–80	—	6.1–12.3	3.3	0–1
Elston and Russell 1985[4]	34	89	6	0	28	22:12	64.0	38–78	97	11	—	—
Savino et al. 1985[17]	15	20	0	15	0	12:3	63.0	40–81	100	12.2	—	—
Frueh and Musch 1986[7]	48	116	42	6	0	31:17	—	38–82	94	11	—	—
Burns et al. 1986[1]	44	—	—	—	—	—	—	—	—	—	—	—
Cohen et al. 1986[2]	75	224	54	0	21	47:28	62.1	28–83	86	12.4	3.6	0.5
Perman et al. 1986[15]	28	56	28	0	0	17:11	55.9	29–80	96	12	—	—
Shore et al. 1986[20]	26	41	21	5	0	15:11	65.0	47–82	96	8.5	—	—
Gonnering 1986[8]	15	41	0	15	0	13:2	69.8	45–85	100	15.6	2.7	0.5
Kristan and Stasior 1987[11]	12	20	—	—	—	—	—	—	100	14.8	—	—
Engstrom et al. 1987[5]	76	220	—	—	—	—	—	—	95	16.7	—	—
Mauriello et al. 1987[14]	100	372	69	21	10	63:37	—	—	97	12.6–17.3	—	—
Dutton and Buckley 1988[3]	232	1044	145	60	27	167:65	62.2	23–88	97	13.3	3.2	0.7
Totals	779	2520	419	133	103	542:247	62.4	23–88	96.5	12.5	3.3	0.7

*Earlier reports which duplicate patients are omitted.
†EB = essential blepharospasm; HS = hemifacial spasm; MS = Meige's syndrome.
‡0 to 4+ scale where 0 = no spasms and 4+ = severe sustained spasms.

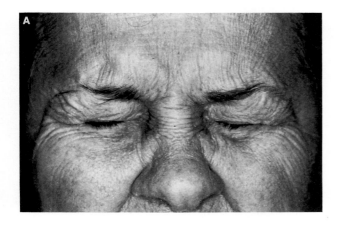

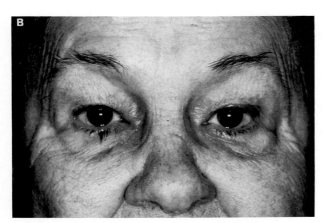

Figure 11-1 A patient with severe essential blepharospasm. *A.* Before treatment. *B.* Five days after injection with botulinum toxin, 25 units on each side.

tomy for blepharospasm does not alter the degree of response to botulinum toxin.[3]

Complications

Complications and side effects are seen in about 20 to 25 percent of all treatments with botulinum toxin, although in some series as many as 65 percent of patients experience adverse side effects. However, in most cases these are mild, local, and transient. The most frequent complications are dry eyes and upper eyelid ptosis (Table 11-2). Dry eyes and corneal exposure result from incomplete blinking caused by orbicularis muscle weakening. The overall rate of symptomatic dry eyes is reported at about 11 percent, although it is probably far more common and many patients are routinely placed on artificial tears after injection.

Upper eyelid ptosis is seen in about 12 percent of all treatments. In most cases it is minimal, amounting to only 1 to 2 mm, but in some cases it may be severe enough to cause visual disability. Ptosis results from weakening of the levator muscle when toxin is injected or diffuses behind the orbital septum. The levator muscle appears to be unusually sensitive to the effects of this toxin, since the superior rectus muscle lying in close approximation to it is almost never involved simultaneously. In all cases, however, the ptosis is transient, resolving over a 2- to 4-week period.

Photophobia and increased lacrimation are seen in 1 to 2 percent of cases. These symptoms seem to result from exposure due to incomplete blinking and to reduction in the efficiency of the lacrimal pump mechanism.

Entropion and ectropion have been reported in less than 1 percent of cases. They result from loss of orbicularis muscle tone, probably in association with excessively lax eyelids

TABLE 11-2　Reported Complications with Botulinum Toxin in the Treatment of Blepharospasm and Hemifacial Spasm (%)

Reference	Ptosis	Dry Eyes	Entropion/Ectropion	Diplopia	Facial Weakness
Lingua[12]	15	—	—	—	23
Scott et al.[19]	14.2	3.9	—	0.7	—
Shorr et al.[21]	—	65	—	—	—
Elston and Russell[4]	32	—	—	—	—
Savino et al.[17]	—	5	5	—	100
Frueh and Musch[7]	19.8	38.8	4.3	17.2	—
Burns et al.[1]	53	—	—	—	—
Cohen et al.[2]	9	3	1	2	—
Perman et al.[15]	—	—	—	—	—
Shore et al.[20]	14.6	9.8	—	—	—
Gonnering[8]	14.6	—	—	—	—
Kristan and Stasior[11]	35	—	—	—	—
Engstrom et al.[5]	—	—	—	—	—
Mauriello et al.[14]	12	12	0.8	0.3	—
Dutton and Buckley[3]	7.3	7.5	0.2	0.5	1.1
Totals	12.1	11.4	0.7	1.5	3.1

seen in many elderly patients. As with other complications, the effect is transient. Facial weakness and mouth droop are seen in less than 1 percent of patients receiving toxin into the orbicularis muscles alone. However, with toxin administration into the mid and lower face for hemifacial spasm and Meige's syndrome, the incidence of facial weakness climbs dramatically to about 11 percent,[3] and in some series is as high as 100 percent.[12,17] This complication can be minimized by injecting very small doses (0.5 to 1.0 unit) into each injection site and by not exceeding 5.0 units into the cheek or perioral region on each side.

Systemic side effects have been reported following toxin injection. These are very uncommon, noted in only 6 of 1044 cases by Dutton and Buckley.[3] These included generalized weakness lasting several weeks, generalized pruritus for 2 weeks, and nausea lasting 3 weeks. Sanders et al. reported measurable electromyographic effects in arm muscles within 24 h of toxin injection into the orbicularis muscles.[16] The significance of this and the long-term effects remain to be determined. No clinically significant long-term systemic effects have been seen in patients treated with up to 22 injections over a 5½-year period.

Conclusions

Botulinum toxin has proved to be a simple, safe, and effective therapy for a variety of facial dystonias. Although 3 to 5 percent of patients will ultimately require surgery for control of their symptoms, botulinum toxin is currently the initial treatment of choice for patients with essential blepharospasm and for those with hemifacial spasm who are not candidates for microvascular decompression of the seventh nerve. Complications are mild, local, and transient. The major drawback with botulinum toxin therapy is the need for repeated treatment (approximately every 3 months) for sustained effect.

References

1. Burns CL, Gammon JA, Gemmill MC. Ptosis associated with botulinum toxin treatment of strabismus and blepharospasm. *Ophthalmology* 1986; 93:1621–1627.

2. Cohen DA, Savino PJ, Stern MB, et al. Botulinum injection therapy for blepharospasm: a review and report of 75 patients. *Clin Neuropharmacol* 1986; 9:415–429.

3. Dutton JJ, Buckley EG. Long-term results and complications of botulinum A toxin in the treatment of blepharospasm. *Ophthalmology* 1988; 95:1529–1534.

4. Elston JS, Russell RWR. Effect of treatment with botulinum toxin on neurogenic blepharospasm. *Br Med J [Clin Res]* 1985; 290:1857–1859.

5. Engstrom PF, Arnoult JB, Mazow ML, et al. Effectiveness of botulinum toxin therapy for essential blepharospasm. *Ophthalmology* 1987; 94:971–975.

6. Fahn S. The varied clinical expressions of dystonia. *Neurol Clin* 1984; 2:541–554.

7. Frueh BR, Musch DC. Treatment of facial spasm with botulinum toxin: an interim report. *Ophthalmology* 1986; 93:917–923.

8. Gonnering RS. Treatment of hemifacial spasm with botulinum A toxin: results and rationale. *Ophthalmic Plast Reconstr Surg* 1986; 2:143–146.

9. Jankovic J, Orman J. Botulinum A toxin for cranial-cervical dystonia: a double-blind, placebo-controlled study. *Neurology* 1987; 37:616–623.

10. Kao I, Drachman DB, Price DL. Botulinum toxin: mechanism of presynaptic blockade. *Science* 1976; 193:1256–1258.

11. Kristan RW, Stasior OG. Treatment of blepharospasm with high dose brow injection of botulinum toxin. *Ophthalmic Plast Reconstr Surg* 1987; 3:25–27.

12. Lingua RW. Sequelae of botulinum toxin injection. *Am J Ophthalmol* 1985; 100:305–307.

13. Loeser JD, Chen J. Hemifacial spasm: treatment by microsurgical facial nerve decompression. *Neurosurgery* 1983; 13:141–146.

14. Mauriello JA Jr, Coniaris H, Haupt EJ. Use of botulinum toxin in the treatment of one hundred patients with facial dyskinesias. *Ophthalmology* 1987; 94:976–979.

15. Perman KI, Bayliss HI, Rosenbaum AL, et al. The use of botu-

linum toxin in the medical management of benign essential blepharospasm. *Ophthalmology* 1986; 93:1–3.

16. Sanders DB, Massey EW, Buckley EG. Botulinum toxin for blepharospasm: single-fiber EMG studies. *Neurology* 1986; 36:545–547.

17. Savino PJ, Sergott RC, Bosley TM, et al. Hemifacial spasm treated with botulinum A toxin injection. *Arch Ophthalmol* 1985; 103:1305–1306.

18. Scott AB. Botulinum toxin injection of eye muscles to correct strabismus. *Trans Am Ophthalmol Soc* 1981; 79:734–770.

19. Scott AB, Kennedy RA, Stubbs HA. Botulinum A toxin injection as a treatment for blepharospasm. *Arch Ophthalmol* 1985; 103:347–350.

20. Shore JW, Leone CR Jr, O'Connor PS, et al. Botulinum toxin for the treatment of essential blepharospasm. *Ophthalmic Surg* 1986; 17:747–753.

21. Shorr N, Seiff SR, Kopelman J. The use of botulinum toxin in blepharospasm. *Am J Ophthalmol* 1985; 99:542–546.

12

Endovascular Therapy of Vascular Lesions of the Central Nervous System

Fernando Viñuela
Jacques E. Dion
Pedro Lylyk
Gary R. Duckwiler

Some intracranial or spinal vascular malformations, aneurysms or tumors may be treated by methods of intravascular catheterization and embolization. The recent manufacturing of soft microcatheters with better control allows navigation beyond the circle of Willis, into cerebral cortical or perforating arteries. Intravascular therapy of some brain and dural arteriovenous malformations and fistulae and/or intracranial aneurysms is a valuable alternative for those cases with a high surgical complication rate.

A thorough angiographic evaluation of intracranial vascular lesions is mandatory before selecting a delivery system or embolic material. The size and the location of the lesion are two important parameters that need to be considered when planning endovascular therapy. The function of the underlying brain is assessed by direct clinical examination and continuous computerized electroencephalographic monitoring. This functional monitoring is complemented by superselective catheterization of cerebral cortical or perforating arteries by a microcatheter, allowing a superselective angiogram and a better delineation of the angioarchitecture of the intracranial vascular lesion.

The purpose of this review is to introduce the techniques of intracranial superselective catheterization for the embolization of intracranial and intraspinal vascular malformations, fistulae, and aneurysms. The discussion will include an overview of delivery systems and embolic materials as well as postembolization morphologic results and technical complications. A section on angioplasty of brachiocephalic vessels and of intracranial angioplasty for treatment of arterial vasospasm will also be included.

Endovascular Therapy of Intracranial Aneurysms

Endovascular occlusion of intracranial aneurysms is an alternative therapy for aneurysms that are difficult to manage surgically. In cases of giant aneurysms it may be necessary to occlude the parent vessel to achieve aneurysm obliteration. Fox et al. reported their experience with the treatment of 68 patients with giant aneurysms by proximal artery occlusion with detachable balloons.[12] Their therapeutic protocol included preembolization assessment of the circle of Willis by angiography and by xenon blood flow studies, with the ultimate evaluation being the temporary test occlusion of the parent vessel under systemic heparinization. They reported a high success rate of aneurysm obliteration (75 percent) with a 1.5 percent permanent morbidity and no mortality.

Other interventional techniques include the insertion of small metallic coils[35] or balloons[22] within the aneurysm, preserving the parent artery (Fig. 12-1). It is important to rule out the presence of a fresh thrombus within the aneurysm before attempting to position the balloon within it. Magnetic resonance (MR) imaging is a suitable technique for assessment of intraluminal contents within giant aneurysms.[39] If fresh thrombus is discovered, the balloon embolization procedure needs to be delayed several weeks to allow clot lysis or organization.[14]

Positioning of the balloon requires gentle maneuvers and excellent fluoroscopy with road mapping capabilities (Fig. 12-2). To obtain permanent occlusion of the aneurysm, it is necessary to exchange the contrast material in the balloon with a polymer that will solidify in a relatively short time (15 to 30 min). Taki et al.[48] and Halbach et al.[14] have used 2-hydroxyethylmethacrylate (HEMA) to solidify the balloon before detachment. This technique of endovascular balloon occlusion of an aneurysm with preservation of the parent artery is attractive and encouraging, but it must be performed by an experienced team to decrease complications such as rupture of the aneurysm by balloon overinflation, balloon rupture with silicon embolization of intracranial vessels, and occlusion of intracranial vessels by a deflated balloon.[14,43] The development of new types of balloons and microcatheters and the centralization of these techniques in neurovascular centers with experience in intravascular intracranial navigation will improve and consolidate this therapeutic alternative for surgically difficult intracranial aneurysms.

Endovascular Therapy of Carotid-Cavernous Arteriovenous Fistulae

Endovascular occlusion of carotid-cavernous arteriovenous fistulae has become the treatment of choice as a result of its excellent clinical results, achieved with a low complication rate.[7] Intravascular occlusion of the fistula may be attempted using detachable balloons via an arterial or venous route or by direct surgical exposure of the cavernous sinus.

The most common approach is via the arterial route. The fistula can be occluded without compromising the flow in

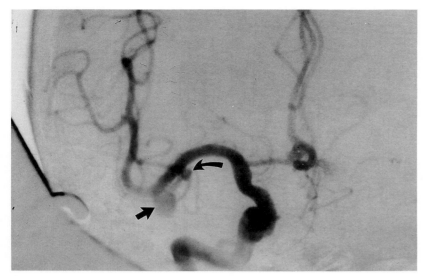

A

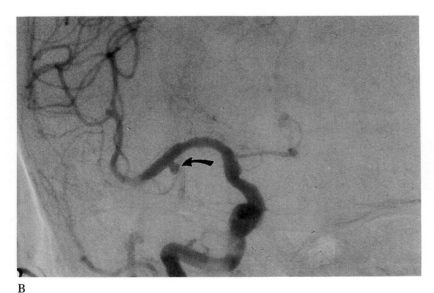

B

Figure 12-1 Balloon occlusion of middle cerebral artery aneurysm. *A*. Right internal carotid angiogram shows a right middle cerebral artery (MCA) trifurcation saccular aneurysm (*straight arrow*) and a smaller proximal aneurysm (*curved arrow*). *B*. Postembolization carotid angiogram shows balloon occlusion of the MCA trifurcation aneurysm with preservation of the MCA lumen and unchanged smaller aneurysm (*curved arrow*).

the internal carotid artery by depositing the detachable balloon in the cavernous sinus, at the fistula site (Fig. 12-3). When the arteriovenous fistula is small, one balloon is sufficient to occlude the fistula. In those cases with a large laceration or an enlarged cavernous sinus, it may be necessary to detach more than one balloon to achieve occlusion of the fistula. The detachment of multiple intracavernous balloons increases pressure in the cavernous sinus and may cause symptoms (cavernous sinus syndrome). These usually subside following the slow deflation of the balloons over the following weeks.[7] When a post-traumatic intimal dissection of the intracavernous portion of the internal carotid artery is identified, it may not be possible to preserve the lumen of the artery; such an intimal dissection is potentially dangerous (Fig. 12-4). The presence of an intraluminal intimal flap may be the source of intracranial embolization of cerebral

arteries. This dissection may be diagnosed by angiography, or it may be suspected if the patient develops severe retro-orbital pain when the balloon is inflated in the carotid lumen near the fistula site.

Intravascular detachment of balloons in a carotid-cavernous fistula by the arterial route may elicit technical complications such as occlusion of the internal carotid artery, intracranial balloon migration by early detachment or deflation, or development of arterial pseudoaneurysms by early balloon deflation.[7] The early balloon deflation may be enough to elicit thrombosis of the cavernous sinus around the balloon, but it leaves a cavity in communication with the arterial lumen.

The transvenous approach to the occlusion of cavernous-carotid fistulae was first described by Manelfe and Berenstein[32] and Debrun et al.[5] This approach may be used when

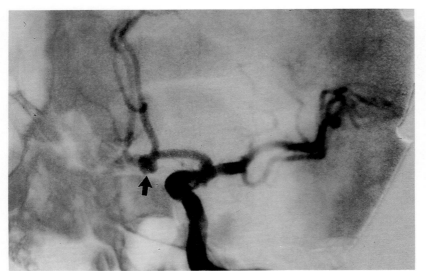

A

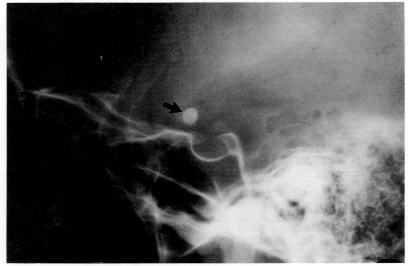

B

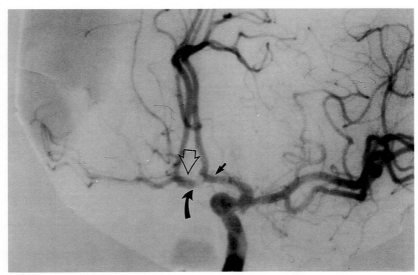

C

Figure 12-2 Balloon occlusion of anterior communicating artery aneurysm. *A.* Oblique left internal carotid angiogram shows a left A-1 anterior communicating artery aneurysm *(arrow)*. *B.* Lateral skull film shows a balloon within the aneurysm *(arrow)*, after detachment. *C.* Postembolization oblique left internal carotid angiogram shows balloon occlusion of the aneurysm *(curved arrow)* with preservation of the left anterior cerebral artery *(straight arrow)* and anterior communicating artery *(open arrow)*.

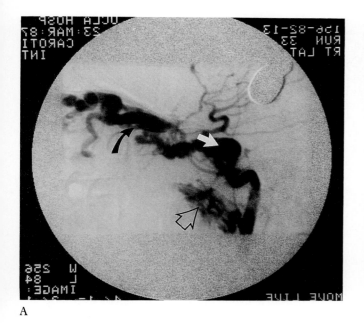
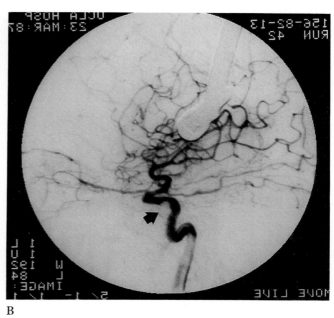

A   B

Figure 12-3 Endovascular occlusion of traumatic carotid-cavernous fistula (c-c fistula). *A.* Preembolization internal carotid angiogram shows a post-traumatic c-c fistula *(straight arrow)* draining through the superior ophthalmic vein *(curved arrow)* and sphenopalatine plexus *(open arrow).* *B.* Postembolization internal carotid angiogram shows balloon occlusion of the c-c fistula *(arrow)* with preservation of the internal carotid artery lumen.

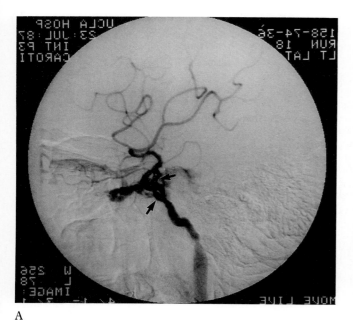
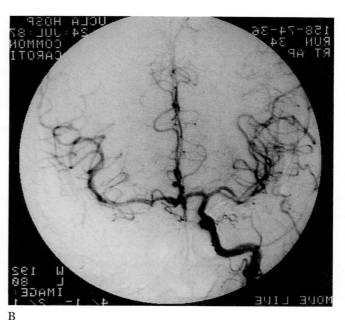

A   B

Figure 12-4 Traumatic carotid-cavernous fistula with arterial dissection. *A.* Preembolization internal carotid angiogram shows a c-c fistula with an irregular lumen of the intracavernous portion of the internal carotid artery. Note the change in caliber of the intrapetrous portion of the internal carotid artery as well as two abnormal communications with the cavernous sinus *(arrows).* The balloon navigation through the intrapetrous and intracavernous portions of the internal carotid artery was painful. *B.* Contralateral common carotid angiogram after balloon occlusion of c-c fistula and internal carotid artery shows nonvisualization of the fistula and satisfactory arterial cross-filling of the cerebral circulation.

the small size of the arterial laceration and the slow arteriovenous shunting preclude the passage of the balloon through the fistula from the arterial side. The inferior petrosal sinus may be selectively catheterized via the femoral vein or by internal jugular puncture in the neck. An introducer is positioned in the jugular bulb, with its tip pointing anteriorly and medially. The inferior petrosal sinus is then catheterized by using a microcatheter with or without a detachable balloon. It is possible to position a microcatheter in the cavernous sinus against the blood flow and deliver a detachable balloon, microcoils, or liquid agents at the fistula site.[16] By using this technique, one must not compromise the lumen of the inferior petrosal sinus without obliterating the arteriovenous fistula. The early occlusion of the inferior petrosal sinus may redirect the arteriovenous shunting into the superior ophthalmic vein and cause increased exophthalmos or into brain cortical veins which may cause intracerebral hemorrhage.[16] The superior ophthalmic vein has also been used to reach the cavernous sinus in cases of traumatic carotid-cavernous fistulae. It may be exposed surgically in the orbit,[49] or it may be catheterized by a transfemoral approach via an enlarged angular vein.[16]

The direct surgical exposure of the cavernous sinus can be used in those cases of failure of the transfemoral arterial or venous approach.[27,34] Various embolic materials may be introduced into the cavernous sinus by direct intraoperative puncture (balloons, coils, silk, muscle, liquid agents).

Traumatic arteriovenous fistulae of vessels in the neck may also be treated by an endovascular route by using detachable balloons or coils. The most frequent vessel involved is the vertebral artery.[11,15] It is possible to occlude the arteriovenous fistula while preserving blood flow in the parent artery. Epidural varices associated with high flow arteriovenous fistulae often cause compression of the spinal cord. This type of fistula may be difficult to occlude because it recruits numerous collaterals from ipsilateral and contralateral branches of the subclavian artery. If a postembolization recruitment of collateral is noted, surgical therapy of the residual arteriovenous fistula should be strongly considered before enlargement of the collateral feeders occurs.[11] Complex spontaneous or traumatic vertebral fistulae may be associated with vascular dysplasias, such as neurofibromatosis[4] or fibromuscular dysplasia.[21] In these cases, it may be difficult to preserve the lumen of the vertebral artery at the fistula site because of the generalized dysplasia of this vessel.

Endovascular Therapy of Spontaneous Intracranial Arteriovenous Fistulae

An arteriovenous fistula is an abnormal communication between an artery and a vein without an intervening capillary network. It may be solitary or it may be associated with other vascular malformations.[59] Clinically, patients have intracranial hemorrhage, mass effect caused by a large varix, brain atrophy, or calcifications. A giant varix is the most noticeable angiographic and pathologic finding.[56]

The most common example of this type of vascular malformation is the aneurysm of the vein of Galen. Its clinical presentation varies with age and includes a loud intracranial

bruit with massive cardiac failure in newborns; moderate heart failure and hydrocephalus in infants and children; and seizures, mild hydrocephalus, and (rarely) subarachnoid hemorrhage in adults. The sudden surgical or endovascular occlusion of the intracranial arteriovenous fistulae can elicit uncontrollable biventricular cardiac failure. This clinical complication may be avoided if the occlusion of the arteriovenous fistulae is achieved in stages.

The angiographic evaluation of vein of Galen aneurysms shows that they may be related to direct arteriovenous fistulae in the wall of the vein of Galen or they may be related to arteriovenous malformations of the diencephalon or mesencephalon. The first group is the one that benefits most from endovascular embolization. It may be performed by the femoral route or by direct surgical exposure of the torcular and catheterization of the straight sinus.

The small size of the femoral artery in newborns and infants may preclude the use of detachable balloon systems. However, Terbrugge et al. described a transfemoral technique capable of using small microcatheters with calibrated-leak balloons to embolize intracranial arteriovenous fistulae with isobutyl-2-cyanoacrylate (IBCA).[50] Vein of Galen aneurysms in children and adults can be treated by using the transfemoral route and detachable balloons. The surgical transtorcular approach was originally described by Hanner and Quisling.[19] Catheterization of the vein of Galen is performed through a small burr hole over the torcular. The vein of Galen is slowly occluded using Gianturco coils (Fig. 12-5). In many cases, more than one procedure is needed to achieve complete obliteration of the arteriovenous fistulae. This type of progressive embolization of vein of Galen aneurysms allows a better medical control of the resulting intracranial and systemic hemodynamic changes.

Giant intracranial varices due to spontaneous high flow arteriovenous fistulae may be found in other areas of the brain. Their most common clinical presentation includes subarachnoid hemorrhage, signs of central nervous system (CNS) compression, or diffuse increased intracranial pressure. They also may be treated by endovascular techniques alone or in combination with surgery.[56]

Endovascular Treatment of Arteriovenous Malformations of the Brain

Luessenhop and Spence reported the first embolization of a large arteriovenous malformation (AVM) of the brain using pellets injected from the cervical portion of the internal carotid artery.[31] This method is technically simple and allows the injection of beads of different caliber depending upon the diameter of the arteries supplying the malformation. Accidental, unpredictable embolization of normal arteries may occur, although the neurologic deficit that has been observed appears to be temporary.[64] This technique was found to be useful before surgery in large cortical AVMs or in those causing intractable seizures or progressive neurologic deficit.[63]

The purpose of endovascular embolization of brain AVMs using superselective catheterization of the arterial feeders is to occlude the nidus of the malformation while

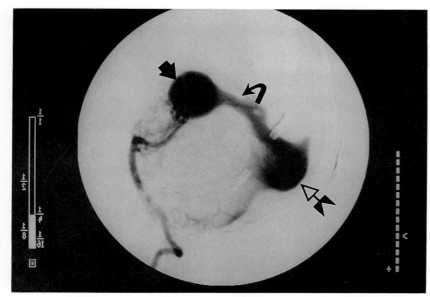

A

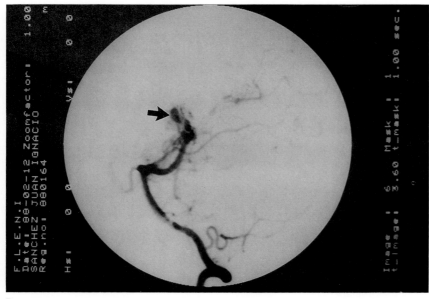

B

Figure 12-5 Transtorcular embolization of vein of Galen aneurysm. *A.* Preembolization left vertebral angiogram shows a vein of Galen aneurysm supplied by posterior choroidal arteries. The dilated vein of Galen *(straight arrow)*, straight sinus *(curved arrow)*, and torcular *(open arrow)* are well identified. Transtorcular deposition of 15 Gianturco coils was performed in two sessions, 2 weeks apart. *B.* Postembolization vertebral angiogram demonstrates obliteration of vein of Galen aneurysm with preservation of local vascular anatomy. Note stagnation *(arrow)* within the aneurysm.

preserving the arteries supplying the blood flow to the brain. The superselective catheterization of arterial feeders is achieved by using microcatheters inserted via the femoral route[55] or via the direct puncture of vessels in the neck,[44] or by craniotomy and direct exposure of the feeding arteries.[3] The patient is awake in most cases, allowing constant evaluation of brain function during the procedure. In AVMs involving eloquent areas of the brain such as motor, sensory, or speech cortex, the clinical evaluation is complemented by monitoring the electrical brain activity with computerized EEG.[8]

A preembolization superselective angiogram of each feeding artery provides anatomic and functional information not available on nonselective cerebral angiograms (Fig. 12-6).[58] A superselective angiogram is followed by a superselective Amytal test, consisting of the injection of 30 mg of amobarbital sodium (Amytal Sodium; Eli Lilly & Company, Indianapolis, IN) through the microcatheter. This test may produce a temporary neurologic deficit if the drug is injected into normal brain tissue. Because of the hemodynamic changes observed after partial obliteration of the AVM nidus, the Amytal injection must be repeated if more than one embolization is performed through the same feeding artery.

Different delivery systems of particles or liquid embolic agents may be used for transfemoral embolization of AVM

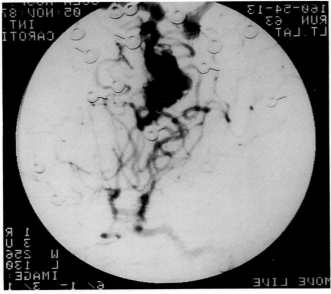

A

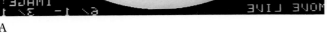

B

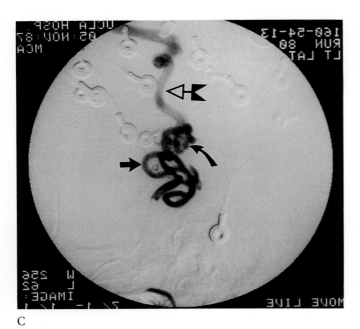

C

Figure 12-6 Embolization of an AVM of the brain. *A.* Internal carotid angiogram shows a posterior frontal AVM. *B.* Preembolization middle cerebral artery angiogram shows two posterior frontal feeders (*straight arrows*) supplying the AVM nidus (*curved arrow*). Two large cortical veins (*open arrows*) drain into the superior sagittal sinus. The AVM was embolized with a mixture of Avitene, PVA, and 30 percent ethanol. *C.* Immediate postembolization superselective angiogram shows obliteration of most of the AVM nidus and the presence of a single arteriovenous fistula. The MCA (*straight arrow*), AV fistula (*curved arrow*), and draining vein (*open arrow*) are well identified. This AV fistula could not be depicted on previous angiograms.

feeders. A Silastic tubing requires a terminal calibrated-leak balloon to be positioned intracranially. New, recently developed exceptionally flexible microcatheters can be used with fine, atraumatic guide wires, and they respond accurately to manual control (Fig. 12-7). It is possible to direct the catheter tip into different cortical vessels by manipulating the microwire.[58] This technical maneuver must be performed carefully to avoid damaging cerebral cortical or deep vessels. Some of these flexible microcatheters also respond promptly to changes in blood flow and they can be used without a guide wire.[8] Overall experience with these new delivery systems is promising. Preliminary results show anatomic improvements with less morbidity and mortality.[8] An important complication associated with the use of calibrated-leak balloons is rupture of an artery caused by balloon overinflation.[6] These new flexible catheters do not require a distal balloon to advance intracranially. The thorough clinical and electrical functional evaluation also plays an important role in the reduction of complications in endovascular embolization of intracranial vascular malformations.

Different embolic materials may be used to occlude an AVM. Preoperative occlusion of large arterial feeders by means of detachable balloons facilitates subsequent surgical removal by decreasing arterial pressure within the AVM

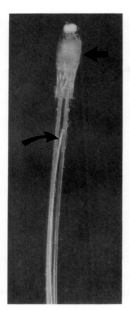

Figure 12-7 New microcatheter and micro-guide wire. Microcatheter from Target Therapeutics (used for super-selective catheterization of intracranial vessels). A small latex balloon (*straight arrow*) has been glued on its tip to make the catheter more sensitive to flow changes. This balloon cannot be inflated. A micro-guide wire is seen within the lumen of the microcatheter (*curved arrows*). This micro-guide wire is atraumatic and can be advanced intracranially.

nidus, therefore reducing blood loss and reducing the risk of postoperative breakthrough phenomena.[18,45] Spetzler et al. described the "normal perfusion pressure breakthrough theory" based on experimental findings: according to this, arteries around an AVM may be unable to constrict after protracted previous dilation.[46] Arterial pressure would then break through into the capillary bed, probably resulting in brain swelling and/or hemorrhage. These events still are the major complications in endovascular or surgical obliteration of brain AVMs. Arterial feeders may also be occluded by using microcoils delivered through microcatheters.

Other techniques of intravascular embolization of brain AVMs aim to occlude its nidus, which may then be followed by surgical resection. Particles of various substances, such as polyvinyl alcohol (PVA) foam, absorbable gelatin foam (Gelfoam; Upjohn Company, Kalamazoo, MI), or silk; a liquid adhesive such as IBCA; or mixtures such as a combination of particles of PVA foam and microfibrillar collagen (Avitene; Alcon Laboratories, Inc., Fort Worth, TX), and 30 percent ethanol may be injected through the microcatheters. The embolic material must be delivered in the core of the AVM nidus. Endovascular occlusion of an arterial feeder proximal to the location of the AVM nidus may be followed by the rapid development of a rich leptomeningeal, medullary, and transdural collateral circulation.[60] The delivery of the embolic material through the AVM nidus may produce an untoward occlusion of draining veins and lead to pulmonary emboli.

Complete occlusion of a brain AVM can be achieved with endovascular techniques. This mainly occurs in small AVMs with one to three pedicles.[60] In large or giant brain AVMs, the purpose of the embolization is to reduce the size of the lesion and the arteriovenous shunting, making otherwise inoperable AVMs amenable to surgical resection or radiotherapy (Fig. 12-8). Partial endovascular obliteration of large cortical AVMs may also prevent progression of symptoms in those patients presenting with a progressive neurologic deficit.[10] There is no evidence that partial endovascular occlusion of AVMs causing intracranial hemorrhage or intractable seizures produces significant changes in the course of the disease. In a few cases in which a substantial portion of the nidus of the AVM has been occluded, a progressive thrombosis and complete obliteration of the AVM nidus has been observed.[57]

The techniques of endovascular embolization of intracranial vascular malformations need to be performed by an experienced team because they carry an intrinsic risk of morbidity and/or mortality. Complications include rupture of an arterial feeder with consequent intracranial hemorrhage, occlusion of normal cortical arteries with cerebral ischemia or infarction, and the development of postembolization vasogenic edema. The authors' experience includes the endovascular embolization of 213 cerebral AVMs; 172 patients had large or giant cerebral AVMs supplied by multiple pedicles. The overall morbidity rate of the procedure was 12 percent (7 percent mild and 5 percent moderate to severe neurologic deficit). The mortality rate was 2.8 percent. Ninety-three patients had successful surgical removal of the AVM after embolization, with very low morbidity and mortality rates.

Endovascular Therapy of Dural Arteriovenous Malformations

The dura mater is supplied by a complex vascular network arising from meningeal branches of the external carotid, internal carotid, and vertebral arteries.[36,42] Spontaneous dural AVMs may be located anywhere in the dura mater but most commonly involve the cavernous, lateral, sigmoid, and superior sagittal sinuses. Dural AVMs are most frequent in adults and in many cases appear to develop as a result of the occlusion of a dural sinus.[26] The most common clinical presentation includes an intracranial bruit, symptoms related to increased intracranial pressure, and sometimes intracranial hemorrhage.[37] The venous drainage of spontaneous dural AVMs may account for unusual clinical manifestations of this disease. The recruitment of cortical veins increases the possibility of intracranial hemorrhage or compression of the neural axis by pial varices (Fig. 12-9).[13,61]

The techniques of superselective catheterization and embolization of meningeal vessels have improved the anatomic results while decreasing the complications (Fig. 12-10). Clinical improvement may be achieved in many cases, although a complete anatomic cure may be difficult to obtain. The anatomic results may be enhanced by using the transvenous approach. Halbach et al. described complete obliteration of dural AVMs of the cavernous sinus and trans-

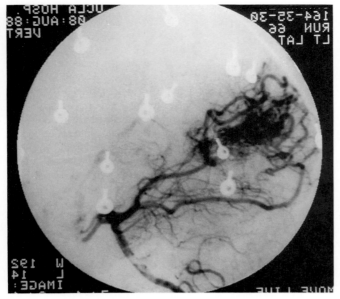

A

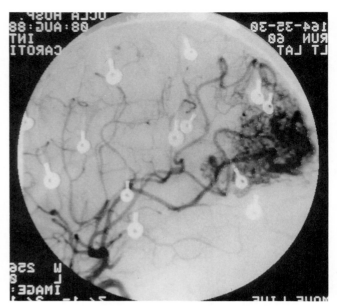

B

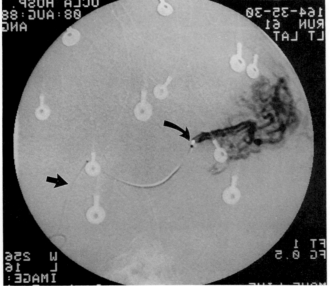

C

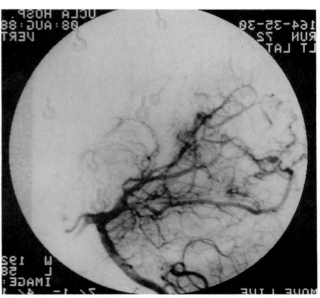

D

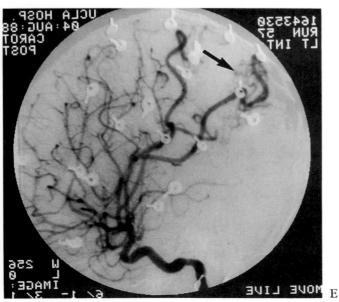

E

Figure 12-8 Presurgical embolization of large cortical AVM. Left vertebral (*A*) and left internal carotid (*B*) angiograms show a large left posterior temporoparietal AVM. *C.* Preembolization left posterior cerebral superselective angiogram shows the microcatheter in the basilar artery (*straight arrow*) with its tip (*curved arrow*) in a posterior temporoparietal feeder. *D.* Postembolization vertebral angiogram shows occlusion of the AVM with preservation of normal vascular anatomy. *E.* Postembolization internal carotid angiogram shows obliteration of most of the lesion with some residual AVM (*straight arrow*) supplied by a posterior parietal feeder. Successful surgical obliteration of the lesion was achieved 2 weeks after embolization.

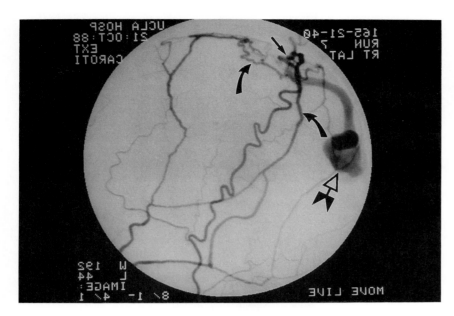

Figure 12-9 Dural AVM of the superior sagittal sinus with pial venous drainage. External carotid angiogram shows a dural arteriovenous fistula (*straight arrow*) between meningeal vessels (*curved arrows*) and a cortical varix (*open arrow*).

verse-sigmoid sinuses by using this route.[17] Catheterization of the cavernous sinus or transverse-sigmoid sinus may be achieved by a femoral route by using microcatheters (Fig. 12-11). Dural AVMs of the cavernous sinus may be embolized with microcoils, silk, or liquid agents.

Endovascular therapy of dural AVMs may cause complications such as blindness and/or stroke due to embolization through external carotid–internal carotid arterial communications.[30] A postembolization cranial nerve palsy may develop due to accidental embolization of neuromeningeal branches of the external carotid artery. These arteries supply the cranial nerves when they pierce the dura mater at the skull base or within the cavernous sinus.[29] Incomplete endovascular occlusion of dural AVMs with cortical venous drainage needs to be followed by a surgical exploration and resection of the residual AVM to eliminate the possibility of an intracranial hemorrhage.[40]

Endovascular Therapy of Spinal AVMs

AVMs of the spinal cord are usually classified according to their localization by selective spinal angiography into cervical, thoracic, and thoracolumbosacral groups. Spinal AVMs may be intramedullary, intradural-extramedullary, dural, or epidural in location.[33] Complete anatomic cure of spinal AVMs can be achieved by endovascular embolization. The most satisfactory results are observed in those patients with dural AVMs with medullary venous drainage.[28] Clinically, this type of AVM presents as a progressive myelopathy in patients 40 to 70 years old. These symptoms are produced by generalized venous hypertension in the spinal cord from recruitment of pedimedullary veins by the AVM. Not infrequently, selective endovascular occlusion of the dural arterial feeders is enough to obtain a clinical cure. These feeders arise from radiculomedullary arteries that can be catheterized selectively by using microcatheters. Small particles of

PVA foam, 100 to 200 μm in diameter, or liquid agents such as IBCA may be injected into the small dural feeders.[33] Surgical excision of the spinal dural AVM may be attempted if embolization is incomplete.[38]

Intramedullary spinal AVMs are also amenable to endovascular therapy. This procedure is regarded as dangerous because serious neurologic deficit may result from occlusion of the anterior spinal artery. Doppman et al. reported a spinal Amytal test as a method of predicting cord blood supply during arteriography or during embolization of critical vessels.[9] This test has the same principles as explained above in relation to the injection of Amytal into the arterial feeders of brain AVMs.

There has been a marked improvement in the techniques of selective catheterization of the anterior spinal artery, followed by temporary balloon occlusion or delivery of particles or liquid embolic agents into the nidus of the AVM. Significant clinical improvement and/or complete anatomic cure of intramedullary spinal AVMs have been reported.[25,41,51] The morbidity of the procedure can be decreased by monitoring somatosensory evoked potentials.[1]

Transluminal Angioplasty in Neuroradiology

Angioplasty can be performed on stenotic lesions of the origins of the main arterial trunks of the aortic arch. Stenotic lesions of the brachiocephalic vessels may be produced by arteriosclerosis and inflammatory lesions such as Takayasu's arteritis. Large balloons (up to 10 mm) are usually required because of the diameter of the vessels to be dilated. Vitek et al.[62] and Thèron[54] advocate the use of a second latex balloon, temporarily inflated distal to the angioplasty balloon, to prevent intracranial migration of plaque debris, usually in lesions of the common carotid or innominate arteries. An-

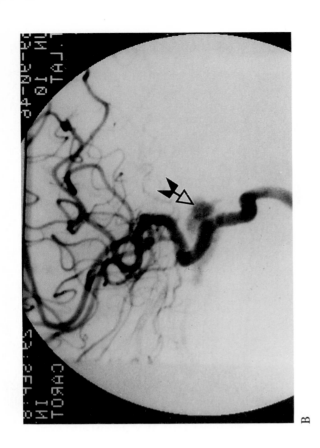

A

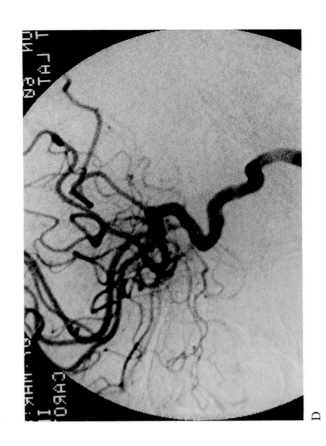

B

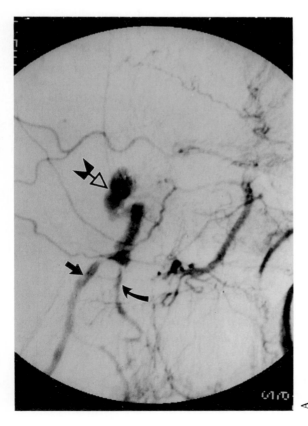

C

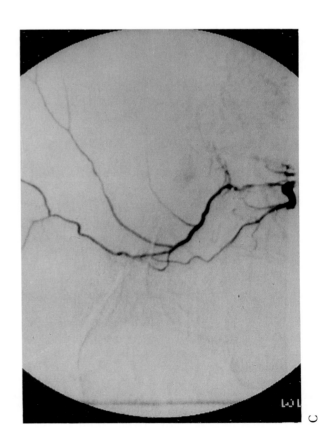

D

Figure 12-10 (*Opposite*) Spontaneous dural AVM of the cavernous sinus. External carotid (*A*) and internal carotid (*B*) angiograms show a spontaneous dural AVM of the cavernous sinus (*open arrow*) with preferential drainage through superior (*straight arrow*) and inferior (*curved arrow*) ophthalmic veins. Endovascular embolization of the external carotid artery branches was performed using PVA foam particles (200 to 300 µm). Postembolization external carotid (*C*) and internal carotid (*D*) angiograms show complete occlusion of the lesion.

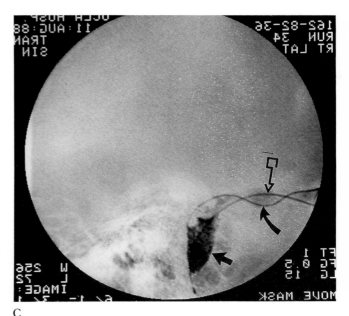

C

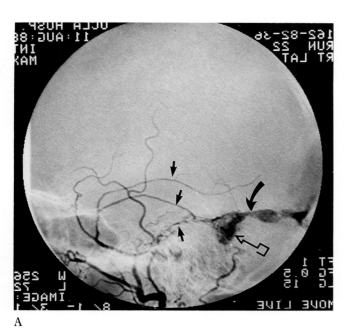

A

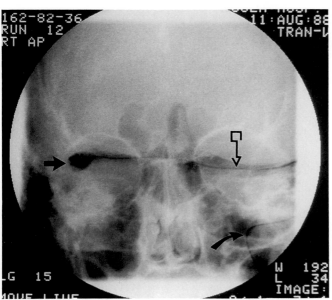

B

D

Figure 12-11 Transvenous embolization of dural AVM of the sigmoid sinus. *A.* Lateral external carotid angiogram shows a spontaneous dural AVM of the right transverse and sigmoid sinuses. Note meningeal feeders (*straight arrows*), stenosis of the transverse sinus (*curved arrow*), and occlusion of the sigmoid sinus (*square arrow*). *B.* A microcatheter has been positioned in the occluded right sigmoid sinus (*straight arrow*) via the left jugular vein (*curved arrow*) and left transverse sinus (*square arrow*). *C.* Right sigmoid sinugram before embolization with microcoils. The occluded right sigmoid sinus is well delineated with contrast material (*straight arrow*). The microcatheter is seen in the left (*curved arrow*) and right (*square arrow*) transverse sinuses. *D.* Postembolization right external carotid angiogram after delivery of 15 microcoils in the occluded sinus shows complete occlusion of the dural AVM.

gioplasty of the left subclavian artery, on the other hand, carries less risk of detachment of atherosclerotic material into the vertebral artery because it is usually associated with reversal of flow in the vertebral artery.[53]

Stenotic ostial lesions of the vertebral arteries are usually of a more fibrous nature and are usually not ulcerated. In cases of vertebrobasilar insufficiency caused by such lesions, these can be successfully and safely dilated. In the series of Courtheoux et al., clinical symptoms disappeared completely in 21 of 24 patients.[2]

Angioplasty of the common carotid artery, the external carotid artery, and the extracranial portion of the internal carotid artery has been performed by a number of groups for the treatment of atherosclerotic stenosis, Takayasu's arteritis, and fibromuscular dysplasia.[20,24,52] Brain protection with a temporarily inflated distal balloon is also recommended.[54]

Dilatation of atherosclerotic lesions of the intracranial vessels is generally considered relatively hazardous,[54] although successful cases have been reported, especially in the vertebrobasilar system.[47]

Zubkov et al. in Russia[65] and Higashida et al.[23] have recently described their excellent results with dilating focal and diffuse areas of vasospasm caused by subarachnoid hemorrhage in the intracranial circulation. They used a balloon composed of a soft silicone elastomer, which allows the balloon to elongate and conform to the vessel contour, without causing rupture. They were able to reverse neurologic deficits induced by spasm, which were refractory to medical therapy.

References

1. Berenstein A, Young W, Ransohoff J, et al. Somatosensory evoked potentials during spinal angiography and therapeutic transvascular embolization. *J Neurosurg* 1984; 60:777–785.
2. Courtheoux P, Tournade A, Thèron J, et al. Transcutaneous angioplasty of vertebral artery atheromatous ostial stricture. *Neuroradiology* 1985; 27:259–264.
3. Cromwell LD, Harris AB. Treatment of cerebral arteriovenous malformations: combined neurosurgical and neuroradiological approach. *J Neurosurg* 1980; 52:705–708.
4. Deans WR, Bloch S, Leibrock L, et al. Arteriovenous fistula in patients with neurofibromatosis. *Radiology* 1982; 144:103–107.
5. Debrun G, Lacour P, Viñuela F, et al. Treatment of 54 traumatic carotid-cavernous fistulas. *J Neurosurg* 1981; 55:678–692.
6. Debrun G, Viñuela F, Fox A, et al. Embolization of cerebral arteriovenous malformations with bucrylate: experience in 46 cases. *J Neurosurg* 1982; 56:615–627.
7. Debrun GM, Viñuela F, Fox AJ, et al. Indications for treatment and classification of 132 carotid-cavernous fistulas. *Neurosurgery* 1988; 22:285–289.
8. Dion JE, Viñuela F, Lylyk P, et al. Impact of recent technological advances on endovascular therapy of brain arteriovenous malformations and fistulas. Presented at the annual meeting of the Western Neuroradiological Society, Rancho Bernardo, CA, October 1988.
9. Doppman JL, Girton M, Oldfield EJ. Spinal Wada test. *Radiology* 1986; 161:319–321.
10. Fox AJ, Girvin JP, Viñuela F, et al. Rolandic arteriovenous malformations: improvement in limb function by IBC embolization. *AJNR* 1985; 6:575–582.
11. Fox AJ, Viñuela F, Pelz DM, et al. Vertebral and external carotid fistulas. *Semin Intervent Radiol* 1987; 4:249–260.
12. Fox AJ, Viñuela F, Pelz DM, et al. Use of detachable balloons for proximal artery occlusion in the treatment of unclippable cerebral aneurysms. *J Neurosurg* 1987; 66:40–46.
13. Gaston A, Chiras J, Bourbotte G, et al. Fistules artérioveineuses méningées à drainage veineux cortical. *J Neuroradiol* 1984; 11:161–177.
14. Halbach VV, Hieshima GB, Higashida RT. Treatment of intracranial aneurysms by balloon embolization. *Semin Intervent Radiol* 1987; 4:261–268.
15. Halbach VV, Higashida RT, Hieshima GB. Treatment of vertebral arteriovenous fistulas. *AJNR* 1987; 8:1121–1128.
16. Halbach VV, Higashida RT, Hieshima GB, et al. Transvenous embolization of direct carotid cavernous fistulas. *AJNR* 1988; 9:741–747.
17. Halbach VV, Higashida RT, Hieshima GB, et al. Transvenous embolization of dural AVMs. Presented at the annual meeting of the Western Neuroradiological Society. Rancho Bernardo, CA, October 1988.
18. Halbach VV, Higashida RT, Yang P, et al. Preoperative balloon occlusion of arteriovenous malformations. *Neurosurgery* 1988; 22:301–308.
19. Hanner JS, Quisling RG. Gianturco coil embolization of vein of Galen aneurysms: technical aspects. *Radiographics* 1988; 8:935–946.
20. Hasso AN, Bird CR, Zinke DE, et al. Fibromuscular dysplasia of the internal carotid artery: percutaneous transluminal angioplasty. *AJNR* 1981; 2:175–180.
21. Hieshima GB, Cahan LD, Mehringer CM, et al. Spontaneous arteriovenous fistulas of cerebral vessels in association with fibromuscular dysplasia. *Neurosurgery* 1986; 18:454–458.
22. Hieshima GB, Higashida RT, Halbach VV, et al. Intravascular balloon embolization of a carotid-ophthalmic artery aneurysm with preservation of the parent vessel. *AJNR* 1986; 7:916–918.
23. Higashida RT, Halbach VV, Brant-Zawadzki B, et al. Percutaneous transluminal angioplasty of arterial vasospasm using a new silicone microballoon device. Presented at the annual meeting of the Western Neuroradiological Society, Rancho Bernardo, CA, October 1988.
24. Higashida RT, Hieshima GB, Tsai FY, et al. Transluminal angioplasty of the vertebral and basilar artery. *AJNR* 1987; 8:745–749.
25. Horton JA, Latchaw RE, Gold LHA, et al. Embolization of intramedullary arteriovenous malformations of the spinal cord. *AJNR* 1986; 7:113–118.
26. Houser OW, Baker HL Jr, Rhoton AL Jr, et al. Intracranial dural arteriovenous malformations. *Radiology* 1972; 105:55–64.
27. Isamat F, Ferrer E, Twose J. Direct intracavernous obliteration of high-flow carotid-cavernous fistulas. *J Neurosurg* 1986; 65:770–775.
28. Kendall BE, Logue V. Spinal epidural angiomatous malformations draining into intrathecal veins. *Neuroradiology* 1977; 13:181–189.
29. Lasjaunias P. Aspect angiographique de la vascularisation des nerfs craniens. Presented at 4ème Congrès Annuel de la Société Française de Neuroradiologie, Toulouse, 1979.
30. Lasjaunias P, Merland JJ, Thèron J, et al. Vascularisation méningées de la fossa cérébrale moyenne. *J Neuroradiol* 1977; 4:361–384.
31. Luessenhop AJ, Spence WT. Artificial embolization of cerebral arteries: report of use in a case of arteriovenous malformation. *JAMA* 1960; 172:1153–1155.
32. Manelfe C, Berenstein A. Treatment of carotid-cavernous fistulas by venous approach: report of one case. *J Neuroradiol* 1980; 7:13–19.

33. Merland JJ, Reizine D. Treatment of arteriovenous spinal cord malformations. *Semin Intervent Radiol* 1987; 4:281–290.
34. Mullan S. Treatment of carotid-cavernous fistulas by cavernous sinus occlusion. *J Neurosurg* 1979; 50:131–144.
35. Mullan S, Raimondi AJ, Dobben V, et al. Electrically induced thrombosis in intracranial aneurysms. *J Neurosurg* 1965; 22:539–547.
36. Newton TH, Cronqvist S. Involvement of dural arteries in intracranial arteriovenous malformations. *Radiology* 1969; 93:1071–1078.
37. Obrador S, Soto M, Silvela J. Clinical syndromes of arteriovenous malformations of the transverse-sigmoid sinus. *J Neurol Neurosurg Psychiatry* 1975; 38:436–451.
38. Oldfield EH, Di Chiro G, Quindlen EA, et al. Successful treatment of a group of spinal cord arteriovenous malformations by interruption of dural fistula. *J Neurosurg* 1983; 59:1019–1030.
39. Olsen WL, Brant-Zawadzki M, Hodes J, et al. Giant intracranial aneurysms: MR imaging. *Radiology* 1987; 163:431–435.
40. Picard L, Bracard S, Moret J, et al. Spontaneous dural arteriovenous fistulas. *Semin Intervent Radiol* 1987; 4:219–241.
41. Riché MC, Melki JP, Merland JJ. Embolization of spinal cord vascular malformations via the anterior spinal artery. *AJNR* 1983; 4:378–381.
42. Roland J, Bernard C, Bracard S, et al. Microvascularization of the intracranial dura mater. *Surg Radiol Anat* 1987; 9:43–49.
43. Romodanov AP, Shcheglov VI. Intravascular occlusion of saccular aneurysms of the cerebral arteries by means of a detachable balloon catheter. In: Krayenbuhl H, Brihaye J, Loew F, et al. (eds.), *Advances and Technical Standards in Neurosurgery.* New York: Springer-Verlag, 1982; 9:25–49.
44. Rufenacht D, Merland JJ. Superselective catheterization using very flexible, formed catheters. *Acta Radiol [Suppl] (Stockh)* 1986; 369:600–602.
45. Serbinenko FA. Six hundred endovascular neurosurgical procedures in vascular pathology: a ten-year experience. *Acta Neurochir [Suppl] (Wien)* 1979; 28:310–311.
46. Spetzler RF, Wilson CB, Weinstein P, et al. Normal perfusion pressure breakthrough theory. *Clin Neurosurg* 1978; 25:651–672.
47. Sundt TM Jr, Smith HC, Campbell JK, et al. Transluminal angioplasty for basilar artery stenosis. *Mayo Clin Proc* 1980; 55:673–680.
48. Taki W, Handa H, Yamagata S, et al. Radiopaque solidifying liquids for releasable balloon technique: a technical note. *Surg Neurol* 1980; 13:140–142.
49. Teng MMH, Guo WY, Huang CI, et al. Occlusion of arteriovenous malformations of the cavernous sinus via the superior ophthalmic vein. *AJNR* 1988; 9:539–546.
50. Terbrugge K, Lasjaunias P, Chiu M, et al. Pediatric surgical neuroangiography: a multicentre approach. *Acta Radiol [Suppl] (Stockh)* 1986; 369:692–693.
51. Théron J, Cosgrove R, Melanson D, et al. Spinal arteriovenous malformations: advances in therapeutic embolization. *Radiology* 1986; 158:163–169.
52. Théron J, Courtheoux P, Henriet JP, et al. Angioplasty of supra-aortic arteries. *J Neuroradiol* 1984; 11:187–200.
53. Théron J, Melançon D, Ethier R. "Pre" subclavian steal syndromes and their treatment by angioplasty: hemodynamic classification of subclavian artery stenoses. *Neuroradiology* 1985; 27:265–270.
54. Théron JG. Angioplasty of supra-aortic arteries. *Semin Intervent Radiol* 1987; 4:331–342.
55. Viñuela F. Endovascular therapy of brain arteriovenous malformations. *Semin Intervent Radiol* 1987; 4:269–280.
56. Viñuela F, Drake CG, Fox AJ, et al. Giant intracranial varices secondary to high-flow arteriovenous fistulae. *J Neurosurg* 1987; 66:198–203.
57. Viñuela F, Fox AJ, Debrun G, et al. Progressive thrombosis of brain arteriovenous malformations after embolization with isobutyl-2-cyanoacrylate. *AJNR* 1983; 4:1233–1238.
58. Viñuela F, Fox AJ, Debrun G, et al. Preembolization superselective angiography: role in the treatment of brain arteriovenous malformations with isobutyl-2-cyanoacrylate. *AJNR* 1984; 5:765–769.
59. Viñuela F, Fox AJ, Pelz DM. Identification of arteriovenous fistulae in cerebral arteriovenous malformations: important therapeutic implications. *Acta Radiol [Suppl] (Stockh)* 1986; 369:770 (abstr.).
60. Viñuela F, Fox AJ, Pelz D, et al. Angiographic follow-up of large cerebral AVMs incompletely embolized with isobutyl-2-cyanoacrylate. *AJNR* 1986; 7:919–925.
61. Viñuela F, Fox AJ, Pelz DM, et al. Unusual clinical manifestations of dural arteriovenous malformations. *J Neurosurg* 1986; 64:554–558.
62. Vitek JJ, Raymon BC, Oh SJ. Innominate artery angioplasty. *AJNR* 1984; 5:113–114.
63. Wolpert SM, Barnett FJ, Prager RJ. Benefits of embolization without surgery for cerebral arteriovenous malformations. *AJNR* 1981; 2:535–538.
64. Wolpert SM, Stein BM. Factors governing the course of emboli in the therapeutic embolization of cerebral arteriovenous malformations. *Radiology* 1979; 131:125–131.
65. Zubkov YN, Nikiforov BM, Shustin VA. Balloon catheter technique for dilatation of constricted cerebral arteries after aneurysmal SAH. *Acta Neurochir (Wien)* 1984; 70:65–79.

13

Neurological Applications of Implanted Drug Pumps

Richard D. Penn

Drug pump technology provides a new mode of treatment for central nervous system (CNS) diseases. By implanting pumps with catheters going directly into the cerebrospinal fluid (CSF) or brain tissue, selective long-term regional perfusion can be achieved. Neurotransmitters and modulators, their agonists and antagonists, neurotrophic factors, immunomodulators, and many other substances which are potentially useful for treatment but which do not penetrate the blood-brain barrier can be utilized. The marked advantage of this method has been demonstrated clinically with the spinal perfusion of morphine for pain and baclofen (Lioresal; CIBA-Geigy Corp., Ardsley, NY) for spasticity. Other applications for Parkinson's disease and Alzheimer's disease are being actively investigated. As the biochemical bases of these and other diseases are better understood, the rationale for further drug trials will be developed. It is likely that neurosurgeons will have to become knowledgeable about these new treatments. The primary objective of this chapter is to present the basic principles of drug distribution in the CSF and brain tissues which underlie all the diverse applications and then present the two most successful applications, both of which illustrate these principles. Then future applications will be considered.

Advantages and Disadvantages of Implanted Pumps

Implantable drug pumps represent a convergence of two recent trends in drug administration. The first is continuous, long-term treatment outside the hospital, and the second is regional perfusion. The patient benefits from steady delivery of medication unrelated to the variables of absorption and the peaks and valleys of intermittent dosage, as well as from the direct delivery of the medicine to the target organ. In the case of CNS applications, another major ad-

vantage is circumventing the blood-brain barrier. The tight junctions between the endothelial cells of the brain capillaries effectively exclude any water-soluble drugs from penetrating. Only lipophilic agents readily cross these endothelial membranes. Some specific carrier-mediated systems also exist, but they are rarely important for drug delivery. One of the exceptions is L-dopa transport, but in this case competition from other amino acids in the blood results in variable penetration.[36]

The delivery of drug directly to the brain-CNS side of the barrier means that the route of distribution will be in CSF or brain tissue and elimination will be into capillaries and the superior sagittal sinus. In this brain-to-blood direction, lipid solubility again is important and lipophilic drugs will rapidly be absorbed before they are distributed in brain tissue.[11] Therefore, a criterion for choosing candidate drugs for CNS perfusion is low lipid solubility. The important point is that this is just what is needed, because water-soluble drugs are precisely the ones which cannot be effectively given systemically. They include many short neuropeptides and CNS transmitter agonists and antagonists. One strategy for introducing water-soluble drugs has been opening the blood-brain barrier with osmotic disruption. Because this is a nonselective technique, all substances which can diffuse down their concentration gradients from the blood into the brain are admitted. The use of a drug pump and catheter system achieves a way around the barrier which is selective.

Other advantages of implanted pumps relate to drug activity and toxicity. Direct CNS perfusion avoids many adverse factors such as metabolism and inactivation by peripheral organs and serum protein binding. Furthermore, the total dose is dramatically reduced and therefore the systemic toxicity is greatly reduced. As will be detailed when considering specific applications, the CNS concentration can be orders of magnitude higher when a drug is given directly rather than systemically. The infused CNS dose is usually eliminated into the venous circulation, so the total systemic dose will equal the amount directly perfused. For most applications this means that the systemic toxicity can be neglected because the dose is so low.

The converse is that direct perfusion of the CNS achieves a very high local concentration and can be neurotoxic when systemic administration is not. This is of particular concern with chemotherapy for brain tumors but may also be important for other drug therapies. However, even drugs which may seem innocuous may produce adverse CNS effects. Practically, this means that any new drug considered for direct infusion into the CNS must be studied carefully for neurotoxicity in animal models before human trials. Furthermore, a high concentration of a drug may produce unpredicted or previously undocumented physiologic effects. These may be useful therapeutically or may be deleterious. An example is a patient who developed severe dysesthesias and myoclonus with long-term intrathecal morphine administration but who had none of these side effects with oral morphine. Only intrathecal morphine helped his pain significantly, but the intrathecal therapy had to be stopped because of side effects due to high concentrations of spinal morphine.

Another disadvantage of direct perfusion is that it relies on catheter systems and mechanical pumps. These systems are bound to fail occasionally, and only surgical intervention can correct the problem. Although changing a pump or a catheter is an easy procedure under local anesthesia, it does have associated discomforts and risks, particularly that of infection. Obviously, any infected system has to be removed and meningitis is always a worry. Although experience has shown these risks to be low, the benefit from using a drug pump versus using a systemic treatment must be substantial to warrant its use.

Principles of Drug Distribution

Proper use of catheter systems to provide drugs to the CNS requires an understanding of the transportation of substances in the CSF and brain tissue. This is a complex subject, but a number of basic principles are well established. To simplify the presentation, distribution in the CSF will be considered first and distribution in tissue second. Ultimately, what is essential for an effect is the presence of the drug at its site of action at the receptor site, be it synaptic junction, neuronal or glial membrane, or endothelial cell. Details of these local sites of action vary with each drug and, if known, will be mentioned with specific applications later.

CSF

The rate of production of CSF in human beings is 0.3 ml/min into a ventricular and subarachnoid space of approximately 125 ml, so on the average the whole volume of CSF turns over five times a day.[12] This means that any drug placed in the CSF will rapidly be distributed and then eliminated into the systemic circulation. Good mixing occurs within the CSF due to the continuous arterial pulsations. This quickly distributes drugs from a point source such as a catheter.

When an inert water-soluble marker like ^{111}In is placed in the CSF, these flow characteristics are easily demonstrated by radionuclide scanning, as shown in Fig. 13-1. The marker was injected into the left lateral ventricle in a patient with Alzheimer's disease who was receiving bethanechol; it moved into both lateral ventricles and then down through the third and fourth ventricles and over the brain stem and convexities before being eliminated into the blood. A small amount was also seen in the spinal CSF (Fig. 13-1A). If the marker is introduced via a lumbar subarachnoid catheter (see Fig. 13-1B, the scan of a patient with severe spasticity with a lumbar subarachnoid catheter), the flow goes throughout the lumbar sac, then upward to the cisterna magna in approximately 3 h, and then over the convexities. As would be expected using this route, relatively little ^{111}In goes into the ventricular system. Although less is known about the kinetics of spinal CSF flow, it can be considered a slightly slower distributor than the ventricular system. Unless there is a block, one can assume that a drug introduced into the lumbar space will disperse along the whole cord within hours. This movement can be followed after a bolus of morphine; the dermatomal spread upward can be monitored by careful pinprick examination, and brain stem

effects such as drowsiness or vomiting usually occur at 2 to 4 h.

The flow pattern just described is what one would predict due to the bulk transport of CSF. This is a swift and effective means of distribution. However, there is a major difference between the concentration gradients achieved, depending upon whether the drug is introduced by bolus or by continuous infusion. A bolus injection produces enormously high local drug concentrations for many minutes until bulk flow results in a significant redistribution. The magnitude of this effect has been determined for a number of drugs, including morphine,[35] methotrexate,[2] and baclofen.[33] For example, an injection of 0.25 mg morphine will result in a local lumbar CSF concentration of 5 μg/ml, which then decreases with an initial half-life of 60 to 90 min, followed by a slower removal after 4 h with a 300- to 400-min half-life. Another aspect of the bolus injection is that the drug remains at high concentrations as it moves in bulk up the spinal canal. Figure 13-2 shows this phenomenon. After lumbar injection, serial cervical sampling demonstrated a peak concentration of morphine 3 h later.[39] Thus, a bolus introduced in the lumbar area can arrive in concentrated form at the brain stem. The situation is quite different with the slow continuous infusion that can be obtained with a drug pump. After an initial period of gradual buildup in concentration (approximately five times the half-life of the drug), a uniform level is maintained.[29] The concentration in the steady state is equal to the rate of infusion divided by the rate of removal, e.g., the bulk flow clearance. For CSF this clearance is equal to the rate of production of CSF. If the rate of infusion of a drug is doubled, the steady state concentration will double. The relationship holds true irrespective of the amount of CSF. If more CSF is present, such as with cerebral atrophy, a longer time is needed to reach the steady state, but the final concentration will be determined exclusively by the infusion rate and clearance.

The above analysis so far has emphasized substances which are removed from the CSF primarily by bulk clearance. In fact, other removal processes exist. The more lipid-soluble the drug, the faster it will be taken up by the brain tissue and cross the dura. These uptake and elimination characteristics of the drug have important consequences. In the extreme case with a very lipid-soluble drug, all of it that encounters the surface of the brain or spinal cord or reaches the dura will be lost immediately from the CSF. This is true for lidocaine and methadone.[39] Consequently, the only effect they can have is close to the site of infusion. Morphine and baclofen are several hundred times less lipid-soluble and so are not removed nearly as rapidly. With lumbar infusion, a steady state concentration distribution is created which is highest in the lumbar area and gradually decreases with distance from the catheter tip. The few measurements that are available in patients indicate a cervical-to-lumbar concentration gradient of 1:5, with a wide variance between patients.[6,29] This distribution pattern is shown in Fig. 13-2.

The flow principles just outlined have a number of practical consequences: (1) Bolus injections create very high local concentrations, and bulk flow can continue to maintain relatively high concentrations as the CSF is carried along the CSF pathways. Therefore, bolus injections should be

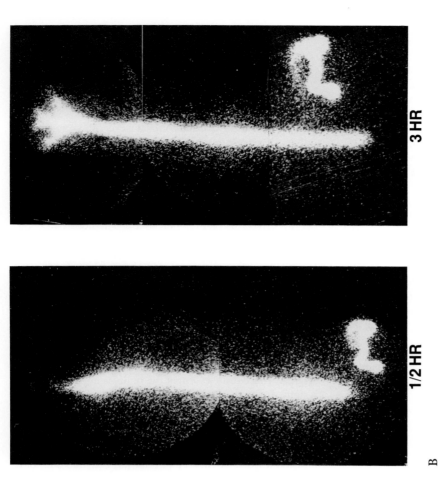

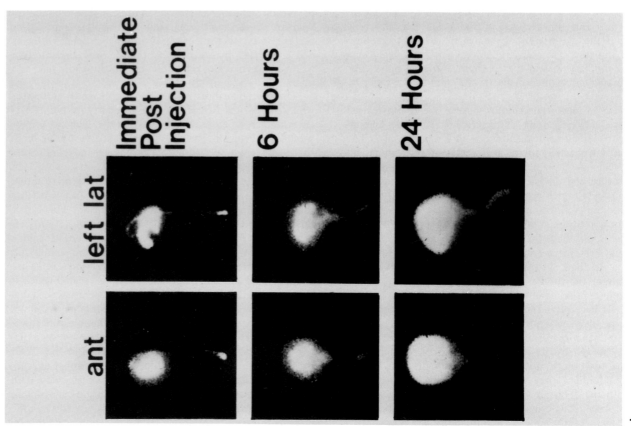

Figure 13-1 Distribution of an ¹¹¹In marker in the CSF after intraventricular injection (*A*) or lumbar intrathecal injection (*B*) from an implanted drug pump, as shown by radionuclide scans. In *A*, the intraventricular spread is first to one lateral ventricle, then to the entire ventricular system, and finally over the convexities and down the spinal canal by 24 h. Note in *B* the rostral redistribution which reaches the brain stem by 3 h after lumbar injection.

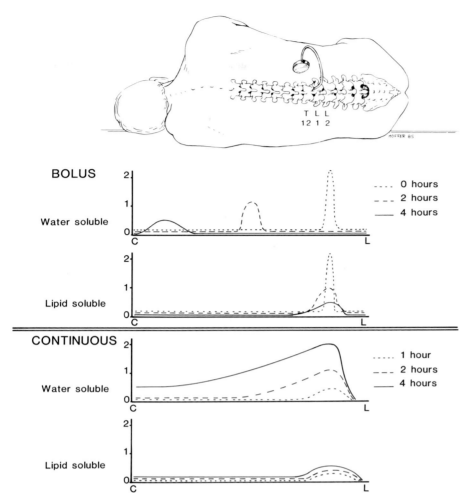

Figure 13-2 Distribution of intrathecal medication over time with continuous perfusion or bolus injection by the lumbar route. Lipid-soluble drugs do not redistribute rostrally. A bolus injection of a water-soluble drug is carried by bulk flow to the brain stem, whereas a continuous infusion creates a concentration gradient from the lumbar to the cervical area. The scale on the ordinate is in relative units rather than actual units.

avoided, or if used, potential side effects must be anticipated. For example, the bolus injection of morphine may cause respiratory depression several hours after lumbar injection, and patients should be monitored for this and other side effects. (2) Continuous infusion results in the gradual buildup of concentration over many hours, and then the level is maintained. The final concentration will be directly related to infusion rate but not total CSF volume. One need not worry about cerebral CSF volume in calculating dosage, so a patient with atrophy will not have differing rate vs. concentration characteristics. (3) A sudden increase in the rate of infusion will result in only a gradual increase in CSF concentration. Therefore, it makes no sense with a drug like morphine or baclofen to change the rate of infusion more than one or two times a day. One has to be patient in adjusting the dosage. (4) The more lipid-soluble a drug, the smaller the distribution will be, and with slightly lipid-soluble drugs, a gradient along the path of bulk flow is created. Therefore, catheter placement is most important with more lipid-soluble drugs and gradients can be utilized to produce proper drug distribution. For example, a lumbar catheter giving baclofen will affect the legs more than the arms. For the upper extremities, a higher placement may be necessary, but this drives the concentration gradient toward

the brain stem. (5) Finally, patients may differ widely in drug clearance rates and absorption. The consequence is that each patient has to be titrated individually. The necessary rate of infusion to achieve a given concentration cannot be easily predicted. Predetermined dosage rates to achieve a given concentration cannot be given, but the necessary levels are easily determined by incremental increases once a pump is implanted and infusion begun.

Neural Tissue

The next step in drug administration which must be considered is the flow from CSF into the neural tissue where the medication has its pharmacologic actions. Less is known about how this occurs. Evidence from horseradish peroxidase tracer studies suggests a rapid passage of marker from the CSF along perivascular spaces deep into the brain parenchyma.[3] This is again a bulk flow phenomenon which is aided by arteriolar pulsations.[45] These numerous conduits for flow probably deliver drugs to within 1.5 to 2.0 cm from any brain region.

The transport system beyond these perivascular channels is the spaces between neurons and glia, the extracellular space (ECS) of the brain. The ECS varies from 15 to 30 percent of brain mass, depending on the area. The pathways along cells are tortuous and narrow. Under normal conditions, there is no evidence of bulk flow in these spaces, and experiments have shown that the major transport mechanism is diffusion.[34] The rate of diffusion is approximately 12 times slower in brain tissue than in simple agar solutions because of the tortuosity of the course and the cells reducing the area of diffusion. Unlike bulk flow, diffusion is an inefficient means of distribution. Just how poor has been demonstrated by experiments in which stable, small molecular weight markers were introduced into the ventricles, and concentration gradients from the surface into the brain tissue were determined.[1,11] The ventricular surface is relatively free of large penetrating vessels, so the diffusion from the ventricular surface into the tissue is via the ECS only. Even with long perfusion times, the distance these markers moved was only millimeters. For example, methotrexate infused for 4 h had a decrease in concentration of 10-fold every 2 mm. This lack of penetration explains why intrinsic brain tumors cannot be adequately treated by intraventricular perfusion.

The drugs which diffuse the farthest in neural tissue are the ones which stay within the ECS. If a drug is bound or taken up by cells or is absorbed into the capillary system, it has little chance for diffusion. Lipid-soluble molecules are the worst in this regard, because they rapidly penetrate cells and endothelial membranes. Diffusion studies have shown that 1,3-bis(2-chloroethyl)-1-nitrosourea (BCNU) is unable to penetrate more than a few millimeters and that this distance does not increase even if the perfusion times are increased. Thus, BCNU would be a poor candidate for CSF or interstitial infusion to treat tumors which have a large volume. On the other hand, if a very limited region is to be treated, a somewhat lipid-soluble drug might be appropriate.

In summary, the following properties have to be considered for any candidate drug for chronic infusion: (1) degree of lipid solubility and size of the region to be treated; (2) stability of the drug [(a) in the drug pump at 37°C, (b) in the catheter tubing, (c) in the CSF, and (d) in the ECS)]; (3) neurotoxicity at high concentrations; and (4) enzymatic and metabolic conversion and degradation in the CSF and brain tissue. So far, the two drugs which best meet these criteria have been the most successful in clinical use, namely morphine and baclofen. Other drugs will have to be carefully selected if they are to be as effective.

Equipment for Drug Perfusion

Drug pump technology is evolving, and it is quite likely that the systems in use now will be modified and improved. As more companies introduce their products, more "bells and whistles" will be added and it will take considerable time to sort out whether these additional features are necessary. The situation will very likely become similar to that of cardiac pacemakers in that many different models will be available and the physician will have to choose the system best suited for the patient considering factors of safety, reliability, complexity, maintenance, longevity, and cost.

At present, three basic types of implantable pumps are available. The first type is passive, with no internal energy source. Typically, such a device uses a one-way compressible pump, like a shunt, combined with a refillable drug reservoir. Such a system can be put together from existing hardware or be obtained as a unit. The Cordis Secor pump (Cordis Corp., Miami, FL) is widely used in Europe.[22] It is designed to deliver one 0.1-ml bolus at a time (Fig. 13-3A). A double valve requires digital compression in two separate steps to avoid inadvertent drug delivery. The patient controls the drug administration and is instructed on the number of compressions to perform. The reservoir holds 12 ml, so approximately 100 boluses can be given before a refill is necessary. The advantages of the pump are its simplicity, low cost, and patient control. The precision of the device in patients has not been determined, but it is unlikely to be extremely accurate. There is no bacteriostatic filter in-line, and an infection in the reservoir can spread to the CSF. The incidence of meningitis is not known; it would depend on whether the drug is likely to be a good culture medium (a chemotherapeutic agent might not be, for example), the number of refills required, the care taken in refilling the device, and the length of time the device is in place.

The second level of pump complexity is represented by the constant flow system manufactured by Shiley Infusaid, Inc. (Norwood, MA) (Fig. 13-3B).[20] A metal bellows reservoir is compressed by Freon gas (E.I. du Pont de Nemours & Co., Wilmington, DE), the internal energy source. At body temperature the gas exerts 1.5 atmospheres of pressure (7 psi), which pushes the liquid in the reservoir through a long metal tube. The resistance of the tubing is so great that it slows the flow to 1 to 3 mm/day. When the reservoir is refilled, the gas is compressed again. The consequence of this design is that changes in atmospheric pressure or body temperature will result in changes in flow rate. In practice, these variations are small unless a patient has a high fever or goes to a markedly different altitude. In our patients, the pumps' average variation has been less than 15 percent once implanted. The pump reservoir can hold up to 50 ml, so it usually has to be refilled every 3 weeks. For CNS use, the pump comes with an in-line bacteriostatic filter and a side port for bolus injections. Its straightforward mechanical design and sturdy construction have made it quite reliable. The major drawback to this type of pump is that in order to change the dosage, the medicine in the reservoir has to be emptied and a new concentration of the drug injected. If frequent dosage adjustments are needed, this becomes a problem.

The most complex pump systems are those that employ mechanical pumps controlled by a computer and powered by batteries. They usually have optional bacteriostatic filters. The Medtronic SynchroMed pump (Medtronic, Inc., Minneapolis, MN) (Fig. 13-3C) has been most widely tested,[17] and other companies are introducing similar versions.[27] The key concept is to provide flexible delivery. Thus, the Medtronic pump can be programmed for continuous, intermittent, or complex patterns depending on the application. Dosage can be changed without refilling the reservoir. The system has the potential for patient-controlled dosage with limits set by the physician or via phone instruction to the pump control unit. Complexity has

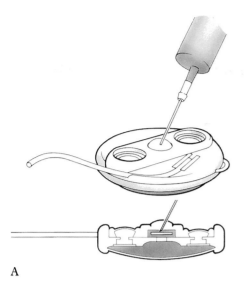

A

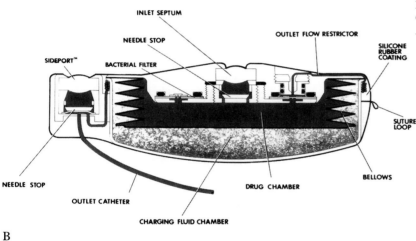

INLET SEPTUM

NEEDLE STOP

OUTLET FLOW RESTRICTOR

SILICONE RUBBER COATING

SIDEPORT™

BACTERIAL FILTER

SUTURE LOOP

NEEDLE STOP

BELLOWS

OUTLET CATHETER

DRUG CHAMBER

CHARGING FLUID CHAMBER

B

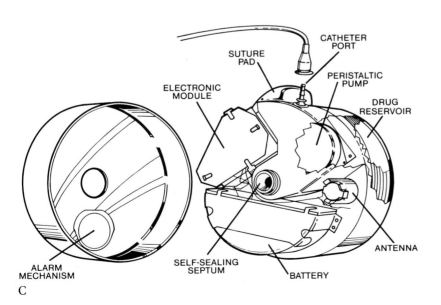

CATHETER PORT

SUTURE PAD

PERISTALTIC PUMP

ELECTRONIC MODULE

DRUG RESERVOIR

ANTENNA

ALARM MECHANISM

SELF-SEALING SEPTUM

BATTERY

C

Figure 13-3 The three basic types of implanted drug pumps. *A.* A passive system with no internal energy source. The Cordis Secor pump has a reservoir and a pumping system that requires digital compression in two separate steps to release a 0.1-ml bolus. *B.* A constant rate infusion device powered by compressed gas. The Shiley-Infusaid Model 400 pump uses Freon gas to compress a metal bellows containing the drug. The flow is slowed to 1 to 3 ml/day by resistance from coiled metal tubing. A side port provides access to the distal catheters. *C.* A programmable, battery-powered pump. The Medtronics SynchroMed pump contains a drug reservoir, rotary peristaltic pump, computer, battery, and communication link (radiofrequency antenna) for external programming. Continuous, intermittent, and complex cycles of medication can be programmed. (Diagrams courtesy of Cordis, Inc., Shiley-Infusaid, Inc., and Medtronic, Inc., respectively.)

its price, and it remains to be seen which devices will be most reliable. The limited life span of the battery is a drawback for long-term use. At present, the battery life is estimated to be 3 to 5 years. In our experience, the accuracy of the Medtronic pump is better than 7 percent. As such, it may be the most precise way ever developed to give medication. Whether this sophistication is needed depends on the application. It has been most useful for drugs like baclofen in which a small difference in a dose may have a major effect on muscle tone, or in which a variation in dose during the day is important. For morphine administration, a simpler patient-activated device may be sufficient.

The pumps must be connected to a catheter which will be compatible with long-term CNS use. Experience with shunts suggests that soft Silastic (Dow Chemical Co., Midland, MI) catheters will be well tolerated. Other materials like polyethylene tubing should not be used until they are demonstrated to be safe and nonkinking. For lumbar subarachnoid placement, the catheter can easily be positioned percutaneously under fluoroscopic control. Using a guide wire, the catheter tip can usually be threaded to the thoracic or cervical area as required. A laminectomy is not necessary. To deliver medication to the ventricle, shunt tubing is satisfactory. Intraparenchymal delivery is much more difficult and requires specialized catheters and stereotactic placement.

Although the present equipment is not perfect, it meets most needs. The operations to implant the units are straightforward and can be done in most patients under local anesthesia. The real challenge is the proper utilization of these new tools, as well as future applications.

Current Clinical Applications

Pain

The use of intraspinal narcotics for pain relief is based on the neuropharmacologic finding that opiate receptors are located in the spinal cord. Recent detailed studies reveal a number of receptor types at different cord regions.[49] Although a complex picture is emerging, the main point is that morphine and its agonists bind to specific mu receptors in Layers I, II, and III of the spinal gray matter. Activation of the mu receptors inhibits the transmission of nociceptive information and accounts for most of the analgesic effect of spinal morphine. The proximity of the receptor sites to the CSF is also important. Morphine molecules introduced into the spinal fluid can rapidly diffuse to their sites of action. Animal experiments show that the diffusion time to Layer II and the onset of analgesia are the same. This same phenomenon is seen in human beings. After the bolus injection of intrathecal morphine, pain relief does not begin for 20 to 30 min. Furthermore, the analgesic effect well outlasts the presence of the drug in the CSF. This sustained action of up to 8 to 12 h is due to the slow diffusion of morphine out of the cord tissue.

The most extensive use of intraspinal morphine has been for postoperative pain control. Most often, an epidural catheter is placed at the time of surgery and an external drug pump is used to deliver morphine. Many studies have demonstrated the effectiveness of the technique, the principal advantage being good pain relief without significant sedation. A number of excellent measurements on the distribution and pharmacokinetics of epidural and intrathecal morphine have been performed.[35]

Several findings are relevant to the chronic infusion of morphine using an implanted drug pump. The first is that epidurally placed morphine goes primarily into the systemic circulation (only 5 to 10 percent crosses the dura and arachnoid to reach the CSF). This means that epidural morphine may have a significant systemic distribution to the whole brain as well as a regional effect on spinal neurons. For chronic epidural infusion, one has to remember that redistribution; in effect, one is giving an intrathecal and systemic drug together. A second characteristic of the epidural bolus is its time course. The process of crossing the dura is slow, and a bolus injection does not reach peak concentration in the CSF for 10 to 20 min. In contrast, a subarachnoid injection of one-tenth the dose gives immediate extremely high concentrations that then decrease in time with the same 1.5- to 2-h half-life of the epidural bolus. If intermittent epidural bolus injections are used in chronic pain therapy, it takes the diffusion time across the dura plus the diffusion time into the spinal cord tissue for the drug to work. This can be 30 to 40 min. Therefore, boluses should not be repeated in short intervals because of the danger of building up a much higher dose than necessary for pain relief, resulting in central side effects. Both epidural and subarachnoid boluses ascend upward with the CSF bulk flow. There is also the possibility that the plexus of epidural veins might carry morphine immediately to the brain stem regions when a rapid epidural bolus is given. This type of redistribution does not seem to occur with slow infusion.

The natural extension of the postoperative use of intraspinal morphine is chronic infusion for intractable pain. Here again, the major advantage is blocking nociceptive information at the spinal level and avoiding central side effects. The first report of a pump implant for spinal infusion was in 1981 in a patient with severe sacral pain due to a chordoma.[37] The pain relief with 1.2 mg/day of intrathecal morphine from a constant flow pump was excellent, and the patient became ambulatory and was discharged without systemic narcotics.

Following this report, many others have appeared.[7,9,14,23,43,46] The great majority of patients in these studies were treated for intractable pain due to cancer and had failed to obtain adequate relief with oral narcotics or could not tolerate their central side effects. The results from these reports are difficult to summarize because of the different patient populations, the various categories used to judge response, and the length of time the patients were treated. Even though the procedure has been experimental and over 3000 pumps have been implanted in the United States alone, no series has more than 50 patients. In spite of this, a number of generalizations can be made.

A majority of patients have good to excellent pain relief (as many as 75 percent of well-selected candidates).[43] The technique has been used primarily to treat midline or lower extremity pain, but some authors remark on good results in pain syndromes as high as the brachial plexus. Severe episodic pain is more difficult to control than chronic boring or burning pain. The best way to tell if the technique will work is to perform a trial with chronic epidural or subarachnoid morphine. Sometimes "neurogenic" pain, such as occurs after herpes zoster or deafferentation, will respond, although oral morphine is usually unsuccessful. As a number of authors have remarked, an advantage of a screening period with epidural morphine and an external pump is that one can judge objectively if oral narcotic needs decrease and activities of daily living improve. Psychogenic factors may also be assessed during this trial period.

The objective of reducing central side effects has been achieved in most patients. The initial fear was that intrathecal infusion would cause respiratory depression and somnolence. This has not happened with any chronic infusion, and the only problems have been due to large bolus test injections. The initial intrathecal dose can be as low as 0.2 to 0.5 mg/day in sensitive individuals, to 2 to 4 mg/day in patients who have had prior exposure to high-dose oral narcotics (5 to 10 times the dose is needed for epidural infusion). By 6 to 12 months, the patient may need 10 to 50 mg/day and yet show no central side effects. A few patients remain on low doses long-term.

Although chronic lumbar infusion has relatively few side effects, it does interfere with micturition. The bladder becomes hypoactive, and especially in older males with obstructions to flow, voiding difficulties can develop. Usually adaptation occurs with time, but sometimes long-term catheterization is necessary. Nausea, vomiting, or pruritus can be produced with the initiation of treatment but is almost always self-limited. Myoclonus and hyperalgesia from high intrathecal doses have been reported in a few cases.

One has to be aware that spinal narcotics do not necessarily provide enough central morphine to avoid withdrawal symptoms. With the introduction of spinal narcotics, acute central withdrawal effects such as sweating, anxiety, diarrhea, and tremors can occur due to too abrupt a decrease in systemic narcotics. Once the patient is withdrawn, small doses of oral narcotics which would not have been effective before are again useful. Thus oral narcotics are a good means of managing brief increases of pain in pump patients. If oral intake increases substantially, then the intrathecal dose should be increased at a refill. No specific spinal withdrawal effects have been recorded other than an increase of pain when spinal morphine is stopped. With very high spinal dosage, cessation of infusion will result in central withdrawal, probably because the narcotic has been redistributed via the systemic circulation to the brain.

The major drawback to spinal morphine is the same as with systemic narcotics, the gradual development of tolerance. Several animal experiments suggested that tolerance to spinal opiates could develop as rapidly as within 1 week.[49] Fortunately, this is not the case for human beings. Most patients need progressively more morphine over months, not days.[14,46] This tolerance can be due to true biologic changes at the receptor level or increased cancer pain. It is often difficult to differentiate the two. In some series, tolerance has been a frequent cause for late failure at 6 months and beyond, but in others, only 20 percent or fewer patients have shown this effect.[43] As long as the morphine is significantly reducing pain, there is no reason not to increase the dose as required. When the dose is higher than can be reasonably delivered via the pump, then a management problem emerges. At that point, the technique has to be abandoned and a destructive procedure has to be used. As an alternative, the patient can be withdrawn from intraspinal morphine and in 1 or 2 weeks it can be restarted at a much lower dose. Cycles of withdrawal may even be necessary.

The development of tolerance has led to a search for other drugs which do not cross-react with morphine. Morphine agonists like hydromorphone and sufentanil are not suitable. They share the same mu receptors, and once mu receptor tolerance has occurred to any one of these agonists, it will be present for the others. The most promising new drug possibilities are intrathecal D-ala-2-D-leu-5 enkephalin (DADL), clonidine, and somatostatin. DADL is a delta receptor opiate agonist, which in animal testing shows only minimal cross-tolerance with morphine.[49] In human trials, it appears to be as potent an analgesic as morphine, and in several patients who have shown morphine tolerance, DADL has been effective.[24,30] Much more testing is required before its range of clinical usefulness as well as its level of toxicity will be known.

Alpha-2 agonists may provide a totally nonopiate way to control pain because nociceptive spinal circuits are inhibited by descending adrenergic neurons. Animal experiments confirm the lack of cross-tolerance between morphine and several alpha-2 agonists.[49] Limited trials in human beings with the alpha-2 agonist clonidine have demonstrated this effect. Morphine-tolerant patients were infused with clonidine and four of six had sufficient relief of pain to allow the intraspinal morphine dose to be lowered.[5] The major side effect of such agents is likely to be hypotension, and this was noted in the trial but could be managed adequately.

Intrathecal somatostatin has also been tried for cancer pain. Much more controversy surrounds this agonist because some animal experiments have demonstrated analgesia and others have not, and one experiment found marked neurotoxicity at levels close to those producing analgesia.[4] It has been used in human beings, and in one series of patients, some of whom were already tolerant to morphine, bolus injections provided excellent pain relief. In addition, it has been tried epidurally for postoperative pain and been found effective.

If any of these newer agents prove to be safe and effective, the major drawback to chronic morphine infusion would disappear. Alternation of agents which work on different receptor sites would eliminate tolerance problems. This would open the door to long-term treatment of cancer pain as well as benign pain by intraspinal agents. The issue of whether certain types of benign pain should be treated before another agent is available is unresolved. Some successes have been reported in benign pain conditions, but low back pain patients failed to benefit in a carefully designed study.[8] Until more experience with specific well-defined benign pain syndromes is available, one should be very cautious in using the technique.

Several other points need to be made. The drug pumps and catheters are far from perfect. Kinks, catheter dislodgments, and rare pump failures have marred all of the reported series. Transient CSF leaks and spinal headaches occur in 5 to 10 percent of patients with intrathecal catheter placement, and scarring in the epidural space can prevent proper diffusion if the epidural space is used.

A final point should be made—that intraspinal morphine solves the problem of midline and bilateral pain. Unilateral pain can often be handled satisfactorily with a percutaneous cordotomy. Unfortunately, most of the true cancer pain is not limited to one side. Even when the pain appears to be unilateral, a cordotomy may unmask midline or contralateral pain. The destructive procedures for bilateral pain almost uniformly cause problems with bowel and bladder function and so are rarely employed. The result has been that the neurosurgeon has had little to offer to alleviate suffering. Intraspinal morphine administration has changed the situation. Furthermore, it is nondestructive and the implant can be inserted under local anesthesia. This explains the rapid application and acceptance of the procedure.

Spasticity

Intraspinal morphine injection is effective for cancer pain because it minimizes the central side effects of oral administration while achieving high tissue levels at spinal opiate receptors. A parallel situation exists for intraspinal baclofen administration for spasticity. Oral baclofen, the best drug for reducing spasms and muscle rigidity, frequently produces drowsiness, confusion, and memory loss as the dose is increased. For patients with severe spasticity, it most often is inadequate, and destructive neurosurgical or chemical procedures are necessary.

For a long time it has been evident that oral baclofen's site of action is the spinal cord. The clinical proof is that even patients with complete transection of the spinal cord respond. The precise location of the baclofen receptors within the spinal cord has recently been demonstrated by autoradiography. The gamma aminobutyric acid-B (GABA-B) receptors are found in Layers I, II, and III in the dorsal horn, the same general region as the mu receptors for morphine.[44] Experiments on animals have shown that baclofen can have a local effect on a small region of the cord. Small lumbar intrathecal doses of baclofen selectively reduced polysynaptic reflexes in the hindlimbs without producing an effect in the forelimbs.[25] A series of animal infusions showed no neurotoxicity.

The first intrathecal trials of baclofen were performed in 1983.[40] As little as 25 μg produced profound decreases in spasticity, and no sedation was encountered. Following the response to bolus injections, chronic infusion using an implantable drug pump began in the United States and Europe. To date, more than 200 patients have been treated, and these numbers are rapidly expanding. Enough is now known about the treatment to assess its effectiveness and side effects.

All the clinical studies to date confirm the initial observations that intrathecal baclofen has a profound effect on spasticity, much more than has been achieved by oral agents.[32,33,41] Electrophysiologic studies demonstrate that intrathecal baclofen not only reduces polysynaptic reflexes, as does oral baclofen, but also can eliminate monosynaptic ones. Central side effects with chronic infusion are rarely seen. This parallels the experience with intraspinal mor-

phine injection and is due in fact to the lumbar-to-cervical gradient of approximately 3 to 1. However, a large bolus injection can cause somnolence and respiratory depression, and in a lesser dose, lightheadedness, nystagmus, and nausea. The bulk flow of spinal CSF redistributes baclofen to the brain stem level in several hours. Although no specific antagonist to baclofen is available to reverse these effects, physostigmine (1 to 2 mg given intravenously over 10 min) has been shown to rapidly reverse coma and respiratory depression in these patients with bolus overdoses.

The long-term effects of baclofen on rigidity and muscle tone are shown in Fig. 13-4, as well as the dose required to maintain clinical improvement. Very mild spasms have been purposely allowed to avoid venous stasis in the lower extremities. Although these graphs demonstrate continued effect, they do not show the most important aspects of the therapy for the patient. The decrease in spasms eliminates associated pain and allows normal sleep. Activities of daily living are significantly improved. Many paraplegic patients are able to dress themselves, perform transfers, and even drive vans. Self-catheterization programs can be initiated, since severe adductor spasms are no longer present.[38] Urodynamic studies reveal increased bladder capacity and lessened sphincter tone, and these findings are reflected in functional improvement of bladder control.[13] Spasms which cause incontinence are eliminated.

The dose of baclofen has varied widely, from 17 to 850 μg/day. In most patients, a gradual increase in dose is necessary for 6 to 12 months. In the majority of patients, this seems to stabilize after a year. However, several cases of tolerance have been encountered. If baclofen is stopped for several weeks, when it is restarted a much lower dose is again effective. This "drug holiday" strategy or substituting intrathecal morphine for baclofen has been useful in these cases of tolerance. Mechanical problems of catheter kinks, dislodgment, and pump failure have occurred, and all of these patients have undergone surgical correction of the problems. The worst side effects were large baclofen overdoses causing coma and respiratory depression in two patients.[41] Both patients survived without sequelae and continued on intrathecal baclofen. The reason for the overdose was a design failure in the programmable pump. After the problem was corrected, no further overdoses have occurred. Obviously, a failure of the pump which results in an overdose is life-threatening, and the pump manufacturers are well aware of the consequences.

Precise adjustment of dose is needed in some patients, especially those that use extensor rigidity for ambulation. Furthermore, many patients prefer to have a higher dose at night to control spasms fully and less during the day so some tone can be maintained. For that reason, a programmable pump is a great advantage. Because long-term chronic use is anticipated in every patient, a pump system with a bacteriostatic filter should be used and great care taken in refills to use sterile technique. Meningitis has not yet been reported but is of considerable concern, and the patient must be aware of the symptoms.

An alternate drug for spasticity is morphine. In treating a pain patient, intrathecal morphine injection was noted to markedly relieve his spasticity. This observation has been confirmed by others, and a series of spastic patients without

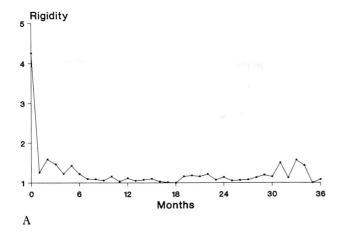

A

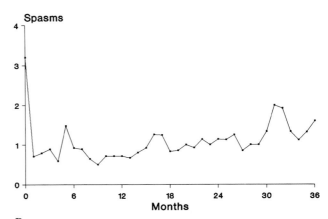

B

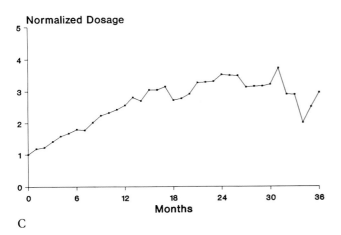

C

Figure 13-4 The results of continuous infusion of intrathecal baclofen for severe spasticity of spinal origin. The average scores for 18 patients treated for 12 to 36 months. *A.* Rigidity (Ashworth scale) is markedly decreased. *B.* Spasms are reduced to a clinically insignificant level. *C.* The average dose to produce these effects increased slowly over the first year and then seemed to stabilize in most patients. The Ashworth rigidity scale is: 1, no increase in tone; 2, slight increase in tone; 3, more marked increase in tone but affected part is easily flexed; 4, passive movement is difficult; 5, rigid in flexion or extension. The spasm scale is: 0, no spasms; 1, mild spasms induced by stimulation; 2, infrequent full spasms (<1/h); 3, spasms occurring >1/h; 4, spasms occurring >10/h. The scale on the ordinate in *C* is in relative units rather than actual units. [From Penn RD, Kroin JS. Intrathecal baclofen in the long-term management of severe spasticity. In: Park TS (ed.), *Management of Spasticity.* Philadelphia: Hanley & Belfus (in press.)]

pain are now being studied.[14] Because morphine acts on different receptor sites than baclofen, cross-tolerance does not develop. This means that baclofen tolerance can be managed by morphine substitution and vice versa. In fact, one patient in Europe with rapid tolerance is now being managed by alternating the two drugs at monthly pump refills. Whether morphine is as effective as baclofen is not yet known.

Most of the patients that have been treated with intrathecal baclofen have had spinal spasticity due to multiple sclerosis or cord injury.[10] In this group, there have been no reported failures of baclofen to reduce spasms and muscle tone. Patients with other types of spasticity have been implanted but not in great enough numbers to know if the technique will be as useful in spasticity of cerebral origin, cerebral palsy and dystonias.

Another application of intrathecal baclofen has been for tetanus.[31] Several patients with overwhelming spasms have been treated with large lumbar intrathecal doses, 1 to 2 mg/day, using an external pump, and the spasms have partially cleared, making management much easier and possibly reducing mortality. This interesting observation may

point to the usefulness of acute management of severe spasms by an external pump.

Other Applications of Drug Pumps

Alzheimer's Disease

Alzheimer's disease appears to be a condition in which the selective CNS infusion of a suitable drug might be of considerable clinical benefit.[16,18] Neurochemical studies have demonstrated a marked reduction in acetylcholine production, which parallels the development of dementia. Loss of cholinergic neurons in the basal nuclei which project widely to the cerebral cortex and hippocampus is an early pathologic finding in the disease. Furthermore, several studies with oral physostigmine suggested that inhibition of acetylcholine breakdown may help some Alzheimer's patients. Because the cholinergic deficit is thought to be primarily on the presynaptic side, transmitter replacement seems to be a good approach. The problem is having a method to get acetylcholine agonists into the brain. Oral precursor treatment with lecithin was tried and failed,[26] and long-acting physostigmine-like drugs are currently being studied.[47]

A more direct approach can be taken using an implanted drug pump. After suitable experiments to test toxicity in dogs, bethanechol, a stable acetylcholine agonist, was given intraventricularly to four patients with Alzheimer's disease using a ventricular catheter attached to a constant infusion pump. A single-blind study was done first.[15] The families of the patients reported no change when placebo was infused, and decreased confusion, increased initiative, and improvement in activities of daily living when bethanechol was given. The preliminary finding was very encouraging and led to a multicenter double-blind trial. Unlike the first study, only a small improvement in mental status, 1 point on a scale of 25, was documented in the full controlled trial. The conclusion is that bethanechol was not effective enough to warrant its use.

A number of reasons might account for the minimal clinical effect. No studies were done on the distribution of bethanechol in brain tissue after chronic infusion. The drug may not diffuse to the site where it is needed. Furthermore, it has primarily M2 as opposed to M1 acetylcholine receptor affinity and just the opposite affinity may be needed. Another reason might be that the incorrect dose was used. This hypothesis was tested in a smaller study on 11 patients.[42] A U-shaped dose response curve with the peak effect at 1 to 1.5 μg/day was shown. Significant behavioral improvements were seen at these doses, which were 3 to 5 times that of the multicenter trials. However, no changes in cognition were achieved at any dose. The lesson is that in intraventricular drug studies, dose response curves have to be run before double-blind trials. CSF clearance values, and consequently concentrations of drug per unit of drug infused, vary from patient to patient. Dose optimization is necessary for each subject.

The search for more active cholinergic agents is continuing in animal experiments. Most cholinergic drugs do not readily penetrate the blood-brain barrier, so it is likely that further intraventricular drug pump studies will be necessary. Another possible neurotransmitter to be tested is somatostatin or a somatostatin analog. Newer biochemical analyses have demonstrated that somatostatin is decreased in Alzheimer's disease and that the parietal and temporal lobes which account for the cognitive deficits in the disease are most affected.[48] Human trials have yet to be performed.

It can be concluded from this research on Alzheimer's disease that studies can be easily blinded using drug pumps and that the problems with drug administration and compliance are eliminated. The small clinical improvements with bethanechol may represent an important step in the right direction or perhaps the best we can ever do with transmitter therapy with Alzheimer's disease—time will tell.

Parkinson's Disease

Neurotransmitter replacement is the hallmark of Parkinson's disease therapy today. The discovery of the relatively selective loss in substantia nigra neurons and the subsequent marked decrease in striatal dopamine content provides the rationale for the most successful treatment available for a chronic neurodegenerative disease. However, chronic L-dopa therapy leads eventually to the serious side effects of dyskinesias and the "on-off" phenomenon of markedly variable clinical response. One theory to account for these phenomena is variable transport of L-dopa by its blood-brain barrier carrier mechanism.[36]

A possible solution to this problem would be direct steady infusion of a dopamine agonist or dopamine itself. Since good experimental models of Parkinson's disease exist, this line of research is being actively pursued. In the rat unilateral lesion model, direct chronic infusion of dopamine into the striatum reverses the abnormal rotations induced by apomorphine. The number of induced rotations represent the degree of the parkinsonian biochemical abnormality, so the reverse is an encouraging sign that infusion helps. The problem is that an infusion of dopamine into the ventricles has no such effect.[21] The reason is that dopamine diffuses less than a millimeter in brain tissue. Thus, the intraventricular route is bound to fail. Furthermore, intraventricular infusion produces undesirable side effects in primates. Levodopa might be an alternative but it is too insoluble to be infused. A more soluble methyl ester has been tried recently. Preliminary experiments in a 1-methyl-1-phenyl-1,2,3,6-tetrahydropyridine (MPTP) model of parkinsonism in primates have demonstrated marked improvement in bradykinesia and improved feeding after bolus injection of L-dopa methyl ester.[19] Dopamine metabolites, a measure of dopamine turnover, increased. One potential clinical problem is that the methyl ester is metabolized to methanol in the brain and may be neurotoxic. Whether this or other drugs will be of use intraventricularly will depend on their receptor site activity and diffusion characteristics.

Another approach would be regional perfusion using multiple catheters. This would concentrate the medication in specific areas and greatly decrease the overall dose. Because the diffusion distances are small even for the best candidate, in human beings 10 to 100 drug sources might have to be used on each striatum. The mechanical and stereotaxic placement problems are considerable; they are solvable and may be a direction to consider if an intraventricular agent does not work.

The reported success with adrenal medullary tissue transplants for Parkinson's disease has led to speculation that the graft acts as a biologic minipump.[28] So far, what the transplant produces is not known. The original animal experiments showed that the adrenal cells in a neural environment changed their enzymatic activity and secreted substantial amounts of dopamine. The intrastriatal infusion of dopamine by pump was to mimic this effect, and dopamine improved signs of Parkinson's disease in the rat rotational model.

In the human transplants, biochemical analysis of the CSF has not revealed dopamine production. Furthermore, dopamine could not be effective because of its lack of diffusion through brain tissue. Current speculation, based on recent animal experiments, attributes the improvements seen after human transplantation to neurotropic factors. A number of interleukins or specific dopaminergic neurotropic factors are possibilities. If such a factor exists and can be isolated, it may be possible to infuse it without resort to transplantation. This area of research is proceeding rapidly, and the use of drug pumps to deliver neurotropic factors may be an important application in the future.

References

1. Blasberg RG, Patlak C, Fenstermacher JD. Intrathecal chemotherapy: brain tissue profiles after ventriculocisternal perfusion. *J Pharmacol Exp Ther* 1975; 195:73–83.
2. Bleyer WA, Dedrick RL. Clinical pharmacology of intrathecal methotrexate. I. Pharmacokinetics in nontoxic patients after lumbar injection. *Cancer Treat Rep* 1977; 61:703–708.
3. Borison HL, Borison R, McCarthy LE. Brain stem penetration by horseradish peroxidase from the cerebrospinal fluid spaces in the cat. *Exp Neurol* 1980; 69:271–289.
4. Chrubasik J. Intrathecal somatostatin. *Ann NY Acad Sci* 1988; 531:133–145.
5. Coombs DW. Intraspinal analgesic infusion by an implanted pump. *Ann NY Acad Sci* 1988; 531:108–122.
6. Coombs DW, Fratkin JD, Meier FA, et al. Neuropathologic lesions and CSF morphine concentrations during chronic continuous intraspinal morphine infusion: a clinical and postmortem study. *Pain* 1985; 22:337–351.
7. Coombs DW, Maurer LH, Saunders RL, et al. Outcomes and complications of continuous intraspinal narcotic analgesia for cancer pain control. *J Clin Oncol* 1984; 2:1414–1420.
8. Coombs DW, Saunders RL, Gaylor MS, et al. Relief of continuous chronic pain by intraspinal narcotics infusion via an implanted reservoir, *JAMA* 1983; 250:2336–2339 (letter).
9. Delhaas EM, Lip H, Boskma RJ, et al. Low-dose epidural morphine by infusion pump. *Lancet* 1984; 1(8378):690.
10. Erickson DL, Blacklock JB, Michaelson M, et al. Control of spasticity by implantable continuous flow morphine pump. *Neurosurgery* 1985; 16:215–217.
11. Fenstermacher J, Kaye T. Drug "diffusion" within the brain. *Ann NY Acad Sci* 1988; 531:29–39.
12. Fishman RA. *Cerebrospinal Fluid in Diseases of the Nervous System*. Philadelphia: Saunders, 1980.
13. Frost FS, Nanninga JB. Effect of intrathecal baclofen on bladder and sphincter function. *J Urol* 1989; 142:101–105.
14. Greenberg HS, Taren J, Ensminger WD, et al. Benefit from and tolerance to continuous intrathecal infusion of morphine for intractable cancer pain. *J Neurosurg* 1982; 57:360–364.
15. Harbaugh RE. Intracerebroventricular bethanechol chloride administration in Alzheimer's disease. *Ann NY Acad Sci* 1988; 531:174–179.
16. Harbaugh RE, Roberts DW, Coombs DW, et al. Preliminary report: intracranial cholinergic drug infusion in patients with Alzheimer's disease. *Neurosurgery* 1984; 15:514–518.
17. Heruth KT. Medtronic SynchroMed drug administration system. *Ann NY Acad Sci* 1988; 531:72–75.
18. Hollander E, Mohs RC, Davis KL. Cholinergic approaches to the treatment of Alzheimer's disease. *Br Med Bull* 1986; 42:97–100.
19. Hood TW, Domino EF, Greenberg HS. Possible treatment of Parkinson's disease with intrathecal medication in the MPTP model. *Ann NY Acad Sci* 1988; 531:200–205.
20. Johnston J, Reich S, Bailey A, et al. Shiley infusaid pump technology. *Ann NY Acad Sci* 1988; 531:57–65.
21. Kao LC, Garvey PM, Kroin JS, et al. The effect of intraventricular DA infusion on rotation and striatal biochemistry in the rat. *Soc Neurosci Abstr* 1988; 5:1.
22. Koning G, Feith F. A new implantable drug delivery system for patient-controlled analgesia. *Ann NY Acad Sci* 1988; 531:48–56.
23. Krames ES, Gershow J, Glassberg A, et al. Continuous infusion of spinally administered narcotics for the relief of pain due to malignant disorders. *Cancer* 1985; 56:696–702.
24. Krames ES, Wilkie DJ, Gershow J. Intrathecal D-ala^2-D-leu^5-enkephalin (DADL) restores analgesia in a patient analgetically tolerant to intrathecal morphine sulfate. *Pain* 1986; 24: 205–209.
25. Kroin JS, Penn RD, Beissinger RL, et al. Reduced spinal reflexes following intrathecal baclofen in the rabbit. *Exp Brain Res* 1984; 54:191–194.
26. Little A, Levy R, Chuaqui-Kidd P, et al. A double-blind, placebo controlled trial of high-dose lecithin in Alzheimer's disease. *J Neurol Neurosurg Psychiatry* 1985; 48:736–742.
27. Lord P, Allami H, Davis M, et al. MiniMed technologies programmable implantable infusion system. *Ann NY Acad Sci* 1988; 531:66–71.
28. Madrazo I, Drucker-Colin R, Diaz V, et al. Open microsurgical autograft of adrenal medulla to the right caudate nucleus in two patients with intractable Parkinson's disease. *N Engl J Med* 1987; 316:831–834.
29. Moulin DE, Inturrisi CE, Foley KM. Cerebrospinal fluid pharmacokinetics of intrathecal morphine sulfate and D-Ala^2-D-Leu^5-enkephalin. *Ann Neurol* 1986; 20:218–222.
30. Moulin DE, Max MB, Kaiko RF, et al. The analgesic efficacy of intrathecal D-ala^2-D-leu^5-enkephalin in cancer patients with chronic pain. *Pain* 1985; 23:213–221.
31. Müller H, Zierski J, Börner U, et al. Intrathecal baclofen in tetanus. *Ann NY Acad Sci* 1988; 531:167–173.
32. Müller H, Zierski J, Dralle D, et al. Intrathecal baclofen in spasticity. In: Müller H, Zierski J, Penn RD (eds.), *Local-Spinal Therapy of Spasticity*. Berlin: Springer-Verlag, 1988: 155–214.
33. Müller H, Zierski J, Dralle D, et al. Pharmacokinetics of intrathecal baclofen. In: Müller H, Zierski J, Penn RD (eds.), *Local-Spinal Therapy of Spasticity*. Berlin: Springer-Verlag, 1988: 223–244.
34. Nicholson C, Phillips JM. Ion diffusion modified by tortuosity and volume fraction in the extracellular microenvironment of the rat cerebellum. *J Physiol (Lond)* 1981; 321:225–257.
35. Nordberg G, Hedner T, Mellstrand T, et al. Pharmacokinetic aspects of intrathecal morphine analgesia. *Anesthesiology* 1984; 60:448–454.
36. Nutt JG, Woodward WR, Hammerstad JP, et al. The "on-off" phenomenon in Parkinson's disease: relation to levodopa absorption and transport. *N Engl J Med* 1984; 310:483–488.
37. Onofrio BM, Yaksh TL, Arnold PC. Continuous low-dose intrathecal morphine administration in the treatment of chronic pain of malignant origin. *Mayo Clin Proc* 1981; 56:516–520.
38. Parke B, Penn RD, Savoy SM. Functional outcome following delivery of intrathecal baclofen in patients with multiple sclerosis or spinal cord injury. *Arch Phys Med Rehabil* 1989; 70:30–32.
39. Payne R, Inturrisi CE. CSF distribution of morphine, methadone and sucrose after intrathecal injection. *Life Sci* 1985; 37:1137–1144.
40. Penn RD, Kroin JS. Intrathecal baclofen alleviates spinal cord spasticity, *Lancet* 1984; 1:1078 (letter).
41. Penn RD, Kroin JS. Long-term intrathecal baclofen infusion for treatment of spasticity. *J Neurosurg* 1987; 66:181–185.
42. Penn RD, Martin EM, Wilson RS, et al. Intraventricular bethanechol infusion for Alzheimer's disease: results of double-blind and escalating dose trials. *Neurology* 1988; 38:219–222.

43. Penn RD, Paice JA. Chronic intrathecal morphine for intractable pain. *J Neurosurg* 1987; 67:182–186.

44. Price GW, Wilkin GP, Turnbull MJ, et al. Are baclofen-sensitive GABA$_B$ receptors present on primary afferent terminals of the spinal cord? *Nature* 1984; 307:71–74.

45. Rennels ML, Gregory TF, Blaumanis OR, et al. Evidence for a 'paravascular' fluid circulation in the mammalian central nervous system, provided by the rapid distribution of tracer protein throughout the brain from the subarachnoid space. *Brain Res* 1985; 326:47–63.

46. Shetter AG. Administration of intraspinal morphine sulfate for the treatment of intractable cancer pain. *Neurosurgery* 1986; 18:740–747.

47. Summers WK, Majovski LV, Marsh GM, et al. Oral tetrahydroaminoacridine in long-term treatment of senile dementia, Alzheimer type. *N Engl J Med* 1986; 315:1241–1245.

48. Tamminga CA, Foster NL, Fedio P, et al. Alzheimer's disease: low cerebral somatostatin levels correlate with impaired cognitive function and cortical metabolism. *Neurology* 1987; 37:161–165.

49. Yaksh TL. Opioid receptor systems and the endorphins: a review of their spinal organization. *J Neurosurg* 1987; 67:157–176.

14

Intraoperative Monitoring of Evoked Potentials: An Update

Aage R. Møller

The main purpose of intraoperative monitoring of evoked potentials during neurosurgical procedures is to reduce postoperative neurologic deficits, but more recently it has become apparent that intraoperative recording of evoked potentials can also aid the surgeon in many operations. The use of intraoperative monitoring of evoked potentials to reduce postoperative permanent deficits is based on the assumption that changes in recordable electrical responses occur as a result of injury and that the injury is still reversible at the time of detection if proper surgical intervention occurs. Monitoring of brain stem auditory evoked potentials (BAEPs) during operations in which the auditory nerve may be manipulated is now widespread, and the use of monitoring to reduce the incidence of hearing loss due to surgical manipulation of the eighth cranial nerve is steadily increasing.[5,6,17,18,22,27,28] Intraoperative monitoring of somatosensory evoked potentials (SSEPs) in operations involving the spinal cord is also on the increase.[13–15,17,23,25,27] However, intraoperative monitoring of visual evoked potentials (VEPs)[6,27,33] has not gained similar acceptance, mainly because of the technical problems involved in generating a suitable stimulus.[1,17]

More recently, intraoperative recording of evoked potentials from the motor system has been introduced to reduce intraoperative injuries to the spinal cord.[11,12] Recording responses from muscles has been shown to be valuable in identifying cranial motor nerves during operations to remove tumors when the anatomy has been altered by the tumor or by previous operations; this is particularly true for operations to remove acoustic tumors,[3,17,19,26] and it has more recently been shown to be of value also in operations to remove large tumors of the skull base.[16,17,29] It has been possible in a few types of operations to use electrophysiologic methods to guide the surgeon in the operation and to ensure,

before the operation is ended, that the therapeutic goal of the operation has been achieved.[17,21]

The objective of intraoperative monitoring of evoked potentials (BAEPs, SSEPs, and VEPs) is to detect changes that occur during the operation. This differs from the goal of the use of evoked potentials for diagnostic purposes, in which it is a deviation from a normal value that is of interest. In intraoperative monitoring, normal values are of little interest; instead, it is important to obtain a baseline recording from an individual patient and then to compare the potentials that are recorded during the operation to that baseline recording. Such a baseline can usually be obtained after the patient has been anesthetized but before the operation has begun.[17]

Preservation of Facial Function during Operations in the Cerebellopontine Angle

Monitoring of contractions of the facial muscles is performed during operations in the cerebellopontine angle to help locate the facial nerve when it is not visually identifiable. Currently most such monitoring involves the surgeon using a hand-held stimulating electrode, which carries short pulses of electric current, to probe the surgical field to identify the facial nerve. Various methods are used to record the subsequent contractions of the facial musculature. Earlier, it was customary to have an assistant observe any movement of the face and then to communicate that movement to the surgeon. More recently, recording electromyographic (EMG) potentials from the facial musculature[3,17,19] and recording movements of the face using electronic sensors[31,32] have become more commonly used to verify that the facial nerve has been stimulated. These more modern methods represent a more quantitative way to assess the degree of facial muscle contraction than visual observation of movements of the face. In addition, it is possible to make recorded EMG potentials audible so that the surgeon can hear when the facial nerve has been stimulated.[19,26] Further, oscillographic display of the recorded EMG potentials is advantageous, in that it allows assessment of the amplitudes and latencies of the recorded EMG potentials.[17] When the movements of the face are recorded by electronic sensors, the movements can be made to elicit a sound (horn).[31]

Since the facial nerve is often split into several fascicles when a large acoustic tumor has displaced it, it is important that recordings are made from the entire face. If only portions of the facial musculature (e.g., the lower face or the upper face) are monitored, failure to locate all parts of the facial nerve could result in inadvertent removal of or injury to portions of the facial nerve; this would result in postoperative paralysis of part of the face. We record EMG activity between two electrodes, one placed on the forehead and one on the lower face (Fig. 14-1A), to reduce the likelihood of postoperative facial paralysis. In addition to recording activity from all muscles on the side of the face on which the electrodes have been placed, this particular arrangement of the electrodes will record contractions of the masseter and temporal muscles. Since these muscles are innervated by the

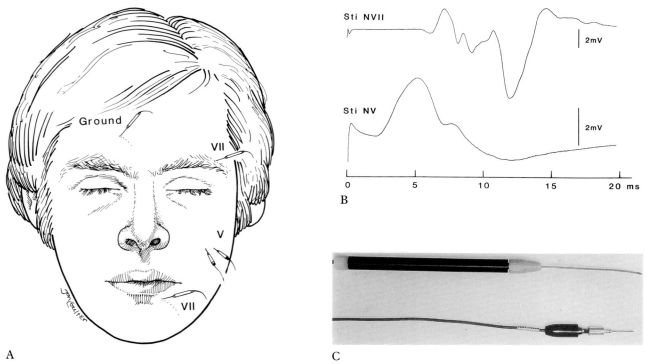

A   C

Figure 14-1 *A.* Schematic illustration of electrode placement for recording EMG potentials from facial muscles and a separate recording of the response from the masseter muscle. *B.* EMG potentials recorded from the electrodes, placed as shown in *A*, to electrical stimulation of CN V and CN VII in the cerebellopontine angle. *C.* Hand-held stimulating electrode (with a hypodermic needle used as the return electrode) for intracranial localization of cranial nerves (Grass Instrument Company). (From Møller.[17])

motor portion of the trigeminal nerve (portio minor), there is the possible risk of mistaking the fifth (motor) nerve for the seventh nerve when probing the cerebellopontine angle for the facial nerve in operations to remove large acoustic tumors that have progressed rostral to the trigeminal nerve. The EMG response to stimulation of the trigeminal nerve, recorded as illustrated in Fig. 14-1*A*, however, can easily be distinguished from the response to stimulation of the facial nerve, because the latency of the recorded EMG potentials differs in the two situations (1.5 ms and 5 to 6 ms, respectively; see Fig. 14-1*B*). An alternative way to distinguish between the response to facial nerve stimulation and that to stimulation of the motor portion of the trigeminal nerve is to record from a muscle innervated by the trigeminal nerve (e.g., the masseter muscle) using a pair of electrodes connected to a separate differential EMG amplifier (Fig. 14-1*A*).

There are several advantages to using EMG recordings as a measure of muscle contraction rather than using a single sensor that records movements of the face. First, EMG potentials from practically all of the facial muscles can be recorded on a single channel (Fig. 14-1*A*), while several sensors are needed to cover the entire face when movements are being recorded.[32] Second, recording EMG potentials makes it possible to measure the latencies of the responses, which

enables one to differentiate between activation of the fifth nerve and activation of the seventh nerve (Fig. 14-1*B*). Third, the amplitude of the EMG response is roughly a measure of how many nerve fibers are functioning, and it therefore provides valuable information about the degree of injury to the facial nerve.

Two types of electrical stimulation of nerves are available for use in recording EMG potentials intraoperatively. Some commercial systems make use of bipolar stimulation, while others offer a choice between bipolar and monopolar stimulation. A monopolar hand-held stimulating electrode is preferable for intraoperative use (Fig. 14-1*C*), mainly because it is easy to use, and because its stimulating power is not affected by its orientation, as is the case for a bipolar stimulating electrode. By using a monopolar hand-held stimulating electrode and having EMG potentials made audible, the surgeon can quickly probe a large area of a tumor and "map" the tumor to locate any portions of the facial nerve that may be in the tumor.[17,19,26]

The electrical stimulation should consist of negative impulses (rectangular) of short duration (0.1 to 0.2 ms), and the stimulus strength should be no greater than necessary to produce a contraction. Some older types of stimulators make use of large current, and some make use of direct current. Such stimulators should not be used because of poor specificity and the risk of injury to the nervous tissue that is being stimulated.

Since shunting of electric current from the stimulating probe can vary widely when the surgical field is wet compared to when it is relatively dry, it is advantageous to use a relatively constant-voltage stimulator rather than the more conventional constant-current type of stimulator. When constant-voltage stimulation is used, the same amount of stimulus current will flow through a specific tissue (e.g., the facial nerve), regardless of how much shunting occurs. If constant-current stimulation is used, then the same total current is delivered, but the amount of current that passes through the tissue depends greatly on how much current is not shunted away; in this case, the stimulus strength depends heavily on whether the field is wet or dry. (Nevertheless, a constant-current stimulator is preferred in situations in which the electrode impedance can vary, as is often the case when, for instance, nerves are to be stimulated through the skin.)

The technique that was just described to record facial EMG responses can also be used to identify regions of a large tumor where no portion of the facial nerve is present. In this case the stimulus strength should be set so that it will activate any facial nerve fibers within a small distance of the tip of a monopolar stimulating electrode. Using this technique can often considerably reduce the time required to remove the tumor, because large portions of the tumor can be removed without risk of causing injury to the facial nerve.[17,19]

When removing large tumors, parts of which may be firmly adherent to the facial nerve, there is a great risk of injuring the facial nerve. Audible monitoring of the spontaneous activity of the facial muscles by means of a loudspeaker provides valuable feedback to the surgeon during the delicate resection of an acoustic tumor.[17,19,26] If the facial nerve is being heated by electrocoagulation, or as a result of the drilling of bone adjacent to the facial nerve, transient or sustained facial muscle activity will result. However, it must be pointed out that the facial nerve can be permanently injured from surgical manipulation, without any change being noticeable in the EMG response; thus, injury from sharp dissection will most likely not result in recordable EMG activity (or movement of the face). For this reason when dissecting near the facial nerve one should not rely on spontaneous EMG activity for assurance that the facial nerve remains intact; in this situation, electrical stimulation should be used frequently to identify the facial nerve so that the surgeon remains aware at all times of the exact location of the nerve.

Monitoring of Cranial Nerves III, IV, VI, and XII in Skull Base Operations

In operations to remove tumors of the skull base, several cranial motor nerves are often in the operative field and are thus at risk of injury from surgical manipulation. This is particularly true in operations within the cavernous sinus, where the nerves that innervate the extraocular muscles [cranial nerve (CN) III, CN IV, CN VI] may be difficult to identify visually. Recording EMG potentials from the extra-

ocular muscles, while the surgical field is probed with a hand-held stimulating electrode (Fig. 14-1C), can make it possible to locate the respective nerves.[16,17] EMG potentials can easily be recorded from these muscles by inserting needle electrodes percutaneously into the respective muscles (Fig. 14-2).

Facial nerve function should also be monitored in these operations, using the methods just described. In addition, identification of CN XII can be facilitated by recording EMG potentials from the tongue (Fig. 14-2A). The potentials recorded from the extraocular muscles in response to electrical stimulation of the respective nerves are easy to distinguish (Fig. 14-3A), as are the potentials recorded from the tongue in response to stimulation of the twelfth cranial nerve (Fig. 14-3B). Continuous recording of EMG potentials from these muscles is also important, because injury to the respective nerves from mechanical manipulation and from heat during electrocoagulation will often result in transient or sustained EMG activity, as was described for the seventh nerve. Thus, such activity can be an important aid in preserving these nerves.

Monitoring of Other Cranial Motor Nerves

CN XI and the motor portions of CN IX and CN X can be monitored, in a way similar to that just described for the facial nerve and the nerves that innervate the extraocular muscles, by stimulating the respective nerves electrically and recording EMG activity from the muscles that these nerves innervate. However, electrical stimulation of CN IX, CN X, and CN XI carries risks. For example, a supramaximal stimulation of CN XI may result in so strong a muscle contraction that dislocation of joints or physical injury to muscles and tendons may result. The risks of electrical stimulation of CN IX and CN X are also not negligible, because of the possible cardiovascular effects.

Hemifacial Spasm

It is generally accepted that hemifacial spasm (HFS) is caused by vascular compression of the facial nerve as it exits the brain stem, and microvascular decompression (MVD) of the root exit zone (REZ) of the facial nerve has long been regarded as the most effective treatment of this disorder.[8–10] However, it is not always obvious from an exploration of the REZ of the facial nerve which of several vessels is causing the spasm, and a certain (small) number of patients who have undergone this operation have experienced spasm postoperatively. Some of these patients had to be reoperated upon, depending on the severity of the spasm.

In our studies of the pathophysiology of HFS, we found that an abnormal muscle response that seems to be characteristic of HFS disappears instantaneously when the offending blood vessel is moved off the intracranial portion of the facial nerve.[20] This abnormal muscle response, which has a

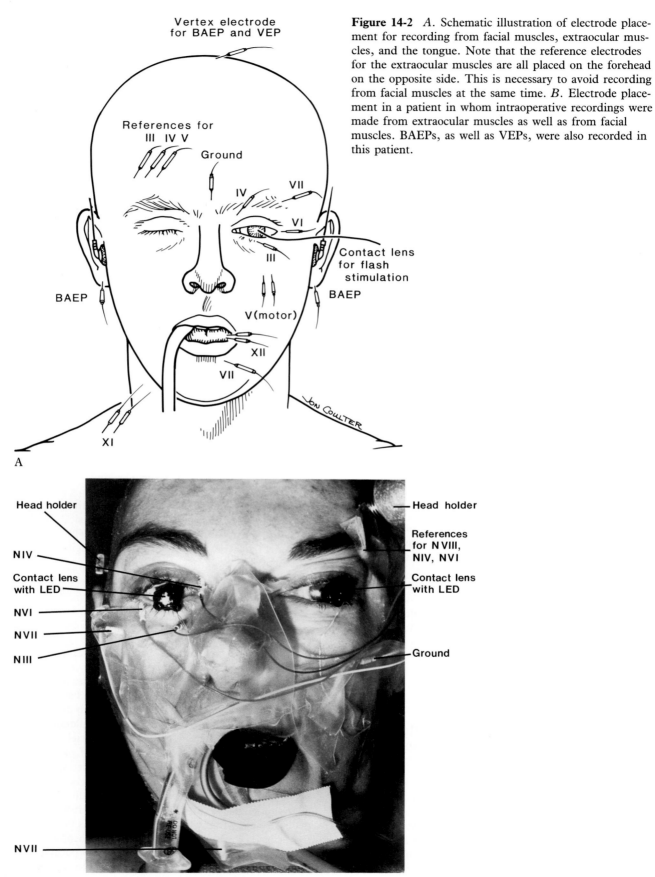

Figure 14-2 *A.* Schematic illustration of electrode placement for recording from facial muscles, extraocular muscles, and the tongue. Note that the reference electrodes for the extraocular muscles are all placed on the forehead on the opposite side. This is necessary to avoid recording from facial muscles at the same time. *B.* Electrode placement in a patient in whom intraoperative recordings were made from extraocular muscles as well as from facial muscles. BAEPs, as well as VEPs, were also recorded in this patient.

latency of about 10 ms, is seen when one branch of the facial nerve is electrically stimulated and recordings are made from muscles that are innervated by other branches of the facial nerve.[4,19,20,24] By monitoring this abnormal muscle response intraoperatively, it is possible to identify the offending blood vessel and to ensure that the nerve has been fully decompressed by watching for the cessation of the abnormal response (Fig. 14-4A and B).[17,21] When using this method, it was found that in many cases there was more than one blood vessel compressing the facial nerve. There are reasons to assume that at least some of the patients who experienced only partial relief from their symptoms before this type of monitoring was introduced, did so because more than one vessel was affecting the facial nerve and only one of

the offending vessels was moved off the facial nerve during the operation.

Monitoring of Visual Evoked Potentials

During operations in which the optic nerve or the optic tract is being manipulated, it would seem to be beneficial to monitor VEPs.[20,33] However, the results of such monitoring have been generally disappointing, since the changes in the recorded potentials correlate poorly with postoperative changes in vision.[1] This is most likely due to limitations inherent in the techniques currently available for intraoperative stimulation, and perhaps to inadequate knowledge of how to interpret the changes in the VEPs that are seen during surgical manipulations of the optic nerve or optic tract; however, essentially there are no practical problems involved in recording VEPs intraoperatively.[17] At present, the most practical type of visual stimulation that can be used intraoperatively is the "flash" type. It has been shown that VEPs elicited by a changing pattern (pattern-reversal checkerboard pattern) are much more diagnostically useful than VEPs recorded in response to flash stimulation[2]; however, eliciting VEPs by the former technique requires that a pattern be focused on the retina, which is not possible to accomplish intraoperatively.

Monitoring of Auditory Evoked Potentials

Intraoperative monitoring of BAEPs is commonly performed to reduce the risk of hearing loss as a result of intraoperative manipulation of the eighth cranial nerve in operations in the cerebellopontine angle.[5,6,17,18,22,27,28] Since the BAEPs are generated by fiber tracts and nuclei in the brain stem (cochlear nucleus, superior olivary complex, inferior colliculus), monitoring of BAEPs may also be of value in operations in which the brain stem is being manipulated or when circulation to the brain stem may be compromised.[16,17] These nuclei are sensitive to manipulation, and there are indications that changes in the BAEPs may occur while an effect is still negligible and before an effect on heart rate and blood pressure becomes noticeable. We therefore find it valuable to monitor BAEPs during operations on the

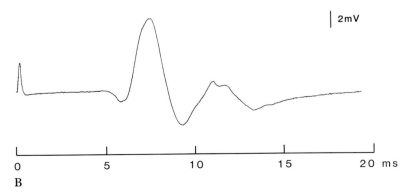

Figure 14-3 *A*. Examples of EMG potentials recorded from the extraocular muscles and the facial muscles in response to intracranial electrical stimulation of the respective cranial nerves using the electrode arrangement shown in Fig. 14-2. *B*. EMG potentials recorded from a pair of electrodes placed on the side of the tongue in response to intracranial electrical stimulation of CN XII. (From Møller.[17])

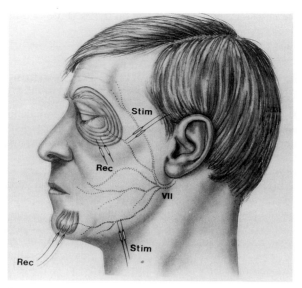

Figure 14-4 *A.* Electrode placement for recording the abnormal muscle response in patients with HFS. (From Møller.[17]) *B.* The abnormal muscle response recorded from the mentalis muscle to electrical stimulation of the temporal branch of the facial nerve. The recordings to the left were obtained before the dura was opened, and they show variable EMG activity in addition to a component with a latency of about 10 ms. After the dura was opened *(right tracings)* only the component with a 10-ms latency is seen. The bottom four tracings were obtained when the offending blood vessel was lifted off the facial nerve. The low-amplitude, spontaneous activity is indicative of slight injury to the facial nerve. (From Møller and Jannetta.[21])

A

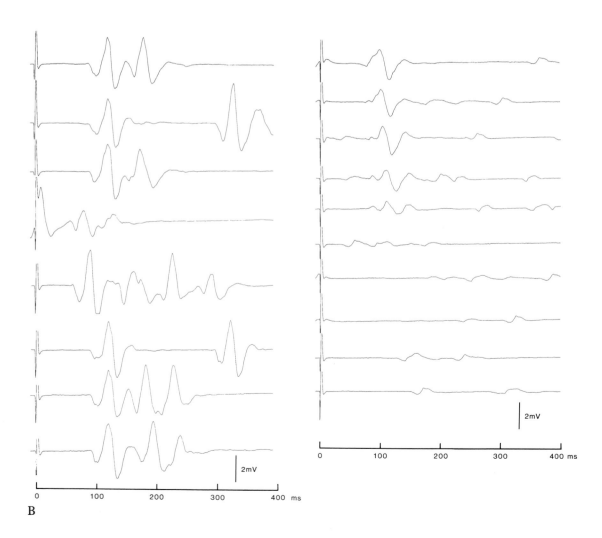

B

skull base and in other situations in which manipulation of the brain stem may occur, such as in operations to remove large acoustic tumors[29] or other tumors of the cerebellopontine angle.

Anesthesia

While recordings of BAEPs are not noticeably affected by any common anesthetic regimen,[25] intraoperative monitoring of cranial motor nerves cannot be done if the patient is paralyzed, because such monitoring depends upon recording of muscle responses. Monitoring of SSEPs is affected by inhalation anesthetics and barbiturates, since it is usually the components generated by cortical activation that are observed. The most commonly used anesthetic regimen for neurosurgical operations involves giving a strong narcotic such as fentanyl for analgesia, together with an inhalation agent, such as nitrous oxide, and small amounts of halogenated agents. As the patient must be kept from moving, he or she must be paralyzed, which is normally done by administering a muscle end-plate blocker (e.g., pancuronium, vecuronium).

Since EMG responses cannot be monitored when a "balanced" anesthesia regimen such as that just described is utilized, a change in the anesthetic regimen must be made if the patient is to be monitored. In our institution, such patients are maintained under inhalation anesthesia, normally using isoflurane and nitrous oxide throughout the operation, possibly with the addition of a small amount of a narcotic agent. Anesthesia is initially induced by thiopental, and muscle relaxation during intubation is achieved by administering succinylcholine, with a small amount (3 mg) of tubocurarine. When EMG monitoring of muscle responses is not required until later in the operation, intubation can be accomplished by using a short-duration end-plate blocker such as atracurium or vecuronium. Even when monitoring of muscle responses will not occur until later in the operation, the use of a long-duration muscle end-plate blocker such as pancuronium bromide is generally not advisable. This regimen has been used in our institution for more than 5 years without any noticeable difficulties or complications.

Preoperative Assessment of Patients for Intraoperative Monitoring

When patients are to undergo intraoperative monitoring of evoked potentials, the systems that are to be monitored should be evaluated quantitatively preoperatively. Thus, if a patient's BAEPs are to be monitored, his or her hearing status should be evaluated preoperatively. Testing should include at least a pure tone audiogram and a determination of speech discrimination scores, and the patient's ears should be checked for obstruction from cerumen, etc. Similarly, if the extraocular muscles are to be monitored, their function should be evaluated preoperatively by state-of-the-art methods. Other factors that may affect neural conduction, such as neuropathies, should be ruled out or measured quantita-

tively, if possible, particularly when SSEPs or facial EMG responses are to be monitored.

Determination of Benefits of Intraoperative Monitoring

Intraoperative monitoring of evoked potentials has only recently been introduced for use in neurosurgical operations, and it is therefore natural that the method has been viewed with skepticism and a demand for proof of the benefits it can provide. As with several other procedures allied to such operations, it has generally been difficult to design studies to provide quantitative estimates of the benefits in terms of reduced postoperative complications. This is largely because many surgeons feel that intraoperative monitoring is valuable in reducing postoperative deficits and therefore will not allow random selection of patients to be monitored. This makes it impossible to study the efficacy of such techniques by a double-blind methodology.

Comparing complications before and after the introduction of intraoperative monitoring thus seems to be the only practical way to assess the value of intraoperative monitoring; however, the results of such evaluations are influenced by any changes in the operative technique introduced at or after the institution of monitoring. Despite this complication, comparisons have been made between the rate of complications (such as facial palsy) of surgical procedures (such as acoustic tumor removal) before and after the introduction of intracranial monitoring of cranial nerve function. These studies have shown a significant decrease in complication rate after the introduction of intraoperative monitoring.[7,30] A similar study of a less frequently performed operation, that to relieve HFS, showed that the efficacy of the operation was higher after intraoperative monitoring was introduced.[21] Further, the number of patients who needed to be reoperated upon because of recurrent or unrelieved spasm decreased from about 15 percent to almost zero. Finally, the frequency of hearing loss as a complication of operations in the cerebellopontine angle decreased radically after the introduction of intraoperative monitoring of auditory evoked potentials during such operations.[22]

Because intraoperative monitoring can many times identify exactly which step in an operation caused an injury likely to result in a permanent neurologic deficit, it has contributed to the development of better and safer operating techniques. In addition, there is little doubt among those who have used intraoperative monitoring in teaching hospitals that such monitoring is of great value in teaching residents. These advantages are difficult to measure quantitatively; nevertheless, they are great enough to lead most surgeons who have operated with the aid of such monitoring to demand that it continue.

References

1. Cedzich C, Schramm J, Fahlbusch R. Are flash-evoked visual potentials useful for intraoperative monitoring of visual pathway function? *Neurosurgery* 1987; 21:709–715.

2. Chiappa KH. Evoked potentials in clinical medicine. In: Baker AB, Joynt RJ (eds.), *Clinical Neurology*, Vol. 1, Chap. 7. Philadelphia: Lippincott, 1987: 1–55.

3. Delgado TE, Buchheit WA, Rosenholtz HR, et al. Intraoperative monitoring of facial muscle evoked responses obtained by intracranial stimulation of the facial nerve: a more accurate technique for facial nerve dissection. *Neurosurgery* 1979; 4:418–421.

4. Esslen E. Der Spasmus facialis: eine Parabioseerscheinung. *Dtsch Z Nervenheilkd* 1957; 176:149–172.

5. Friedman WA, Kaplan BJ, Gravenstein D, et al. Intraoperative brain-stem auditory evoked potentials during posterior fossa microvascular decompression. *J Neurosurg* 1985; 62:552–557.

6. Grundy BL. Monitoring of sensory evoked potentials during neurosurgical operations: methods and applications. *Neurosurgery* 1982; 11:556–575.

7. Harner SG, Daube JR, Beatty CW, et al. Intraoperative monitoring of the facial nerve. *Laryngoscope* 1988; 98:209–212.

8. Jannetta PJ. Observations on the etiology of trigeminal neuralgia, hemifacial spasm, acoustic nerve dysfunction, and glossopharyngeal neuralgia: definitive microsurgical treatment and results in 117 patients. *Neurochirurgia (Stuttg)* 1977; 20: 145–154.

9. Jannetta PJ. Hemifacial spasm. In: Samii M, Jannetta PJ (eds.), *The Cranial Nerves*. Heidelberg, West Germany: Springer-Verlag, 1981: 484–493.

10. Jannetta PJ. Posterior fossa neurovascular compression syndromes other than neuralgias. In: Wilkins RH, Rengachary SS (eds.), *Neurosurgery*. New York: McGraw-Hill, 1985:1901–1906.

11. Levy WJ, McCaffrey M, York DH, et al. Motor evoked potentials from transcranial stimulation of the motor cortex in cats. *Neurosurgery* 1984; 15:214–227.

12. Levy WJ, York DH, McCaffrey M, et al. Motor evoked potentials from transcranial stimulation of the motor cortex in humans. *Neurosurgery* 1984; 15:287–302.

13. Lueders H, Gurd A, Hahn J, et al. A new technique for intraoperative monitoring of spinal cord function: multichannel recording of spinal cord and subcortical evoked potentials. *Spine* 1982; 7:110–115.

14. Lueders H, Lesser R, Hahn J, et al. Subcortical somatosensory evoked potentials to median nerve stimulation. *Brain* 1983; 106:341–372.

15. Maccabee PJ, Levine DB, Pinkhasov EI, et al. Evoked potentials recorded from scalp and spinous processes during spinal column surgery. *Electroencephalogr Clin Neurophysiol* 1983; 56:569–582.

16. Møller AR: Electrophysiological monitoring of cranial nerves in operations in the skull base. In: Sekhar LN, Schramm VL Jr (eds.), *Tumors of the Cranial Base: Diagnosis and Treatment*. Mt Kisco, NY: Futura, 1987: 123–132.

17. Møller AR: *Evoked Potentials in Intraoperative Monitoring*. Baltimore: Williams & Wilkins, 1988.

18. Møller AR, Jannetta PJ. Monitoring auditory functions during cranial nerve microvascular decompression operations by direct recording from the eighth nerve. *J Neurosurg* 1983; 59: 493–499.

19. Møller AR, Jannetta PJ. Preservation of facial function during removal of acoustic neuromas: use of monopolar constant-voltage stimulation and EMG. *J Neurosurg* 1984; 61:757–760.

20. Møller AR, Jannetta PJ. Microvascular decompression in hemifacial spasm: intraoperative electrophysiological observations. *Neurosurgery* 1985; 16:612–618.

21. Møller AR, Jannetta PJ. Monitoring facial EMG responses during microvascular decompression operations for hemifacial spasm. *J Neurosurg* 1987; 66:681–685.

22. Møller AR, Møller MB. Does intraoperative monitoring of auditory evoked potentials reduce incidence of hearing loss as a complication of microvascular decompression of cranial nerves? *Neurosurgery* 1989; 24:257–263.

23. Nash CL, Lorig RA, Schatzinger LA, et al. Spinal cord monitoring during operative treatment of the spine. *Clin Orthop* 1977; 126:100–105.

24. Nielsen VK. Pathophysiology of hemifacial spasm: I. Ephaptic transmission and ectopic excitation. *Neurology* 1984; 34: 418–426.

25. Nuwer MR. *Evoked Potential Monitoring in the Operating Room*. New York: Raven Press, 1986.

26. Prass RL, Lüders H. Acoustic (loudspeaker) facial electromyographic monitoring: Part I. Evoked electromyographic activity during acoustic neuroma resection. *Neurosurgery* 1986; 19:392–400.

27. Raudzens PA. Intraoperative monitoring of evoked potentials. *Ann NY Acad Sci* 1982; 388:308–326.

28. Schramm J, Mokrusch T, Fahlbusch R, et al. Detailed analysis of intraoperative changes monitoring brain stem acoustic evoked potentials. *Neurosurgery* 1988; 22:694–702.

29. Sekhar LN, Møller AR. Operative management of tumors involving the cavernous sinus. *J Neurosurg* 1986; 64:879–889.

30. Shiobara R, Nakatsukasa M, Toya S, et al. Intraoperative monitoring and preservation of the facial nerve in acoustic neuroma surgery. In: Castro D (ed.), *Proceedings, Sixth International Symposium on the Facial Nerve*, (in press).

31. Silverstein H, Norrell H, Hyman SM. Simultaneous use of CO_2 laser with continuous monitoring of eighth cranial nerve action potential during acoustic neuroma surgery. *Otolaryngol Head Neck Surg* 1984; 92:80–84.

32. Sugita K, Kobayashi S. Technical and instrumental improvements in the surgical treatment of acoustic neurinomas. *J Neurosurg* 1982; 57:747–752.

33. Wilson WB, Kirsch WM, Neville H, et al. Monitoring of visual function during parasellar surgery. *Surg Neurol* 1976; 5: 323–329.

15

The Paranasal Sinuses: Neurosurgical Considerations

Joseph C. Farmer, Jr.

Functional Anatomy of the Nose and Paranasal Sinuses

A brief review of the functional anatomy of the nose and paranasal sinus complex is in order to develop a better understanding of how diseases in these structures can become neurosurgically significant. The exact relationship of these structures to human respiration has been long debated; however, the anatomic position at the entrance of the respiratory system plus the unique vasculature, mucus-secreting mechanisms, and innervation suggest that they have a major role in human respiration. Current theories indicate that the nose has the following respiratory functions: (1) air passageway, (2) control systems to match inspired and expired air flows to the needs of alveolar ventilation, (3) humidification and warming of the inspired air for optimum alveolar gas exchange, (4) filtration of inspired air, (5) protective system to resist respiratory tract infections and chemical injury, and (6) olfaction.[13,26] The nasal and sinus mucosal lining consists of ciliated, stratified or pseudostratified columnar respiratory epithelium except for squamous epithelium in the nasal vestibule and olfactory epithelium located on the roof of the nasal vault, the adjacent superior nasal septum, and on an occasionally present superior turbinate. This mucosal lining secretes about 1 liter of mucus per day in the adult; approximately one-half is evaporated by the inspired airstream, and the remaining half is swept by the cilia as a blanket into the nasopharynx and swallowed. This mucous blanket contains an electrostatic charge that attracts particulate matter plus immunoglobulins and lysosymes which react to inspired antigens and microorganisms.

On the sides of each nasal passageway are the inferior, middle, and variably present superior turbinates. The mucosal lamina propria of these turbinates contains large vascular spaces that function as erectile tissue which empty and fill in response to changes in temperature and humidity of the inspired airstream and to emotional stimuli. Inspiration of cold dry air results in an increase in mucosal temperature with hyperemia of the surface vessels and filling of the erectile tissues, whereas exposure to warm moist air results in constriction of the surface vessels, emptying of the erectile tissues, and a decrease in mucosal temperature. Breathing warm air of average relative humidity will result in constriction of the superficial vessels with congestion and filling of the deeper vascular spaces. Surface irritation results in emptying of the vascular spaces but with superficial arterial dilatation and increased mucosal surface temperature. A sympathetic response consisting of vasoconstriction and mucosal shrinkage occurs with fear and terror; however, chronic anxiety, frustration, and anger result in a parasympathetic response with swelling of the vascular spaces and increased nasal secretions.[13,26]

The functions of humidification, warming, and cleansing are performed quite efficiently. Once the inspired airstream has reached the nasopharynx, its temperature and relative humidity are raised to close to body temperature and saturation. Large particulate matter is removed by the nasal hairs, whereas smaller particles are retained in the mucous blanket. The nasal functions are further enhanced by the specific anatomy of the nasal channel, with the anterior nares being smaller than the posterior openings. This results in the inspired airstream passing superiorly in a wide curve past the olfactory epithelium and in eddy currents being produced over the anterior aspects of the middle and inferior turbinates and in the posterior nasal passageways. With expiration, eddy currents fill the entire nasal cavity, thus providing for some retention of moisture.[38]

The function of the paranasal sinuses has been long debated, with some investigators concluding that the sinuses seem to serve no purpose and others concluding that the paranasal sinuses act as "surge tanks" to dampen the surge of pressures caused by the stopping and starting of the respired airstream during each respiratory cycle. A more likely function is that the paranasal sinuses provide an increased surface area for mucous production, thus enhancing the defense systems and the humidification of the inspired airstream.

All of the paranasal sinus ostia open into the middle meatus, located beneath the middle turbinate, except for the ostia of the sphenoid and posterior ethmoid sinuses, which open into the posterosuperior nasal passageway (Fig. 15-1). The maxillary sinuses are the largest and, with some portions of the ethmoid sinus complex, are usually present at birth. The medial wall of the maxillary sinus forms the lateral wall of the nasal cavity; its roof forms the floor of the orbit. The medial walls of the ethmoid air cells are the lateral walls of the upper one-half of the nasal cavity. The lateral wall of the ethmoid complex forms the medial wall of the orbit (the lamina papyracea), whereas the posterior wall forms the lateral aspect of the anterior wall of the sphenoid sinus. The roof of the ethmoid complex and the cribriform area form the anteromedial aspect of the floor of the anterior cranial fossa (Fig. 15-2).

The frontal sinuses are located in the frontal bone and vary greatly in size and shape. They start to develop from the anterior ethmoid sinuses at approximately 8 years of age, with continuing development occurring until approximately 25 years of age. The frontal sinuses are absent or rudimen-

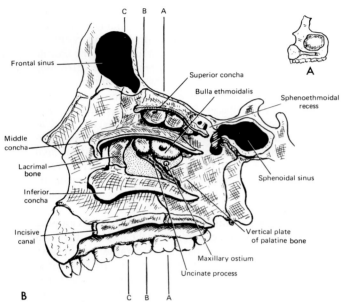

Figure 15-1 *B*, Lateral wall of the nose of an adult, with turbinates removed. *A*. Dry maxilla showing a large ostium. Lines *A*, *B*, and *C* refer to coronal sections in Figure 15-2. [From Davis J. Embryology and anatomy of the head, neck, face, palate, nose, and paranasal sinuses. In: Paparella MM, Shumrick DA (eds.), *Otolaryngology*, 2d ed. Philadelphia: Saunders, 1980; 1:120, with permission.]

tary in about 20 percent of the adult population. The posterior wall of the frontal sinuses forms the inferior aspect of the anterior wall of the anterior cranial fossa. Inferiorly, the frontal sinus posterior wall can extend horizontally along the

floor of the anterior fossa for 1 to 2 cm. This is particularly seen with large frontal sinus cavities.

The sphenoid sinus is located deep in the skull base and begins to pneumatize at about age 8 to 10 years, with pneumatization continuing into the late teens or early adult life. The sphenoid sinus is divided by a central septum, which is in a variable location, with the two lateral cavities opening anteriorly into the posterosuperior aspect of the nasal vault, the sphenoethmoidal recess. These openings are located in a line drawn along the length of the middle turbinate, just posterior to the posterior end of the turbinate. The anatomic relationships of the sphenoid sinus are important (Figs. 15-3 and 15-4). Immediately lateral to the anterior half of the sinus are located the optic foramina, containing the optic nerve and ophthalmic artery plus the contents of the superior orbital fissure including the superior ophthalmic vein, the superior branch of the oculomotor nerve, the nasociliary nerve, the inferior branch of the oculomotor nerve, and the abducens nerve. These structures as well as the contents of the optic foramen are encircled by the fibrous annular ligament of Zinn, which gives origin to the extrinsic ocular muscles. Laterally in the superior orbital fissure are located the lacrimal, frontal, and trochlear nerves. Anteriorly, the lateral bony walls of the sphenoid sinus are of varying thickness. More posteriorly, the superior and posterior bony walls are frequently thin and separate the sinus from the sella turcica, containing the pituitary gland. The cavernous sinuses and internal carotid arteries lie against the lateral walls of the sphenoid sinus. In the cavernous sinus, the abducens nerve is located just lateral to the internal carotid artery; from superior to inferior, are the oculomotor nerve, the trochlear nerve, the ophthalmic nerve, and the maxillary nerve. The anterior roof of the sphenoid sinus forms the posterior floor of the anterior cranial fossa, the planum sphenoidale.

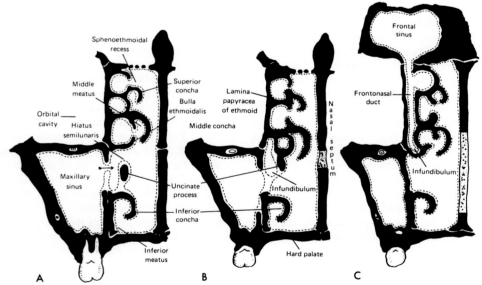

Figure 15-2 Coronal sections along the planes A, B, and C shown in Fig. 15-1. [From Davis J. Embryology and anatomy of the head, neck, face, palate, nose, and paranasal sinuses. In: Paparella MM, Shumrick DA (eds.), *Otolaryngology*, 2d ed. Philadelphia: Saunders, 1980; 1:121, with permission.]

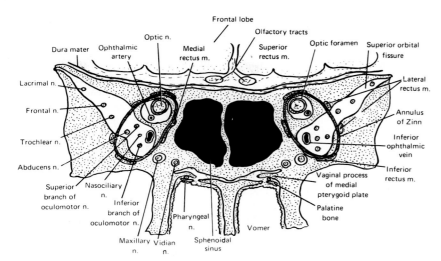

Figure 15-3 Coronal section through the sphenoid sinus at the level of the optic foramina and superior orbital fissures. [From Davis J. Embryology and anatomy of the head, neck, face, palate, nose, and paranasal sinuses. In: Paparella MM, Shumrick DA (eds.), *Otolaryngology*, 2d ed. Philadelphia: Saunders, 1980; 1:122, with permission.]

The Development of Rhinosinusitis

Acute sinus infections by bacteria, viruses, or (rarely) fungi generally result from factors which alter the usually efficient protective nasal physiology described above. Frequently, the alterations caused by common viral rhinitis result in secondary bacterial infection. The common infecting bacteria are *Streptococcus pneumoniae*, group A beta hemolytic streptococci, *Staphylococcus aureus*, and *Haemophilus influenzae*. Sinusitis usually develops from obstruction of the sinus ostia due to mucosal edema and venous engorgement followed by the development of negative pressure from absorption of oxygen. Sinus mucosal congestion with subsequent microorganism invasion, infiltration of leukocytes, venous inflammation, pus formation, and positive pressure then occurs.[6,38]

The common underlying factors which predispose to secondary nasal and sinus infection include:

1. **Allergic rhinosinusitis** The symptoms, which may be seasonal or perennial, include obstruction, sneezing, watery rhinorrhea, and, occasionally, anosmia. Bronchi-tis and asthma may be present. Nasal and sinus polyps occur in the more severe cases, particularly those complicated by secondary infection, and will further compound the problem by producing a mechanical obstruction component.

2. **Chronic nasal irritation** The causative factors include smoking, excessive use of topical nasal adrenergic agents, and, less commonly, industrial fume exposures.

3. **Mechanical nasal obstruction** This is usually related to congenital or trauma-induced internal and external nasal deformities and less frequently to polyps or neoplasia. In children, adenoidal hypertrophy can produce obstruction.

4. **Vasomotor rhinitis** Increased parasympathetic stimulation from emotional stress or medications such as adrenergic blocking agents may result in nonallergic vascular engorgement of the nasal mucosa with sneezing and watery discharge.

Less common causes of rhinosinusitis include:

1. Primary infections such as syphilis, tuberculosis, rhinoscleroma, or leprosy

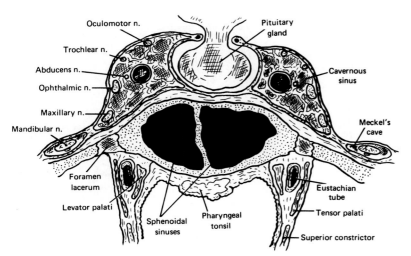

Figure 15-4 Coronal section through the sphenoid sinus at the level of the sella turcica and cavernous sinuses. [From Davis J. Embryology and anatomy of the head, neck, face, palate, nose, and paranasal sinuses. In: Paparella MM, Shumrick DA (eds.), *Otolaryngology*, 2d ed. Philadelphia: Saunders, 1980; 1:122, with permission.]

2. Mycotic infections such as aspergillosis or mucormycosis, which are usually seen in patients who are immunocompromised from other systemic diseases or treatments such as uncontrolled diabetes mellitus, hematologic neoplasia, or chemotherapy

3. Biochemical disorders such as cystic fibrosis

4. Microstructural cilial anomalies such as in Kartagener's syndrome (situs inversus and chronic polypoid rhinosinusitis)

5. Collagen vascular diseases such as necrotizing vasculitis, periarteritis nodosa, relapsing polychondritis, lupus erythematosus, or Sjögren's syndrome

6. Other causes such as Wegener's granulomatosis, lethal midline granuloma, or sarcoidosis

Paranasal sinus infections usually occur secondary to one or several of the above underlying causes. Some patients may have mild chronic problems which are then compounded by secondary infection that develops with exposure to cold, dry air in the winter months.

Intracranial Complications of Rhinosinusitis

The proximity of the paranasal sinuses, particularly the frontal, ethmoid, and sphenoid sinuses, to the orbit, cavernous sinuses, and anterior cranial fossa, plus the shared venous drainage of the sinuses with the diploe of the skull and the intracranial veins, increase the likelihood of orbital and/or intracranial spread of sinus infections (Fig. 15-5).[1,37,44] The development and use of effective antibiotic treatment for purulent sinusitis has been associated with a significant decrease in major orbital and intracranial complications. However, such complications do occur, particularly in immunocompromised patients[2] or with inadequate antibiotic therapy, factors which can mask the clinical picture. Thus, a high index of suspicion with astute clinical judgment is frequently required to recognize and effectively manage these complications.

Sinus infections resulting in intracranial complications usually begin with purulent rhinitis and early involvement of the ethmoid bulla. Rapid spread to the ethmoid, maxillary, and frontal sinuses then occurs because of the close proximity in the middle meatus of the intranasal ostia of these sinuses. Involvement of the posterior ethmoid and sphenoid sinuses also occurs. The purulent inflammatory process results in increased intracavity pressure, disruption and necrosis of the mucosal lining, and subsequent mucoperiosteal inflammation, thrombophlebitis of the venous drainage, and septic thrombosis. Extension into the orbit, cavernous sinus, superior orbital fissure, or cranial cavity then can occur by direct extension through congenital dehiscences, by osteomyelitic breakdown of the bony wall, or by septic thrombophlebitis.[1]

The most common intracranial complications of paranasal sinus infection are meningitis and cavernous sinus thrombosis.[1] The sphenoid sinus has been thought to be the most common site of origin; however, with most intracranial complications of sinusitis there is usually involvement of the frontal, ethmoid, and sphenoid sinuses, and the definition of one sinus as a site of origin can be misleading. Meningitis and CSF rhinorrhea may also follow trauma or sinonasal surgery.[15]

Epidural and subdural abscesses may develop from frontal sinusitis.[32] Cavernous sinus thrombosis and the superior orbital fissure syndrome are thought to usually occur by thrombophlebitis of the nonvalved veins draining the sphenoid and posterior ethmoid sinuses or from extension of ethmoid sinusitis into the orbital apex.[8,39] Frontal lobe abscesses are usually seen with frontal sinusitis but can occur from sphenoid and ethmoid sinusitis.[3] Temporal lobe abscesses are usually related to otologic infections but may occur with sinusitis.[23]

Frontal sinus infection or frontal sinus trauma may lead to osteomyelitis of the frontal bone or infection in a frontal craniotomy bone flap. The causative organism is usually *S. aureus*, but aerobic and anaerobic *Streptococcus* infections can also occur. Initial treatment includes the use of adequate intravenous doses of appropriate antibiotics as determined by culture and sensitivity studies plus surgical drainage of collections of pus in the frontal sinus, pericranial space, and epidural space as localized by computed tomography (CT) scans. Once the acute process is controlled, osteoplastic tissue obliteration of the frontal sinuses using adipose tissue grafts and fascia to plug the frontonasal ducts is usually indicated. Infected or devitalized bone must be removed. The subsequent bone defects are repaired 6 to 12 months later using autogenous rib or iliac bone grafts.[27] The insertion of methyl methacrylate gives a better cosmetic result but increases the risk of a subsequent exacerbation of infection.

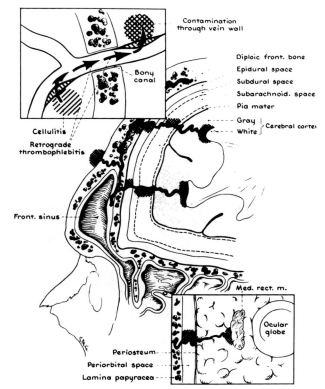

Figure 15-5 Diagrammatic presentation of the venous routes of intracranial spread of sinus infection. (From Adams GL et al.,[1] with permission.)

Paranasal Sinus Mucoceles

A specific lesion of the paranasal sinuses which can lead to intracranial infection is a mucocele. This is a mucus-containing cyst which occurs within the sinus, usually resulting from the trapping of mucus-producing sinus lining by trauma or during an infection. These cysts are benign; they are more commonly seen in the maxillary sinuses, where they are usually innocuous. However, the occurrence of such a cyst in the smaller ethmoid, sphenoid, or frontal sinuses is termed a mucocele and results in pressure atrophy erosion of the surrounding bony walls with extension into the orbit, the anterior soft tissues of the frontal area, or the cranial cavity through the roof of the ethmoid complex or posterior walls of the frontal sinuses. Such cysts can become infected and are then termed mucopyoceles; they are accompanied by more rapid erosion of the surrounding bony walls and increased chances of orbital or intracranial infection.[1]

Mucoceles may present with the symptoms of chronic frontal, vertex, or occipital headache which may be associated with a history suggestive of chronic rhinosinusitis. Commonly, mucoceles occur in the frontoethmoid areas and may present with proptosis or lateral and downward displacement of the eye plus soft tissue swelling from erosion of the adjacent sinus bony walls. Posterior frontal sinus wall erosion may result in meningitis or epidural, subdural, or brain abscess. Sphenoid and posterior ethmoid mucoceles are less frequent and may present with orbital involvement resulting in decreased vision, exophthalmos, or diplopia plus the superior orbital fissure syndrome with ocular palsies and decreased forehead sensation.[7,30,41,44] Radiographic images reveal a shadow density within the involved sinuses, with a smooth dehiscence, thinning, or outward bulging of the surrounding bony walls, suggesting an expanding lesion. The appropriate preoperative evaluations include CT scanning using intravenous contrast administration and bone and soft tissue windows to demonstrate the bony deformities and the extent of the lesion.

The radiographic differentiation of a mucocele from an expanding neoplasm may be difficult. Actual patchy disruption of the adjacent bony architecture would suggest an infiltrating neoplasm. However, such can also be seen with acute sinus infection from a mucocele which has become a mucopyocele or has obstructed the sinus ostium. Neoplasms may also obstruct the sinus ostia, with subsequent infection of the sinus cavity and radiographic disruption or thinning of the sinus walls.[45] Magnetic resonance imaging may offer an improved imaging technique to differentiate paranasal sinus mucoceles from neoplasms and other lesions[19,40]; however, this has not yet been established.

Nasal and Paranasal Sinus Neoplasms

Neoplastic lesions of the nose and paranasal sinuses, particularly those involving the frontal, ethmoid, and sphenoid sinuses plus the upper nasal regions, the cribriform plate area, and the nasopharynx, frequently have neurosurgical significance. These tumors may be classified as benign, intermediate, or malignant.[16]

The most common benign tumors are the squamous cell papillomas, thought to be caused by papovaviruses. They occur as exophytic types or as inverting papillomas which are invasive and can destroy bone but do not metastasize. Malignant degeneration to squamous cell carcinoma occurs in 10 percent of the cases.[38] These occur usually in the lateral wall of the nose and invade the ethmoid and maxillary sinuses.[36] They usually can be removed by resection of the lateral wall of the nasal cavity or through an external ethmoidectomy approach. Less frequent benign tumors which may also have neurosurgical significance include fibromas, neurilemomas, ossifying fibromas, and osteomas. Osteomas are noted more commonly in the frontal sinus or anterior ethmoid regions and may block the nasofrontal duct, producing frontal sinusitis or a mucocele.

Three percent of all malignant tumors of the upper respiratory tract arise in the nose and paranasal sinuses, with 59 percent of such tumors involving the maxillary sinuses; 24 percent, the nasal cavities; 16 percent, the ethmoid sinuses; and less than 1 percent involving the sphenoid or frontal sinuses.[36] The most common malignant neoplasms are squamous cell carcinomas, occurring in 80 percent of the cases.[36] Other malignant tumors which occur less frequently are adenoid cystic carcinoma, mucoepidermoid carcinoma, malignant mixed tumor, adenocarcinoma, melanoma, lymphoma, fibrosarcoma, osteosarcoma, and chondrosarcoma. The most common malignant neoplasm arising elsewhere and metastasizing to the paranasal sinuses is hypernephroma.[36,38] Other metastatic lesions of the paranasal sinuses include undifferentiated tumors arising from the lung, breast, prostate, and pancreas.[36] Regional node involvement from primary squamous cell carcinoma in the paranasal sinuses occurs in about 15 percent of all cases; nodal spread and distant metastasis occur in 8 percent, and distant metastasis only occurs in 9 percent.[43]

The diagnosis of nasal and paranasal sinus cancer is usually made late because the early symptoms of such cancers are similar to those found in patients with acute and chronic sinusitis. Frequently, tumors arising in the maxillary sinus have spread to the ethmoid sinuses, cribriform plate, and orbit by the time the diagnosis is made. Tumors arising in the ethmoid, frontal, and sphenoid sinuses are less common; however, intracranial or orbital involvement are frequently seen at the initial presentation.[43]

Treatment of Paranasal Sinus Mucoceles and Neoplasms

The optimal treatment of expanding mucoceles and neoplasms of the paranasal sinuses is surgical removal; frequently, pre- or postoperative radiation therapy is needed for carcinoma.[27,36] When the preoperative history, physical examination, and appropriate imaging techniques reveal probable or definite intracranial involvement or when the location of a lesion requires an intracranial exposure for *en bloc* removal, a combined effort of the otolaryngology–head and neck surgery and neurosurgical teams is required. The advantages of a combined neurosurgical and head and neck surgical team approach have long been recognized and include (1) a more precise localization of the intracranial extent of the lesion, (2) improved protection of the brain during lesion removal, (3) an increased possibility of *en bloc* removal, and (4) improved capabilities of avoiding CSF fistulas.[4,21,22]

Surgical resections which result in a loss of more than one-half of the posterior wall of the frontal sinus or injury to the frontonasal duct usually require techniques that remove the frontal sinus as an air-containing cavity in order to avoid sequestration and trapping of the sinus mucosa, which may lead to subsequent mucocele formation or sinus infection. A suitable such technique is cranialization of the frontal sinus.[10,28] Cranialization is accomplished by complete removal of the remaining posterior sinus wall and the remaining frontal sinus mucosa using a drill and rotating burrs, plus plugging of the frontonasal ducts with fascia to prevent future mucosal ingrowth and to separate the nasal cavity from the anterior cranial fossa. The dura mater and brain are allowed to expand against the anterior frontal sinus table.

Another technique to remove the frontal sinus as a functioning cavity is obliteration, which is generally considered if the frontal sinus bony walls are largely intact. It is accomplished via a coronal scalp flap or bilateral upper brow and glabella incision and exposure of the frontal sinus complex through an anterior osteoplastic flap which is constructed with the aid of a sterilized x-ray template trimmed from a 6-ft Caldwell roentgenogram. The frontal sinus mucosa is removed completely using a drill and rotating burrs, and the frontonasal ducts are obstructed with fascia. The sinus is then packed with a fat graft obtained from the anterior abdominal wall. The osteoplastic flap is closed and anchored into position with galeal and/or transosseous sutures.[27]

If significant portions of both the anterior and posterior or the anterior frontal sinus bony walls are missing, the frontal sinus may be ablated by removing bone and mucosal fragments completely, plugging the frontonasal ducts, and collapsing the anterior scalp flap against the dura. This leaves an unsightly, depressed forehead, which will require future reconstruction. The techniques of cranialization, obliteration, or ablation of the frontal sinus complex are also used in the management of frontal sinus fractures as discussed below.

If there are only small disruptions of the bony anterior and/or posterior frontal sinus walls and the frontonasal ducts seem to be functional without inflammation or disruption, the frontal sinus cavity may be preserved. The dura is repaired as needed and may be reinforced by a fascial graft placed between the dura and the bony defect. Defects in the roof of the ethmoid sinuses and cribriform complex can be managed by an intracranial fascial graft,[5] an intracranial galeal graft,[34] or an intranasal mucosal flap.[27] Large anterior skull-base defects have been successfully managed by pericranial flaps.[21,22,31] A split-thickness skin graft is used to reinforce the flap from the intranasal side. Defects in the walls of the sphenoid sinus are treated by a trans-septal or external ethmoid approach.[27] The sinus mucosa is removed, and the defect is closed by packing the sinus with adipose and fascia tissue grafts taken from the anterior abdominal wall. A septal mucosal flap may be used with an ethmoidectomy approach. The nose and posterosuperior nasal recess are then packed using antibiotic-impregnated gauze, which can be removed in 4 to 5 days.

Paranasal Sinus and Nasal Fractures Associated with Intracranial Injury

Fractures involving the nasal-ethmoid complex and frontal sinuses may be associated with intracranial complications, particularly pneumocephalus and CSF rhinorrhea.[11,17,25,35,42] These complications frequently occur acutely but may be unrecognized initially, with patients presenting sometime later with meningitis, brain abscess, late pneumocephalus from forceful sneezing, or continuous or intermittent CSF rhinorrhea. Disruption of the frontonasal ducts or entrapment of sinus mucosa may lead to late frontal sinusitis and empyema or a frontoethmoid mucocele or mucopyocele with intracranial involvement. These complications may occur years after the initial injury. The appropriate management of these injuries commonly requires a coordinated effort between the neurosurgical and otolaryngology–head and neck surgery teams. Nasoethmoid fractures, including those occurring with Le Fort II and Le Fort III maxillary fractures with detachment of the midface skeleton from the cranium, may result in acute or delayed pneumocephalus, recurrent meningitis, or other intracranial infection or CSF rhinorrhea. Any patient who complains of clear watery nasal discharge or has a history of recurrent meningitis, particularly those patients with a past history of head trauma, should be suspected of having a break in the mucosal, skeletal, and dural layers which normally separate the CSF and brain from the sinus and nasal cavities. Nasoethmoid fractures also commonly result in disruption of the frontonasal duct; thus, these patients may also present with late frontal sinusitis, frontal sinus empyema, or a frontoethmoid mucocele.

Diagnosis and Surgical Treatment of CSF Rhinorrhea

The diagnosis of CSF rhinorrhea can be difficult, particularly in those patients who have minimal and intermittent watery nasal discharge.[18,27] The classical method of diagnosis by determining the glucose concentration of the collected nasal drainage may be misleading because lacrimal and nasal secretions contain widely varying glucose concentrations.

Patients with a prior history of trauma who develop watery nasal discharge should undergo special studies to determine the presence or absence of a CSF leak. If the CSF leakage is of sufficient volume, it may be detected by the intrathecal injection of a water-soluble contrast agent in combination with a CT scan of the anterior cranial fossa and paranasal sinus complex, with saggital and coronal views. However, small leaks may not be detectable by this method.

A possibly more precise method involves the nasal insertion of separately labeled cotton pledgets into the topically anesthetized posterosuperior sphenoethmoidal recess, the superior nasal passageway above the middle turbinate, and the middle meatus–ethmoid bulla area. Fluorescein diluted with CSF or with Ringer's solution, or radioactive technetium, is then injected intrathecally, and the patient is placed in a head-dependent position. Up to several hours later, depending upon the estimated rate of leakage, the cotton pledgets are removed and analyzed for fluorescence or radioactivity. The appearance of marked fluorescence or radioactivity (1) in the pledget from the posterosuperior sphenoethmoid recess suggests a leak through the ipsilateral sphenoid or posterior ethmoid sinus complex, (2) in the pledget that had been placed above the middle turbinate suggests a leak from the ipsilateral cribriform plate area, or (3) in the pledget that had been placed in the middle meatus–ethmoid bulla region suggests a leak from the ipsilateral anterior ethmoid cells or frontal sinus.

The management of CSF rhinorrhea resulting from nasoethmoidal or frontal fractures is surgical.[18,27] Cribriform, nasoethmoid, or sphenoid sinus leaks are usually repaired by an external frontoethmoid approach; frontal sinus leaks are best managed by an osteoplastic flap approach through a brow-glabella or coronal scalp flap incision.[27] Occasionally, the preoperative leak studies reveal only the side of the leak; then a frontoethmoid approach should be chosen because inspection of the roof of the ethmoid complex, the sphenoid sinus, the cribriform plate, and a large part of the inferior frontal sinus can be accomplished via this approach. The operating microscope is used to appropriately identify the skeletal and dural defects, which are closed with fascia and covered by nasal mucosa that is held in place with intranasal packing for 4 to 7 days. Sphenoid sinus leaks are repaired by removal of the sphenoid sinus mucosa and insertion of fascia plus abdominal wall fat to pack the sinus. Alternative methods of closing the defects include the creation of a nasal septal mucosal flap as described by Montgomery.[27] With large defects involving the floor of the anterior cranial fossa, an approach through a frontal craniotomy with closure intracranially utilizing fascia grafts or fascia-pericranial flaps, as described above, should be considered.

During such extradural operations, the detection of small or intermittent leaks can be difficult. A technique to enhance detection involves the insertion of a lumbar subarachnoid catheter and the instillation of sterile Ringer's solution to increase the pressure and flow of CSF through the defect while one is closely observing the surgically exposed suspect area using the operating microscope. The anesthesia team must carefully monitor the vital signs. Once the leak is identified, the catheter can be used to drain fluid at operation and postoperatively in order to facilitate and enhance closure.[18]

These surgical procedures should be accompanied by the perioperative administration of one or more antibiotics which can penetrate into the CSF space. The nasal packing is usually left in place for 4 to 7 days to allow fixation of fascial flaps and grafts. Defects that are repaired by the application of tissue grafts and flaps from below usually require removal of CSF for several days through a lumbar subarachnoid catheter to reduce the intracranial CSF pressure and enhance the sealing of the defect. However, care must be taken to observe the patient carefully and ensure that a pneumocephalus does not develop because of a less-than-optimal seal and the development of a relatively negative intracranial pressure at the site of the defect due to the removal of a large amount of CSF. Defects that have been repaired by grafts or flaps applied intracranially, above the defect, may be best managed by avoiding drainage of CSF to allow the intracranial pressure to press the graft or flap against the sides of the defect.

Frontal Sinus Fractures

The diagnosis and management of frontal sinus fractures have been controversial and are still evolving. Part of this is due to the relatively small numbers of patients and short follow-up periods in the early reported series. Also, the use of improved imaging techniques has allowed more accurate diagnoses of the extent of the fractures. Classic techniques using plain x-ray films of the skull frequently have not demonstrated these fractures well, particularly those with displacement of the thinner posterior frontal sinus wall which increases the likelihood of dural or intracranial injuries with CSF leakage.[35,42] Although polytomography can improve the delineation of posterior table and anterior fossa floor fractures, CT has evolved to be the optimal imaging technique for the evaluation of frontal sinus fractures.[29,35] CT scanning has the advantage of delineating soft tissue as well as bone injury. The use of intravenous contrast with CT can further delineate inflammation or abscess formation in the late evaluation of these injuries. The optimal evaluation of the frontal sinus walls is obtained with CT scans that utilize thin, 2-mm bone windows.[35] Computer programs which provide three-dimensional reconstructions of bone window CT scans promise to further enhance the preoperative visualization of these fractures.[20]

Recent classifications and recommendations for management of frontal sinus fractures have been published by Duvall et al.,[14] Wallis and Donald,[42] and Shockley et al.[35] Management considerations are discussed according to which walls of the frontal sinus are involved.

Fractures of the anterior frontal sinus table which are linear and minimally displaced are managed by observation. Serial Caldwell x-ray films are used to monitor the clearing of the sinus; a lack of clearing in 2 weeks indicates a frontonasal duct injury and the need for drainage. Such drainage may be approached through an external frontoethmoid incision.[27] The intersinus septum can then be taken down to attempt ventilation and drainage of the involved sinus through the opposite frontonasal duct until function returns to the involved duct. If function does not return, more extensive surgery such as obliteration will be needed.[27]

Anterior table fractures which are depressed should be explored and elevated. The posterior walls and frontonasal ducts can be directly evaluated. Compound fractures with depressed anterior wall fragments are usually approached through the laceration, using a horizontal incision placed in a natural forehead crease to gain additional exposure, if necessary. If no laceration is present, the anterior wall of the frontal sinus can be approached through bilateral brow incisions which are connected across the bridge of the nose or with a coronal scalp flap incision.[27] While the fractures are exposed, the periosteum is preserved as much as possible and the fragments are carefully reapproximated. Frontonasal duct function may be evaluated by observing for the nasal appearance of diluted methylene blue instilled into the frontal sinus. Lack of ductal patency indicates the need for takedown of the intersinus septum or possible obliteration of the sinus. However, if there is no associated fracture of the posterior wall and no obvious ductal injury is present, one may wish to institute temporary external drainage of the sinus with takedown of the intersinus septum. If frontonasal duct function does not develop within 1 to 2 weeks, obliteration of the sinus can then be considered.

To avoid mucosal entrapment at the fracture lines and subsequent mucocele formation, the adjacent sinus mucosa is carefully removed by excision and drilling.[11] Extensively comminuted anterior table fractures require reinserting and wiring of the fragments.[11,12] Duvall et al.[14] and Mathog[25] suggest that unstable anterior wall fractures may be splinted by absorbable gelatin sponges placed within the sinus. However, Donald advises against any form of packing or intrasinus support because of the potential damage to sinus mucosa and enhancement of mucocele formation.[11] Wiring of the fragments and the placement of an external splint over the fracture is suggested. The management of comminuted anterior wall fractures associated with significant segments of missing bone poses additional problems. Large gaps in the anterior wall usually result in retraction of the forehead scalp and significant areas of depression. These can be reconstructed later with bone grafts. Gaps less than 1.5 cm in size usually do not result in unsightly depression.[11] If large areas of anterior frontal sinus wall are destroyed or unstable and cannot be salvaged, the older operative procedure of ablation of the sinus by completely removing the anterior table as well as the mucosal covering of the entire sinus, plugging the frontonasal ducts with muscle or fascia, and collapsing the frontal skin against the denuded posterior bony wall can be considered. However, this results in an unsightly depression of the forehead which will require future reconstruction. The use of bone grafts from the rib, iliac crest, or outer skull table is not recommended in the acute phase because of the greater risks of infection, reabsorption, or extrusion of the graft, especially with compound injuries. After sufficient healing and contraction has occurred, usually by 6 to 12 months, such grafts can be used to repair depressions of the forehead or defects in the superior orbital rim.

The management of posterior wall fractures is controversial. The results of Duvall et al.[14] would suggest that nondisplaced or minimally displaced posterior wall fractures are generally not associated with CSF leaks and can be managed successfully with antibiotic coverage and observation. However, in this series, all the posterior wall fractures were associated with anterior wall fractures, most of which required operative management that allowed direct visualization of the posterior wall fracture with confirmation of minimal bone displacement and the probable lack of dural injury. Donald,[11] Wallis and Donald,[42] and Shockley et al.[35] recommend exploration of all posterior fractures, both displaced and nondisplaced, because of the significant incidence of undiagnosed dural lacerations, involvement of the frontonasal duct in the fracture, and later development of a frontal sinus mucocele, CSF leakage, or intracranial infection. The exploration is approached either through the brow-glabella or coronal scalp incision and an osteoplastic flap of the anterior frontal sinus wall is constructed.[27] The coronal incision is preferred because this will provide exposure for an intracranial procedure, if this is needed, and the subsequent scar is ordinarily hidden behind the hairline. A sterilized template cut from a 6-ft Caldwell x-ray film is used to construct an osteoplastic flap of the anterior frontal sinus wall. Associated anterior wall injuries will require alterations of the oste-

oplastic flap with careful preservation of the periosteal attachment to the remaining bone fragments.

Posterior wall fractures which are minimally displaced or nondisplaced are managed by removal of a small width of mucosa and bone from both sides of the fracture lines to ensure no mucosal entrapment and to allow inspection and repair of any dural lacerations if present. When severe posterior wall displacement with dural tears and CSF leakage are present, neurosurgical involvement is needed for dural closure and perhaps a craniotomy with dural grafting. Donald recommends obliteration for fractures which involve the frontonasal duct, with cranialization for those cases in which a significant portion of the posterior frontal sinus wall is missing.[11] With cranialization, any defects of the anterior sinus wall can often be repaired with removed posterior wall bone fragments. Shockley et al. suggest that posterior frontal sinus wall fractures, both displaced and nondisplaced, as well as those involving frontonasal duct injury can be managed by obliteration.[35] Through-and-through injuries or those involving extensive comminution of the bony walls or significant bony wall loss are handled with either cranialization or ablation.

Wallis and Donald caution against obliteration with fat grafts when a significant portion of the frontal sinus wall is missing, citing animal studies[12] which revealed decreased fat graft survival when placed against a less vascular dural graft or tissues other than the drill-burred bony sinus wall.[42] Subsequent necrosis of the fat graft leads to retraction away from the frontonasal duct and ingrowth of the mucosa with mucocele development. Thus, cranialization is preferred if more than 20 percent of the sinus walls is missing. None of the patients in the series by Shockley et al. required cranialization.[35] The series of Duvall et al. included 20 patients with displaced posterior wall fractures; 7 underwent sinus cranialization and 13 underwent obliteration.[14] In spite of both groups appearing to have similar extents of injury, three of the seven cranialization patients had meningitis or CSF leaks, whereas no serious complications were encountered with patients undergoing obliteration. Wallis and Donald have reported a much smaller incidence of serious complications with cranialization.[42] Thus, the choice as to which operative procedure to perform for displaced posterior wall fractures, where a significant portion of the wall is missing, i.e., obliteration or cranialization, is not clear. These injuries plus those involving the frontonasal duct require the removal of the frontal sinus as a functioning cavity; with both techniques, careful removal of all frontal sinus mucosa, plugging of the frontonasal ducts with frontal muscle or fascia, and adequate dural closure are important. With obliteration, complete filling of the frontal sinus cavity with fat grafts that have been obtained atraumatically, avoiding crushing or cautery, is needed.

Management of the Frontal Sinuses during a Frontal Craniotomy

Frontal craniotomies which involve entry into the frontal sinuses can result in the early or delayed complications of osteomyelitis of the frontal bone flap and surrounding frontal bone; abscess in the subcutaneous, subperiosteal, or epidural compartment; or frontal sinus mucocele or mucopyocele. The incidence of these complications after frontal craniotomy has not been well documented. Montgomery described one case,[27] and Schramm and Maroon reported in 1979 seven patients who developed inflammatory complications from 2 to 20 years after frontal craniotomies performed for tumors, aneurysms, or trauma.[33] In each case, the frontal sinus had been entered at the time of craniotomy. The complications included subperiosteal abscess, osteitis, osteomyelitis, and mucopyocele. Predisposing factors to the development of these complications when the sinus was entered at the time of craniotomy included a prior history of chronic rhinosinusitis or upper respiratory tract allergy; entrapment of the mucosa in the craniotomy osteotomies; migration of mucosa into the gap of the osteotomy or burr hole defect; obstruction of the frontonasal duct by traumatic disruption, foreign bodies, bone wax, or bone fragments; and an inflammatory reaction of the sinus mucosa to the bone wax or bone fragments.

The recommended management of these complications includes adequate radiographic imaging to identify subcutaneous, subperiosteal, or intracranial abscesses as well as the presence of a mucopyocele and the extent of osteomyelitis.[33] High doses of intravenous antibiotics, initially choosing a broad-spectrum antibiotic such as a second- or third-generation cephalosporin and later modifying the choice based on cultures and sensitivities, are administered. Abscesses are immediately incised and drained. The incision site for such drainage is ideally placed through the previous coronal craniotomy incision or through a brow incision. If possible, midforehead incisions are avoided because of future cosmetic defect and interference with flap viability during subsequent surgery. After the initial inflammatory response has subsided, usually after 7 to 14 days of drainage and antibiotic therapy, definitive surgery is performed, ideally through a coronal incision in order to provide adequate exposure of the frontal bone as well as the frontal sinuses. A template of the frontal sinus and previous craniotomy site which has been cut from a 6-ft Caldwell x-ray film and sterilized is used to construct an osteoplastic frontal sinus flap. The upper edge of the osteoplastic flap should not go above the previous craniotomy osteotomy in order to avoid dural injury. Mucosa found in the previous craniotomy flap as well as all frontal sinus mucosa plus osteitic and necrotic bone are removed with a drill. Any mucopyocele or foreign body, including fragments of bone wax, are removed. The sinus is then obliterated with adipose tissue taken from the abdominal wall, as described above. Postoperative intravenous antibiotics for 5 to 7 days and oral antibiotics for 6 to 8 weeks should be administered, particularly if osteomyelitis is present.

Steps can be taken to prevent or significantly lessen the chances of such complications at the time of craniotomy. Planned frontal craniotomies should include preoperative consideration of whether the frontal sinus will have to be entered. A preoperative Caldwell x-ray view can be used to assist in this evaluation. If possible, the frontal sinus should not be entered. However, particularly with a low frontal craniotomy and when a large sinus is present, entry into the frontal sinus may be unavoidable. Denneny and Davidson describe a combined otolaryngological and neurosurgical approach in treating frontal sinus fractures in patients who are known preoperatively to require a frontal craniotomy.[9] This approach utilizes a frontal or bifrontal craniotomy which is constructed so that the inferior border of the bone flap transects the superior frontal sinus. A preoperative x-ray template from a 6-ft Caldwell view is used to precisely locate the lower margin of the craniotomy so that the frontal sinus can be adequately exposed. This allows appropriate management of frontal sinus injuries, and the authors claim that adequate exposure can be obtained for examination of the sinus and frontonasal ducts as well as needed obliteration or cranialization. In these instances, it is important that all the mucosa, including the mucosa of the bone flap, be removed by drill burrs and that the frontonasal ducts are sealed with fascia or muscle grafts. The authors suggest that if obliteration or cranialization is unnecessary, the function of the sinus is undisturbed by this planned approach for trauma patients.

Schramm and Maroon recommend several steps to lessen the chance of future complications if the frontal sinus is entered during craniotomy.[33] These include the use of powdered Gelfoam (absorbable gelatin sponge; The Upjohn Company, Kalamazoo, MI) or Gelfoam paste instead of bone wax to control bone bleeding and the avoidance of entrapment of mucosa in the craniotomy incision by removal of the mucosa with a diamond burr from that part of the sinus, including the bone flap, adjacent to the craniotomy incision. Muscle or fat grafts are then used to cover the remaining localized areas of bare bone. These implants are secured with an absorbable suture to the adjacent periosteum. Wire sutures to secure the craniotomy flap should not be placed through the frontal sinus because these sutures disrupt the mucosa and thereby increase the chances for mucocele formation. Also the wire and suture tracts provide a direct route for mucosal invasion and spread of any frontal sinus infection to the bone flap or intracranially.

Mann et al.[24] compared three approaches to the management of the frontal sinus during craniotomy: (1) In 25 patients, the surgeon obliterated the entire frontal sinus with muscle, but only in 4 was complete obliteration successful. Partial reaeration of the sinus occurred in 16 patients, and in 5 the sinus became infected. (2) In 11 patients, the surgeon bisected the frontal sinus horizontally. The upper portion of the sinus was cranialized. The frontonasal ducts were maintained, and the lower portion of the sinus was covered with a flap of galea and periosteum. Ten of the 11 sinuses remained aerated and draining; 1 became infected. (3) In 3 patients, the surgeon bisected the sinus vertically. Two of the sinuses remained aerated and draining; 1 became infected. Based on their experience, these authors concluded that, in the management of the frontal sinus during craniotomy, the surgeon should preserve the residual mucosa (except in the bone flap) and should preserve the integrity of the frontonasal ducts. The residual portion of the sinus should be covered with fascia but should not be obliterated. In particular, bone wax should not be left within the sinus.

The question remains as to whether all craniotomy patients who must undergo a preoperatively planned entry into the frontal sinus should also undergo a frontal sinus cranialization or fat obliteration when these procedures are not indicated because of trauma or to remove lesions. In one of their five cases, Denneny and Davidson noted normal frontonasal ducts and no other sinus injury after reduction of a superior anterior table fracture; obliteration was not done in this case.[9] However, this patient was lost to follow-up 3 months afterward, an insufficient time for the development of a mucocele or other complications. Others have not reported frequent complications after craniofacial surgery in which the frontal sinus was usually entered.[4,21,22] However, as Schramm and Maroon have pointed out,[33] the possibility of such complications certainly exists and becomes more likely in those craniotomy patients who have a history of significant rhinosinusitis or nasal allergies. For these patients, obliteration or cranialization would seem indicated if the frontal sinus must be entered. For those patients who do not have a history of significant rhinosinusitis or nasal disease who must undergo frontal sinus entry at craniotomy, and in whom obliteration or cranialization would not seem needed because of trauma or lesion removal, the minimum needed steps to lessen the chances for future complications would be those suggested above.

References

1. Adams GL, Boies LR Jr, Paparella MM. *Boies's Fundamentals of Otolaryngology*, 5th ed. Philadelphia: Saunders, 1978: 407–412.
2. Berlinger NT. Sinusitis in immunodeficient and immunosuppressed patients. *Laryngoscope* 1985; 95:29–33.
3. Bradley PJ, Manning KP, Shaw MDM. Brain abscess secondary to paranasal sinusitis. *J Laryngol Otol* 1984; 98:719–725.
4. Bridger GP. Radical surgery for ethmoid cancer. *Arch Otolaryngol* 1980; 106:630–634.
5. Bridger GP, Shaheen AH. Radical surgery for ethmoid cancer. *J Laryngol Otol* 1968; 82:817–824.
6. Carenfelt C, Lundberg C. Purulent and non-purulent maxillary sinus secretions with respect to pO$_2$, pCO$_2$ and pH. *Acta Otolaryngol (Stockh)* 1977; 84:138–144.
7. Chen HJ, Kao LY, Lui CC. Mucocele of the sphenoid sinus with the apex orbitae syndrome. *Surg Neurol* 1986; 25:101–104.
8. Dale BAB, Mackenzie IJ. The complications of sphenoid sinusitis. *J Laryngol Otol* 1983; 97:661–670.
9. Denneny JC, Davidson WD. Combined otolaryngological and neurosurgical approach in treating sinus fractures. *Laryngoscope* 1987; 97:633–637.
10. Donald PJ. Frontal sinus ablation by cranialization: report of 21 cases. *Arch Otolaryngol* 1982; 108:142–146.
11. Donald PJ. Frontal sinus fractures. In: Cummings CW (ed.), *Otolaryngology—Head and Neck Surgery*. St Louis: Mosby, 1986; 1:901–921.
12. Donald PJ, Ettin M. The safety of frontal sinus fat obliteration when sinus walls are missing. *Laryngoscope* 1986; 96:190–193.
13. Drake-Lee AB. Physiology of the nose and paranasal sinuses. In: Kerr AG, Groves J (eds.), *Scott-Brown's Otolaryngology*. 5th ed. London: Butterworths, 1987; 1:162–182.
14. Duvall AJ III, Porto DP, Lyons D, et al. Frontal sinus fractures: analysis of treatment results. *Arch Otolaryngol Head Neck Surg* 1987; 113:933–935.
15. Freedman HM, Kern EB. Complications of intranasal ethmoidectomy: a review of 1000 consecutive operations. *Laryngoscope* 1979; 89:421–434.
16. Goldstein JC, Sisson GA. Tumor of the nose, paranasal sinuses, and nasopharynx. In: Paparella MM, Shumrick DA (eds.), *Otolaryngology*, 2d ed. Philadelphia: Saunders, 1980; 3:2078–2114.
17. Holt GR. Maxillofacial trauma. In: Cummings CW (ed.), *Otolaryngology—Head and Neck Surgery*. St Louis: Mosby, 1986; 1:313–344.
18. Hudson WR, Hughes LA. Cerebrospinal rhinorrhea: diagnosis and management. *South Med J* 1975; 68:1520–1523.
19. Kennedy DW, Zinreich ST, Kumar AJ, et al. Physiologic mucosal changes within the nose and ethmoid sinus: imaging of the nasal cycle by MRI. *Laryngoscope* 1988; 98:928–933.
20. Koltai PJ, Wood GW. Three-dimensional CT reconstruction for the evaluation and surgical planning of facial fractures. *Otolaryngol Head Neck Surg* 1986; 95:10–15.
21. Ketcham AS, Chretien PB, Van Buren JM, et al. The ethmoid sinuses: a re-evaluation of surgical resection. *Am J Surg* 1973; 126:469–476.
22. Ketcham AS, Wilkins RH, Van Buren JM, et al. A combined intracranial facial approach to the paranasal sinuses. *Am J Surg* 1963; 106:698–703.
23. Maniglia AJ, Van Buren JM, Bruce WB, et al. Intracranial abscesses secondary to ear and paranasal sinus infection. *Otolaryngol Head Neck Surg* 1980; 88:670–680.
24. Mann W, Gilsbach JM, Richelmann H, et al. Management of the frontal sinus during craniotomy. Presented at the Fourth International Congress of the Skull Base Study Group, Hannover, Federal Republic of Germany, June 3, 1988.
25. Mathog RH. Frontoethmoid fractures. In: Gates GA (ed.), *Current Therapy in Otolaryngology—Head and Neck Surgery*. Philadelphia: Decker, 1984:100–104.
26. Meyerhoff WL. Physiology of the nose and paranasal sinuses. In: Paparella MM, Shumrick DA (eds.), *Otolaryngology*, 2d ed., Philadelphia: Saunders, 1980; 1:297–318.
27. Montgomery WW. *Surgery of the Upper Respiratory System*, 2d ed. Philadelphia: Lea & Febiger, 1979, vol 1.
28. Nadell J, Kline DG. Primary reconstruction of depressed frontal skull fractures including those involving the sinus, orbit, and cribriform plate. *J Neurosurg* 1974; 41:200–207.
29. Noyek AM, Kassel EE. Computed tomography in frontal sinus fractures. *Arch Otolaryngol* 1982; 108:378–379.
30. Nugent GR, Sprinkle P, Bloor B. Sphenoid sinus mucoceles. *J Neurosurg* 1970; 32:443–451.
31. Price JC, Loury M, Carson B, et al. The pericranial flap for reconstruction of anterior skull base defects. *Laryngoscope* 1988; 98:1159–1164.
32. Remmler D, Boles R. Intracranial complications of frontal sinusitis. *Laryngoscope* 1980; 90:1814–1824.
33. Schramm VL Jr, Maroon JC. Sinus complications of frontal craniotomy. *Laryngoscope* 1979; 89:1436–1445.
34. Schramm VL Jr, Myers EN, Maroon JC. Anterior skull base surgery for benign and malignant disease. *Laryngoscope* 1979; 89:1077–1091.
35. Shockley WW, Stucker FJ Jr, Gage-White L, et al. Frontal sinus fractures: some problems and some solutions. *Laryngoscope* 1988; 98:18–22.
36. Sisson GA, Becker SP. Cancer of the nasal cavity and paranasal sinuses. In: Suen JY, Myers EN (eds.), *Cancer of the Head and Neck*. New York: Churchill Livingstone, 1981:242–279.
37. Small M, Dale BAB. Intracranial suppuration 1968–1982: a 15 year review. *Clin Otolaryngol* 1984; 9:315–321.
38. Snow B Jr. *Introduction to Otorhinolaryngology*. Chicago: Year Book, 1979.
39. Sofferman RA. Cavernous sinus thrombophlebitis secondary to sphenoid sinusitis. *Laryngoscope* 1983; 93:797–800.
40. Som PM, Shugar JMA, Troy KM, et al. The use of magnetic resonance and computed tomography in the management of a patient with intrasinus hemorrhage. *Arch Otolaryngol Head Neck Surg* 1988; 114:200–202.

41. Tew JM, Saul TG, Mayfield FH. Neurosurgery. In: Paparella MM, Shumrick DA (eds.), *Otolaryngology*, 2d ed. Philadelphia: Saunders, 1980; 1:900–950.

42. Wallis A, Donald PJ. Frontal sinus fractures: a review of 72 cases. *Laryngoscope* 1988; 98:593–598.

43. Weber AL, Stanton AC. Malignant tumors of the paranasal sinuses: radiologic, clinical, and histopathologic evaluation of 200 cases. *Head Neck Surg* 1984; 6:761–776.

44. Wilson WR, Montgomery WW. Infections and granulomas of the nasal airway and paranasal sinuses. In: Paparella MM, Shumrick DA (eds.), *Otolaryngology*, 2d ed. Philadelphia: Saunders, 1980; 3:1972–1983.

45. Zizmor J, Noyek AM. Radiology of the nose and paranasal sinuses. In: Paparella MM, Shumrick DA (eds.), *Otolaryngology*, 2d ed. Philadelphia: Saunders, 1980; 1:1010–1066.

16

Intraoperative Use of Topical Hemostatic Agents in Neurosurgery

Arthur G. Arand
Raymond Sawaya

It has been said that the feature which most distinguishes neurosurgery as a surgical specialty is the control of bleeding without ligature. Indeed, since the rediscovery of the principle of ligature in the sixteenth century, multiple forms of the modern hemostat have been devised to hold blood vessels to allow them to be ligated. Today, ligature clips and staples are among the mainstays in surgical hemostasis. However, the bony confinement, sensitive nature, and indispensability of structure intrinsic to neurosurgery make the use of ligature impossible in many instances. These limitations combined with the potentially devastating consequences of intracranial hemorrhage have facilitated the development and utilization of other hemostatic modalities in neurosurgery, namely, thermal and chemical agents.

The use of thermal energy to achieve hemostasis dates to pharaonic Egypt, but this technique did not return to prominence until the work of Bovie and Cushing in the late 1920s. Their work led to the development of the Bovie electric scalpel and ultimately the bipolar electric coagulator in 1940.[6] These devices achieve hemostasis by induction rather than conduction and radiation of heat, thus limiting tissue destruction. The electric current passing through the tissue generates a magnetic field, aligning the molecules of the tissue along its path. As the current alternates direction, tissue molecules alternate orientation 180 degrees, causing internal friction and heat, thus coagulating tissue. In addition, the intrinsic resistance of the tissue to current causes heating and coagulation. The recent development of bipolar coagulators with impedance sensing feedback systems avoids the problems of sparking, charring of coagulated tissues, and unnecessary damage to adjacent tissue, all of which were possible with the previous systems. One of the reasons that lasers have come to the fore in neurosurgical

hemostasis is the thermal reaction induced by their excitation of the vibrational and rotational qualities of matter. Of significance is the neodymium:yttrium-aluminum-garnet (Nd:YAG) laser, whose long extinction length and preferential heme-pigmented tissue absorption results in a pronounced coagulating effect.

Chemical or topical hemostasis, the focus of this chapter, dates to the time of Hippocrates. Initially, these agents consisted of caustic compounds that caused widespread destruction of the protein elements of tissue, thus achieving an often unreliable amorphous hemostatic plug. With the development of bone wax by Horsley in 1892 and the introduction of gelatin by Carrot in 1886,[29] the modern era of chemical hemostasis was begun. The development of the previously described mechanical and thermal modalities, while of great surgical application where identifiable bleeding vessels required coagulation, were not of any use in the control of bleeding from multiple small vessels of the brain and dura. This need to control topical capillary bleeding provided the impetus for the development of today's topical hemostatics. Initially, cotton pads were used; however, their removal was frequently associated with renewed bleeding, leading to the search for an absorbable pad or agent that could be left in place. Cushing introduced an absorbable agent when he used a skeletal muscle patch to stop capillary ooze. Although later discarded, this approach prompted research that led to the development of oxidized cellulose in 1942 and gelatin foam in 1945, two of today's most commonly used topical hemostatic agents. Since the development of these agents, many other topical agents or combinations of agents have been developed, including microfibrillar collagen, chitosan, topical thrombin, cryoprecipitate coagulum, and fibrin glue. Although similar in purpose, these agents often have different mechanisms of action (Fig. 16-1, Table 16-1).

Gelatin Sponge

Gelatin sponge (Gelfoam; The Upjohn Co., Kalamazoo, MI), was first introduced by Correll and Wise in 1945, as an absorbable material created from gelatin solution. Intrinsically inert, Gelfoam was initially suggested as an absorbable solid carrier for thrombin. Its intensely porous structure allows it to absorb 45 times its weight in blood. Thus, when saturated with blood the pressure exerted by the weight of the blood-soaked Gelfoam in contact with the oozing surface assists in hemostasis because of the swelling of this agent associated with blood absorption. Care should be taken when applying this agent within enclosed bony spaces because of its tendency to swell.

Once in position, Gelfoam can be left in place. Precipitation of fibrin and the gluing effect of the platelet plug between the sponge and wound surface provide some adhesion to the surface tissue. However, some studies have shown that Gelfoam can be easily dislodged from a wound surface.[28] The principal advantage of this agent is its large absorptive capability yielding effectively voluminous amounts of sponge without implanting large quantities of material. Gelfoam is supplied in multiple sizes and shapes and is easily

TABLE 16-1   Summary of Topical Hemostatic Agents

Generic Name	Mode of Action	Advantages	Disadvantages	Complications
Absorbable gelatin sponge	Pressure exerted by large volume of blood absorbed by agent	Nonantigenic No excessive tissue reaction Best agent for control of bone bleeding Absorbs large amount of blood	No intrinsic hemostatic ability Increased incidence of wound infection Swells with blood absorption	Easy to dislodge from site of application Pressure on neural structures by the agent as it absorbs blood
Oxidized regenerated cellulose and oxidized cellulose	Acidity of material reacts with blood in a caustic manner to create an artificial clot; pressure is exerted by the pack against the wound	Mild tissue reaction Rapid reabsorption Decreased adhesion formation Bacteriocidal Easy to handle	Not preferable for sealing dural sinuses Retards bone growth Narrowing and stiffening of vessels when used to wrap vessels	Compressive neuropathies and paraplegia have resulted from swelling of these agents left in bony cavities
Microfibrillar collagen	Provides surface to which platelets can adhere and undergo release reaction; accelerates clotting via direct action on platelets that is mediated through factor XI or a similar factor on platelet's surface	Easy to remove an excess of the agent Uses small amount of the agent Low incidence of allergic reaction Excellent wound adherence No interference with bone growth Best agent for coating vascular anastomoses	Intensely hydrophilic; adheres to instruments and surgical gloves Floated off surfaces by brisk bleeding Increases infection	Can exacerbate abscess formation Can cause dehiscence of cutaneous closure May promote hematoma formation in penetrating wound
Thrombin	Enters directly into coagulation cascade and catalyzes conversion of fibrinogen to fibrin	Instant coagulation Shortens duration of bleeding in heparinized patients No intermediate physiologic agent	Easily washed off surfaces Difficult to apply unless on matrix Does not control arterial bleeding if used alone Loses activity over time	Intravenous penetration can cause intravascular thrombosis and death Febrile reaction due to previous exposure and sensitization
Chitosan	Polymerization or cross-linking of the cellular elements of blood	Not dependent on normal clotting Forms gel of heparinized blood Removal of pledget rarely causes rebleeding Mild tissue reaction Useful in patients with coagulopathies	Lack of clinical studies	None reported thus far due to lack of clinical data
Cryoprecipitate coagulum and fibrin seal	Mimics natural clotting cascade by mixing fibrinogen and thrombin together with the necessary activators	Adheres well to wound Rapid coagulation No toxicity Effective in heparinized patients Controls mild arterial bleeding	Inadequate mixing can produce inconsistent clotting Need to change needle between each pause when applying fibrin seal	Absorption into circulation Allergic reaction to bovine thrombin
EACA and aprotinin	Both agents are reversible fibrinolysis inhibitors, which decrease the rate of activation of plasminogen into plasmin	Rapid reversible action Fibrin stabilizing effect	No effect in slowing hemorrhage from disrupted vasculature	Allergic reaction to aprotinin because it is a foreign protein

SOURCE: Modified from: Arand AG, Sawaya R. Intraoperative chemical hemostasis in neurosurgery. *Neurosurgery* 1986; 18:223–233.

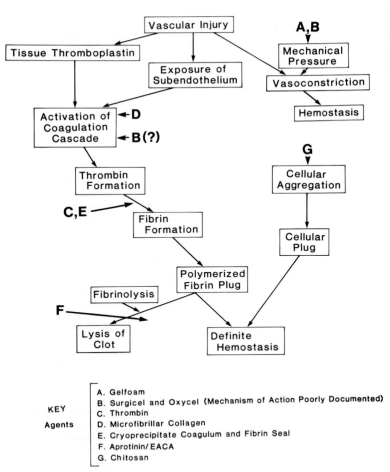

Figure 16-1 Summary of the methods of action of chemical hemostatic agents. (From: Arand AG, Sawaya R. Intraoperative chemical hemostasis in neurosurgery. *Neurosurgery* 1986; 18:223–233.)

KEY
Agents

A. Gelfoam
B. Surgicel and Oxycel (Mechanism of Action Poorly Documented)
C. Thrombin
D. Microfibrillar Collagen
E. Cryoprecipitate Coagulum and Fibrin Seal
F. Aprotinin/EACA
G. Chitosan

shaped by the surgeon at the operating table. Frequently, Gelfoam is soaked with thrombin prior to use to enhance its hemostatic effectiveness. If this is done, the thrombin-soaked Gelfoam should be covered with a cotton pledget and held in place for 10 s with suction, and the pledget then removed.[17] To be maximally effective, blood should absorb through the entire width of the Gelfoam. Failure to accomplish this is due to too much pressure while holding the pledget, too concentrated a thrombin solution, or too thick a piece of Gelfoam. Thus, Gelfoam is minimally effective until coagulation occurs.

If Gelfoam is placed in the epidural space after a laminectomy to control venous bleeding, care must be taken in the interpretation of postoperative magnetic resonance imaging (MRI) scans. The mixture of Gelfoam, blood, and plasma exudate can present as a postoperative mass of inhomogeneous signal that may be confused with a pathologic process, specifically, an epidural hematoma or abscess.[11]

Several studies have attempted to document the histologic reaction of tissue to Gelfoam. Most studies show complete absorption of the Gelfoam between 20 and 45 days after insertion. In one report, a tissue reaction consisting of a leukocytic infiltrate began on about day 6 after implantation and reached a maximum on days 10 to 15.[17] More recent studies have indicated that gelatin sponge is not associated with an increased incidence of postsurgical intraperitoneal adhesion formation.[23]

Gelfoam has been proved to be nonantigenic, despite its animal skin origin, probably due to its lack of aromatic radicals. However, several studies have demonstrated an increase in the rate of infection with implanted Gelfoam, especially in contaminated wounds. In one such study by Dineen, 98 percent of Gelfoam-containing experimentally created and contaminated wounds developed sepsis vs. 96 percent of controls and 3 percent of the Oxycel-implanted group.[10]

Thrombin-soaked Gelfoam reduces bleeding from cancellous bone by up to 75 percent over control values. Furthermore, gelatin foam does not retard bone growth when applied to cancellous bone or fracture surfaces, as do other topical agents. When made into a paste (1 g Gelfoam mixed with 4 ml saline), a reduction in bleeding time of 85 percent is noted, an improvement of 10 percent over thrombin and Gelfoam and far better than that achieved by microfibrillar collagen (47 percent). This effect is thought to be due to better filling of the pores of the bone by the paste, and the lattice structure of the Gelfoam which facilitates clotting. The Cloward procedure often requires controlling such cancellous bone bleeding. Gelfoam can be used in this setting in one of two ways. First, Gelfoam paste may be applied to the side walls during drilling and at the end, after drilling is completed.[32] The second approach utilizes folded sheets of Gelfoam containing thrombin (a 45-cm sheet with 250 units of thrombin) placed into the hole with forceps while drilling to make a pulp and force it into the pores of the bone.[24] Although sufficient to control cancellous ooze, Gelfoam will not control diploic bleeding; bone wax is the agent of choice for this situation.

Compression with Gelfoam can control venous sinus bleeding; however, it is easily dislodged from the sinus tear when the overlying cottonoid is removed. With the increasing development of interventional neuroradiology, new uses for Gelfoam have been found in preoperative embolization of highly vascular lesions such as meningiomas.[27] Other uses of Gelfoam include the control of capillary ooze, the sealing of spinal fluid leaks, the bridging of defects in the dura mater, and the control of bleeding from small arteries.

Oxidized Cellulose and Oxidized Regenerated Cellulose

Oxidized cellulose (OC) (Oxycel; Parke-Davis, Morris Plains, NJ) and oxidized regenerated cellulose (ORC) (Surgicel; Johnson & Johnson Patient Care, New Brunswick, NJ) are absorbable, chemically altered forms of cellulose, a well-studied biopolymer. OC was first described in 1942 and consists of cellulose in the form of cotton or gauze that is subjected to oxidation by nitrous oxide. This oxidation converts certain hydroxyl groups to carboxyl groups and thus solubilizes the material at physiologic pH. Initially, control of bleeding was thought to be mechanical, secondary to exerted pressure by the gauze pack. Later research revealed that oxidation of cellulose causes the resulting product to behave as an organic acid. As such, it behaves as a caustic agent, reacting with blood to produce a reddish-brown mass that functions as an artificial clot. The color change is due to the production of acid hematin.[29] Because of its acidic properties, OC is much more of a chemical agent than Gelfoam, whose mechanism is essentially mechanical. Also, because of its acidic pH, OC is rendered less effective by the addition of the more basic thrombin, which is destroyed by the acidic environment. ORC is made from cellulose that is first dissolved and extruded as a continuous fiber. The fabric made from these fibers has a more uniform composition, and its oxidation can be more closely regulated, resulting in less variation in tissue absorption and in tissue reaction. Mechanistically, Surgicel and Oxycel are identical and are therefore considered together in this discussion. The only significant differences are the superior handling characteristics of the Surgicel and the interference with epithelialization characteristic of Oxycel.

These products come in a wide variety of preparations: Oxycel as a gauze pad, pledget, or cotton-type pledget, and Surgicel in different-sized knitted strips. Their most frequent use is to control topical capillary ooze. They can be placed under osteoplastic flaps to control epidural oozing or control oozing from dural surfaces. In spinal procedures, they are frequently used to control bleeding from the lateral veins of the extradural plexus. Used alone, neither of these materials will stop oozing from a large or medium-sized artery, nor will they control dural sinus bleeding,[20] something better achieved with Gelfoam.

Several earlier studies demonstrated that the tissue reaction to OC was very mild. There was no delay in wound healing, no evidence of rebleeding on removal of the brown gelatinous mass, and no evidence of a foreign-body reaction. The rate of absorption of the material varied from 2 days to 6 weeks, depending on the amount implanted, the nature of the tissue, and the degree of oxidation. In general, there was a direct correlation between oxidation, acidity, and tissue reaction. When implanted into the cortex of cats, total absorption of the material was noted within 3 to 6 weeks, with a minimum of glial reaction.[13] A recent study of OC implanted into the rabbit cortex showed oxidized cellulose to be resorbed from the outer border inward; it did induce the formation of giant cells, but was ultimately resorbed.[34]

Recent studies indicate that, in vivo, Surgicel consists of two components, a uremic acid component and a fibrous component.[22] Nearly complete absorption of the uremic acid component occurred within 48 h of implantation. The fibrous residue was then phagocytized by macrophages, but the material did not appear to be easily processed by the cell, as evidenced by large phagosomes present within the macrophages. These results confirm earlier studies that showed residual Surgicel found at implantation sites. Several studies have shown that Surgicel actually reduces adhesion formation in intraperitoneal insertion models.[23,31]

One major advantage of the cellulose products over other topical agents is their potent action against a wide variety of pathogenic organisms.[30] This effect is immediate and is due to the acidic nature of the cellulose (it can be reversed by the addition of sodium hydroxide).[10] It is thought that OC reduces the effective initial inoculum, allowing the host's natural defense to overcome the organisms. Many studies have shown that OC is more effective than gelatin sponge or microfibrillar collagen in preventing artificially inoculated wounds from becoming infected.[30] This antibacterial action can be overcome by very large amounts of OC, which then acts more like a typical foreign body; in that circumstance, there is a higher incidence of wound infection.

Among the major disadvantages associated with oxidized cellulose include its tendency to retard bone growth. When implanted in bone resection sites, OC has been associated with a lack of bone formation and increasing calcification.[21] Histologically, a dense fibrous tissue mass was noted at the Oxycel insertion site when compared to the microfibrillar collagen insertion site, where a minimal inflammatory reaction was noted. Also, when used as a hemostatic agent to wrap vascular anastomoses, progressive narrowing and stiffening of the wrapped artery has occurred over time.[1] These changes were associated with a greater periadventitial inflammatory response and fibrous tissue response in the cellulose-wrapped vessels. The manufacturer warns against such wrapping because of the possibility of stricture formation. Finally, there have been reports of compressive neuropathy resulting from placement of cellulose in areas of bony confinement. These neuropathies were thought to result from a swelling of cellulose when in contact with blood in a closed space. Potential sites of difficulty include the epidural space in laminectomies or around the optic nerve and chiasm, where swelling could produce unwanted pressure.

Microfibrillar Collagen

This polymeric product was first reported as a hemostatic agent in 1969. It is a water-insoluble salt of natural collagen in the form of fibers containing microcrystals 1 μm in length, prepared from purified bovine dermal collagen. Microfibrillar collagen (MFC) is presumed to act through two mechanisms. The first of these is through enhancement of platelet activity, as natural collagen does, facilitating platelet adhesion to fibrin and subsequent platelet aggregation and release of intraplatelet substances. This is based on studies that revealed that MFC can accelerate the coagulation of blood and produce adhesion and aggregation of platelets in native, citrated, and heparinized blood.[18] In addition, microfibrillar collagen reduced the number of free platelets in normal subjects, those with coagulation abnormalities, and those with moderate thrombocytopenia; however, it lost its effectiveness in the presence of severe thrombocytopenia (<10,000/ml).[2] It does not accelerate the clotting time, as measured by prothrombin time or partial thromboplastin time tests. There are more recent studies which suggest that MFC, when applied to incised surfaces, may be cross-linked to the forming fibrin matrices by factor XIIIa, and may form more compact matrices.[15] Taken together, these results suggest that MFC promotes platelet aggregation and release through platelet trapping but also participates in the formation of large, stable hemostatic plugs.

Microfibrillar collagen (Avitene; Avicon, Inc., Fort Worth, TX) is available in flour form and should be kept dry before use because moisture impairs its hemostatic capacity. Since MFC is intensely hydrophilic, dry, smooth, sterile forceps should be used for handling it. Excess agent should be removed, because MFC is a foreign protein and may exacerbate infection and abscess formation. When applied, MFC should be held on the applied surface for 30 s because brisk bleeding tends to float it off. If bleeding recurs, more collagen is added. As a flour, 1 g of MFC will control 50 cm^2 of topical bleeding. Additional methods of application include using a 10-ml syringe, cutting off the tip, removing the plunger and packing it partially full with MFC, reinserting the plunger and compressing the MFC into a wafer which can be applied topically.[3] Alternately, sheets of Oxycel may be filled with MFC and folded to form a sandwich that can be applied to the area of concern.[26] In addition to the control of topical bleeding, MFC can be used to control sinus bleeding, bleeding from cancellous bone, hemorrhage from vascular anastomoses, and, like Gelfoam, as a transcatheter embolization agent.[9]

In the control of cancellous bone bleeding, MFC has shown a decrease in blood loss of up to 73 percent over controls. It is significantly better than thrombin powder alone (40 percent), comparable to thrombin-soaked gelatin foam (61 percent), but not as effective as thrombin-soaked gelatin sponge and gelatin paste (75 to 85 percent). MFC shows no interference with bone healing or increased foreign body reaction, as do Oxycel or bone wax.[8,34] MFC is more difficult to use than gelatin sponge but does adhere better to bone. If used to control bone bleeding, MFC should be packed into the bone surface and pressure applied for 5 to 10 min.

When placed around vascular anastomoses, MFC is more effective than OC and has resulted in a lower percentage of angiographic abnormalities postoperatively (55 vs. 90 percent).[1] In comparison with Gelfoam in the control of bleeding from sagittal sinus lacerations, MFC has been found to be equally effective.[20] Although Gelfoam was easier to apply, MFC offered excellent wound adherence and demonstrated no rebleeding after inadvertent removal, and an excess of the material was easily removed without the reinitiation of bleeding.

Cortical bleeding in dogs and rabbits was easily controlled by MFC in half the time necessary for OC to be effective and required only half the amount of material.[14,34] Adhesion formation was similar, but the cellular response differed, MFC being absorbed faster. Histologically, MFC caused a mild inflammatory reaction and was shown to be completely assimilated within 7 weeks. When it was implanted into the canine cortex, there was a moderate inflammatory cell infiltrate at 4 months, but by 6 months there were only a few inflammatory cells noted. MFC has been noted to cause an increase in the rate of intraperitoneal adhesion formation, but no significant differences were noted in wound closure rates or the breaking strength of wounds versus controls.

Because MFC is an exogenous material, it can potentiate allergic reactions. To date, however, no systemic reactions to beef antibody have been reported. Because beef albumin remains intercalated with the collagen, some weak reaction to these antigens has been reported, but no serious reactions have been noted. In addition, absolute eosinophil counts over 3 postoperative days showed no difference between patients with MFC implanted and those without.[7]

Earlier reports suggested that implanted MFC did not cause any alteration in blood chemistries up to 84 days after implantation. However, with the advent of cell-saving devices, several studies have demonstrated that when it is used topically, MFC can pass through the filters used in these blood-collecting circuits and be reintroduced into the patient's systemic circulation, thus potentially causing organ damage via embolization.[25] In addition, other work has demonstrated that the aggregating ability of platelets exposed to MFC filtrates was 18 to 40 percent of the maximum response induced by adenosine-5'-diphosphate.[19] Both studies support the position that blood contaminated with MFC should not be returned to the patient's circulation.

Finally, as a foreign protein, MFC has the tendency to increase the rate or severity of infection. Versus control animals, animals with MFC and artificially inoculated wounds had a much higher incidence of infection (90 vs 0 percent). Infection occurred even when as little as 5 to 10 mg of agent was used. MFC may also cause hematoma formation in penetrating wounds due to the sealing of surfaces.

Thrombin

The first relatively pure preparation of thrombin in the laboratory was described in 1933. It is produced via a conversion reaction in which bovine prothrombin is activated to thrombin by tissue thromboplastin and $CaCl_2$. It is then standardized, dried, and aseptically sealed. Thrombin (Thrombostat; Parke-Davis) (Thrombinar; Armour Pharmaceutical Co., Blue Bell, PA) is produced in vials containing 100 to 10,000 NIH units. Each unit is equivalent to the amount of thrombin needed to clot 1 ml of a standardized fibrinogen solution in 15 s. Thrombin can be applied as a powder made into a solution and applied directly (Thrombostat spray) or combined with gelatin sponge on a cottonoid patty. Although it causes nearly instant coagulation when it is applied directly, thrombin is easily washed off surfaces if bleeding is severe. Thus, gelatin sponge is the preferred carrier for thrombin, as MFC and OC cannot be used for the reasons discussed above.

Thrombin does shorten the duration of bleeding from puncture sites in heparinized patients. It is not dependent on intermediate agents and thus clots fibrinogen, whole blood, or plasma directly. Its speed of action is concentration-dependent, and it is only ineffective in the absence of fibrinogen. It is not effective alone in the control of arterial bleeding, but it has been used alone in the control of bleeding from cancellous bone. Used in this fashion, however, it is less effective than other topical agents.[8]

Thrombin as a foreign protein is antigenic and should be avoided in patients sensitive to its components. If injected directly into large vessels it can lead to thrombosis and death. In solution, loss of activity occurs within 8 h at room temperature or within 48 h if refrigerated. After these time periods, it should be discarded. When used in neurosurgical procedures, a 100 U/ml concentration is usually effective. This is obtained by mixing 10 ml diluent with the contents of a 1000-U package. If bleeding is more severe, up to 2000 U/ml can be used.

Additional Agents

There are several other topical hemostatic agents whose uses within neurosurgery are still evolving. The first of these is *cryoprecipitate coagulum*. This agent was first described in 1943. At that time, it was successfully used to remove single or multiple calculi from the renal pelvis. Its use declined due to the complexity of the technique, anaphylactic reactions, and a high risk of contracting hepatitis. Since then, the replacement of bovine fibrinogen by autologous plasma has resolved the problem caused by anaphylactic reactions on second exposure. Subsequent studies indicated that human single-donor cryoprecipitate and bovine thrombin-$CaCl_2$ in a 1-ml:2-U:1-mg ratio formed a clot of consistent and comparable strength. Single-donor cryoprecipitate has solved many of the above-mentioned problems. It is stable for up to 2 years, can be thawed in 15 min, and is hepatitis-B antigen screened. Autologous cryoprecipitate can be used, but 10 days are required to yield 25 to 40 ml of concentrate.[12] Although initially used to treat renal calculi,[5,12] there have been more recent reports of its use as a topical hemostatic agent in neurosurgery, with excellent results.[16] A slight modification of this technique is known as the fibrin seal. This technique, which is described in detail in the following chapter, involves mixing cryoprecipitate (or fibrinogen)

with bovine thrombin, $CaCl_2$, and aprotinin, thus mimicking the end stage of plasmatic coagulation. Obviously, this agent could be of great use in neurosurgery.

Chitosan is another potential topical hemostat. It is a polymerized and partially deacetylated derivative of arthropod chitosan, the structural polymer of arthropods. As a hemostatic agent, it is not dependent on normal clotting mechanisms and is rapidly active. It will form a coagulum when it comes in contact with defibrinated blood, heparinized blood, or washed red blood cells. The clot that is formed does not retract, and thus the supposed mechanism of action implies polymerization or cross-linking of the cellular elements of blood. Chitosan is obtained as a solid but can be made into a solution that must be refrigerated to maintain effectiveness. Histologic studies did not reveal any significant differences between chitosan and other topical agents in tissue biocompatibility.[4] However, to date no studies have sought to further evaluate this agent's potential use in neurosurgery as a topical hemostatic agent.

Antifibrinolytic agents, which exert their effect by the inhibition of plasmin, the effector substance in fibrinolysis, can be used systemically or topically. Epsilon-aminocaproic acid (EACA) (Amicar; Lederle Laboratories, Pearl River, NY) acts by competitive inhibition of plasmin activators which split peptides from plasminogen to form plasmin. This agent is given systemically for the control of fibrinolytic hemorrhage. Aprotinin (Trasylol; FBA Pharmaceuticals, Inc., New York, NY) is not currently licensed for use in the United States. It is a polypeptide derived from bovine salivary glands that inhibits plasmin by forming a stable complex with the free enzyme. Aprotinin has been used in the control of fibrinolytic hemorrhage and in high concentration has been used in the fibrin glue technique to create a fibrin-stabilizing effect. This effect has also been demonstrated by intraoperative application topically on swabs of film foam.[33] Early studies report no complications or intolerances due to the use of aprotinin.

Conclusions

There are currently a wide variety of topical agents available in neurosurgery. The fundamental knowledge concerning these agents at both clinical and scientific levels varies considerably from agent to agent, but based on research done to date, several conclusions can be drawn. First, Gelfoam is clearly the best agent for the control of bone bleeding and is useful as a vehicle for other agents. Surgicel and Oxycel show a clear advantage for the control of topical bleeding in patients in whom the risk of infection is high. Their tendency to retard bone growth and induce occlusion of vessels in microvascular surgery and their capacity to swell, causing potential neuropathies, limits their use. Microfibrillar collagen is the superior agent for the control of bleeding from vascular anastomoses and is of great use in stopping capillary ooze and bone bleeding. But it is easily floated off surfaces and can promote abscess formation, especially in penetrating wounds. Chitosan shows potential in the treatment of patients with coagulopathies, but there is a lack of clinical data. Antifibrinolytic agents and agents such as fibrin glue, which is discussed in the following chapter, show great potential in neurosurgical practice, but more data are needed.

Clearly, the trend is toward the development of agents whose mechanisms of action are known by design and whose effect is due to augmentation of the coagulation cascade or interference with fibrinolysis. This biochemical targeting of agents will undoubtedly produce more effective topical hemostatics, but until then, the agents in use today can be of great benefit when their use is based on a sound knowledge of the agent's mechanism of action and its limitations.

References

1. Abbott WM, Austen WG. Microcrystalline collagen as a topical hemostatic agent for vascular surgery. *Surgery* 1974; 75:925–933.

2. Abbott WM, Austen WG. The effectiveness and mechanism of collagen-induced topical hemostasis. *Surgery* 1975; 78:723–729.

3. Allavie JJ, Kalina RE. Microfibrillar collagen hemostat in ophthalmic surgery. *Ophthalmology* 1981; 88:443–444.

4. Brandenberg G, Leibrock LG, Shuman R, et al. Chitosan: a new topical hemostatic agent for diffuse capillary bleeding in brain tissue. *Neurosurgery* 1984; 15:9–13.

5. Broecker BH, Hackler RH. Simplified coagulum pyelolithotomy using cryoprecipitate. *Urology* 1979; 14:143–144.

6. Caffee HH, Ward D. Bipolar coagulation in microvascular surgery. *Plast Reconstr Surg* 1986; 78:374–377.

7. Cameron WJ. A new topical hemostatic agent in gynecologic surgery. *Obstet Gynecol* 1978; 51:118–122.

8. Cobden RH, Thrasher EL, Harris WH. Topical hemostatic agents to reduce bleeding from cancellous bone: a comparison of microcrystalline collagen, thrombin, and thrombin-soaked gelatin foam. *J Bone Joint Surg [Am]* 1976; 58A:70–73.

9. Diamond NG, Casarella WJ, Bachman DM, et al. Microfibrillar collagen hemostat: a new transcatheter embolization agent. *Radiology* 1979; 133:775–779.

10. Dineen P. The effect of oxidized regenerated cellulose on experimental intravascular infection. *Surgery* 1977; 82:576–579.

11. Dubin LM, Quencer RM, Green BA. A mimicker of postoperative spinal mass: Gelfoam® in a laminectomy site. *AJNR* 1988; 9:217–218.

12. Fischer CP, Sonda LP III. Cryoprecipitate: its use and effects in canine coagulum pyelolithotomy. *Invest Urol* 1979; 16:266–269.

13. Frantz VK. Absorbable cotton, paper and gauze (oxidized cellulose). *Ann Surg* 1943; 118:116–126.

14. Hait MR, Robb CA, Baxter CR, et al. Comparative evaluation of Avitene microcrystalline collagen hemostat in experimental animal wounds. *Am J Surg* 1973; 125:284–287.

15. Hatsuoka M, Seiki M, Sasaki K, et al. Hemostatic effects of microfibrillar collagen hemostat (MCH) in experimental coagu-lopathy model and its mechanism of hemostasis. *Thromb Res* 1986; 42:407–412.

16. Kennedy JG, Saunders RL. Use of cryoprecipitate coagulum to control tumor-bed bleeding: case report. *J Neurosurg* 1984; 60:1099–1101.

17. Light RU, Prentice HR. Surgical investigation of a new absorbable sponge derived from gelatin for use in hemostasis. *J Neurosurg* 1945; 2:435–455.

18. Mason RG, Read MS. Some effects of a microcrystalline collagen preparation on blood. *Haemostasis* 1974; 3:31–45.

19. McClure M, Duncan GD, Born GV, et al. *In vitro* effect of a microfibrillar collagen hemostat on platelets. *Haemostasis* 1987; 17:349–352.

20. Murphy DJ, Clough CA. A new microcrystalline collagen hemostatic agent. *Surg Neurol* 1974; 2:77–79.

21. Nappi JF, Lehman JA Jr. The effects of Surgicel® on bone formation. *Cleft Palate J* 1980; 17:291–296.

22. Pierce A, Wilson D, Wiebkin O. Surgicel®: macrophage processing of the fibrous component. *Int J Oral Maxillofac Surg* 1987; 16:338–345.

23. Raftery AT. Absorbable haemostatic materials and intraperitoneal adhesion formation. *Br J Surg* 1980; 67:57–58.

24. Rengachary SS, Manguoglu AB. Control of bone bleeding during Cloward procedure: technical note. *J Neurosurg* 1980; 52:138–139.

25. Robicsek F, Duncan GD, Born GVR, et al. Inherent dangers of simultaneous application of microfibrillar collagen hemostat and blood-saving devices. *J Thorac Cardiovasc Surg* 1986; 92:766–770.

26. Rush DS, Bivins BA. The Avitene sandwich method for handling hemostatic agents. *Surg Gynecol Obstet* 1982; 154:729–730.

27. Rutka J, Muller PJ, Chui M. Preoperative Gelfoam® embolization of supratentorial meningiomas. *Can J Surg* 1985; 28:441–443.

28. Rybock JD, Long DM. Use of microfibrillar collagen as a topical hemostatic agent in brain tissue. *J Neurosurg* 1977; 46:501–505.

29. Schechter DC. History of the evolution of methods of hemostasis and the study of blood coagulation. In: Ulin AW, Gollub SS (eds.), *Surgical Bleeding: Handbook for Medicine, Surgery and Specialties*. New York: McGraw-Hill, 1966:1–11.

30. Scher KS, Coil JA Jr. Effects of oxidized cellulose and microfibrillar collagen on infection. *Surgery* 1982; 91:301–304.

31. Shimanuki T, Nishimura K, Montz FJ, et al. Localized prevention of postsurgical adhesion formation and reformation with oxidized regenerated cellulose. *J Biomed Mater Res* 1987; 21:173–185.

32. Taheri ZE. The use of Gelfoam® paste in anterior cervical fusion. *J Neurosurg* 1971; 34:438.

33. Tzonos T, Giromini D. Aprotinin for intraoperative haemostasis. *Neurosurg Rev* 1981; 4:193–194.

34. Voormolen JHC, Ringers J, Bots GTAM, et al. Hemostatic agents: brain tissue reaction and effectiveness: a comparative animal study using collagen fleece and oxidized cellulose. *Neurosurgery* 1987; 20:702–709.

17

The Use of Fibrin Glue in Neurosurgery

Eugene Rossitch, Jr.
Robert H. Wilkins

Historical Aspects

The use of substances containing fibrin for wound management and hemostasis began as early as World War I. At that time, Grey[6] and Harvey[10] used fibrin tampons and patches to control surgical bleeding. In 1940, Young and Medawar reported the sealing of severed peripheral nerves with blood plasma in the laboratory.[21] This was duplicated 3 years later by Tarlov et al.[19]

In spite of the many advantages to using a biomaterial for wound management, these early attempts met with a high degree of failure due to the poor adhesive strength and durability of the sealing material. Because of these unsatisfactory results, the technique was not pursued further until the 1970s. At that time, the initial experiments by Matras et al. led to the development of a two-component fibrin sealant.[16]

Basic Principles

The process of wound healing begins with the formation of hemostatic blood clots. These clots contain fibrinogen as well as platelets and red blood cells. Healing proceeds as fibrin is cross-linked due to the action of factor XIII. This healing process is simulated by the fibrin sealant system.

Use of the two-component fibrin sealant system consists of mixing two solutions. One solution contains fibrinogen, factor XIII, fibronectin, aprotinin, and plasminogen. The second solution contains thrombin and calcium. After mixing these two components, fibrinogen is converted to fibrin monomers which aggregate and form a gel. Simultaneously, thrombin converts factor XIII to factor XIII', which in the presence of calcium ions forms the active enzyme XIIIa. This enzyme cross-links the aggregated fibrin monomers to a high-molecular-weight polymer. Factor XIIIa also cross-links the fibronectin and probably cross-links fibrin and fibronectin with collagen.[17]

During the healing process, plasminogen activators derived from surrounding tissue convert the small amount of plasminogen present in the sealing solution to plasmin, by which the cross-linked fibrin is eventually lysed. To inhibit premature fibrin degradation, aprotinin, a fibrinolysis inhibitor, is added to the solution in order to stabilize the sealing until natural wound healing is sufficiently advanced.

General Use

Because of its three main effects, hemostasis, tissue sealing, and wound healing enhancement, many uses have been found for fibrin sealing in surgery. The hemostatic properties have been employed successfully in numerous clinical situations. In the operating room, fibrin glue has been helpful in stopping diffuse parenchymal bleeding as well as capillary oozing. This function has been especially beneficial to patients with bleeding disorders. In addition, the sealant can be used to preclot porous vascular prostheses in cardiovascular surgery.[12]

Multiple applications have also been found for the tissue-sealing properties of fibrin glue. The glue can reinforce sutures and make a suture line impervious to liquids or gas. This reinforcement is especially useful with suture lines placed in intestinal[5] or microvascular[4] anastomoses. The sealant can also fix osteochondral fragments without requiring artificial implants,[1] treat the premature rupture of the membranes in pregnancy,[3] and fill in bone cavities and defects.[15]

Finally, fibrin sealing can enhance wound healing. It has been employed in the management of skin necrosis and ulceration.[18] In plastic surgery, the sealant has proved to be beneficial when skin is grafted, especially to devascularized or infected recipient sites.[2]

Neurosurgical Uses

We have discussed just some of the general uses for fibrin glue. This list is by no means comprehensive. In neurosurgery, as in the other surgical specialties, multiple applications have also been developed.

Dural defects located at the base of the skull, over the cortical convexity, and along the spinal canal have all been repaired successfully with fibrin sealant. This is done using a suturing-sealing technique in combination with fascia or lyophilized dura. In this situation, the glue simplifies the surgical technique and provides a leakproof dural seal. Using a canine model, Hadley et al. found that a fibrin glue patch method provided a more effective dural closure after a transoral operation than did a primary suture closure or a laser patch weld technique.[9]

Fibrin glue has proved useful in the anastomosis of nerves and nerve grafts in cases in which nerves have been injured by trauma or by tumor excision.[20] Its main advantage over sutures is that the procedure is shorter and the anastomosis is easier to perform, especially in areas where access is difficult.

Fibrin sealant can help provide hemostasis during the operative treatment of large vascular tumors,[7] intracerebral hematomas, or frontobasal injuries.[13] The glue has been used to reinforce cerebral saccular aneurysms[8] and to seal intracranial microvascular anastomoses.[14] Carotid-cavernous fistulas have been repaired using a fibrin adhesive system.[11] In addition, the two-component fibrin system can be employed in the fixation of bone fragments or in a fibrin–bone dust mixture to repair small skull defects. However, more clinical experience must be accumulated before the efficacy of fibrin glue can be assessed adequately. So far, few studies have compared the sealant with traditional treatment options. Yet there is little question that fibrin glue offers many advantages and carries with it a great deal of potential.

Product Information

Fibrin sealant is manufactured under the registered trade names of Tisseel and Tissucol by Immuno AG of Vienna. It is prepared from pooled human plasma obtained exclusively from licensed plasmapheresis centers in central Europe. Only plasma units which have been found to be unreactive in tests for hepatitis B antigen and human immunodeficiency virus (HIV) antibodies are used.

Side effects and contraindications are as yet unknown. However, intravenous administration should be avoided, as thromboembolic complications may occur.

When this chapter was prepared, the fibrin sealant was not yet approved for use in the United States but was available for use in Canada.

References

1. Albrecht FA, Roessner A, Zimmermann E. Closure of osteochondral lesions using chondral fragments and fibrin adhesive. *Arch Orthop Trauma Surg* 1983; 101:213–217.
2. Azzolini A, Bocchi A. Fibrin sealing in plastic surgery. In: Schlag G, Redl H (eds.), *Fibrin Sealant in Operative Medicine: Plastic Surgery—Maxillofacial and Dental Surgery*, Vol 4. Berlin: Springer-Verlag, 1986: 71–78.
3. Baumgarten K, Moser S. The technique of fibrin adhesion for premature rupture of the membranes during pregnancy. *J Perinat Med* 1986; 14:43–49.
4. Fundaro P, Velardi AR, Santoli C. Fibrin gluing a valid aid in coronary artery bypass graft surgery. In: Schlag G, Redl H (eds.), *Fibrin Sealant in Operative Medicine: Thoracic Surgery—Cardiovascular Surgery*, Vol 5. Berlin: Springer-Verlag, 1986: 152–154.
5. Giardino R, Brulatti M, Franchinni A. Colonic anastomoses protected with fibrin sealant. In: Schlag G, Redl H (eds.), *Fibrin Sealant in Operative Medicine: General Surgery and Abdominal Surgery*, Vol 6. Berlin: Springer-Verlag, 1986: 155–158.
6. Grey EG. Fibrin as a haemostatic in cerebral surgery. *Surg Gynecol Obstet* 1915; 21:452–454.
7. Haase J. Fibrin sealing in a case of intractable bleeding from a glioblastoma. In: Skjoldborg H (ed.), *Scientific Workshop 82: Tisseel Tissucol Symposium*. Vienna: Immuno AG, 1982: 75–77.
8. Haase J, Falk E, Find-Madsen F, et al. Experimental and clinical use of Tisseel and muscle to reinforce rat arteries and human cerebral saccular aneurysms. In: Schlag G, Redl H (eds.), *Fibrin Sealant in Operative Medicine: Ophthalmology—Neurosurgery*, Vol 2. Berlin: Springer-Verlag, 1986: 172–175.
9. Hadley MN, Martin NA, Spetzler RF, et al. Comparative transoral dural closure techniques: a canine model. *Neurosurgery* 1988; 22:392–397.
10. Harvey SC. The use of fibrin paper and forms in surgery. *Bost Med Surg J* 1916; 174:658–659.
11. Hasegawa H, Bitoh S, Obashi J, et al. Closure of carotid-cavernous fistulae by use of a fibrin adhesive system. *Surg Neurol* 1985; 24:23–26.
12. Haverich A, Maatz W, Stegman T, et al. Experimental and clinical experiences with double-velour woven dacron prostheses. *Thorac Cardiovasc Surg* 1986; 34:52–53.
13. Kletter G. The use of fibrin adhesive in neurotraumatology. In: Schlag G, Redl H (eds.), *Fibrin Sealant in Operative Medicine: Ophthalmology—Neurosurgery*, Vol 2. Berlin: Springer-Verlag, 1986: 116–122.
14. Kletter G. Fibrin adhesives in intracranial microvascular surgery. In: Schlag G, Redl H (eds.), *Fibrin Sealant in Operative Medicine: Ophthalmology—Neurosurgery*, Vol 2. Berlin: Springer-Verlag, 1986: 129–138.
15. Lucht U, Bünger C, Møller JT, et al. Fibrin sealant in bone transplantation: No effects on blood flow and bone formation in dogs. *Acta Orthop Scand* 1986; 57:19–24.
16. Matras H, Dinges HP, Mamoli B, et al. Non-sutured transplantation: a report on animal experiments. *J Maxillofac Surg* 1973; 1:37–40.
17. Mosher DF, Schad PE. Cross-linking of fibronectin to collagen by blood coagulation factor XIIIa. *J Clin Invest* 1979; 64:781–787.
18. Pers M, Snorrason K, Nielsen IM. Primary results following surgical treatment of pressure sores. *Scand J Plast Reconstr Surg Hand Surg* 1986; 20:123–124.
19. Tarlov IM, Denslow C, Swarz S, et al. Plasma clot suture of nerves. *Arch Surg* 1943; 47:44–58.
20. Wigand ME, Thumfart W. Neurosynthesis of the facial nerve: electrical vs. clinical results. In: Samii M, Jannetta PJ (eds.), *The Cranial Nerves: Anatomy, Pathology, Pathophysiology, Diagnosis, Treatment*. Berlin: Springer-Verlag, 1981: 463–468.
21. Young JZ, Medawar PB. Fibrin suture of peripheral nerves: measurement of the rate of regeneration. *Lancet* 1940; 2:126–128.

18

High Speed Drills

Fremont P. Wirth

Historical Perspective

The application of power tools in surgical procedures is not new. Dr. George F. Green, an English dentist, is credited with having developed the first power instrument in 1869. His foot-powered pneumatic engine preceded the development in the 1920s of a pneumatic osteotome by Dr. Horace C. Pitkin at the Massachusetts General Hospital. Sir Heneage Ogilvie, at Guys Hospital in London, is credited with having developed an air-powered drill and osteotome for use in neurosurgery in 1928. Modern drills with which we are familiar were developed in the 1950s. Dr. Robert J. Nelson, an American Dental Association research fellow at the National Bureau of Standards, developed a high-speed turbine handpiece in 1953.[4] Dr. Robert M. Hall, an oral surgeon in Pittsburgh, developed a high speed drill for dental surgery in 1959 and adapted this to the Hall Surgairtome, a turbine motor-operated drill, in 1963. Dr. Forest C. Barber initiated the development of a high-speed power tool for cranial surgery in the 1950s and after many modifications and refinements produced a vane-type motor in 1967. This motor, the Midas Rex pneumatic drill (Midas Rex Pneumatic Tools, Fort Worth, TX), remains the standard against which all other high-powered pneumatic systems are measured.[5] The Hall (Hall Surgical, Santa Barbara, CA) and Anspach (The Anspach Effort, Inc., Lake Park, FL) companies have more recently introduced similar devices.

Mechanics of High Speed Drills

The vane-type motor is the hallmark of modern high speed drills. These motors incorporate a rotor spindle which is smaller than the inner diameter of the rotor housing and is placed eccentrically. Lengthwise slots in the rotor spindle permit the installation of vanes (Fig 18-1). The vanes move in and out of their slots to trap air as the rotor turns in its eccentric position. Air, which enters the entrance hole, pushes the rotor vane, and centrifugal force pushes the vane outward against the inner casing of the rotor housing, creating a closed chamber. This creates a small pressure chamber, which collects air and holds it until it is dumped at the exhaust port. On occasion, the motor will not start because of this feature, when a vane is positioned over the air en-

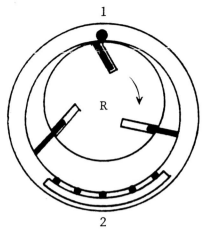

Figure 18-1 Cross section of a vane-type pneumatic motor. Air enters at point 1 and exits through exhaust ports 2. The motor rotates clockwise, and the vanes are held against the rotor housing by centrifugal force. R, rotor.

trance port. In this instance, rotating the motor spindle slightly will allow the motor to start. This type of motor allows speeds of up to 100,000 rpm.[5] The Midas Rex motor is designed to operate at 75,000 rpm but will operate at up to 100,000 rpm. The Surgairtome II drill, marketed by Hall, operates at 90,000 rpm, and the Anspach 65K System operates at approximately 65,000 rpm.

The advantages of high speed drill motors are many. These devices operate with virtually no torque, which minimizes their tendency to shift in position with starting and stopping or with changes of speed. This allows much greater control and hence safety in application of the drill to areas where great precision is required. The high speed and power of these drills combined with specially designed cutting tools allows very rapid bone removal. Furthermore, the cutting tools designed by Midas Rex, and perhaps other manufacturers as well, resist dissection of soft tissue.

These vane-type motors are small and lightweight. The Midas Rex motor is $\frac{3}{4}$ in. in diameter and 3 in. in length, and weighs 3 oz. The Anspach motor is similar. Both of these motors are activated by a foot switch. This allows the hands to be used exclusively for control of the drill. The Hall Surgairtome II is operated by a hand switch attached to the motor. In certain instances this may limit delicate control in operating this motor. Because of the speed, the lack of torque, and the light weight of these devices, they may be used as a bone scalpel with great precision. The power available from the vane-type motor also allows cutting of metal and acrylic where necessary.

Attachments

A variety of cutting tools are available with each of the high speed drills. The broadest selection of dissecting tools is marketed with the Midas Rex drill (Fig. 18-2). A variety of

197

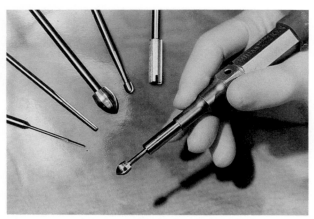

Figure 18-2 A selection of burrs for use with the Midas Rex drill.

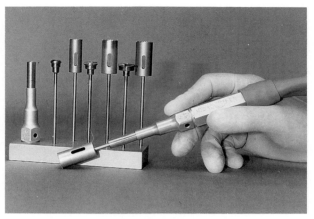

Figure 18-4 Drills and matching hole saws for anterior cervical discectomy and fusion with the Midas Rex drill.

acorn-shaped burrs in different sizes are available for creating burr holes, and smaller cutting drill bits are available to create holes for wiring bone flaps or facets, as well as for removing bone from facet joints, the sphenoid ridge, the anterior clinoid process, the acoustic meatus, and other areas. For the latter applications, longer small drills with delicate sleeves are designed to allow access to deep structures with minimal obstruction of vision.

A craniotome is available with a fine dissecting foot which separates the dura from the inner table of the skull with facility (Fig. 18-3). This suffers from the limitations of all other devices in the elderly patient with thin, adherent dura and an irregular inner table of the skull. It is possible even with this device to cut the dura in these individuals. In the author's experience, however, the use of this craniotome is superior to other methods of bone flap separation. Furthermore, the dissecting ability of the Midas Rex craniotome is adequate for cutting bone over the superior sagittal sinus with safety in most individuals. This same craniotome blade is adaptable for cervical and upper thoracic laminectomy. A

larger version, with a larger footplate and longer cutting blade, is available for use in lumbar and lower thoracic laminectomy. All three manufacturers listed above offer a craniotome blade suitable for craniotomy and cervical and upper thoracic laminectomy. The larger blade and footplate are available from Midas Rex and Anspach for lumbar and lower thoracic laminectomy. The long dissecting tools for posterior fossa or deep cranial work are not available with the Hall Surgairtome II.

In 1981, the author, with technical assistance from engineers at Midas Rex, developed tools for anterior cervical discectomy and fusion, which have been modified and improved over the past 7 years (Fig. 18-4). These tools are not available with the Hall system, and the newest design, offering greater safety, is available only through Midas Rex.

A number of other specially designed tools are also available. These include right-angle drills, pediatric-sized craniotome drills, and various small burrs for craniofacial work. Most manufacturers offer these devices. Various large barrel-shaped burrs are also available from Midas Rex which facilitate corpectomy during anterior operations on the spine. These tools allow rapid bone removal. Many orthopedic attachments are available, but these are of limited interest to the neurosurgeon.

Applications

For cranial work, the high speed drill may be used for virtually every procedure. Burr holes may be created with minimal pressure using the high speed drill which cuts rapidly with light pressure application as opposed to lower speed drills which require application of up to 20 lb pressure for cutting. It is also possible to make a very small bony opening, sufficient to allow access of the 3 × 8 mm footplate of the craniotome, for the creation of a bone flap. The cosmetic advantages of this as compared to the standard four-burr-hole cranial flap are obvious. When properly wired in place, this type of bone flap leaves virtually no visible evidence of a craniotomy. The availability of the small footplate with the

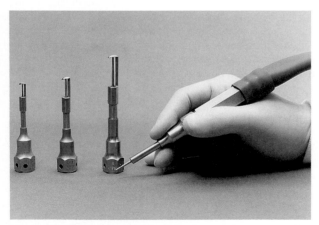

Figure 18-3 Pediatric- and adult-size craniotomy attachments and large sternal cutting tool for the Midas Rex drill.

capability of separating the dura from the inner table of the bone makes this type of flap feasible.

The high speed drill has unique application for the treatment of craniosynostosis. The rapid bone cutting and tendency to seal the cut bony margin greatly decreases blood loss in these cases.[6] As already noted, specially designed drills with various tip sizes and lengths allow removal of bone from the medial sphenoid wing, the anterior clinoid process, the optic canal, the acoustic meatus, and clival structures with the high speed drill. The high speed and tendency to resist capture by soft tissue allow precise control in these areas and greatly enhance the safety of drilling. It is important to recognize, however, that these drills will snare cottonoids, with potentially harmful consequences. For this reason, it is important to use a collagen sponge (e.g., BICOL; Codman & Shurtleff, Inc., Randolph, MA) or similar material, which will not adhere to the drill, to protect critical structures while drilling.[2] Special applications for thick bone and unusual craniofacial anomalies have also been reported with the Midas Rex drill.[3]

The small size of the motor assembly and craniotomy footplate also allows the excision of a posterior fossa bone flap for hemispheric cerebellar tumors, eighth nerve tumors, and microvascular decompression procedures. Replacement of the bone allowed by this technique not only results in improved cosmetics but enhances a sense of security on the patient's part by avoiding the cranial defect over the posterior fossa. This may also decrease the incidence of spinal fluid leakage associated with these procedures by further eliminating the initial dead space associated with these incisions. It is not recommended that an attempt be made to cross the midline or enter the foramen magnum when performing a posterior fossa craniotomy with this device. It has been possible to safely remove bone over the transverse sinus with this device but not over the torcular.

Applications of high speed drills to spinal bone work are many. Use of the craniotome for cervical and upper thoracic laminectomy has already been mentioned. The larger sternal cutting tool may also be used for lumbar laminectomy. For tumors where extensive exposure is necessary, this technique has the obvious advantage of decreasing markedly the surgeon's effort required for bone removal. Bone removal is also much more rapidly accomplished with this method than with rongeurs. By facilitating bone removal in this fashion, the surgeon is more rested and capable of the delicate dissection necessary for intraspinal lesions.

Laminectomy for spinal stenosis is also much easier with the craniotome or sternal-type cutting tools. The lamina in these situations is frequently thickened and harder than normal. Older techniques which require the repeated placement of the rongeur foot beneath the lamina increase both the probability of neural element compression and the risk of dural injury and spinal fluid leakage. In the author's experience, using the high speed drill for cervical, thoracic, and lumbar laminectomy in over 100 cases of spinal stenosis, neither spinal fluid leakage nor neural injury has occurred. In only one case has the dura been partially incised.

The nature of the facets, even in the normal lumbar and thoracic spine, prevent sufficient lateral cutting with the drill to allow entrapment of nerve roots by the device. Especially in lumbar laminectomies, after removal of lamina and spinous process, additional lateral bone removal is generally necessary with a variety of techniques including the dissecting burrs of the high speed drill. In the cervical region where a relatively wider laminectomy is possible, the anterior direction of the nerve roots and their lateral position protect them from entrapment in the cutting tool.

This laminectomy technique allows replacement of the lamina, which may be particularly important in the pediatric patient in prevention of the later development of a spinal deformity. The craniotomy or sternal cutting tools also allow removal of laminar elements in an unstable spine. The high speed and ability of these devices to cut with minimal application of pressure renders this feasible.

It is important, however, to recognize some limitations in the application of the craniotome-type cutting tool for laminectomy. It is critical that the footplate of the device be maintained against the undersurface of the bone. It is also essential that the footplate be below the ligamentum flavum to establish cutting. Irrigation while cutting is important to decrease the heating of adjacent structures. Use of the device on the lamina of C1 and C2 is not recommended because of the variable position of the vertebral artery in this area. In certain other instances, laminectomy with the craniotomy-type cutting tool is also contraindicated. These include patients with a previous hemilaminectomy or other surgery which might be expected to cause scarring of critical structures to the undersurface of the lamina or ligamentum flavum. Likewise, patients with either a penetrating injury, potentially resulting in an open dura and protruding nerve roots, or a dysraphic state where open dura and abnormal adhesions between bony and soft tissue structures might exist are not candidates for laminectomy by this method.

In addition to the use of small cutting burrs for foraminotomy, these same burrs may be used for anterior spinal approaches to remove osteophytes via the disc space after anterior discectomy or to enlarge the disc space in anterior cervical fusion for easier access to osteophytes or to allow the placement of a Smith-Robinson type of bone graft where desired. The cutting tool may also be used to shape the bone for either Smith-Robinson or corpectomy replacement bone grafts.

For anterior cervical discectomy and fusion by a modified Cloward technique, instruments developed by the author in conjunction with Midas Rex offer a number of advantages. Use of the high speed drill for drilling out the interspace allows visual control of drilling depth, avoiding the blind drilling procedure of the hand drill. It also allows angle control for seating of the bone plug in other than a vertical position if desired. Because of the cutting ability of these tools with relatively little pressure, this technique may be used on fractured and otherwise unstable vertebral bodies where application of the pressure necessary to use the hand drill might have unfortunate consequences. The hole saw, with its small size and high speed, greatly facilitates removal of an iliac crest bone dowel with minimal dissection through a muscle-splitting incision. This technique is very rapid relative to the hand drill. Not only is operating time decreased but donor site pain is significantly reduced as well. The author has had experience with this technique in 111 patients at 162 levels with a 95 percent rate of fusion.

In addition to these applications, the high speed drill may

be used for bone decortication prior to fusion, for removal of acrylic, and for a variety of drill hole placements for reconstruction of cranial bones or facial bones after trauma. Vertebral body excision via the anterior approach is greatly enhanced by use of the large burrs with the high speed drill.

Training

The high speed drill is a relatively new tool for neurosurgeons. Few neurosurgical training programs provide laboratory experience and instruction in the use of these devices. For this reason, hands-on workshops are important for the development of appropriate skills and the understanding of the capabilities and limitations of this type of instrumentation. It is unlikely that a surgeon unfamiliar with the capabilities of these drills would recognize their full potential by initiating their use in the operating room setting without prior experience in the laboratory. The implications for patient safety should be obvious. The Midas Rex Institute offers several excellent courses annually; these courses are highly recommended by the author and others for the development of appropriate skills in the use of the drill.[1]

Costs

The Midas Rex drill is the most expensive and costs approximately $25,000. This includes the drill motor and basic attachment set for neurosurgical use. Special attachments are available at additional costs. Burrs and other cutting tools are one-time-use items and cost approximately $75 each. The drill carries a 1-year warranty. The drill has a record of high reliability in the experience of the author and his colleagues. Service is excellent and prompt.

The Hall Surgairtome II, manufactured by Hall Surgical, sells for approximately $2300. Various burr guards and other adaptations are not included in the basic price and are additional-charge items. Burrs are largely single-use items. The Surgairtome II does not include as many attachments as the Midas Rex instrument. Long burrs for this device are one-half the length of the Midas Rex A series tools and are approximately 3.7 in., maximum. An angled attachment is available. Large dissecting burrs for vertebral corpectomy and modified Cloward-type anterior cervical discectomy and fusion cutting tools are not available.

The Anspach 65K system is an adaptation of a drill designed for orthopedic use and has not enjoyed wide acceptance among neurosurgeons to date. The system sells for $15,000, including the drill and basic attachments. The drill has a 2-year warranty. Individual dissecting tools, which are one-time-use items, sell for approximately $65 each.

References

1. Kaufman HH, Wiegand RL, Tunick RH. Teaching surgeons to operate: principles of psychomotor skills training. *Acta Neurochir (Wien)* 1987; 87:1–7.
2. Kurze T. The surgical removal of acoustic tumors. In: Ransohoff J (ed.), *Modern Technics in Surgery: Neurosurgery.* New York: Futura, 1984.
3. Monroe IR, Lauritzen CG, Hoffman HJ, et al. Craniometaphyseal dysplasia, correction of a giant head. In: *Transactions, International Congress of Plastic and Reconstructive Surgery.* Montreal: The Congress, 1988: 323–324.
4. Nelsen RJ, Pelander CE, Kumpula JW. Hydraulic turbine contra-angle handpiece. *J Am Dental Assoc* 1953; 47:324–329.
5. Stillwell WT, Barber FC, Mitchell SB. Instrumentation for total hip arthroplasty. In: Stillwell WT (ed.), *The Art of Total Hip Arthroplasty.* Orlando, FL: Grune & Stratton, 1987: 97–122.
6. Winston KR. Craniosynostosis. In: Wilkins RH, Rengachary SS (eds.), *Neurosurgery.* New York: McGraw-Hill, 1985: 2173–2191.

19

Calcium Phosphate Ceramics as Bone Substitutes

Charles E. Rawlings III
Robert H. Wilkins

Periodically in neurosurgical practice there is a need to fill bony defects in the skull or spine or to fuse bony elements of the spine. Autogeneic (autologous) bone from the iliac crest, calvarium, or rib is often used for these purposes and usually provides a satisfactory result. However, its use necessitates the removal of the graft from another site, adding time, discomfort, and usually a second incision to the operative procedure. In the circumstance of a cranioplasty, unless it involves the simple replacement of a previously removed bone flap, the surgeon may find it difficult to shape the donor bone exactly in order to provide an excellent cosmetic result, especially along the supraorbital rim or at the nasion. Furthermore, grafts of autogeneic bone may be resorbed to a significant degree with time.

Two developments in recent decades have provided the possibility of using a synthetic material both to fill a bony defect and to simultaneously permit or stimulate the regrowth of endogenous bone in the same defect. The first of these developments has been the extraordinary growth of interest and experience in the use of various materials and devices to replace or augment human tissues and organs. The second has been the testing, standardization, and regulation of such materials and devices to ensure their efficacy and safety.[6,22]

The inclination to fill bony defects in the skull has a long history.[34,39] Trephination was performed in many parts of the world as early as the New Stone Age. Some of the trephined skulls from that time and later also showed evidence of attempted cranioplasty, with pieces of gourd, shell, bone, bark, gold, or silver being present in the cranial defect. Toward the end of the nineteenth century, some surgeons used small fragments or larger pieces of autogeneic bone from the skull as free grafts to fill cranial defects, and the use of osteoperiosteal flaps from adjacent skull was introduced in 1890.[30,34,39] Subsequently, other sources of autogeneic bone were tried, such as tibia, rib, ilium, scapula, and sternum.

Autogeneic bone dust has also been used. Since the end of the nineteenth century, numerous other materials have also been used to fill cranial defects and to obliterate the frontal sinus. The list includes autogeneic cartilage, autogeneic fat, allogeneic (homogenous) bone, xenogeneic (heterogenous) bone, decalcified or boiled xenogeneic bone, horn, ivory, rubber, gutta percha, plaster of Paris, mica, celluloid, gum, cork, silver, gold, lead, aluminum, platinum, tantalum, Vitallium, titanium, ticonium, stainless steel, stainless steel wire mesh (alone or with acrylic), methyl methacrylate, polypropylene-polyester, polyethylene, polytetrafluoroethylene-carbon composite, polyethylene terephthalate mesh plus polyetherurethane elastomer (used in association with autogeneic bone and bone paste), silicon rubber, tetrafluoroethylene fluorocarbon polymer, alumina ceramic, epoxy resin–impregnated porous ceramic, and polyacryl.[30,34,39]

In similar fashion, over the years numerous materials and devices have been introduced to provide internal stabilization and fusion of the spine, and to fill bony cavities resulting from tumor removal, etc. Many of the materials that were tried in the skull or spine were found to provoke antigenic or foreign body reactions of varying severity or occasionally to become infected. Even the more refined metal or plastic implants have had problems such as corrosion, fatigue fracturing, and loosening because of the formation of a boundary layer of connective tissue between the implant and the adjacent bone.[21]

These experiences have stimulated a search for biocompatible materials that will temporarily fill bony defects while simultaneously encouraging the restoration of endogenous bone. This search has naturally focused attention on the composition and structure of normal bone and its mechanisms of regeneration.

Normal Bone and Bone Regeneration

Normal bone contains bone cells (osteoblasts, osteocytes, and osteoclasts), collagen, and basic bone substance (which has both organic components such as proteoglycans, hyaluronic acid, and glycogenic proteins and inorganic components such as various calcium salts and water).[9,21] Collagen comprises about 90 to 95 percent of the organic bone matrix. The main inorganic component of bone is hydroxyapatite. The typical mineral composition of bone is 36.7% Ca, 16.0% P, 8.0% CO_3, 0.77% Na, 0.46% Mg, and 0.04% F. The Ca:P ratio is 1.77.[41]

All bone growth is the result of bone deposition on some preexisting surface; bone grows entirely by apposition, one layer at a time. In most bones, osteogenesis occurs by the ossification of a cartilaginous forerunner (endochondral ossification). However, the flat bones of the cranium and face are formed by ossification within an embryonic connective tissue membrane (intramembranous ossification).[9]

By either process, bone can be formed into a cancellous or compact pattern. Cancellous bone is arranged as a lattice of trabeculae, the intervening spaces being filled with marrow. Cortical bone consists of a dense collection of osteons, with each osteon composed of lamellae of bone arranged concentrically around a vascular (haversian) canal. In addition to longitudinal haversian canals, the cortical bone is crossed in a transverse or oblique direction by Volkmann's vascular channels.[9,21,28]

If a bone is fractured but the fracture line is stable and no significant gap exists between the two bone edges, primary healing occurs. New, longitudinally oriented osteons are formed to bridge the fracture cleft. In the more usual circumstance in which a significant gap exists or the fracture is unstable, callus is formed and secondary healing takes place; initially a hematoma collects between the bone edges, and it is then replaced in turn by granulation tissue, fibrous connective tissue or fibrous cartilage, osteoid, and new bone.[9,21]

After the removal of a portion of the calvarium, regeneration of bone originates from the remaining periosteum. When a cranioplasty is performed with a transplant (tissue) or an implant (denatured tissue or a synthetically produced or treated substance), the material inserted and the bed into which it is inserted have a mutual influence on each other.[21] Both are important to the success of the procedure.

If autogeneic cortical bone is inserted as a graft into a bony defect, the osteocytes in the graft undergo necrosis, fibrovascular tissue invades the haversian canals, osteons are resorbed, and apposition of new bone occurs in the spaces formed by this resorption (a process referred to as creeping substitution).[16] However, the formation of new bone may be incomplete. When a free skull flap is replaced at the end of a craniotomy or after a period of sterile storage, the sequential dynamics of skull revitalization are revascularization, resorption, and accretion of new bone. Prolo has noted that the speed and success of bone reincorporation depends upon the rate of revascularization.[31]

Bone Replacement Materials

Numerous types of metal or plastic constructs have been used to replace destroyed segments of bone and diseased joints and to provide skeletal stability. Other materials have been used not only to fill bony defects but also to stimulate the restoration of bone. These have included various organic or inorganic components of bone, or combinations of them. Among the denatured organic substances that have been produced and tested have been collagen and decalcified allogeneic bone matrix, and among the biomaterials of mineral origin that have been developed and tried have been the calcium phosphate ceramics.[21]

A ceramic has been defined as a product made by the baking or firing of a nonmetallic mineral[29] and as a product formed by the combination of one or more metallic elements with one or more nonmetallic elements to form partially ionic, partially covalent compounds.[41] Ceramics of various types were introduced into biomedical use because of the basic idea that since ceramics are materials in an oxidized state, they should not degrade in the human body or tend to be included in biologic reactions, as is true of metals.[12] Biomedical ceramics vary in their solubility, with aluminum oxide ceramics being among the most insoluble and calcium phosphate ceramics being among the most soluble. Intermediate in solubility between these are the glass ceramics.[21]

An important consideration in the replacement of bone

by an artificial substitute is that of implant porosity. Despite the fact that initially it will be weaker from a structural standpoint, a porous material should have an advantage over a solid substance in that the pores should facilitate the ingrowth of fibrovascular tissue that will then ossify.[32] Experiments by Hulbert and Klawitter and their associates have established some guidelines about critical pore size.[18,19,23,24] Klawitter and Hulbert found that mineralized bone growth into porous calcium aluminate skeletal implants required a minimum interconnection pore size of 100 μm, the ingrowth of osteoid tissue required a minimum pore size between 40 and 100 μm, and the ingrowth of fibrous tissue required a minimum pore size between 5 and 15 μm.[23]

Calcium Phosphate Ceramics

Chemical, Physical, and Biologic Properties

A calcium phosphate (CaP) bioceramic is a CaP structure attained by sintering (agglomerating a powder at a temperature below the melting point), coating, thermal conversion, or some other high-temperature process.[11] Virtually all current CaP biomaterials are polycrystalline ceramics which consist of a $CaO \cdot P_2O_5 \cdot H_2O$ system.[20,41] There are six principal calcium salts of orthophosphoric acid; three are too soluble for use in the preparation of biomaterials, and a fourth is difficult to synthesize.[15]

However, CaP ceramics are not a collection of discrete structures. There is, instead, a continuous spectrum of materials of varying Ca:P ratio, hydration, crystalline structure, and stoichiometry that, in the human or animal body, are in dynamic equilibrium with aqueous environments such as serum.[5,10,27,41] CaPs with a Ca:P ratio of 1 or less are soluble in aqueous media and will resorb upon implantation.[41]

Chief among the synthetic calcium phosphates that have been investigated as bone implants have been hydroxyapatite (HA) with the chemical formula of $Ca_{10}(PO_4)_6(OH)_2$ and Ca:P ratio of 1.67, and beta tricalcium phosphate (TCP) having the chemical formula of $Ca_3(PO_4)_2$ and Ca:P ratio of 1.50.[15] TCP ceramics have been found to have exceptionally good tissue compatibility and bond directly to bone without an intermediary layer of connective tissue. However, porous TCP ceramics are dissolved and resorbed relatively quickly and do not have good mechanical stability. With HA ceramics, resorption is considerably slower.[21]

Both TCP and HA have several different crystallographic forms as well as variations in stoichiometry. TCP can have at least six different structures, and HA, with a hexagonal system of loosely held ionic components, routinely has molecular substitutions such as carbonate for hydroxyl groups or carbonate for phosphate groups.[15] In the presence of water, TCP converts to HA via hydroxylation, i.e.,[41]

$$H_2O + 4\ Ca_3(PO_4)_2$$
$$\rightarrow Ca_{10}(PO_4)_6(OH)_2 + 2\ Ca^{2+} + 2\ HPO_4$$

The physical forms and properties of TCP and HA are determined primarily by their methods of manufacture. Either can be solid or porous with varying degrees of porosity.

Several methods are available for the preparation of solid CaP ceramics. The majority involve the sintering of either wet slurries or compacted powders.[41]

The shaping and sintering of a CaP slurry produces a "green body," which has form but poor strength. The green body is then heated further to the firing temperature at which almost complete fusion of the CaP crystals occurs. However, the finished ceramic contains random micropores varying up to 5 μm in size. To obtain a denser product with increased strength and stability, dry CaP powder can be compressed and sintered either in sequence or simultaneously, thus producing a material with less than 5 percent microporosity.[20,21,41]

The term *macroporous* is used to describe a material containing pores varying from 100 to 500 μm in size, a form that enhances the ingrowth of vessels, fibrous tissue, and new bone. There are several methods used to prepare this type of porous CaP ceramic.[20,21,41] If the CaP slurry is made with a powder and an aqueous solution of hydrogen peroxide, oxygen is released at elevated temperatures and leaves behind interconnecting pores up to 100 μm in diameter. As an alternative, an organic structure such as naphthalene or cellulose can be incorporated with the CaP powder before it is compacted and fired, thus yielding a macroporous material. In recent years, it has been noted that the reef-building sea corals have a skeleton that is microscopically similar to an osteon-evacuated bone graft.[16,17] White et al. showed that the porous coral structure can be duplicated by the replamineform process in ceramic, metal, or polymer,[40] and Roy and Linnehan demonstrated that, by another method involving hydrothermal exchange, the calcium carbonate exoskeleton of the coral can be converted directly to hydroxyapatite.[35]

Because of their mechanical properties, discussed below, CaP ceramics are not by themselves good structural materials. They are not prepared as monolithic dense solids for major bony replacement but rather as granules or a porous block for insertion into bony cavities.

The biologic properties of CaP materials are well known and to a large part are based on the fact that calcium and phosphate ions are freely diffusible at the surface of the implant and are identical to those ions found in natural bone. This allows for the accumulation of calcium and phosphate ions on the surface of the implant, and these take part in the formation of new bone directly adjacent to that surface. It has been shown that CaP bioceramics are well tolerated by the body; they cause no inflammation and cause no systemic toxicity. There is no foreign body response nor any evidence of rejection. Moreover, there is excellent bonding to bone, and in porous varieties, ingrowth of new bone occurs. Abnormal calcifications do not occur nor is there elevation of calcium and phosphorous levels in the serum. Around the implant site, the Ca:P ratio slowly rises toward that of normal bone. In other words, biologically, implantation of a CaP biomaterial is much like implantation of a piece of natural bone.[4,8,13,16,17,20,21,32,37]

Factors Governing Biostability

The factors governing the biostability are bioresorbability of CaP ceramics are complex and, even now, are not fully understood. There do, however, appear to be three major factors governing the stability of a bioceramic. These include the chemical structure of the substance, the physical structure of the substance, and the biologic processes active in resorption.[20,27,41]

Chemically, a low Ca:P ratio is associated with high resorbability, whereas a high ratio is associated with greater stability. This, however, is affected by both the density and form of the material. Acidity, the presence of various cations and anions (e.g., Mg^{2+}), and surface charge are also chemical factors affecting absorption. A physical structure with a large degree of porosity is generally associated with a high degree of bioresorbability, whereas a dense ceramic is considered stable. This is mainly a consequence of the increased amount of surface area associated with porosity. Biologic factors such as osteoclasts, macrophages, and the complement system also seem to have a role in the resorption of bioceramics.

Based on his review of the available evidence, Jarcho formulated three guiding rules concerning the bioresorption of CaP implant materials: (1) High density implants of TCP, HA, or mixtures of the two show little tendency to resorb. (2) Porous TCP implants will resorb much more rapidly than porous HA implants. (3) The presence of microporosity may promote bioresorption.[20]

Biomechanical Properties

As has been noted in vitro and confirmed by in vivo trials, the major drawbacks to the use of CaP ceramics are their adverse mechanical properties. They are brittle, have low impact resistance, and have low tensile strength; consequently, they fail when used in a structural capacity. Since both TCP and HA are similar in composition, their mechanical properties depend on their physical structure, primarily their porosity. As mentioned previously, porosity varies from that of a dense material, with a maximum of 5 percent microporosity; to microporous, containing more numerous micropores of up to 5 μm in size; to macroporous, containing pores of 100 to 500 μm in size. As porosity increases, strength decreases.[10] In fact, compressive strength is inversely proportional to the volume percentage of porosity.[41]

Compressive strength has been measured for most forms of CaP material.[41] In macroporous TCP or HA, it varies from 6 to 60 MN/m^2; in microporous phosphates, it varies from 200 to 600 MN/m^2. In the dense form of HA, compressive strength is approximately 900 MN/m^2. On the average, in all CaP materials, tensile strength is only 20 percent of the compressive strength. The flexural strength (e.g., the ability to resist alternating bending moments) of CaP materials varies from 25 to 45 MN/m^2.[21]

Compressive strength of bone varies from 40 to 60 MN/m^2 for cancellous bone to 160 MN/m^2 for cortical bone, but the flexural strength of bone is 100 MN/m^2.[21] Therefore, although calcium phosphates compare favorably to bone with regard to compressive strength, they have poor tensile and flexural strength. It is only with external support, until adequate bony ingrowth occurs, that they can be used as a structural material.

Histologic Events after Ceramic Implantation

The histologic sequelae of bioceramic implantation including the response of both soft tissue and bone are well documented.[4,7,8,13,16,17,20,21,32,36–38] The soft tissue response to implantation is relatively simple histologically and remains that way over time. After implantation, there is fibrous encapsulation of the ceramic along the soft tissue interface, associated with minimal numbers of macrophages and giant cells. This appearance remains stable throughout the life of the implant. There is no evidence of hematologic, immunologic, or systemic perturbations associated with this.

The processes which occur along the ceramic-bone interface, however, are vastly different, much more dynamic, and more crucial to the ultimate fate of the implant. These responses of bone vary according to the degree of porosity of the implant.

After the implantation of a dense or microporous TCA or HA implant, the CaP material becomes incorporated within the bony defect and is directly bonded to the bone without an intervening fibrous layer. By 3 to 5 months, it is solidly encased by new bone. In addition, the Ca:P ratio rises to near that of normal bone (approximately 1.67 to 1.75) during this period of incorporation. This is due to the ionic exchange of calcium and phosphorous and the subsequent deposition of new bone.

On closer examination, the direct bond first appears in the form of an amorphous, electron-dense band concurrent with the appearance of acellular bone matrix. This "bonding zone" shrinks after several months to a width of 500 to 2000 nm. Throughout this zone of amorphous ground substance that appears similar to natural bone-cementing substance, there are perpendicularly palisaded mineral crystals which attach the ceramic to the natural bone. The bonding zone results in an extremely strong attachment between bone and ceramic to the point that an applied shear force normally fractures either the bone or the ceramic rather than the bone-ceramic interface.[20]

Macroporous CaP materials involve a somewhat different type of response. Recently, several authors have reviewed the histologic events that follow the implantation of a porous CaP material. Although the time frame and amount of final bone deposition differ according to the specific chemical, physical, and biologic factors involved, the general sequence is essentially the same. The general pattern of bone bonding described above eventually occurs along the outer surfaces and pores of the material, but initially there is a fibrous response. After implantation, the material is quickly surrounded by fibrous connective tissue which extends into the peripheral pores. This tissue infiltration becomes denser and more organized and extends deeper into the implant until all pores and tunnels are filled. There is no evidence of an inflammatory response, and cellular differentiation is osteoblastic rather than fibroblastic. Accompanying this ingrowth of connective tissue are sprouting capillaries which follow the pores. Beginning at 1 week to 1 month after implantation, osteoid and then new bone are deposited along the implant-fibrous tissue interface throughout the maze of interconnecting pores. With time, the connective tissue within the implant pores is replaced by bone and bone marrow.

Between 2 weeks and 5 months, the implant, if it is of the bioresorbable type, shows increasing signs of resorption. From 4 to 8 months after implantation, the graft is completely infiltrated with new mature bone. The appositional lamellar bone has a stress-strain orientation. There are mature osteons with haversian canals as well as mature bone marrow and vessels. As with the dense implants, the new bone is bonded directly to the implant material without any intervening fibrous tissue.

As noted previously, pore size is critical in determining the amount of ingrowth. A minimum pore size of 5 to 15 μm is needed for fibrous ingrowth, 100 μm is needed for new bone regeneration, and a minimum size of 200 μm is needed for mature osteons to form. Finally, depending upon the pore size and the biologic system studied, the eventual content of new bone in porous CaP implants has been found to range from 60 to 80 percent.

Potential Uses and Limitations of Calcium Phosphate Ceramics

The initial studies of calcium and phosphate compounds in bone regeneration arose from the idea that a locally available supply of calcium and phosphorus might hasten the regrowth of bone after a fracture or the removal of bone.[1,14] The properties of plaster of Paris (calcium sulfate hemihydrate) have been studied in numerous animal models, and it has been used as a bone substitute in human patients since at least 1892.[32] Its rate of absorption closely coincides with the rate at which new bone can grow into a defect, but it does not seem to hasten bone regeneration.

In 1920, Albee and Morrison reported the results of experiments in which they injected a TCP solution into a surgically created defect in the rabbit radius.[1] They found that the defects so treated healed more quickly than those not treated. Other investigators studied the injection or insertion of such salts as tricalcium phosphate, dicalcium phosphate, monocalcium phosphate, calcium glycerophosphate, calcium hexose phosphate, calcium carbonate, calcium in gelatin, and secondary sodium phosphate in animals and humans.[14] These studies seemed to indicate that the local presence of calcium and phosphate salts accelerates the rate of bony union. However, Haldeman and Moore concluded from their own experiments that although the addition of TCP at the site of a fracture could accelerate previously delayed healing, in the normal healing of a fracture under favorable conditions, the continued presence of a local excess of calcium and phosphorus either did not influence the rate of union or retarded it.[14]

Synthetic HA was first prepared in 1951 and was studied by Ray and Ward at that time as implants in surgically created defects in the long bones and iliac wings of dogs and the skulls of cats and monkeys.[33] This study showed that appositional bone formation occurred around the synthetic HA crystals, that they were gradually replaced in the process of ossification, and that they functioned as a matrix for new bone growth. Small defects seemed to heal more rapidly after implantation of the crystals compared with untreated control defects, but healing was not as rapid as when the defects were filled with fresh autogenous cancellous bone chips.

Since 1952, many other studies have been performed that have led to our present understanding of CaP biomaterials.[12,20,21,28] Their possible uses range from augmenting atrophic alveolar ridges to repairing long-bone defects and ununited fractures. In neurosurgical practice, there are several areas where the CaP biomaterials have potential use.[11,26] These include cranioplasty, craniofacial repair, and vertebral fusions.

During the past 5 years, there have been several animal studies that have shown the efficacy of various forms of CaP bioceramics for cranioplasty (Holmes RE. Cranial reconstruction with porous hydroxyapatite implants and split rib autografts: A histometric study. Presented at the 31st Annual Meeting, Plastic Surgery Research Council, Norfolk, Virginia, May 20, 1986).[32,37,38] All indicate that there is no systemic or local toxicity or inflammation associated with the graft. There are no infections or neurologic insults attributable to the material. There is excellent bony regeneration into and around porous graft material, as well as bony incorporation of solid grafts. The material becomes firmly embedded in the cranial defect, shows good stability, and gives excellent cosmetic results.

Recently, several reports have detailed the initial use of CaP bioceramics in human cranioplasty. Koyama and Handa in 1986 presented three forms of porous HA for use in neurosurgery.[26] One form was a wedge used to fit the craniotomy or cranioplasty flap securely in place. They had used the wedges in 60 patients without complications and with good results. In 1987, Zide et al. reported the repair of frontal bone defects in seven patients using dense HA particles with (three patients) or without (four patients) autogeneic bone.[43] Two patients had superficial postoperative hematomas which were evacuated, and both required slight recontouring of the material. Other cases had slight undercontouring, and one defect was overfilled, with slight migration of the particles. The longest follow-up was $3\frac{1}{2}$ years, and there was no evidence of inflammation, rejection, or resorption. Aronin and Matukas also reported the use of particulate HA as an adjunct to the bone grafting of cranial defects in nine children; no infections or extrusion of the graft material were encountered, and the cosmetic results were good during a follow-up period of 1 to 4 years.[3] Most recently, Yamashima reported the use of dense HA in the form of a button for burr-hole defects or as particles for filling linear skull defects.[42] He used these materials in 100 patients, and after a follow-up period of up to 2 years, he noted no signs of inflammation, resorption, or extrusion. All patients had good cosmetic results; one had scattering of the HA particles because of incomplete suturing of the dura mater.

The repair of orbital defects, especially the reconstruction of the supraorbital rim, is a technical challenge for the surgeon because of the irregular contours in this area and the presence of the frontal sinus with its bacterial contamination. The best current materials for repair either are difficult to shape (autogeneic bone), are resorbed to some extent (autogeneic bone), or may become infected (methyl methacrylate, autogeneic bone). Consequently, better materials are being sought. Chuang and Bensinger implanted porous TCP into surgically created defects in the infraorbital rims of 18 rabbits.[7] They showed that there was progressive replacement of the substance with new bone, with no infection, migration, or rejection of the implant. After 40 weeks, mature cortical bone with an extensive haversian canal system was present. Allard and Swart, using a porous HA plate, reconstructed the orbital roof in a patient who had undergone resection of a cyst involving the frontal sinus.[2] The postoperative course was good; no infection was noted, and the cosmetic result was excellent after 18 months.

The need for bony fusion following a spinal procedure is another circumstance in which CaP bioceramics may be utilized. Shima et al. investigated the use of TCP as a possible bone substitute in anterior cervical discectomy.[36] They implanted dowels of TCP in 20 dogs at the C_3-C_4 level and showed that, at the end of 22 weeks, all ceramic implants were infiltrated by vessels, osteoid, and new bone. Unfortunately, anterior or posterior displacement occurred in 70 percent of the implants and, by the end of 6 weeks, all grafts had suffered compression. The authors concluded that TCP will adequately fuse with bone but with its high incidence of compression and extrusion and its inherently poor biomechanical properties, it is unacceptable as cervical graft material. Cook et al., in 1985, using porous HA as cervical grafting material in dogs showed essentially the same problems.[8] There was bony regeneration and fusion with the passage of time, but 39 percent of all grafts developed both fracture and extrusion and most of the other 61 percent showed fracture without extrusion. The authors concluded that, due to the brittleness of the ceramic, it could not be used alone as a fusion graft, and they suggested a composite system.

In contrast, Flatley et al., using a porous ceramic containing approximately equal amounts of HA and TCP as an implant between lumbar vertebrae in rabbits, showed excellent fusion; there was no mention of graft fracture or migration.[13] In addition, Koyama and Handa used porous HA beads in patients undergoing cervical laminoplasty for stenosis.[25,26] Sixty patients were operated upon; the anteroposterior diameter of the spinal canal was enlarged and maintained by the interpostion of the HA beads between the cut laminal surfaces. There were no complications from the implants such as inflammation or dislodgement or crushing of the beads.

References

1. Albee FH, Morrison HF. Studies in bone growth: triple calcium phosphate as a stimulus to osteogenesis. *Ann Surg* 1920; 71:32–39.
2. Allard RHB, Swart JGN. Orbital roof reconstruction with a hydroxyapatite implant. *J Oral Maxillofac Surg* 1982; 40:237–239.
3. Aronin P, Matukas V. The use of hydroxylapatite for cranioplasty in children. *Childs Nerv Syst* 1988; 4:168.
4. Bhaskar SN, Brady JM, Getter L, et al. Biodegradable ceramic implants in bone: electron and light microscopic analysis. *Oral Surg Oral Med Oral Pathol* 1971; 32:336–346.

5. Bonel G, Heughebaert JC, Heughebaert M, et al. Apatitic calcium orthophosphates and related compounds for biomaterials preparation. *Ann NY Acad Sci* 1988; 523:115–130.

6. Burton CV, McFadden JT. Neurosurgical materials and devices: report on regulatory agencies and advisory groups. *J Neurosurg* 1976; 45:251–258.

7. Chuang EL, Bensinger RE. Resorbable implant for orbital defects. *Am J Ophthalmol* 1982; 94:547–549.

8. Cook SD, Reynolds MC, Whitecloud TS, et al. Evaluation of hydroxylapatite graft materials in canine cervical spine fusions. *Spine* 1986; 11:305–309.

9. Cormack DH. *Ham's Histology*, 9th ed. New York: Lippincott, 1987: 273–323.

10. de Groot K. Effect of porosity and physicochemical properties on the stability, resorption, and strength of calcium phosphate ceramics. *Ann NY Acad Sci* 1988; 523:227–233.

11. de Groot K, Tencer A, Waite P, et al. Significance of the porosity and physical chemistry of calcium phosphate ceramics: dental and other head and neck uses. *Ann NY Acad Sci* 1988; 523:272–277.

12. Ducheyne P. Introduction. *Ann NY Acad Sci* 1988; 523:1–3.

13. Flatley TJ, Lynch KL, Benson M. Tissue response to implants of calcium phosphate ceramic in the rabbit spine. *Clin Orthop* 1983; 179:246–252.

14. Haldeman KO, Moore JM. Influence of a local excess of calcium and phosphorus on the healing of fractures: an experimental study. *Arch Surg* 1934; 29:385–396.

15. Heughebaert JC, Bonel G. Composition, structures and properties of calcium phosphates of biological interest. In: Christel P, Meunier A, Lee AJC (eds.), *Biological and Biomechanical Performance of Biomaterials*. Amsterdam: Elsevier, 1986: 9–14.

16. Holmes RE. Bone regeneration within a coralline hydroxyapatite implant. *Plast Reconstr Surg* 1979; 63:626–633.

17. Holmes R, Mooney V, Bucholz R, et al. A coralline hydroxyapatite bone graft substitute: Preliminary report. *Clin Orthop* 1984; 188:252–262.

18. Hulbert SF. Biomaterials: the case for ceramics. In: Hulbert SF, Young FA (eds.), *Use of Ceramics in Surgical Implants*. New York: Gordon and Breach, 1978: 1–53.

19. Hulbert SF, Young FA, Mathews RA, et al. Potential of ceramic materials as permanently implantable skeletal prostheses. *J Biomed Mater Res* 1970; 4:433–456.

20. Jarcho M. Calcium phosphate ceramics as hard tissue prosthetics. *Clin Orthop* 1981; 157:259–278.

21. Katthagen BD. *Bone Regeneration with Bone Substitutes: An Animal Study*. Berlin: Springer-Verlag, 1986.

22. Kaufman HH. Voluntary standardization of medical devices and procedures. *Neurosurgery* 1983; 13:464–470.

23. Klawitter JJ, Hulbert SF. Applications of porous ceramics for the attachment of load bearing internal orthopedic applications. *J Biomed Mater Res* 1972; 5(6) (symposium 2):161–229.

24. Klawitter JJ, Talbert CD, Hulbert SF, et al. Artifical bones. In: Hulbert SF, Young FA (eds.), *Use of Ceramics in Surgical Implants*. New York: Gordon and Breach, 1978: 95–114.

25. Koyama T, Handa J. Cervical laminoplasty using apatite beads as implants: experiences in 31 patients with compressive myelopathy due to developmental canal stenosis. *Surg Neurol* 1985; 24:663–667.

26. Koyama T, Handa J. Porous hydroxyapatite ceramics for use in neurosurgical practice. *Surg Neurol* 1986; 25:71–73.

27. LeGeros RZ, Parsons JR, Daculsi G, et al. Significance of the porosity and physical chemistry of calcium phosphate ceramics: biodegradation-bioresorption. *Ann NY Acad Sci* 1988; 523:268–271.

28. Niesz DE, Tennery VJ. *Ceramics for Prosthetic Applications—Orthopedic, Dental and Cardiovascular*. Columbus, Ohio: Metals and Ceramics Information Center, 1974.

29. Parker SP (ed.), *Dictionary of Scientific and Technical Terms*, 3d ed. New York: McGraw-Hill, 1984: 272.

30. Prolo DJ. Cranial defects and cranioplasty. In: Wilkins RH, Rengachary SS (eds.), *Neurosurgery*. New York: McGraw-Hill, 1985: 1647–1656.

31. Prolo DJ, Burres KP, McLaughlin WT, et al. Autogenous skull cranioplasty: fresh and preserved (frozen), with consideration of the cellular response. *Neurosurgery* 1979; 4:18–29.

32. Rawlings CE III, Wilkins RH, Hanker JS, et al. Evaluation in cats of a new material for cranioplasty: a composite of plaster of Paris and hydroxylapatite. *J Neurosurg* 1988; 69:269–275.

33. Ray RD, Ward AA Jr. A preliminary report on studies of basic calcium phosphate in bone replacement. *Surg Forum* 1951; 2:429–434.

34. Reeves DL: *Cranioplasty*. Springfield, Illinois: Charles C Thomas, 1950.

35. Roy DM, Linnehan SK. Hydroxyapatite formed from coral skeletal carbonate by hydrothermal exchange. *Nature* 1974; 247:220–222.

36. Shima T, Keller JT, Alvira MM, et al. Anterior cervical discectomy and interbody fusion: an experimental study using a synthetic tricalcium phosphate. *J Neurosurg* 1979; 51:533–538.

37. Uchida A, Nade SML, McCartney ER, et al. The use of ceramics for bone replacement: a comparative study of three different porous ceramics. *J Bone Joint Surg [Br]* 1984; 66B:269–275.

38. Urist MR, Nilsson O, Rasmussen J, et al. Bone regeneration under the influence of a bone morphogenetic protein (BMP) beta tricalcium phosphate (TCP) composite in skull trephine defects in dogs. *Clin Orthop* 1987; 214:295–304.

39. Walker AE (ed.), *A History of Neurological Surgery*. Baltimore: Williams & Wilkins, 1951: 240–247.

40. White RA, Weber JN, White EW. Replamineform: a new process for preparing porous ceramic, metal, and polymer prosthetic materials. *Science* 1972; 176:922–924.

41. Williams DF. The biocompatibility and clinical uses of calcium phosphate ceramics. In: Williams DF (ed.), *Biocompatability of Tissue Analogs*, vol. II. Boca Raton, FL: CRC Press, 1985: 43–69.

42. Yamashima T. Reconstruction of surgical skull defects with hydroxylapatite ceramic buttons and granules. *Acta Neurochir (Wien)* 1988; 90:157–162.

43. Zide MF, Kent JN, Machado L. Hydroxylapatite cranioplasty directly over dura. *J Oral Maxillofac Surg* 1987; 45:481–486.

20

Nutrition and Parenteral Therapy

Guy L. Clifton
Hope Turner

Nutritional Support in Neurosurgical Patients

Energy Requirements

After Trauma or Sepsis

The metabolic response of uninjured human beings to starvation is a marked decrease in energy requirements and protein utilization. With starvation, energy requirements may decrease by as much as 30 percent. After trauma, however, the body is unable to adapt to starvation, and energy requirements rise whether feeding is instituted or not. In patients suffering injury or sepsis, hypercatabolism has been demonstrated by the technique of indirect calorimetry. The extent of elevation in caloric requirements is related to the severity of injury and the time after injury. Energy requirements may vary from minimal elevation after elective abdominal surgery to values of 100 to 150 percent above baseline in severe burns.[16,24,26] A similar hypercatabolic response has been found after brain injury. The body's inability to economize in its need for nutrients makes hyperalimentation essential after injury.

After Neurologic Injury

Recent publications have dealt with energy requirements after head injury.[7-9,14,19,21,26,32,33,42] Studies by the first author (GLC) of patients with altered Glasgow coma scale (GCS) scores from subarachnoid hemorrhage or intracerebral hemorrhage have shown almost exactly the same response as found in head injury. Data from all these investigators have yielded a mean increase in metabolic expenditure of approximately 140 percent of normal requirements in comatose patients with an isolated head injury. This is 3500 kcal/24 h in a 70-kg rested human being. Variations in metabolic expenditure of 120 to 250 percent of expected values were seen in these patients. Data in non-steroid-treated patients are in agreement with calorimetric data in steroid-treated patients.[42]

The duration of the hypermetabolic response and the cause of the wide variations in its intensity among patients have been the subjects of recent investigations to enable a more accurate estimation of caloric needs. Metabolic expenditure using indirect calorimetry was measured 312 times during the first 2 weeks in 57 patients with severe head injury without other major injuries.[7] Data were taken when patients were lying still in bed or slightly moving, were not paralyzed with pancuronium bromide, and, if sedated, were only lightly so with morphine. At the time of measurement, heart rate, temperature, blood pressure, and GCS score were recorded. By multiple regression analysis, a significant relationship was found between heart rate (HR), day since injury (DSI), and GCS in patients with a GCS $\leq$ 7 according to this relationship:

$$\% \text{ RME} = 152 - 13 \text{ (GCS)} + 0.4 \text{ (HR)} + 7 \text{ (DSI)}$$
$$(n = 111, r = 0.7, p < 0.0001)$$

where % RME is the resting metabolic expenditure as a percent of normal. This formula can be used to predict caloric requirements of the comatose patient in the first 2 weeks after injury. Energy requirements after the first 2 weeks after brain injury have not been investigated.

The duration of this hypermetabolic response and the contribution of muscle tone and activity to it have been investigated. A major part of the response is related to muscle tone as shown by the finding in head-injured patients that paralysis with pancuronium bromide or the use of barbiturate coma decreased metabolic expenditure from a mean of 160 percent of expected to 100 to 120 percent.[9] Even with paralysis, energy expenditure remained 20 to 30 percent elevated in some patients.

In contrast to the hypermetabolic response to brain injury, caloric requirements in quadriplegic and paraplegic patients are not increased over those of uninjured rested human beings.[6,11,23] Caloric requirements of alert patients with a focal brain injury have not been measured.

Nitrogen Metabolism

Nitrogen Balance

Nitrogen balance is defined as the difference between nitrogen intake and nitrogen excretion. Nitrogen excretion is measured by analyzing urinary nitrogen or urea and adding a factor of 2 to 3 g for fecal and cutaneous nitrogen loss. Urinary urea can be readily measured in any hospital's clinical laboratory and on the average comprises 85 percent of total urinary nitrogen. Because urea can vary from 60 to 95 percent of urinary nitrogen, direct measurement of urinary nitrogen by the chemiluminescent or micro-Kjeldahl techniques is preferable.[9] In nutritional management, the term *nitrogen* is used interchangeably with *protein*, since measured nitrogen has a constant relationship to protein which is taken in or catabolized:

$$\frac{1 \text{ g protein}}{6.25} = 1 \text{ g nitrogen}$$

For each gram of nitrogen measured in the urine (plus fecal loss), 6.25 g of protein has been catabolized.

Urinary nitrogen excretion normally lags from 3 to 8 days behind the intake or metabolic event which influenced it. Normal human beings oscillate from positive to negative nitrogen balance with a periodicity of 3 to 4 days.[4] For these reasons, balance periods of at least 4 days are required to accurately reflect metabolic status. In normal human beings, optimal protein utilization has been found to be heavily dependent upon the adequacy of caloric intake. Catabolism of protein, which yields only 4 kcal/g (as opposed to fat, which yields 8 kcal/g), makes up 10 percent or less of consumed calories normally.[16] The minimal nitrogen requirement for active adults with full replacement of expended calories has been found to be 3 to 5 g/day or 20 to 30 g of protein.[4]

Nitrogen Metabolism after Injury

After major injury, not only do energy requirements rise greatly but so also does nitrogen excretion. Cuthbertson first reported increased nitrogen excretion in the urine of patients with skeletal trauma, and this response has been a hallmark of hypermetabolism.[12] The contribution of protein to consumed calories after trauma reaches levels three times those of normal human beings (given 10 g/day nitrogen intake and full caloric replacement).[16] The elevated urinary nitrogen reflects catabolism of amino acids derived primarily from muscle tissue. In starved normal human beings, the ratio of loss of lean body mass to fat is 0.5:1. After injury, the ratio is markedly shifted, with a ratio of loss of lean body mass to fat of 2:1 to 4:1.[17]

The extent of the nitrogen excretion which occurs after trauma varies with the severity of the injury and, as will be noted, with the level of nitrogen intake. Comparative data of Long et al. are shown in Table 20-1 with the addition of the first author's data for head injury.[8,26] The highest levels of nitrogen excretion have been found in patients with sepsis, burns, and multiple injuries. Kinney concluded that, in general, the extent of protein catabolism was proportional to the increase in energy expenditure and found nitrogen excretion to peak at about the same time after injury that energy expenditure reached its peak (10 days to 2 weeks).[24]

Nitrogen Metabolism after Neurologic Injury

Available data on nitrogen excretion in neurosurgical patients are from patients with severe head injury or spinal cord injury and from patients having elective neurosurgical procedures. Perhaps the first publication regarding nitrogen excretion in neurosurgical patients is that of Drew et al., who performed nitrogen balance studies on 12 patients after elective craniotomy (most were ambulatory).[15] At normal levels of nitrogen intake (8 g/24 h) no patient was in nitrogen balance during the first 5 days, but in an enterally hyperalimented group, nitrogen balance was achieved in most patients with intakes of 17 g/24 h. This was in a time before steroid usage. Cooper et al. attempted hormonal management of catabolism in this group of patients.[10] These data are consistent with nitrogen balance studies of patients after elective abdominal surgery.[16] In postoperative patients after elective surgery, nutritional replacement beyond the ordinary has not been considered important to outcome, since the negative nitrogen balance found has been transitory and mild.

Head injury has received extensive study in the last 5 years. All studies in comatose, head-injured patients have shown an elevation in nitrogen excretion seemingly varying with the level of nitrogen intake. Unlike metabolic expenditure, nitrogen balance is profoundly affected by both the level of caloric intake and the level of nitrogen intake, so that comparison of nitrogen balance data among patient groups is only possible with the same protein intakes and full caloric replacement. The level of nitrogen wasting after head injury is similar to that of the most hypermetabolic patients. In 10 comatose head-injured patients, studies within the first 2 weeks after head injury (with steroid treatment, 16 mg/day of dexamethasone), nitrogen excretion was 26.8 g/day (0.36 g/kg/day) with 18 g/day nitrogen intake.[8] These data are comparable with those of Long et al. in Table 20-1 for burned and septic patients in which there was a 20 g/day nitrogen intake.[25] In fasted patients with severe head injury, moderately elevated levels of nitrogen excretion of 0.199 g/kg/day have been found.[19] At levels of nitrogen intake of 10 g/24 h, values of 0.28 g/kg/day and 0.214 g/kg/day have been found.[8,42] A peak in nitrogen excretion appears to occur in the second week, with improvement in nitrogen retention by the third week. It is only after the third week that achievement of nitrogen balance becomes possible.

All investigators have noted a wide variability in nitrogen excretion among patients who are similar clinically. The relationship of a number of factors to nitrogen excretion has been examined by the first author in head-injured patients to determine the sources of this variability. It has not been possible to relate the degree of nitrogen excretion to GCS score or other variables as was done for caloric expenditure.

The question of steroid effect has been addressed in two publications. Robertson et al. compared nitrogen balance in two matched groups of 10 comatose patients fasted for 3 days and then fed at full caloric replacement with 15 g nitrogen/day.[32] Steroids resulted in a 30 percent increase in nitrogen excretion during fasting, but the difference was lost during feeding. Young et al., in a series of head-injured pa-

TABLE 20-1 Nitrogen Catabolism after Injury and Illness as Shown by Urinary Nitrogen Excretion, g/kg/day*

Elective Surgery	Skeletal Trauma	Blunt Trauma	Trauma with Steroid Treatment	Sepsis	Burns	Head Injury (GCS < 8)	Normals
0.214 ± 0.027†	0.317 ± 0.018	0.322 ± 0.055	0.338 ± 0.106	0.366 ± 0.060	0.369 ± 0.035	0.36 ± 0.08	0.085 ± 0.002

*Nitrogen intake, 20 g/day or greater.
†Mean ± SEM.

tients who were not treated with steroids and who were fed 15 g nitrogen/day, found nitrogen excretion of 0.24 g/day, consistent with previously published data in steroid-treated patients.[42] The increased nitrogen excretion of neurologic injury cannot then be attributed to steroid administration.

Spinal cord injury demonstrates a fundamentally different metabolic response from head injury. Metabolic expenditure is below normal almost from the moment of injury. A massive wasting of nitrogen occurs in the first 10 days, with nitrogen excretion of 0.24 g/day with only 5 g/day intake.[23] This exceeds the levels of excretion found in fasted head-injured patients. At some point in the chronic phase of spinal cord injury, nitrogen excretion falls well below normal, reflecting a reduced body muscle mass. This is consistent with the known relationship between creatinine-height index and nitrogen excretion.

Nutritional Management of the Neurosurgical Patient

Use of Anthropometric Indices for Assessment of Nutritional Status

A variety of anthropometric and biochemical indices have been described as methods of monitoring nutritional status. These include weight, arm muscle circumference, triceps skin-fold thickness, serum albumin level, transferrin value, and lymphocyte count. Severe levels of nutritional depletion, as judged by these anthropometric indices, have clearly been shown to be associated with impairment of wound healing and increased morbidity. Limitations of these indices in the first few weeks after injury are that they are sensitive to factors other than nutrition as shown by a high incidence of abnormalities in albumin level, lymphocyte count, and skin test reactivity in well-nourished trauma patients.[36] In head-injured patients, despite hyperalimentation, 15 percent weight loss occurred during the first 3 weeks after injury and serum albumin levels drifted to chronically low values.[8] By the time severe anthropometric changes occur, malnutrition is advanced, making the indices of limited value in nutritional management of the acutely injured patient. These indices are of value in assessing the nutritional status of patients after the third week of injury, however.

Weight may be the most valuable anthropometric index of nutritional status. The most clear relationship to outcome of all anthropometric indices exists for weight loss. Studley showed in patients who were to have a gastrectomy for ulcer treatment that a 30 percent weight loss preoperatively resulted in a tenfold increase in operative mortality.[39] It is generally considered that levels of weight loss of 10 to 15 percent are not of great consequence, 20 percent increases susceptibility to stress, and 30 percent increases morbidity and mortality appreciably. A 20-g nitrogen loss for 7 days is equivalent to a loss of 7 to 10 percent of muscle mass in a 70-kg human being. Therefore, an unreplaced nitrogen loss of 20 g for 2 weeks could result in a 20 to 30 percent weight loss. This is an expected degree of nitrogen loss in some hypermetabolic neurosurgical patients who are underalimented. Changes in weight are not accurate until the sec-

TABLE 20-2 Caloric Replacement of Patients with Acute Neurologic Dysfunction, Based on Metabolic Expenditure

Patient	Caloric Replacement, kcal/kg
Resting 70-kg male (normal)	26
Postoperative craniotomy (best estimate)	26
Posturing (GCS 4–5), first week	40–50
Posturing (GCS 4–5), second week	50–60
Localizing or flexor withdrawal (GCS 6–7), first week	30–40
Localizing or flexor withdrawal (GCS 6–7), second week	40–50
GCS 8–12	30–35
Paraplegia	27
Quadriplegia	23

ond week after injury due to intravenous fluids and to the water and sodium retention after trauma.

Objectives for Caloric Replacement

Full replacement of expended calories is the objective of nutritional management, since without full energy replacement, protein is wasted. Since values for caloric expenditure of injured patients have been done at rest, clinical investigators have recommended the addition of 20 percent to the values obtained at rest by indirect calorimetry to estimate total energy expenditure.[25] In neurologically injured patients, this has not been found necessary and feeding can best be estimated by existing predictive formulas.[7]

Feeding at levels over actual caloric expenditure is not desirable. Overfeeding may result in hyperglycemia, uremia, and increased carbon dioxide production. In one study of head-injured patients which attempted to achieve nitrogen balance by hyperalimentation, levels of caloric replacement of 40 percent over measured metabolic expenditure were administered. Increased carbon dioxide production was the only systemic complication.[8] Table 20-2 lists the recommended range of caloric intake based on measured metabolic expenditure for different categories of neurosurgical patients.

Objectives for Protein Replacement

Whereas replacement of expended calories is a clear goal of nutritional management, the desired level of reduction of nitrogen loss is less well quantified. The rise in nitrogen excretion which occurs with feeding in head-injured patients demonstrates a defect in utilization of nitrogen, as illustrated by this example: Two matched groups of 10 comatose head-injured patients each were treated enterally with intakes of 17.6 ± 3.6 g nitrogen/day (Traumacal; Mead Johnson Laboratories, Evansville, IN) and 29.0 ± 5.3 g nitrogen/day (Magnacal: Organon, Inc., West Orange, NJ), respectively, at 140 percent replacement of expended calories.[8] Data are from 7-day balance periods within the first 2 weeks after injury. A nitrogen balance of -9.2 ± 6.7 g/day was found in the lower-protein group, and a balance of -5.3 ± 5.0 g/day in the higher-protein group. These data suggest that at a high range of nitrogen intake after head injury (>17 g/day), less than 50 percent of administered nitrogen is retained. Despite a higher protein intake in the group treated with Traumacal, the difference in nitrogen balance was not statistically significant due to wide variability in retention of nitrogen among patients. It is because of this wide variability that the routine measurement of nitrogen balance is advocated in patient management. Urinary nitrogen measurement can be made available through the clinical laboratory of any hospital.

The problem of nitrogen content in feeding formulas is somewhat simplified for the physician, since in both parenteral and enteral formulas there is an upper limit of protein beyond which one may not go given full caloric replacement. In enteral formulas, more than 20 percent of protein by weight produces sufficient viscosity that the formulation cannot be fed by tube. Existing enteral formulas contain maximally a ratio of nonprotein calories to grams of nitrogen of 104:1. A ratio of 130:1 has been recommended for the most hypermetabolic patients, and given full caloric replacement, this provides a protein intake of 2.0 to 2.5 g/kg/day.[17,29] This level of protein intake, either enterally or parenterally, has been recommended by the first author and by other investigators for head-injured patients.

Enteral Alimentation

Nutritional support may be administered either enterally or parenterally. There are advantages to enteral alimentation if it can be used. The major one is avoidance of a central venous catheter and its associated septic complications. There has been no evidence that superior nutrition is achieved by enteral alimentation as compared to prolonged intravenous alimentation. One major advantage of enteral alimentation, however, is maintenance of gut mucosal integrity and the intestinal mucosal barrier to bacteria.[13,35,41] This barrier may be lost with prolonged parenteral alimentation.[1] Recent studies have indicated that when gut mucosal atrophy occurs, there is bacterial translocation to the mesenteric lymph nodes and subsequent systemic bacterial translocation with septicemia.[41] The three major mechanisms that influence bacterial translocation are thought to be (1) altered permeability of gut mucosa, (2) decreased host defense secondary to protein depletion, and (3) increased enteral bacterial flora secondary to antibiotic therapy and gut stasis.[1,13,35,41]

Experience has shown that 20 to 30 percent of patients after acute neural injury will not tolerate gastric feedings, primarily due to impaired gastric emptying. Patients treated with morphine will usually have impaired gastric emptying. Patients treated with broad-spectrum antibiotics will often develop diarrhea which does not respond to slowing of feedings. To avoid the problems of gut atrophy from prolonged parenteral hyperalimentation and of gastric intolerance of enteral feedings, we are evaluating percutaneously placed or nasally inserted jejunal feeding tubes as a routine method. This technique appears to permit early enteral feeding of all patients. By either method, at least 3 days are taken to

achieve full replacement. Slow advancement of feedings maximizes tolerance by either the jejunal or gastric route.

Most marketed formulas contain insufficient water for the hypermetabolic patient and, if 30 to 60 cc/h of water is not given enterally or intravenously, hypernatremia commonly results. Rapid administration of enteral feedings will almost always result in diarrhea. Experience has shown that by slow advancement of feeding over several days, enteral alimentation will be tolerated in many patients, dependent on the location of the feeding tube (stomach, duodenum, jejunum). One recommended schedule is to use a continuous infusion beginning at 25 to 50 cc/h of full-strength formula and advancing it by 25 cc every 12 h until full intake is achieved, allowing for the stomach or duodenum to adjust to increased volumes and decreased resultant hypermotility and diarrhea. The optimal final infusion rate is 100 to 150 cc/h. Some prefer to use diluted formulas as a method of advancing intake in the stomach or duodenum.

For gastric feeding, the gastric contents are aspirated every 4 h and feedings decreased for residual volumes of >200 cc. For nasojejunal feedings, which bypass the stomach, the feeding is directly absorbed and is not dependent on gastric motility. To prevent aspiration, a nasogastric tube should still be placed initially when nasoduodenal or nasojejunal feedings are used to check for reflux or slipping of the tube back into the stomach. Psyllium hydrophilic colloid (Metamucil; Searle Laboratories, Chicago, IL) can be placed down a nasogastric tube and will increase stool bulk. For diarrhea, diphenoxylate hydrochloride with atropine (Lomotil; Searle Laboratories) or kaolin and pectin (Kaopectate; The Upjohn Company, Kalamazoo, MI) can be used. Persistent diarrhea indicates malabsorption and is an indication for decreasing or discontinuing enteral feedings.

The choice of enteral formulas is wide. The proteins of most formulas are egg- and milk-based. Egg is the most biologically available protein source.[28] Biologic availability refers to the extent to which a given protein source is retained rather than catabolized. Proteins with poor biologic availability are excreted as urea. In general, the higher the amount of essential amino acids, the more biologically available is a protein. Vegetable oils make up the fat component, and sucrose and corn starch the carbohydrate sources of most enteral feedings. There are differences among formulas in the percentages of calories derived from glucose, fat, and protein. This and the calorie/nitrogen ratio are the primary factors to be considered in selecting a formula for the hypermetabolic patient. Formulas containing nonhydrolyzed proteins and a nonprotein calorie/nitrogen ratio of at least 130:1, such as Traumacal or Ensure Plus (Ross Laboratories, Columbus, OH), are recommended for gastric feeding. For jejunal feeding, hydrolyzed proteins or free amino acids are required to avoid malabsorption, and formulas such as Vital HN (Ross Laboratories, Columbus, OH) or Vivonex HN (Norwich-Eaton Laboratories, Norwich, NY) are recommended.

Parenteral Alimentation

What are the indications for parenteral nutrition in the neurosurgical patient? In many respects, with the sophisticated nutritional support available in most hospitals, it is simpler to administer parenteral than enteral formulas. There is no question of tolerance, fewer adjustments of rate are necessary, and higher rates of intake are often achieved earlier in many patients. Nursing personnel may be more tolerant of giving intravenous solutions than enteral feeding. For these reasons, parenteral alimentation has received wide use in neurosurgical patients. If a method of enteral feeding (such as jejunal) can be developed, which all patients tolerate early after injury, parenteral alimentation should not be necessary.

Standard parenteral formulations are available through the hospital pharmacy. Failure of delivery of full caloric requirements by enteral feedings by the fifth to seventh day after neurologic injury in a patient who will require prolonged nutritional support constitutes an indication for parenteral hyperalimentation. Another indication would be diarrhea resulting from antibiotic therapy which cannot be controlled by an appropriate antidiarrheal agent (based on tube location).

One potential contraindication to parenteral therapy is cerebral edema. Waters et al. have shown aggravation of edema in a cold lesion model with parenteral alimentation.[40] In the very acute phase of neurologic injury when intracranial pressure is elevated and where mannitol is required, the use of parenteral therapy is difficult. In the patient without elevated intracranial pressure, there is no evidence to suggest that parenteral hyperalimentation induces or aggravates cerebral edema. Based on data showing exacerbation of cerebral ischemia by elevated serum glucose levels, the avoidance of hyperglycemia by insulin usage is strongly recommended.[3,30]

The methodology of parenteral nutrition is well described, and recent texts provide excellent accounts.[34] Several aspects as they apply to neurosurgical patients deserve emphasis. Several parameters can be varied to improve the efficiency of parenteral nutrition, just as enteral formulations may be selected. Parenteral nutrition may be varied by calorie source, amount of calories, amino acid pattern, and calorie/nitrogen ratio. There has been considerable debate about whether glucose or fat is the optimal caloric source. Glucose has been reported in some studies to be more effective than fat in promoting nitrogen anabolism.[2] More than 50 percent fat as a calorie source can result in fat deposition

in the liver.[37] Recent data indicate that fat is preferentially used as a calorie source in stress states, though not in nonstress conditions, and that the limiting factor in fat utilization after trauma is hepatic function.[18,22,38] Without fat, essential fatty acid deficiencies occur. High quantities of glucose may produce fat synthesis and result in respiratory quotients of over 1.0 with increased carbon dioxide production. This can be a problem in the management of the patient who requires hyperventilation for intracranial pressure control and is, perhaps, the major complication of early hyperalimentation in the neurologically injured patient. This complication is reduced with fat as a calorie source. A mixed caloric source with approximately 50 percent fat in the acute state, decreasing to 30 percent as stress resolves, has been recommended in head injury.[14]

The amino acid mixture in parenteral and enteral alimentation may also be varied. Eight amino acids are essential: the branched-chain amino acids (leucine, isoleucine, and valine), lysine, methionine, phenylalanine, tryptophan, and threonine. There are very few differences in amino acid content of most commercially available solutions. As in most enteral formulations, branched-chain amino acids make up 20 percent of the total amino acid content in parenteral solutions. Increasing the percentage of branched-chain amino acids to 40 percent has been reported to improve nitrogen retention after trauma.[5,20] The applicability of this concept to the neurologically injured patient has not been investigated. Commercial formulations with high branched-chain amino acid content are now available for use in stress states (FreAmine HBC; McGaw Laboratories, Santa Ana, CA).

Nonprotein calorie/nitrogen ratio is the third variable to be selected in the use of parenteral nutrition. Studies of nitrogen retention in stressed patients have shown significantly better nitrogen retention with higher nonprotein calorie/nitrogen ratios, as noted. For states of severe stress, a ratio of 130:1 has been found optimal. As in enteral preparations, there is an absolute limit of protein which may be given with parenteral solutions. Nitrogen intakes of more than 30 g/day are generally not possible in 3 liters of parenteral solution without interfering with the adequacy of caloric intake. Examples of various formulations which would provide a range of calorie/nitrogen ratios, amino acid mixtures, and sources of nonprotein calories are shown in Table 20-3.

TABLE 20-3 Examples of Individualized Parenteral Formulas for Hypermetabolic Patients*

	3 Units 750 ml 6.9% FreAmine HBC† Plus 3 Units 250 ml 70% Dextrose Injection USP		3 Units 750 ml 8.5% Aminosyn‡ Plus 3 Units 250 ml 70% Dextrose Injection USP
	+1 Unit (500 ml) 10% Lipid	+1 Unit (500 ml) 20% Lipid	+1 Unit (500 ml) 20% Lipid
Total nitrogen (g)	21.9	21.9	29.3
Total amino acids (g)	150	150	192
Total protein equivalent (g)	138	138	183
Nonprotein calories (kcal)	2336	2885	2785
Nonprotein calorie/nitrogen ratio	107:1	131:1	95:1
Nonprotein calories from fat (%)	23	35	36
Nonprotein calories from carbohydrates (%)	77	65	64

*Tolerance of lipid emulsions must be verified by daily plasma triglyceride analysis.
†McGaw Laboratories, Santa Ana, CA.
‡Abbott Laboratories, North Chicago, IL.

Vitamins and Minerals

Vitamin and mineral deficiency complicating chronic alimentation has not been a major problem in enteral alimentation. Since existing formulas are composed of commonly available foodstuffs, a range of vitamins and minerals is included in the formulations. With long periods of parenteral alimentation, a variety of deficiency states have been identified. Since vitamin deficiencies may develop in normal individuals within 1 to 2 weeks, vitamins are routinely added to parenteral solutions. The vitamin and mineral requirements of stressed patients are not known; however, recent data would suggest increased requirements of zinc and of ascorbic acid in trauma. Increased zinc excretion has been documented in severe head injury.[27] Until recently, trace minerals were provided in parenteral alimentation as incidental contaminants of the solutions. With clinical reports of parenteral alimentation–induced deficiencies of copper, zinc, chromium, and selenium, solutions of trace minerals for addition to parenteral solutions have recently been approved. Standards for vitamin and mineral replacement in total parenteral nutrition are established in most hospitals.

The Consequences of Underalimentation

Despite many studies, no clear relationship of the extent of nutritional support to outcome has been documented except at the extremes. It was for this reason that aggressive attempts to achieve nitrogen equilibrium were largely abandoned in most hypermetabolic patients. One important comparative study has been done in neurosurgical patients by Rapp et al.[31] Eighteen head-injured patients were treated with parenteral nutrition and 17 with enteral nutrition via the nasogastric route. A significant improvement in outcome was found in the parenterally alimented group. Analysis of these data shows that this was a study of what has probably been common neurosurgical management (severe undernutrition) versus nutrition. Unreplaced nitrogen losses of 14 to 22 g occurred for 2 weeks in the enterally alimented group with caloric intakes of 200 to 1000 kcal/day. In the parenterally alimented group, nitrogen losses due to greater nitrogen intake were reduced to 10 to 12 g/day with caloric intakes of 1800 to 2000 kcal/day. This study documented the consequence of one extreme of management, failure of nutritional support, and is important in verifying the need to replace expended calories and to provide a level of nitrogen intake likely to reduce daily nitrogen losses to below 10 g. A major clinical objective is to develop a method of early enteral alimentation which provides full caloric replacement and reduces nitrogen loss to less than 10 g/day for all patients within the first 3 days after brain injury.

References

1. Alverdy JC, Aoys E, Moss GS. Total parenteral nutrition promotes bacterial translocation from the gut. *Surgery* 1988; 104:185–190.

2. Ang SD, Leskiw MJ, Stein TP. Effect of increasing total parenteral nutrition on protein metabolism. *J Parenter Enteral Nutr* 1983; 7:525–529.

3. Berger L, Hakin AM. The association of hyperglycemia with cerebral edema in stroke. *Stroke* 1986; 17:865–871.

4. Calloway DH, Margen S. Variation in endogenous nitrogen excretion and dietary nitrogen utilization as determinants of human protein requirement. *J Nutr* 1971; 101:205–216.

5. Cerra FB, Mazuski JE, Chute E, et al. Branched chain metabolic support: a prospective, randomized, double-blind trial in surgical stress. *Ann Surg* 1984; 199:286–291.

6. Clarke KS. Caloric costs of activity in paraplegic persons. *Arch Phys Med Rehabil* 1966; 47:427–435.

7. Clifton GL, Robertson CS, Choi SC. Assessment of nutritional requirements of head-injured patients. *J Neurosurg* 1986; 64:895–901.

8. Clifton GL, Robertson CS, Contant CF. Enteral hyperalimentation in head injury. *J Neurosurg* 1985; 62:186–193.

9. Clifton GL, Robertson CS, Grossman RG, et al. The metabolic response to severe head injury. *J Neurosurg* 1984; 60:687–696.

10. Cooper IS, Rynearson EH, MacCarty CS, et al. The catabolic effect of craniotomy and its investigative treatment with testosterone propionate. *J Neurosurg* 1951; 8:295–299.

11. Cox SAR, Weiss SM, Posuniak DO, et al. Energy expenditure after spinal cord injury: an evaluation of stable rehabilitating patients. *J Trauma* 1985; 25:419–423.

12. Cuthbertson DP. Observations on the disturbance of metabolism produced by injury to the limbs. *Q J Med* 1932; 2:233–246.

13. Deitch EA, Winterton J, Berg R. The gut as a portal of entry for bacteremia: role of protein malnutrition *Ann Surg* 1987; 205:681–692.

14. Deutschman CS, Konstantinides FN, Raup S, et al. Physiological and metabolic response to isolated closed head injury. Part 1: Basal metabolic state: correlations of metabolic and physiological parameters with fasting and stressed controls. *J Neurosurg* 1986; 64:89–98.

15. Drew JH, Koop CE, Grigger RP. A nutritional study of neurosurgical patients with special reference to nitrogen balance and convalescence in the postoperative period. *J Neurosurg* 1947; 4:7–15.

16. Duke JH Jr, Jorgensen SB, Broell JR, et al. Contribution of protein to caloric expenditure following injury. *Surgery* 1970; 68:168–174.

17. Elwyn DH. Nutritional requirements of adult surgical patients. *Crit Care Med* 1980; 8:9–20.

18. Freund HR, Yoshimura N, Fischer JE. Does intravenous fat spare nitrogen in the injured rat? *Am J Surg* 1980; 140:377–383.

19. Gadisseux P, Ward JD, Young HF, et al. Nutrition and the neurosurgical patient. *J Neurosurg* 1984; 60:219–232.

20. Gazzaniga AB, Waxman K, Day AT, et al. Nitrogen balance in adult hospitalized patients with the use of a pediatric amino acid model. *Arch Surg* 1988; 123:1275–1279.

21. Haider W, Lackner F, Schlick W, et al. Metabolic changes in the course of severe acute brain damage. *Eur J Intensive Care Med* 1975; 1:9–26.

22. Jeejeebhoy KN, Anderson GH, Nakhooda AF, et al. Metabolic studies in total parenteral nutrition with lipid in man: comparison with glucose. *J Clin Invest* 1976; 57:125–136.

23. Kearns PJ Jr, Pipp TL, Quirk M, et al. Nutritional requirements in quadriplegics. *J Parenter Enteral Nutr* 1982; 6:577(abstr).

24. Kinney JM. Energy deficits in acute illness and injury. In: Morgan AP (ed.), *Proceedings of the Conference on Energy Metabolism and Body Fuel Utilization*. Cambridge, MA: Harvard University Printing Office, 1966:167–179.

25. Long CL, Blakemore WS. Energy and protein requirements in the hospitalized patient. *J Parenter Enteral Nutr* 1979; 3:69–71.

26. Long CL, Schaffel N, Geiger JW, et al. Metabolic response to injury and illness: estimation of energy and protein needs from indirect calorimetry and nitrogen balance. *J Parenter Enteral Nutr* 1979; 3:452–456.

27. McClain CJ, Twyman DL, Ott LG, et al. Serum and urine zinc response in head injured patients. *J Neurosurg* 1986; 64:224–230.

28. Mitchell HH, Carman GG. The biological value of the nitrogen of mixtures of patent white flour and animal foods. *J Biol Chem* 1926; 68:183–215.

29. Peters C, Fischer JE. Studies on calorie to nitrogen ratio for total parenteral nutrition. *Surg Gynecol Obstet* 1980; 151:1–8.

30. Pulsinelli WA, Waldman S, Rawlinson D, et al. Moderate hyperglycemia augments ischemic brain damage: a neuropathologic study in the rat. *Neurology* 1982; 32:1239–1246.

31. Rapp RP, Young B, Twyman D, et al. The favorable effect of early parenteral feeding on survival in head-injured patients. *J Neurosurg* 1983; 58:906–912.

32. Robertson CS, Clifton GL, Goodman JC. Steroid administration and nitrogen excretion in the head-injured patient. *J Neurosurg* 1985; 63:714–718.

33. Robertson CS, Clifton GL, Grossman RG. Oxygen utilization and cardiovascular function in head-injured patients. *Neurosurgery* 1984; 15:307–314.

34. Rombeau JL, Caldwell MD. *Parenteral Nutrition*. Philadelphia: Saunders, 1986.

35. Saito H, Trocki O, Alexander JW, et al. The effect of route of nutrient administration on the nutritional state, metabolic hormone secretion and gut mucosal integrity after burn injury. *J Parenter Enteral Nutr* 1987; 11:1–7.

36. Silberman H, Eisenberg D, Shofler R, et al. Nutrition-related factors in acutely injured patient. *J Trauma* 1982; 22:907–909.

37. Stein TP, Buzby GP, Leskiw MJ, et al. Protein and fat metabolism in rats during repletion with total parenteral nutrition (TPN). *J Nutr* 1981; 111:154–165.

38. Stoner HB, Little RA, Frayn KN, et al. The effect of sepsis on the oxidation of carbohydrate and fat. *Br J Surg* 1983; 70:32–35.

39. Studley HO. Percentage of weight loss: a basic indicator of surgical risk in patients with chronic peptic ulcer. *JAMA* 1936; 106:458–460.

40. Waters DC, Hoff JT, Black KL. Effect of parenteral nutrition on cold-induced vasogenic edema in cats. *J Neurosurg* 1986; 64:460–465.

41. Wilmore DW, Smith RJ, O'Dwyer ST, et al. The gut: a central organ after surgical stress. *Surgery* 1988; 104:917–923.

42. Young B, Ott L, Norton J, et al. Metabolic and nutritional sequelae in the non-steroid treated head injury patient. *Neurosurgery* 1985; 17:784–791.

21
Restorative Neurology

Larry B. Goldstein
James N. Davis

The last decade has seen major advances in our understanding of the neurobiologic basis of functional recovery after brain injury. Fundamental laboratory investigations indicate that the rate and degree of recovery may be influenced by a variety of factors including drugs (Table 21-1). These studies have led to an appreciation of the potential for the pharmacologic management of patients after brain damage. This is particularly important since patients suffering stroke or head injury may already be receiving drugs which influence the recovery of function. In fact, more than 150 different drugs have been reported to be of benefit to patients recovering from stroke and head trauma. This chapter will provide a theoretical framework based on these basic and clinical studies which may help to organize this diverse literature. Three themes are emphasized:

1. Our current understanding of the fundamental neurobiologic processes which underlie functional recovery
2. The variety of mechanisms through which diverse drugs may act to enhance or impair recovery of function
3. The possibility that some drugs might facilitate recovery through one mechanism, but could delay recovery through a different mechanism

Biologic and Environmental Factors

The initial deficit and ultimate recovery after brain damage are influenced by both biologic and environmental factors (Table 21-2). Investigations with laboratory animals show that the animal's sex, nutritional status, age (the so-called Kennard principle), the rate of development of the lesion, the presence of prior lesions, previous experience and envi-

TABLE 21-1 Mechanisms Determining Rate and Extent of Functional Recovery after Brain Injury

Biologic and environmental factors
The brain's responses to injury
Adaptive responses (synaptic plasticity)
Neuronal rearrangements (neuronal plasticity)

TABLE 21-2 Biologic and Environmental Factors

Lesion location
Presence of and time since prior brain lesions
Previous experience or training
Nutritional status
Age
Sex

ronment, and the lesion's location in the brain are critical to the ultimate rate and extent of recovery.[15]

These same factors seem to be important in human beings, but only limited data are available for comparison with the animal studies. For example, the importance of lesion location on recovery was demonstrated in a clinical study correlating infarct size measured radiographically with degree of motor deficit after stroke.[28] The site (subcortical vs. cortical), but not the size of the lesion, correlated with ultimate recovery. Several studies have suggested that lesion location is also important for recovery of language in aphasics. Although patients with small lesions recovered fluency whereas those with large lesions had poorer outcomes,[24] the larger lesions involved subcortical as well as cortical areas. Language recovery in patients with intermediate-sized lesions showed a clear relationship with lesion location. Finally, the importance of preinjury "experience" is suggested by a study comparing preinjury intelligence and education, brain-tissue volume loss, and lesion location to the persistence of cognitive deficits after penetrating brain wounds.[18] Preinjury intelligence and education were the most important predictors of postinjury performance.

Thus, each of these biologic and environmental factors appears to be important predictors of recovery of function in animals and probably play important roles in humans. The identification of these factors is analogous to defining the risk factors for stroke or heart disease. In clinical studies of the effects of any intervention on recovery of function, it is important to know how these biologic and environmental factors are distributed between experimental and control groups of patients.

The Brain's Responses to Injury

In addition to biologic and environmental factors, the type and extent of the brain's response to injury is an important determinant of eventual recovery. Current pharmacologic approaches to the treatment of stroke and head injury are designed to limit the amount of damage at the time of injury. Table 21-3 lists some of the mechanisms that may underlie secondary injury caused by responses to injury in the central nervous system (CNS).

TABLE 21-3 The Brain's Responses to Injury

Cerebral edema
Secondary neuronal death
Diaschisis
Inhibition and excitation

Recently, attention has been directed to the phenomenon of selective neuronal death associated with transient ischemia. Increased extracellular levels of excitatory neurotransmitters, especially glutamate, have been implicated in mediating selective neuronal injury.[19,21,34] A specific glutamate receptor subtype, the N-methyl-D-aspartate (NMDA) receptor, is activated by glutamate during periods of sustained stimulation. NMDA receptor activation allows entry of Na^+ and Ca^{2+} ions into neurons. Na^+ entry leads to acute cell swelling and cytotoxicity.[33] Ca^{2+} entry may lead to delayed neuronal death by a different mechanism.[7]

The availability of specific drugs which competitively and noncompetitively block NMDA responses has stimulated trials of these agents in experimental ischemia.[25] MK-801 is a highly potent NMDA channel blocker and is a good example of this type of drug. Although controversial, MK-801 treatment appears to reduce brain injury after transient[16] and focal[25,31] ischemia. MK-801 is also an example of a drug that promotes recovery of function by one mechanism but could have adverse effects through a second mechanism. MK-801 interferes with brain functions including learning and memory and thus may disrupt the adaptive responses which seem to play an important role in recovery (see below).

Cerebral edema is the most widely recognized and studied response to brain injury.[6] Edema contributes to the functional deficit after injury, and resolution of edema may underlie some spontaneous recovery. There appear to be several different forms of cerebral edema accompanying different forms of injury. Controversy remains about the role of glucocorticoids in reducing such cerebral edema. Although glucocorticoids have been shown to reduce edema in experimental and clinical studies of brain tumors or other mass lesions, they do not appear to influence the edema accompanying head injury and stroke.[2,30] New drugs aimed at interrupting cellular processes responsible for astrocytic and other cellular swelling such as GM1-ganglioside may become more important in the future.[23]

An appreciation of the potential role of calcium ions in the ischemic cascade[20] has led to clinical trials of calcium channel antagonists and experimental studies of phenothiazines in ischemic stroke. Cytidine 5'-diphosphocholine (CDP-choline) accelerates phospholipid synthesis and may suppress the release of free fatty acids by ischemic neurons. Administration of CDP-choline to rats after ischemia lessens the resultant neurologic deficit.[22] A recent double-blind multicenter trial indicates that CDP-choline may improve functional outcome in patients with ischemic stroke.[40]

Diaschisis, a term originated by Von Monakow,[42] refers to sudden remote functional depression of brain regions distant from the site of injury.[12] Von Monakow believed that diaschisis was due to loss of excitation in the remote area. Today, it is clear that sudden changes of function in uninjured brain can result from changes in either excitation or inhibition by projections from the injured area. Others have attributed diaschisis to injury-evoked changes in cerebral blood flow. Reductions of blood flow and metabolism following unilateral cerebral hemisphere injury have been demonstrated by positron emission tomography in the noninjured ipsilateral cerebral hemisphere, contralateral cerebral hemisphere, and contralateral cerebellum.[27,29]

These alterations of blood flow may simply reflect changes in excitation or inhibition, or they could directly lead to loss of function. Alternatively, blood flow changes could be the direct result of the primary injury.

Adaptive Responses

Adaptive responses refer to the mechanisms that uninjured brain uses to "take over" functions that were performed by the damaged brain. An important assumption in understanding these responses is that the basic cellular mechanisms that underlie normal learning and memory may also be responsible for adaptation after injury. It is almost as if the uninjured brain must "learn" the functions that were lost during the injury. It is not surprising that drugs which affect learning and memory also have dramatic effects on the adaptive responses after brain injury.

Hypotheses of the neural basis of learning and memory are the subject of a recent review.[41] A variety of theories have developed concerning the physiologic and cellular basis of learning. Perhaps the best understood and most compelling cellular mechanism is long-term potentiation (LTP). LTP has been best characterized in the hippocampus, where a train of stimuli can alter normal synaptic relationships. After such a stimulus train, a subsequent single stimulus results in a greater postsynaptic response. This potentiation of a single stimulus is long-lasting. LTP is one of the mechanisms by which a transient stimulus can have a long-lasting effect on neuronal function.[39,41]

The phenomenon of LTP appears to be mediated by the NMDA receptor[3] (see above). LTP is regulated by a number of neurotransmitters and may vary among brain regions. Blockers of NMDA receptor activation disrupt learning and memory. Other cellular mechanisms which may play a role in learning and memory as well as in adaptive responses have not been as well characterized as LTP. Examples include receptor up- and down-regulation[36,43] and unmasking.[1]

Neurotransmitters can influence the development of LTP and have been implicated in memory processes. The same neurotransmitters also have an impact on functional recovery after brain injury. Norepinephrine is a good example of this type of neurotransmitter. Central noradrenergic neurons may be critical to memory and learning,[9,11,32,38] and norepinephrine can influence the development of LTP.[37,39] Amphetamine's capacity to facilitate motor recovery after brain injury appears to be mediated through central noradrenergic neurons.[14] Amphetamine-facilitated recovery is mimicked by an intraventricular infusion of norepinephrine but not dopamine.[4] Lesions of the nucleus locus ceruleus, the major source of central noradrenergic projections, influence motor recovery.[26] Active motor experience during the period of drug intoxication is required for amphetamine-facilitated recovery to occur. The effect may be blocked by restraining the animals after administration of the drug.[13] These data are consistent with the hypothesis that amphetamines facilitate "relearning" after brain injury. A study of a small group of highly selected stroke patients suggested that amphetamine administration coupled with physical therapy could also promote motor recovery in humans.[8]

Drugs which inhibit neuronal firing could impair the development of LTP and may prolong the functional deficit after cortical brain injury. Local administration of gamma-aminobutyric acid (GABA), a central inhibitory neurotransmitter, increases hemiplegia produced by a small motor cortex lesion in rats.[5] The systemic administration of the benzodiazepine, diazepam, causes recovery from a sensory cortex lesion in rats to be delayed indefinitely.[35]

Acetylcholine is another central neurotransmitter with putative effects on memory processes which may also influence functional recovery. Much of the data concerning the impact of cholinergic agents on recovery of function is old and inadequate by current standards (for review, see Ref. 14). However, acetylcholine appears to enhance recovery of function. It should be recognized that the putative effect of cholinergic agents on recovery may be mediated by the influence of these drugs on the firing of locus ceruleus neurons. Also, the effect of CDP-choline on recovery in both animals[22] and human beings[40] could be due to an enhancement of cholinergic function associated with the administration of the drug.

Neuronal Rearrangements

In the past two decades, a variety of morphologic and neuronal rearrangements have been demonstrated in many brain injuries (Fig. 21-1). This area of neuroscience is expanding rapidly and reaching the stage where the "rules" regulating these rearrangements are beginning to be understood.[10] It is clear that not all rearrangements lead to recovery; at least some neuronal rearrangements are maladaptive and may contribute to the final functional deficit. It is also clear that these rearrangements do not happen at the same time; some begin as early as 8 h after the injury, while others take months to develop. Although little is known of the

pharmacology of these rearrangements, greater understanding could ultimately lead to powerful agents for facilitating recovery. Clinical trials with a putative neurotrophic drug, GM1-ganglioside, are currently being carried out in the United States and Europe.

The classification of neuronal rearrangements used here should be viewed as an organizing hypothesis open to change in the future.[10] This scheme fits well with available animal studies of rearrangements in different regions of the CNS.

Regeneration refers to the extension of an injured neuron's axon proximal to the level of injury and extending to eventually reinnervate the denervated target. This type of rearrangement probably does not occur in the CNS. It would be the ideal rearrangement to restore function and would probably take several weeks to months depending on the distance to be covered by the growing neurites.

Pruning occurs in highly collateralized neurons. When one axon is injured, nearby uninjured collaterals expand to reinnervate the vacant target. This phenomenon does occur in the CNS and may be responsible for many of the outgrowths described in central neurons. It should be an adaptive rearrangement leading to restored function and usually takes months to reach completion.

In contrast to regeneration and pruning, collateral sprouting is a response of an uninjured neuron to the loss of nearby axons from injured neurons. Collateral sprouting has been studied extensively in the septal nucleus, hippocampus, and peripheral nervous system. It occurs rapidly, being first identified within as little as 8 h and becoming complete within 7 to 14 days. Since collateral sprouting usually results in the hyperinnervation of a target, it seems reasonable to hypothesize that it could be maladaptive in some cases, resulting in a functional deficit instead of recovery.

Ingrowth is the least well-known of the rearrangements. It is the response of an uninjured nerve to a remote injury. In this form of rearrangement the neuron grows to innervate a foreign target in response to loss of fibers at that target. The best studied example of this rearrangement is sympathetic ingrowth. Sympathetic fibers arising in the superior cervical ganglion and normally innervating blood vessels on the surface of the brain grow into brain regions in response to the loss of forebrain cholinergic neurons. Hippocampal sympathetic ingrowth has been most extensively studied. It appears to result from the production of a tropic factor, nerve growth factor, in the hippocampus. This factor is normally transported away by cholinergic neurons, but when they are injured, it may accumulate and attract sympathetic neurons. Sympathetic ingrowth seems particularly anomalous and probably is maladaptive. It takes about 1 month to become apparent.

It should be noted that the same cellular behaviors underlie each of these rearrangements. In all cases, the neuronal plasma membrane must bud, a growth cone must form, and the neurite must extend and be guided. Appropriate targets must be recognized, and finally a permanent neuronal-target relationship must be established. This relationship is often synaptic. In the intact brain, these cellular events are regulated differently depending on the specific type of neuronal rearrangement.

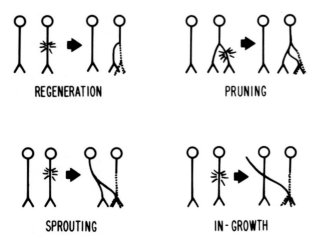

Figure 21-1 Hypothetical models of different types of neuronal rearrangements after injury. (Adapted from Davis.[10])

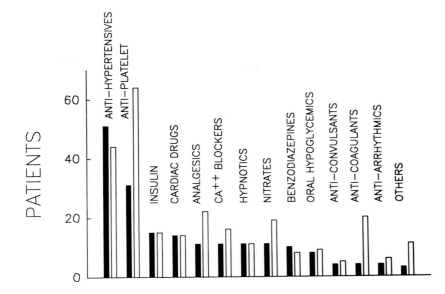

Figure 21-2 Physician prescribing patterns before and after cerebral infarction. Classes of drugs are specified above the bars. Each bar represents the numbers of patients receiving a drug in that class. The closed bars represent drugs prescribed at the time of hospital admission, while the open bars represent drugs prescribed on discharge. (Data from Goldstein and Davis.[17])

Clinical Implications and Future Directions

Drugs currently used after stroke or brain injury such as some centrally acting antihypertensives, anticonvulsants, and sedative-hypnotics could have profound effects on recovery of function in human beings as they do in animals. A recent review of physician prescribing patterns for patients after ischemic stroke indicated that over 80 percent of these individuals were taking drugs at the time of the stroke.[17] Antihypertensives and sedative-hypnotics were among the most commonly used classes of drugs (Fig. 21-2). It may not be surprising that recovery of function varies from patient to patient even when lesion location and type are similar. The initial deficit and recovery are influenced by a variety of biologic and environmental factors. In addition, drugs prescribed for coincident medical problems may have dramatic effects on recovery. It seems prudent to recommend that most drugs be discontinued whenever medically possible during the recovery period. An appreciation of the impact of pharmacologic agents on recovery may lead to effective new therapeutic strategies for stroke and head-injury patients in the future.

References

1. Bach-y-Rita P. Central nervous system lesions: sprouting and unmasking in rehabilitation. *Arch Phys Med Rehabil* 1981; 62:413–417.
2. Bauer RB, Tellez H. Dexamethasone as treatment in cerebrovascular disease: 2. A controlled study in acute cerebral infarction. *Stroke* 1973; 4:547–555.
3. Bliss TVP, Dolphin AC. What is the mechanism of long-term potentiation in the hippocampus? *Trends Neurosci* 1982; 5: 289–290.
4. Boyeson MG, Feeney DM. The role of norepinephrine in recovery from brain injury. *Soc Neurosci Abs* 1984; 10:68 (abstr).
5. Brailowsky S, Knight RT, Blood K, et al. Gamma-aminobutyric acid-induced potentiation of cortical hemiplegia. *Brain Res* 1986; 362:322–330.
6. Cervós-Navarro J, Ferszt R (eds). *Brain Edema: Pathology, Diagnosis, and Therapy.* (*Advances in Neurology*, vol. 28.) New York: Raven Press, 1980.
7. Choi DW. Calcium-mediated neurotoxicity: relationship to specific channel types and role in ischemic damage. *Trends Neurosci* 1988; 11:465–469.
8. Crisostomo EA, Duncan PW, Propst M, et al. Evidence that amphetamine coupled with physical therapy promotes recovery of motor function in stroke patients. *Ann Neurol* 1988; 23: 94–97.
9. Crow TJ, Wedlandt S. Impaired acquisition of a passive avoidance response after lesions induced in the locus coeruleus by 6-OH-dopamine. *Nature* 1976; 259:42–44.
10. Davis JN. Neuronal rearrangements after brain injury: a proposed classification. In: Becker DP, Povlishock JT (eds.), *Central Nervous System Trauma Status Report*. Bethesda, MD: National Institute of Neurological and Communicative Disorders and Stroke, 1985: 491–501.
11. Everitt BJ, Robbins TW, Gaskin M, et al. The effects of lesions to ascending noradrenergic neurons on discrimination learning and performance in the rat. *Neuroscience* 1983; 10:397–410.
12. Feeney DM, Baron J-C. Diaschisis. *Stroke* 1986; 17:817–830.
13. Feeney DM, Gonzalez A, Law WA. Amphetamine, haloperidol, and experience interact to affect rate of recovery after motor cortex injury. *Science* 1985; 217:855–857.
14. Feeney DM, Sutton RL. Pharmacotherapy for recovery of function after brain injury. *Crit Rev Neurobiol* 1987; 3:135–197.
15. Finger S, Stein DG. *Brain Damage and Recovery*. New York: Academic Press, 1982.
16. Gill R, Foster AC, Woodruff GN. Systemic administration of MK-801 protects against ischemia-induced hippocampal neurodegeneration in the gerbil. *J Neurosci* 1987; 7:3343–3349.
17. Goldstein LB, Davis JN. Physician prescribing patterns after ischemic stroke. *Neurology* 1988; 38:1806–1809.

18. Grafman J, Salazar A, Weingartner H, et al. The relationship of brain-tissue loss volume and lesion location to cognitive deficit. *J Neurosci* 1986; 6:301–307.

19. Greenamyre JT. The role of glutamate in neurotransmission and in neurologic disease. *Arch Neurol* 1986; 43:1058–1063.

20. Hass WK. The cerebral ischemic cascade. *Neurol Clin* 1983; 1:345–353.

21. Jørgensen MB, Diemer NH. Selective neuron loss after cerebral ischemia in the rat: possible role of the neurotransmitter glutamate. *Acta Neurol Scand* 1982; 66:536–546.

22. Kakihana M, Fukuda N, Suno M, et al. Effects of CDP-choline on neurologic deficits and cerebral glucose metabolism in a rat model of cerebral ischemia. *Stroke* 1988; 19:217–222.

23. Karpiak SE, Li YS, Mahadik SP. Gangliosides (G$_{M1}$ and AGF2) reduce mortality due to ischemia: protection of membrane function. *Stroke* 1987; 18:184–187.

24. Knopman DS, Selnes OA, Niccum N, et al. A longitudinal study of speech fluency in aphasia: CT correlates of recovery and persistent nonfluency. *Neurology* 1983; 33:1170–1178.

25. Kochhar A, Zivin JA, Lyden PD, et al. Glutamate antagonist therapy reduces neurologic deficits produced by focal central nervous system ischemia. *Arch Neurol* 1988; 45:148–153.

26. Krobert KA, Boyeson MG, Scherer PJ. The role of the locus ceruleus in recovery of function from sensorimotor cortex injury. *Soc Neurosci Abs* 1987; 13:1664 (abstr).

27. Lenzi GL, Frackowiak RSJ, Jones T. Cerebral oxygen metabolism and blood flow in human cerebral infarction. *J Cereb Blood Flow Metab* 1982; 2:321–335.

28. Lundgren J, Flodström K, Sjögren K, et al. Site of brain lesion and functional capacity in rehabilitated hemiplegics. *Scand J Rehabil Med* 1982; 14:141–143.

29. Martin WRW, Raichle ME. Cerebellar blood flow and metabolism in cerebral hemisphere infarction. *Ann Neurol* 1983; 4:168–176.

30. Norris JW, Hachinski VC. High dose steroid treatment in cerebral infarction. *Br Med J* 1986; 292:21–23.

31. Park CK, Nehls DG, Graham DI, et al. The glutamate antago-nist MK-801 reduces focal ischemic brain damage in the rat. *Ann Neurol* 1988; 24:543–551.

32. Prado de Carvalho L, Zornetzer SF. The involvement of the locus coeruleus in memory. *Behav Neural Biol* 1981; 31:173–186.

33. Rothman SM. The neurotoxicity of excitatory amino acids is produced by passive chloride influx. *J Neurosci* 1985; 5:1483–1489.

34. Rothman SM, Olney JW. Glutamate and the pathophysiology of hypoxic-ischemic brain damage. *Ann Neurol* 1986; 19:105–111.

35. Schallert T, Hernandez TD, Barth TM. Recovery of function after brain damage: severe and chronic disruption by diazepam. *Brain Res* 1986; 379:104–111.

36. Sibley DR, Lefkowitz RJ. Molecular mechanisms of receptor desensitization using the β-adrenergic receptor-coupled adenylate cyclase system as a model. *Nature* 1985; 317:124–129.

37. Stanton PK, Sarvey JM. Blockade of norepinephrine-induced long-lasting potentiation in the hippocampal dentate gyrus by an inhibitor of protein synthesis. *Brain Res* 1985; 361:276–283.

38. Stein L, Beluzzi JD, Wise CD. Memory enhancement by central administration of norepinephrine. *Brain Res* 1975; 84:329–335.

39. Swanson LW, Teyler TJ, Thompson RF. Hippocampal long-term potentiation: mechanisms and implications for memory. *Neurosci Res Program Bull* 1982; 20:601–769.

40. Tazaki Y, Sakai F, Otomo E, et al. Treatment of acute cerebral infarction with a choline precursor in a multicenter double-blind placebo controlled study. *Stroke* 1988; 19:211–216.

41. Thompson RF. The neurobiology of learning and memory. *Science* 1986; 233:941–947.

42. Von Monakow C. Diaschisis. In: Pribram KH (ed.), *Brain and Behavior I: Mood States and Mind*. Baltimore: Penguin Books, 1969.

43. Wagner HR, Davis JN. β-Adrenergic receptor regulation by agonists and membrane depolarization in rat brain slices. *Proc Natl Acad Sci USA* 1979; 76:2057–2061.

22

Advances in Molecular Genetics in Relation to Neurogenetic Diseases

Mark J. Alberts
Allen D. Roses

TABLE 22-1 Chromosomal Location of the Defective Gene in Inherited Neurologic Diseases

Disease	Chromosome	Gene/Protein*
Familial Alzheimer's disease[†]	21	U
Huntington's disease	4	U
Duchenne's dystrophy	X	Dystrophin
Becker's dystrophy	X	Dystrophin
Myotonic dystrophy	19	U
Neurofibromatosis		
Peripheral form	17	U
Central form	22	U
Tuberous sclerosis[†]	9,11	U
Lesch-Nyhan disease	X	HGPRT deficiency
Friedreich's ataxia	9	U
Spinocerebellar ataxia[†]	6	U
Familial amyloidotic neuropathy	18	U
Charcot-Marie-Tooth (CMT) disease[†]	1,17	U
X-linked CMT disease	X	U
Manic-depressive illness[†]	11	U

*U indicates that the gene and protein are unknown.
[†]Genetic heterogeneity is proved or suspected, indicating that all cases may not be linked to the same locus.

Molecular genetic research is having a growing impact on the understanding of the etiology, pathogenesis, and potential therapy of neurogenetic diseases. Molecular genetics uses the techniques of molecular biology to determine the order and topography of genes on chromosomes and the genetic defects responsible for inherited diseases.[29] Since its application in the early 1980s, these techniques have led to the discovery of the genetic defect underlying several disorders such as Duchenne's muscular dystrophy and cystic fibrosis.[18,28] The defects for many other neurogenetic diseases have been localized to specific chromosomes or subregions of a chromosome, although the causative genes have not been identified (Table 22-1). In this chapter we will review the commonly used techniques of molecular genetics and highlight new findings in several neurogenetic diseases.

General Principles and Techniques

Each human cell contains approximately 3 billion base pairs of deoxyribonucleic acid (DNA), organized into 23 pairs of chromosomes. The DNA is functionally classified into introns and exons. Introns are segments of DNA that are not ultimately translated into proteins, although introns may be transcribed and may have a role in transcriptional regulation. Exons are portions of DNA that code for sequences of messenger ribonucleic acid (mRNA) that are translated into proteins.

There are approximately 100,000 genes expressed in humans, although not every cell expresses every gene. The brain expresses approximately 50,000 genes, the vast majority of which code for unknown proteins. As cells specialize, their repertoire of expressed genes may vary. For example, neurons may express the gene for neuron-specific enolase and tubulin, whereas glial cells express the gene for glial fibrillary acidic protein. The precise mechanisms which control specific gene expression are unclear, although various growth factors and oncogenes appear to be important. The isolation of a defective gene from among billions of bases of DNA or tens of thousands of normal genes involves the assignment of the defective locus to a chromosome, then to a chromosomal subregion, and finally to a small segment of DNA which can be sequenced.

Two general disease-oriented research approaches will be outlined, although in practice many more are in use. In the first approach, the defective protein is known, but the causative gene is unknown (Fig. 22-1). Once the defective protein is isolated and purified, its amino acid sequence can be determined. Because specific triplets (codons) of RNA code for corresponding amino acids, the probable sequence of the RNA and the original DNA can be determined. A synthetic DNA probe can be constructed corresponding to all or part of the protein of interest. This probe can be used to isolate the gene of interest. Once the gene is isolated, it can be localized to a chromosome, sequenced, and compared to the gene from normal individuals to determine the exact underlying genetic defect. This approach can also be used when the normal gene is isolated and then compared to the abnormal gene. This general approach has been used to isolate the genes responsible for sickle cell anemia, hemophilia, and other diseases.

The second approach is sometimes termed *reverse genetics* and is useful when the defective protein is unknown, as is the case for most neurogenetic diseases (Fig. 22-2). The technique most widely used is genetic linkage analysis. Ge-

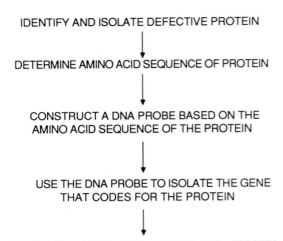

IDENTIFY AND ISOLATE DEFECTIVE PROTEIN

↓

DETERMINE AMINO ACID SEQUENCE OF PROTEIN

↓

CONSTRUCT A DNA PROBE BASED ON THE
AMINO ACID SEQUENCE OF THE PROTEIN

↓

USE THE DNA PROBE TO ISOLATE THE GENE
THAT CODES FOR THE PROTEIN

↓

COMPARE THE GENE FROM NORMAL AND AFFECTED
INDIVIDUALS TO IDENTIFY ABNORMALITIES;
DETERMINE THE CHROMOSOMAL LOCATION OF THE GENE

Figure 22-1 Research scheme for a genetic disease where
the defective protein has been identified.

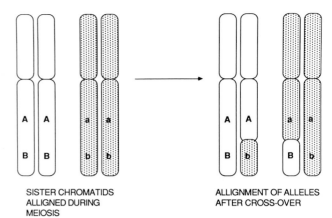

SISTER CHROMATIDS
ALLIGNED DURING
MEIOSIS

ALLIGNMENT OF ALLELES
AFTER CROSS-OVER

Figure 22-3 Diagrammatic representation of crossing-
over during meiosis. Allelles A and B were inherited
from one parent, whereas allelles a and b were inherited
from the other parent. Note that loci closer together have
a reduced chance of being separated during crossing-over
than loci farther apart.

netic linkage occurs when two loci (or genes) are so close
together on the same chromosome that they are inherited as
a unit. Because chromosomes frequently exchange material
during meiosis in a process called *crossing-over*, those loci
close together will have less chance of being separated than
those loci farther apart (Fig. 22-3). The odds of linkage are
commonly expressed as a lod score, "lod" meaning *log of the
odds of linkage*. Lod scores ≥ 3 (i.e., $\geq 1000:1$ odds of linkage) indicate linkage, whereas lod scores ≤ -2 (i.e., $100:1$
odds against linkage) indicate nonlinkage. Linkage is statistical, because the probability of crossing-over between two
loci is proportional to the distance between the two loci. The

actual linkage calculations are performed by computer programs.[23] The distances between two loci are often expressed
as centimorgans (cM); 1 cM is equivalent to approximately
1 million bases of DNA. Centimorgans also provide a measure of recombination frequency. For example, two loci
10 cM apart have a 10 percent frequency of crossing-over.
Finding a marker closely linked to a disease locus greatly
narrows the search from several billion bases to a few million bases of DNA.

Several expressed markers such as blood types and isoen-
zymes have been used for linkage analysis. However, these
markers are few in number and do not adequately span the
human genome. Most inherited diseases have been tested for
linkage to these markers with negative results. The new
markers for linkage analysis are restriction fragment length
polymorphisms (RFLPs).[7] An RFLP is produced when differences in the genomic DNA sequence result in the creation
or deletion of an enzymatic cut site (Fig. 22-4). Differences

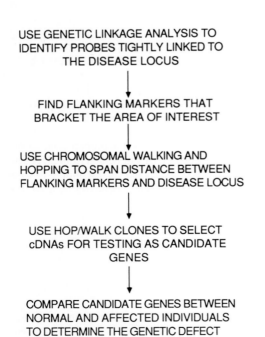

USE GENETIC LINKAGE ANALYSIS TO
IDENTIFY PROBES TIGHTLY LINKED TO
THE DISEASE LOCUS

↓

FIND FLANKING MARKERS THAT
BRACKET THE AREA OF INTEREST

↓

USE CHROMOSOMAL WALKING AND
HOPPING TO SPAN DISTANCE BETWEEN
FLANKING MARKERS AND DISEASE LOCUS

↓

USE HOP/WALK CLONES TO SELECT
cDNAs FOR TESTING AS CANDIDATE
GENES

↓

COMPARE CANDIDATE GENES BETWEEN
NORMAL AND AFFECTED INDIVIDUALS
TO DETERMINE THE GENETIC DEFECT

Figure 22-2 Research scheme for a genetic disease where
the defective protein is unknown.

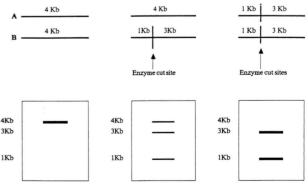

Figure 22-4 Different restriction fragment length polymorphism (RFLP) patterns expected after enzyme diges-
tion and gel electrophoresis of DNA from an individual.
A and B represent different haplotypes inherited from
each parent.

in DNA sequence among individuals are quite common, occurring every 200 to 500 base pairs. Because RFLPs are inherited as mendelian traits, they can be used as markers for linkage testing. The enzymes that cut the DNA are restriction endonucleases. These enzymes cut DNA only at specific base sequences. For example, the enzyme Eco RI will recognize the DNA sequence GAATTC, and cut it between the G and A. If a DNA sequence (a probe) that recognizes the resulting DNA fragments is available, variations in the restriction fragment lengths can be detected. An optimal RFLP is one which is readily detectable, occurs commonly, and has several variants throughout the population.

Once the DNA is cut, it is electrophoresed on an agarose gel (which separates the DNA based on size) and transferred onto a nylon or nitrocellulose filter in a process called *Southern blotting*.[35] The blot is then hybridized to a radioactive probe (segment of DNA) which will detect the cut fragments. The blot is washed and exposed to x-ray film in a process called *autoradiography*. The band pattern is then read, and the segregation of the RFLP and disease locus through a family can be determined. Hundreds of RFLPs have been described over the past 5 years, allowing linkage to be tested with many markers throughout the genome.

Once a closely linked marker (i.e., within 1 to 2 million bases of the disease locus) is identified, physical means of genetic analysis such as chromosomal walking or jumping can be used to identify the defective gene. Chromosome walking involves the successive cloning of adjacent segments of DNA which bridge the gap between the linked marker and the disease gene. Each walking clone can be tested for linkage (if an appropriate polymorphism exists or is discovered) and can be tested as a possible candidate gene by determining if that clone is expressed in the tissue of interest.

Chromosome jumping is accomplished by using a restriction enzyme that cuts at an infrequent site, thereby producing large DNA fragments averaging several hundred thousand bases. Because these large DNA fragments cannot be cloned in existing vectors, they are reduced in size by deleting much of the internal DNA, while saving the ends. Because the ends of some clones will share sequences with other jump clones, they can be used to isolate adjacent segments of DNA. Successive jump clones are examined to determine the direction of the last jump. In this manner, one to two million bases of DNA can be *jumped over* relatively easily. Clones of interest can be tested for linkage to the disease locus to determine if the jumping is going in the proper direction, and to ascertain if further walks or jumps are necessary. These techniques have been used successfully to identify the genes responsible for several diseases, including Duchenne's muscular dystrophy and cystic fibrosis.[18,28]

Another valuable tool in molecular genetics is a complementary DNA (cDNA) library. A cDNA library is made by isolating the messenger RNA from an organ (which represents the genes expressed in the organ) and synthesizing single-stranded cDNA using the enzyme reverse transcriptase. It is preferable to work with DNA instead of RNA because the latter is quite labile and can be degraded by ubiquitous RNAses. Once the single-stranded cDNA is synthesized, it can be made double-stranded and ligated into a vector (usually a bacteriophage). The phage then infects bacteria and multiplies, producing billions of copies of each

phage (which contains the cDNA insert). The resulting library contains billions of copies of each cDNA, which represents each gene expressed in the organ of interest. Once a walking or hopping clone of interest is isolated, it can be used to screen a cDNA library. Any positive clone would be of interest as a candidate gene, and would be localized to a chromosome and studied by linkage analysis. Once a putative disease gene is identified, its DNA sequence can be determined and compared to normal genes for any gross abnormalities such as deletions, insertions, and point mutations. If the disease gene codes for a previously unknown protein, it can be studied in a cell system which will transcribe and translate the gene and produce the protein. This novel protein can be studied; localized to particular organs, cells, and subcellular regions; and compared in normal and diseased individuals to determine if any quantitative, structural, or functional differences exist.

Clinical Advances

Genetic linkage analysis has been used to determine the chromosomal location of the defective gene in many neurogenetic diseases (Table 22-1). Even though the actual gene and genetic defect has yet to be determined for most diseases, the establishment of closely linked markers is significant for these reasons: (1) it greatly advances the search for the actual gene, (2) it allows for more accurate genetic counseling, and (3) it establishes a genetic etiology for the disease. Several prevalent neurogenetic diseases will be discussed, although it must be remembered that several thousands exist.

Alzheimer's Disease

Alzheimer's disease (AD) is the most common cause of dementia and a tremendous social and financial burden upon society, patients, and families. It is characterized by the slow onset and insidious progression of memory disturbance and loss of higher cortical functions.

Several groups have described numerous families with an apparently inherited form of AD with autosomal dominant transmission.[8,36] It was initially thought that familial AD (FAD) was a disease of predominantly young patients with disease onset before age 65. However, recent studies have documented late-onset familial AD (onset >65 years) with a pattern of inheritance consistent with autosomal dominant transmission.[8,15] In fact, this form of late-onset FAD appears to have a peak penetrance at age 90. Therefore, unless family members live to an advanced age, the genotype of AD will not be expressed. The percentage of AD cases that are genetic is subject to debate, but it has been estimated that between 40 and 90 percent of AD cases may be inherited. Since the late-onset form of AD is far more common than early-onset AD, clues about its etiology may have significant implications for large numbers of the elderly.

In 1986, cerebral amyloid (β-amyloid) was investigated as a candidate protein in the etiology of AD. This type of amyloid is found in the senile plaques and cerebral vessels of patients with AD. Because the amino acid sequence of β-amyloid had been determined previously, Goldgaber and colleagues were able to construct a DNA probe for the β-amyloid gene.[11] After the gene was isolated, it was localized to chromosome 21 (CH 21). This was of note because CH 21 had received much attention as the possible location for the AD gene. This interest was based on several findings, including the increased incidence of Down's syndrome (trisomy 21) in families with AD, and the similarity of the pathologic changes seen in the brains of individuals with AD or Down's syndrome.

Linkage studies were performed using the β-amyloid gene and other CH 21 probes. However, there were crossovers between the FAD locus and β-amyloid, indicating that β-amyloid was not the gene responsible for FAD.[38] Initial reports of triplication of the amyloid gene were refuted.[37] Other probes on CH 21 have been linked to FAD, and it now appears that the gene for at least one type of FAD may be on the proximal long arm of CH 21, near the centromere.[36] It has been suggested that all forms of FAD are linked to a locus on CH 21.[10] However, two groups have presented data indicating that late-onset FAD may not be linked to this CH 21 locus.[26,30] These findings may suggest genetic heterogeneity among FAD pedigrees.

Huntington's Disease

Huntington's disease (HD) is an autosomal dominant disorder marked by progressive choreiform movements and dementia. It was one of the first neurogenetic diseases for which linkage was found. Gusella and colleagues began linkage testing on a large Venezuelan family in 1983, planning to test hundreds of random probes.[12] However, the eighth probe (G8) was found to be linked to the HD gene and was localized to chromosome 4. Further studies have isolated more closely linked probes, and genetic counseling can now be given with greater than 99 percent accuracy to individuals who are affected or at risk.[21,41] The causative gene for HD has not been identified, perhaps because the HD locus is close to the tip of CH 4, thereby making isolation of a flanking marker and walking experiments difficult.

Duchenne's Muscular Dystrophy and Becker's Muscular Dystrophy

Duchenne's muscular dystrophy (DMD) is an X-linked recessive disorder which causes progressive muscle weakness. It usually has its onset by 5 years, and most children are confined to a wheelchair by adolescence. In a series of elegant experiments, Kunkel and colleagues noted the presence of deletions of part of the X chromosome in males with Duchenne's muscular dystrophy and translocations of the X chromosome in rare females with DMD.[19] They then performed a subtraction hybridization experiment, in which the X chromosomes containing the deletions were hybridized to normal X chromosomes. This allowed the isolation of segments of DNA that were missing in some male patients with DMD, but present in normal individuals. These clones were

then used for chromosome walking experiments to isolate the entire gene.[18]

The DMD gene was found to be extremely large, spanning 2 million bases and having 8 major exons and many more minor exons. The gene was then placed into an expression system and the end protein was produced. This protein, dystrophin, accounts for only 0.002 percent of muscle proteins but appears to have a vital membrane function.[13] Patients with DMD have little or no measurable dystrophin in their muscle, probably because a deletion in the first part of the gene shifts the reading frame and terminates transcription or translation.[14] As many as 65 percent of males with DMD may have a detectable deletion in some part of the DMD gene.[2] Patients with a milder form of muscular dystrophy, Becker's muscular dystrophy (BMD), appear to have a defect in the same gene, but one which is smaller or does not alter the reading frame. Patients with BMD have moderately low levels of dystrophin.[14] Therefore, a high correlation exists between the underlying genetic defect, the protein defect, and the clinical syndrome.

Genetic counseling for individuals at risk for DMD in families with detectable deletions can now be performed accurately and easily. Through the use of chorionic villus biopsy in the eighth to tenth week of pregnancy, the genetic status of the fetus can be determined early in the pregnancy. Pilot experiments are now under way to test the feasibility of transplanting myoblasts containing the normal dystrophin gene into affected patients.

Myotonic Muscular Dystrophy

Myotonic muscular dystrophy (DM) is an autosomal dominant dystrophy with myotonia, distal muscle wasting, and systemic involvement. The gene for DM has been localized to the proximal long arm of CH 19, and linkage studies have found close linkage with several markers including apolipoprotein C2, creatine kinase band M (CKMM), and an anonymous probe, LDR 152.[3,43] Recent studies have identified a number of possible flanking markers in this region that are being tested. Experiments are under way to identify possible candidate genes. In particular, genes related to intrinsic membrane ion channel proteins are being evaluated. The availability of closely linked markers has made genetic counseling possible with 98 to 99 percent accuracy in an informative situation.

Neuropathies

Charcot-Marie-Tooth disease (CMT) is an autosomal dominant neuropathy characterized by distal atrophy of leg muscles, loss of deep tendon reflexes, and mild sensory changes. Several different varieties of CMT have been described based upon clinical, nerve conduction, pathologic, and genetic findings. CMT 1 was linked initially to the Duffy blood group on CH 1.[4] However, most families do not show linkage to this locus.[5] Vance and colleagues found linkage of six large CMT 1 families to two CH 17 markers.[39] It is unclear what percentage of CMT 1 cases will be linked to this CH 17 locus.

Several Portuguese families with inherited amyloidotic neuropathy have been described and studied for genetic linkage. Linkage was found with a probe on CH 18.

Phakomatoses

The phakomatoses such as neurofibromatosis (NF), tuberous sclerosis (TS), and von Hippel-Lindau disease (VHL) have been the focus of intense genetic research. These diseases are of primary interest to neurosurgeons because all have prominent CNS manifestations and may present for neurosurgical evaluation and treatment.

The peripheral form of NF (NF1) is an autosomal dominant disorder with neurofibromas, café au lait spots, and Lisch nodules. The gene for NF1 has been mapped through linkage and physical mapping studies to the pericentromeric region of CH 17.[1,31] The isolation of flanking markers and chromosomal translocations have narrowed the search for the NF1 gene to a small region of CH 17.[31] The central form of NF, characterized by bilateral acoustic neurinomas, meningiomas, and other CNS tumors, has been linked to a locus on chromosome 22 near the center of the long arm.[42]

TS is an autosomal dominant disease with cutaneous and central nervous system involvement. Initial studies found linkage of TS to the ABO blood group locus on CH 9. One recent study failed to detect linkage of TS to any part of CH 9, but another group found linkage to CH 9 in some families and CH 11 in others.[17,33] These results appear to indicate genetic heterogeneity.

VHL is an autosomal dominant disorder characterized by CNS hemangioblastomas and a susceptibility to various forms of cancer. VHL was linked to the locus encoding the RAF1 oncogene located on CH 3.[32] Because crossovers were detected between the VHL and RAF1 loci, it is unlikely that the RAF1 oncogene is directly responsible for the VHL phenotype. It has been postulated that inactivation of a nearby tumor suppressor could account for some of the cancers seen in VHL, but there are no supporting data.

Inherited Ataxias

Two forms of inherited ataxias have recently been linked. Friedreich's ataxia, an autosomal recessive disease, was linked to chromosome 9 using an anonymous probe and the interferon-β gene probe.[9] An autosomal dominant form of spinocerebellar ataxia has been linked to chromosome 6, within 15 cM of HLA-A.[27]

Vascular Disease

Atherosclerosis of the carotid artery is the underlying lesion in many cases of stroke. Although lipid metabolism is under multigenic control, several genetic defects in lipid metabolism have been described which predispose to premature and clinically significant atherosclerosis. These include hypercholesterolemia, elevated triglycerides, and lipid transport defects.[22]

There are numerous inherited disorders resulting in co-agulopathies associated with an increased risk of cerebrovascular and systemic complications. Deficiencies in antithrombin III, tissue plasminogen activator (tPA), and proteins C have been described.[22] The chromosomal location of some of these factors has been determined. Homocysteinuria is an autosomal recessive disorder causing premature stroke and myocardial infarction.[6] Recombinant DNA techniques have made possible the production of pharmacologic quantities of tPA to treat myocardial infarction and other thrombotic occlusions.

The Icelandic form of intracerebral hemorrhage is an autosomal dominant disorder characterized by the deposition of cystatin C in cerebral vessels which leads to cerebral hemorrhages and death. Cystatin C is a cysteine protease inhibitor, and its function in the brain is unclear. The gene for cystatin C has been isolated and sequenced, and a mutation has been found in patients with this disorder.[20,24]

An autosomal dominant form of cerebral amyloid angiopathy has been found in Dutch families. Patients present with cerebral hemorrhages that are most common in the parietal and occipital lobes. Up to 50 percent may have clinical or pathologic changes of Alzheimer's disease. The vascular deposits of amyloid stain with antisera against the amyloid found in AD brains. It is possible that this form of familial amyloid angiopathy will be linked to the amyloid gene on CH 21, although this has not been proved.

Several cases with a familial occurrence of intracranial aneurysms and arteriovenous malformations, with or without other anomalies such as connective tissue disorders, have been reported.[34]

Epilepsy

Epilepsy is not commonly thought of as an inherited disease, but there is evidence of significant genetic influences in different types of epilepsy. Although 10 percent of all epilepsies arise on a clearly inherited basis, perhaps 2 to 3 times as many cases have significant genetic components. Epilepsy syndromes can be divided into those with epilepsy as part of another illness with diverse CNS or systemic manifestations, and those with isolated epilepsy (i.e., idiopathic epilepsy). Several of the inherited disorders with epilepsy have been linked to various loci; however, none of the idiopathic epilepsies have been linked. Numerous murine models of single locus mutants with epilepsy (both major motor seizures and spike-wave discharges with behavioral arrest) have been described.

Gene Therapy

While a full discussion of gene therapy is beyond the scope of this chapter, several points deserve mention. The therapy of genetic disorders can include either systemic treatments, in which medications are given to blunt the effects of the underlying genetic defect, or genetic treatments, in which either new genetic material is added to cells or genes already in the patient are modified and regulated to produce more or less of a specific protein. The introduction of new genetic material into either somatic or germ cells is possible, especially if stem cells are available (such as bone marrow cells) which can serve as a perpetual supplier of genetically altered cells.[16] However, the introduction of new genetic material into cells by retroviruses is complicated by the potential for malignant transformation of the cells and difficulty regulating gene expression.[40] Although preliminary experiments in animal models have proved encouraging, technical problems remain, especially for the introduction of new genes into cells of the CNS.[25]

Conclusion

Through the use of molecular genetics, our understanding of many neurogenetic diseases has been advanced tremendously over the past 10 years. The chromosomal locus of the defect for many diseases has been determined, and in some cases the defective gene and protein have been isolated. Accurate genetic counseling is widely available for many inherited diseases. The future challenge will be to devise safe and effective techniques for somatic or genetic therapy.

References

1. Barker D, Wright E, Nguyen K, et al. Gene for von Recklinghausen neurofibromatosis is in the pericentromeric region of chromosome 17. *Science* 1987; 236:1100–1102.
2. Bartlett RJ, Pericak-Vance MA, Koh J, et al. Duchenne muscular dystrophy: high frequency of deletions. *Neurology* 1988; 38:1–4.
3. Bartlett RJ, Pericak-Vance MA, Yamaoka L, et al. A new probe for the diagnosis of myotonic muscular dystrophy. *Science* 1987; 235:1648–1650.
4. Bird TD, Ott J, Giblett ER. Evidence for linkage of Charcot-Marie-Tooth neuropathy to the Duffy locus on chromosome 1. *Am J Hum Genet* 1982; 34:388–394.
5. Bird TD, Ott J, Giblett ER, et al. Genetic linkage evidence for heterogeneity in Charcot-Marie-Tooth neuropathy (HMSN type 1). *Ann Neurol* 1983; 14:679–684.
6. Boers GHJ, Smals AGH, Trijbels F, et al. Heterozygosity for homocystinuria in premature peripheral and cerebral occlusive arterial disease. *N Engl J Med* 1985; 313:709–715.
7. Botstein D, White RL, Skolnick M, et al. Construction of a genetic linkage map in man using restriction fragment length polymorphisms. *Am J Hum Genet* 1980; 32:314–331.
8. Breitner JCS, Silverman JM, Mohs RC, et al. Familial aggregation in Alzheimer's disease: comparison of risk among relatives of early- and late-onset cases, and among male and female relatives in successive generations. *Neurology* 1988; 38:207–212.
9. Chamberlain S, Shaw J, Rowland A, et al. Mapping of mutation causing Friedreich's ataxia to human chromosome 9. *Nature* 1988; 334:248–250.
10. Goate AM, Owen MJ, James LA, et al. Predisposing locus for Alzheimer's disease on chromosome 21. *Lancet* 1989; 1:352–355.
11. Goldgaber D, Lerman MI, McBride OW, et al. Characterization and chromosomal localization of a cDNA encoding brain amyloid of Alzheimer's disease. *Science* 1987; 235:877–880.
12. Gusella JF, Wexler NS, Conneally PM, et al. A polymorphic DNA marker genetically linked to Huntington's disease. *Nature* 1983; 306:234–238.
13. Hoffman EP, Brown RHJ, Kunkel LM, et al. Dystrophin: the protein product of the Duchenne muscular dystrophy locus. *Cell* 1987; 51:919–928.
14. Hoffman EP, Fischbeck KM, Brown RH, et al. Characterization of dystrophin in muscle-biopsy specimens from patients with Duchenne's or Becker's muscular dystrophy. *N Engl J Med* 1988; 318:1363–1368.
15. Huff FJ, Auerbach J, Chakravarti A, et al. Risk of dementia in relatives of patients with Alzheimer's disease. *Neurology* 1988; 38:786–790.
16. Jähner D, Haase K, Mulligan R, et al. Insertion of the bacterial gpt gene into the germ line of mice by retroviral infection. *Proc Natl Acad Sci USA* 1985; 82:6927–6931.
17. Kandt RS, Pericak-Vance MA, Hung W-Y, et al. Multilocus linkage analysis in tuberous sclerosis. *Am J Hum Genet* 1989; 104:223–228.
18. Koenig M, Hoffman EP, Bertelson CJ, et al. Complete cloning of the Duchenne muscular dystrophy (DMD) cDNA and preliminary genomic organization of the DMD gene in normal and affected individuals. *Cell* 1987; 50:509–517.
19. Kunkel LM, Monaco AP, Middlesworth W, et al. Specific cloning of DNA fragments absent from the DNA of a male patient with an X-chromosome deletion. *Proc Natl Acad Sci USA* 1985; 82:4778–4782.
20. Levy E, Lopez-Otin C, Ghiso J, et al. Stroke in Icelandic amyloid angiopathy is related to a mutation in the cystatin C gene, an inhibitor of cysteine proteases. *J Exp Med* 1989; 169:1771–1778.
21. Meissen GJ, Myers RH, Mastromauro CA, et al. Predictive testing for Huntington's disease with use of a linked DNA marker. *N Engl J Med* 1988; 318:535–542.
22. Natowicz M, Kelley RI. Mendelian etiologies of stroke. *Ann Neurol* 1987; 22:175–192.
23. Ott J. Estimation of the recombination fraction in human pedigrees: efficient computation of the likelihood for human linkage studies. *Am J Hum Genet* 1974; 26:588–597.
24. Palsdottir A, Abrahamson M, Thorsteinsson L, et al. Mutation in cystatin C gene causes hereditary brain hemorrhage. *Lancet* 1988; 2:603–605.
25. Parkman R. The application of bone marrow transplantation to the treatment of genetic diseases. *Science* 1986; 232:1373–1378.
26. Pericak-Vance MA, Yamaoka LH, Haynes CS, et al. Genetic linkage studies in Alzheimer's disease families. *Exp Neurol* 1988; 102:271–279.
27. Rich SS, Wilkie P, Schut L, et al. Spinocerebellar ataxia: localization of an autosomal dominant locus between two markers on human chromosome 6. *Am J Hum Genet* 1987; 41:524–531.
28. Rommens JM, Iannuzzi MC, Bat-Sheva K, et al. Identification of the cystic fibrosis gene: chromosome walking and jumping. *Science* 1989; 245:1059–1065.
29. Roses AD, Pericak-Vance MA, Yamaoka LH, et al. Recombinant DNA strategies in genetic neurological diseases. *Muscle Nerve* 1983; 6:339–355.
30. Schellenberg GD, Bird TD, Wijsman EM, et al. Absence of linkage of chromosome 21q21 markers to familial Alzheimer's disease. *Science* 1988; 241:1507–1510.
31. Seizinger BR, Farmer GE, Haines JL, et al. Flanking markers for the gene causing von Recklinghausen neurofibromatosis (NF1). *Am J Hum Genet* 1989; 44:30–32.
32. Seizinger BR, Rouleau GA, Ozelius LJ, et al. Von Hippel-Lindau disease maps to the region of chromosome 3 associated with renal cell carcinoma. *Nature* 1988; 332:268–269.

33. Smith M, Dumars K, Bauman R, et al. Evidence for genetic heterogeneity in tuberous sclerosis: one gene maps to the 9q34 region and a second gene maps in the 11q22-11q23 region. Program of the 10th International Human Gene Mapping Workshop, New Haven, CT. 1989:14.

34. Snead OC, Acker JD, Morawetz R. Familial arteriovenous malformation. *Ann Neurol* 1979; 5:585–587.

35. Southern EM. Detection of specific sequences among DNA fragments separated by gel electrophoresis. *J Mol Biol* 1975; 98:503–517.

36. St. George-Hyslop PH, Tanzi RE, Polinsky RJ, et al. The genetic defect causing familial Alzheimer's disease maps on chromosome 21. *Science* 1987; 235:885–890.

37. Tanzi RE, Bird ED, Latt SA, et al. The amyloid β protein gene is not duplicated in brains from patients with Alzheimer's disease. *Science* 1987; 238:666–669.

38. Tanzi RE, St. George-Hyslop PH, Haines JL, et al. The genetic defect in familial Alzheimer's disease is not tightly linked to the amyloid β-protein gene. *Nature* 1987; 329:156–157.

39. Vance JM, Nicholson GA, Yamaoka LH, et al. Linkage of Charcot-Marie-Tooth neuropathy type la to chromosome 17. *Exp Neurol* 1989; 104:186–189.

40. Van der Putten H, Botteri FM, Miller AD, et al. Efficient insertion of genes into the mouse germ line via retroviral vectors. *Proc Natl Acad Sci USA* 1985; 82:6148–6152.

41. Wasmuth JJ, Hewitt J, Smith B, et al. A highly polymorphic locus very tightly linked to the Huntington's disease gene. *Nature* 1988; 332:734–738.

42. Wertelecki W, Rouleau GA, Superneau DW, et al. Neurofibromatosis 2: clinical and DNA linkage studies of a large kindred. *N Engl J Med* 1988; 319:278–283.

43. Yamaoka LH, Pericak-Vance MA, Speer MC, et al. Tight linkage of creatine kinase (CKMM) to myotonic dystrophy on chromsome 19. *Neurology* 1989 (in press).

23

Oncogenes and Nervous System Tumors

H. Earl Ruley
Henry H. Schmidek

At a cellular level, neoplasia is a heritably altered, relatively autonomous growth of tissue. Most neoplasms are clonal in origin and thus apparently arise from a single altered cell whose genetic abnormalities provide a selective growth advantage as compared to normal cells. In recent years, certain molecular mechanisms contributing to neoplastic change have been elucidated. In particular, two classes of genes (oncogenes and tumor suppressor genes) have been identified, which, when altered by mutation, help to sustain the growth autonomy of tumor cells.[7,23,39,40]

Oncogenes express proteins which promote the growth of susceptible cell types, while the tumor-suppressor genes (also referred to as antioncogenes or emerogenes) apparently function to restrain growth. Tumor progression (i.e., the tendency of tumors to become more malignant with time) can result from multiple genetic changes within the neoplastic clone of cells, giving rise to subpopulations of cells with increasingly aggressive characteristics.[30] At least some of these changes involve mutations that activate oncogenes or inactivate antioncogenes, thus abolishing controls necessary to maintain normal patterns of growth and differentiation. The current concepts in this field will be discussed with special reference to nervous system tumors.[38]

Chromosomal Abnormalities in Nervous System Neoplasms

For many years, it has been known that chromosomal abnormalities occur in malignant cells, and more specifically that such abnormalities are present among some nervous system neoplasms.[34,35,46,47] Cytogenetic analyses carried out on direct preparations and short-term cultures of gliomas by a number of investigators have revealed nonrandom, numerical and structural abnormalities involving chromosomes 1, 6, 7, 8, 9, 10, 17, and 22.[3-5]

Genotypic changes in various other tumor types have been described in the absence of gross chromosomal aberra-

tions by comparing restriction fragment length polymorphisms (RFLPs) in DNA isolated from constitutional and neoplastic tissues from affected individuals. While the list of tumor-associated chromosome aberrations revealed by this type of analysis is expanding rapidly, it is generally unclear whether these aberrations are linked to tumor initiation or tumor progression. In some cases (retinoblastoma, neuroblastoma, meningioma, neurofibromatosis, acoustic neuroma with Recklinghausen's disease), the underlying mechanism suggests that recessive mutations are involved in the etiology of the disease. As will be discussed later, loss of a single genetic locus appears sufficient for tumorigenesis.[2,15]

James and colleagues have analyzed gliomas consisting of a mixture of glial cell subtypes spanning the grades of histologic malignancy.[21] RFLP analysis indicates that loss of part or all of chromosome 10 is specifically associated with glioblastoma, while nonrandom aberrations involving other chromosomes can be detected across the other grades of gliomas. These results also indicate that, irrespective of the pathologic heterogeneity noted in a glioblastoma, this tumor is clonal in nature and that its cells demonstrate a homozygous loss of alleles on chromosome 10.

In a similar study of lower-grade gliomas, James et al. compared allelic combinations at seven loci on human chromosome 17 in tumor and normal tissues from 35 patients.[22] Loss of constitutional heterozygosity at one or more of these loci was observed in 8 of 24 tumors displaying astrocytic differentiation and in a single neuroectodermal tumor. In contrast, tumors of oligodendrocytic, ependymal, or mixed cellular differentiation did not exhibit loss of alleles at any of the loci examined. These data suggest that the loss of a gene on chromosome 17p may contribute to the oncogenesis of nervous system tumors, particularly those showing solely astrocytic differentiation.

In summary, chromosome abnormalities are common in neural tumors. Nonrandom changes probably have etiologic significance and are not simply manifestations of the genetic instability characteristic of tumor cells. In most cases, the underlying genetic targets are unknown. However, as with other tumors, some are likely to reveal instances in which oncogenes and tumor-suppressor genes have been activated and inactivated, respectively.

Isolation of Oncogenes

Oncogenes were first discovered associated with infectious retroviruses capable of transmitting malignant disease from one animal to another.[43] The oncogenic potential of these viruses generally results from additional gene segments incorporated and expressed as part of the virus. Homologues of most viral oncogenes (proto-oncogenes) are present in normal cells. The viral oncogenes arise from rare events in which the virus has captured portions of the cellular proto-oncogene. The pathogenic potential of the captured gene is unmasked as a result of mutations, ectopic expression of the gene under viral controls, and physical linkage to a transmissible virus.

Retroviruses which lack captured oncogenes can also activate cellular proto-oncogenes if the retrovirus integrates near the gene and disrupts cellular controls that regulate normal expression.[43] However, given the low probability of these events, the carcinogenic process requires longer than when the virus already carries an activated oncogene.

With a few exceptions, retroviruses do not contribute to naturally occurring tumors in human beings. Nevertheless, retroviral carcinogenesis demonstrates that events which deregulate the expression or activity of normal cellular genes can contribute to malignant change. Indeed, with the discovery that DNA purified from tumor cells can induce cultured cells to express malignant phenotypes, cellular oncogenes have been detected and isolated directly from human tumor cells.

The first oncogene isolated from human tumor cells was the human homologue of the H-*ras* oncogene, initially characterized as a gene segment captured by the Harvey murine sarcoma virus. Subsequent transfection experiments have isolated additional cellular genes previously encountered as oncogenes captured by retroviruses. As with the retroviral oncogenes, the oncogenic potential of the cellular oncogenes was unmasked by mutations.

While oncogenes carried by retroviruses are often not detected by transferring tumor DNA, these studies demonstrated that genes identified in association with animal retroviruses may also be involved in human cancer. In retrospect, this is not surprising, since proto-oncogene sequences are highly conserved across large phylogenetic distances and thus may regulate activities fundamental to metazoan organisms.

Conservation of nucleic acid sequence has also allowed retroviral oncogenes to be used as probes to analyze human tumor cells for alterations in related genes. In several instances, proto-oncogenes activated by retroviruses are associated with several types of tumor-specific chromosome abnormalities. These include translocations of chromosomal segments and chromosomal structures that result from tandem amplifications of specific gene loci, known as double minutes and homogenous staining regions. For example, virtually all African Burkitt's lymphoma tumors contain translocations involving the *myc* gene on chromosome 8 and segments of the immunoglobin heavy and light chain genes, located on chromosomes 14, 22, and 2; and in greater than 90 percent of chronic myelogenous leukemia, the *abl* proto-oncogene on chromosome 9 is translocated to a region on chromosome 22. Likewise, amplifications involving c-*myc*, N-*myc*, *myb*, and *erb*B have been observed in human tumors.

Oncogene Classes

Growth of metazoan cells is tightly regulated so that cell division keeps pace with the need for additional cells associated with embryonic development, tissue renewal, or increased demand for cellular functions. Extracellular signals play an essential role, alerting stem cells of the number of new cells required by the tissue or organism. Many, and perhaps all, proto-oncogenes encode components of the signal transduction pathways by which extracellular factors regulate cell growth and differentiation (Fig. 23-1). Somatic mutations and virus associations circumvent controls that regulate proto-oncogene function or expression in normal cells, thus promoting the growth autonomy characteristic of tumor cells.

Table 23-1 lists retroviral and cellular oncogenes classified according to their likely roles in a generalized signal transduction pathway (reviewed by Bishop,[7] Heldin and Westermark,[19] and Weinberg[44]). In addition to the oncogenes identified associated with oncogenic retroviruses or by gene transfer, Table 23-1 includes cellular genes or gene products experimentally found to have oncogenic potential in animals following activation by in vitro genetic manipula-

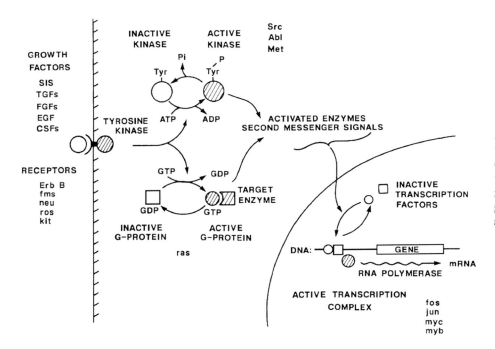

Figure 23-1 Oncogenes and signal transduction. Many proto-oncogenes encode components of the signal transduction pathways by which extracellular factors regulate cell growth and differentiation. Oncogenes may function as growth factors, growth factor receptors, intermediaries (kinases or G-proteins) that transduce or amplify second messenger signals, and as genes whose transcription is activated by growth factors.

TABLE 23-1 Classification of Viral/Cellular Oncogenes

Gene	Discovery*	Function or Activity	Activation in Human Tumors
Growth Factors			
sis	RC	B-chain PDGF	Increased expression
PDGF A chain	H, EA	A-chain PDGF	Amplification
EGF	EA	Epidermal growth factor	Increased expression
TGFα	EA	EGF-like growth factor	Increased expression
GM-CSF	EA	Granulocyte-macrophage colony stimulating factor	
M-CSF	EA	Macrophage-colony stimulating factor	
IL-2	EA	T-cell growth factor	
IL-3	IA, EA	Multi-CSF	
A-FGF	EA	Acidic FGF	Increased expression
B-FGF	EA	Basic FGF	
hst/Kfgf	TX	FGF-like growth factor	
int-2	IA	FGF-like growth factor	
FGF-5	EA	FGF-like growth factor	
Growth Factor Receptors			
erbB	RC, IA	CSF-1 receptor	
neu	TX	EGF receptor-like	Amplification
kit	RC	Ligand unknown	
ros(mcf3)	RC, TX	Ligand unknown	Amplification
trk	TX	Ligand unknown	
Nonreceptor Tyrosine Kinases			
src	RC		Increased expression
yes	RC	src-like kinase	
fgr	RC	src-like kinase	
fyn	H, EA	src-like kinase	
lck	IA, EA	src-like kinase	
fps/fes	RC		
abl	RC		Translocation
sea	RC		
lsk/tck	TX		
slk	H, EA		
met	TX		
hsc	TX		

Gene	Discovery*	Function or Activity	Activation in Human Tumors
Serine Threonine Protein Kinases			
mil/raf	RC, TX		
mos	RC, IA		
Guanine Nucleotide Binding Proteins			
Ha-ras	RC, TX		Point mutations
Ki-ras	RC, TX		Point mutations
N-ras	TX		Increased expression Point mutations
Nuclear Location			
c-myc	RC, IA	?	Translocation, amplification
N-myc	H, EA	?	Amplification
L-myc	H, EA	?	Amplification
myb	RC	Binds DNA	Amplification
fos	RC	Binds transcription factor AP-1/jun	
ski	RC	?	
p53	EA	? Binds SV40 T antigen	Increased expression
jun	RC	Transcription factor AP-1	
Other Receptors			
erbA	RC	T3/T4 receptor	
mas	TX	Angiotensin receptor	
Presently Unclassified			
ets	RC		
rel	RC, TX		
mcf2	TX		
ret	TX		
dbl	TX		
lca	TX		
int-1	IA, EA	A secreted factor	
crk	RC	Similar to non-kinase domains of src and phospholipase C	
Bcl-2	CT, EA		Translocation

*CT = tumor-specific chromosome translocation; EA = experimental activation; H = homology to other oncogenes; IA = insertional activation; RC = retrovirus capture; TX = DNA transfection.

tions. Finally, Table 23-1 indicates instances where oncogenes are known to be activated in human tumors as a result of chromosome translocation, gene amplification, and somatic mutation. Instances of increased proto-oncogene expression are also noted, but these do not necessarily reflect mutational activation, since elevated expression of certain proto-oncogenes [e.g., sis, transforming growth factor a (TGF-a)] can accompany transformation by other oncogenes. In addition, tumor cells may simply maintain high levels found in nonmalignant cells at an earlier developmental stage.

Growth Factors

Growth factors are polypeptides which can stimulate cell proliferation upon binding to cell surface receptors. That oncogenes can encode growth factors was established when the protein sequence of the B chain of platelet-derived growth factor (PDGF) proved to be homologous to the *sis* oncogene of the simian sarcoma virus.

The number of known growth factor oncogenes has expanded as genes encoding growth factors have been cloned and tested for transforming activity. The growth factor genes are activated to become oncogenes by events which allow the factor to be expressed continuously in responsive cell types. The resulting ectopic production of growth factor enables cells to proliferate in the absence of appropriate environmental stimuli.

Glial cells can both produce and respond to PDGF provided they express PDGF receptors. Extracts of brain tumors have been found to contain high levels of mRNA encoding either the A or B chain of PDGF. Some tumors produce both mRNAs, but expression of each appears to be regulated independently. Likewise, glial tumors of fibroblastic morphology contain relatively high levels of mRNA encoding the PDGF receptor. Human glioblastoma cells secrete PDGF, but expression of the growth factor alone does not transform glial cells.[19] Several brain tumor extracts also secrete TGF-β. TGF-β is present at increased levels in astrocytomas, anaplastic astrocytomas, and glioblastomas but not in meningiomas or ependymomas.[29]

Growth Factor Receptors and Tyrosine Kinases

A majority of oncogenes identified in association with oncogenic retroviruses encode proteins with tyrosine kinase activities. Several are derived from genes which encode known growth factor receptors (*erb*B, *fms*) or receptor-like proteins (*neu, kit, ros,* and *trk*). Protein sequencing also established the oncogenic potential of growth factor receptors when the sequence of the epidermal growth factor receptor and the *erb*B oncogene of avian erythroblastosis virus proved to be related.

Growth factor receptors span the plasma membrane such that the growth factor binding domain is located outside the cell while an enzymatic (tyrosine kinase) domain resides inside the cell. Binding extracellular growth factor activates the receptor tyrosine kinase within the cell and initiates a signaling process which stimulates the proliferation of susceptible cell types. Interactions between growth factors and receptors are tight and highly specific; thus, minute quantities of growth factor are sufficient to elicit cellular responses.

Receptor oncogenes are activated by mutations which deregulate the tyrosine kinase activity of the receptor, thus stimulating cells in the absence of environmental growth factors. Other tyrosine kinase oncogenes (e.g., *src*) lack sequences characteristic of membrane-spanning receptors. The functions of nonreceptor tyrosine kinases are unknown; however, all apparently function near the plasma membrane or within the cytoplasm of cells.

That most growth factor receptors and many oncogene proteins are tyrosine kinases is significant given that phosphorylations on tyrosine constitute only a small fraction (0.1 percent) of the total protein phosphate. Thus, tyrosine phosphorylation appears to be tightly linked to pathways regulating cell growth and differentiation. Mutations which deregulate protein tyrosine kinases are thought to contribute to malignant change by activating these pathways.

Receptor-like tyrosine kinase oncogenes are frequently activated in both spontaneous and carcinogen-induced neural tumors. *Erb*B encodes the receptor for both epidermal growth factor and TGF-α. Amplification and overexpression of the epidermal growth factor receptor (EGFR) gene has been demonstrated in a number of human brain tumors.[28] For example, in one study 4 of 10 freshly resected human gliomas expressed increased EGFR activity, highest among high-grade gliomas and lower in neuroblastomas and meningiomas.[28]

Glioblastomas can be induced in the offspring of pregnant rats treated with ethylnitrosourea. The DNA from these tumors can transform 3T3 cells, an activity associated with mutationally activated *neu* oncogenes. A single amino acid change in the transmembrane domain of the receptor is sufficient to convert *neu* to an activated oncogene. Finally, amplified *neu* oncogenes have been detected in glioblastomas and gliosarcomas induced in the offspring of pregnant rats injected with nitrosourea.[37]

ras: A Family of GTP Binding Proteins

The *ras* oncogenes encode four closely related proteins that appear to transduce or amplify intracellular signals activated by cell surface receptors. Thus, *ras* proteins share both structural and functional similarities with several guanine nucleotide-regulated signal transducers, and inhibiting *ras* proto-oncogene products in normal cells prevents growth factors from stimulating proliferation.

Little is known about upstream receptors expected to activate *ras* proteins or about downstream targets presumably regulated by *ras*. However, binding and hydrolysis of guanosine triphosphate (GTP) have been shown experimentally to regulate normal *ras* functions. Moreover, point mutations which activate the oncogene deregulate p21 activities, thus locking *ras* in a functionally active state.

In a wide variety of tumors, *ras* genes activated by point mutations can be detected.[6] Gene transfer experiments suggest that 10 to 20 percent of all human tumors harbor activated *ras* genes, although in pancreatic tumors the frequency approaches 100 percent. K-*ras* is activated preferentially in carcinoma of the colon and lung, while N-*ras* activation is more frequent in leukemia and in neuroblastoma.

Oncogenes and Transcriptional Control

Upon binding to cell surface receptors, growth factors affect many biochemical processes within cells; however, stable changes in cell growth and differentiation ultimately depend on changes in cellular gene expression. Several proto-oncogene products are localized to the cell nucleus and function as distal targets of signal transduction pathways in at least two different ways.

First, transcription of several proto-oncogenes (for example, *fos*, c-*myc* and *jun*) is induced in cells stimulated by growth factors. Transcriptional regulation of these proto-oncogenes is important in growth control, since activating mutations allow the genes to be expressed continuously in the absence of growth factors and also enable cells to proliferate with fewer exogenous growth factors.

Second, several oncogene protein products (e.g., *fos*, *jun*) bind DNA and actively regulate the transcription of growth factor–induced genes. Thus, AP-1, initially characterized as a protein involved in the transcriptional control of genes induced by tumor-promoting phorbol esters and growth factors, unexpectedly proved to be the c-*jun* gene product.[8] Moreover, c-*jun* and c-*fos* proteins form stable complexes and interact with similar DNA sequences, at least when bound together.[33] Oncogenic activation of *fos* and *jun* may therefore affect the expression of similar genes involved in malignant change. How *fos* and *jun* regulate transcription is presently unknown. However, as illustrated in Fig. 23-2, cytoplasmic second messenger signals are thought to direct the assembly of transcription factors into DNA-protein complexes and thus promote the transcription of genes by RNA polymerase.

Although located in the nucleus, the functions of the *myc* proteins are unknown; c-*myc* belongs to this family of genes, each member of which appears to be expressed in a tissue-specific manner. N-*myc* amplification has been observed in approximately 40 percent of neuroblastomas and in medulloblastomas.[24] Among neuroblastomas, there is a direct relationship between the clinical prognosis and the extent of N-*myc* amplification.[10,11]

The *tat* gene of human T-cell leukemia virus (HTLV-I) also activates transcription of both viral and cellular genes. Although not a transduced cellular oncogene, *tat* deserves special mention, since transgenic mice harboring the gene develop tumors with the morphologic and biologic properties of neurofibromatosis.[20] Most of these tumors are benign, although in some cases the tumors exhibit some malignant features. When autopsied, these animals all prove to have tumors arising from cranial nerves, and in some of these, the trigeminal nerve ganglion is involved. These animals also develop tumors on their peripheral nerves between 90 and 130 days of age and malignant tumors considerably later in their lives.

Oncogenes and Multistep Carcinogenesis

Carcinogenesis is typically a multistep process; thus, conversion of normal cells to a fully malignant state probably requires multiple genetic alterations affecting several levels of growth control.[25] Therefore, it is not surprising that activated oncogenes, acting alone, are generally unable to convert normal cells to a tumorigenic state. Gene transfer experiments have demonstrated that two different oncogenes (for example, *myc* and *ras*) can act in a complementary fashion to convert normal cells to a tumorigenic state, and in the process, the two oncogenes elicit phenotypes induced by neither oncogene alone.[36,44] Cooperation between oncogenes has been reported in a variety of cell types, including human embryonic retinoblasts.[12]

The cooperative effects of *myc* and *ras* have also been demonstrated in transgenic mice.[41] Thus, mice harboring both *myc* and H-*ras* oncogenes develop more mammary adenocarcinomas and nonmalignant Harderian gland tumors than animals harboring either oncogene alone. The increase in tumor incidence exceeds the additive effect of each oncogene acting separately, and the tumors arise sooner. Nevertheless, the tumors emerge as discrete foci, suggesting that other genetic or epigenetic events are required for malignant transformation.

Oncogenes may also influence both early and late stages of tumor progression, affecting not only growth autonomy but also the acquisition of properties essential for invasion and metastasis. For example, mutated *ras* genes contribute to premalignant skin and colon lesions[1,9,16]; whereas, *myc* amplification has been observed in advanced neuroblastoma and carcinoma of the lung. In some cases, the presence of mutated oncogenes in tumor cells correlates with disease prognosis.[10,11,42]

Antioncogenes

Carcinogenesis can involve the loss of genes that otherwise preclude tumor cell growth.[23] These suppressor genes (also termed antioncogenes or emerogenes) were first characterized as loci responsible for inherited susceptibility to several childhood tumors, namely, retinoblastoma, neuroblastoma, and Wilms' tumor.

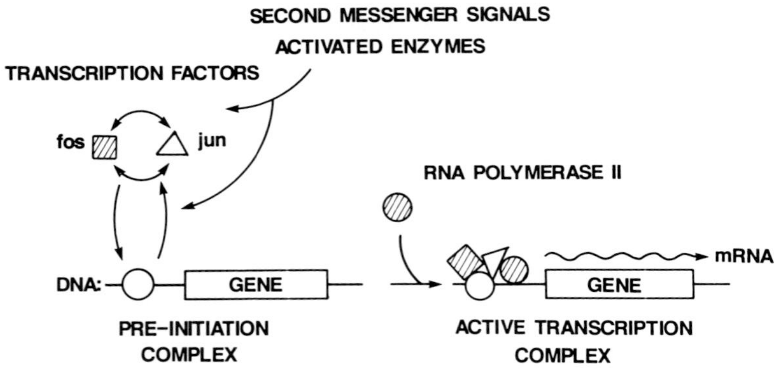

Figure 23-2 Regulation of transcription by oncogenes. Activated enzymes, such as kinases, or second messenger signals direct the binding of transcription factors to DNA, thereby influencing the transcription of genes by RNA polymerase. Transcription factors include the protein products of the *fos* and *jun* proto-oncogenes. Oncogenic activation of *fos* and *jun* by mutation enhances the expression of genes normally expressed in cells stimulated by growth factors.

Retinoblastoma is prototypical of neoplasms associated with loss of an antioncogene arising from neural tissues. Sixty percent of cases are sporadic and the remainder are familial. Familial cases involve the deletion of a gene (RB) normally present on chromosome 13.[13,17] This deletion represents a recessive trait. If later during development a second alteration occurs in the same region of the other chromosome, the cell becomes refractory to normal differentiation signals, continues to divide, and acquires other hallmarks of a malignant neoplasm.

While loss of RB in cells of the fetal or infant retina is probably sufficient to cause retinoblastoma, loss of the gene also confers susceptibility to other tumor types, including osteosarcoma, carcinoma of the breast, and small cell lung carcinoma. However, the risk of developing these other tumors is much lower, suggesting that further changes, in addition to the loss of RB, are required for malignant transformation. Factors that dictate whether the loss of RB will affect cell growth are not understood, but there is no reason to assume that the probability of losing the normal gene copy is particularly high in retinoblasts.

Small cell lung cancer, unlike retinoblastoma, does not appear to have a hereditary component but is associated with heavy cigarette smoking. It may be that carcinogen exposure from tobacco increases mutation rates in the bronchial epithelium, while large genes such as RB may be especially susceptible to mutational inactivation.[18]

It is important to note that the lower penetrance associated with RB loss in cells outside the embryonic retina is more typical of antioncogenes in general. Thus, antioncogenes are likely to play a much larger role in carcinogenesis than might be predicted from the special situations in which cancer susceptibility is clearly inherited. Indeed, as the list of potential antioncogenes increases,[32] loss of gene functions may prove to play a greater role in carcinogenesis than gene activations.

The biochemical functions of the antioncogenes are unknown. RB encodes a nuclear phosphoprotein ($pp110^{RB}$) that binds DNA and may therefore be a transcription factor.[26] Indeed, one suspects that, like oncogenes, the products encoded by antioncogenes will function in signal transduction pathways. However, while oncogenes activate genes involved in cell cycle progression, the antioncogenes are likely to regulate genes required for remodeling postmitotic cells and for terminal differentiation.

Oncogenes of the DNA Tumor Viruses

Several DNA viruses, including adenoviruses, papilloma viruses, simian virus 40, and polyoma virus, carry genes that transform cultured cells and induce tumors in animals.[27] The DNA viral oncogenes are all expressed early after infection, prior to DNA replication, and encode activities necessary for the expression and replication of viral DNA. Since these small viruses depend on the host cell for most of the biochemical functions required for viral DNA replication, it is likely that the viral oncogenes mimic or activate cellular functions required during cell division. This notion is supported by the fact that several proteins encoded by the viral

oncogenes bind tightly to cellular proteins encoded by both oncogenes and antioncogenes.[14,27,45]

For example, the polyoma virus middle tumor (T) antigen binds and activates several tyrosine kinases (src, yes, and fyn), while the simian virus 40 large T antigen and a protein expressed from adenovirus early region 1B each bind (and stabilize) the same cellular proto-oncogene product (termed p53). The adenovirus early region 1A proteins and SV40 large T antigen each bind the protein product of RB, the retinoblastoma susceptibility gene. In short, these viral early region proteins appear to transform cells by interacting with the same types of cellular targets that are mutationally activated in naturally occurring tumors.

DNA viruses induce a variety of neuronal tumors in animals when injected into young animals prior to the development of a functional immune system or when injected into immunologically tolerant sites such as the brain. Brain tumors have been induced in rats, hamsters, mice, and baboons using human type 12 adenovirus. Adenoviruses are known to cause cancerous transformation of a wide variety of mammalian cells. Adenovirus E1A proteins participate in transformation by immortalizing cells, thereby giving them the ability to divide indefinitely in culture. As mentioned above, the RB and E1A proteins bind, and the complex requires a region of E1A necessary for E1A transforming activities.[45] While loss of RB leads to malignant transformation of retinoblasts in vivo, E1A enables E1B and ras oncogenes to transform human retinoblasts in vitro,[12] suggesting that by binding to RB, E1A inactivates RB functions.

The papovaviruses (including SV40, polyoma virus, and papilloma viruses) are a second category of DNA viruses which have been associated with a variety of experimental brain tumors induced in mice, rats, rabbits, and hamsters. These tumors have included a variety of gliomatous tumors as well as meningiomas, fibrosarcomas, and medulloblastomas.

The effects of SV40 large T antigen has been studied in transgenic animals. These animals develop choroid plexus tumors.[31] The tumor formation in this tissue is dependent on the presence of the SV40 enhancer. Southern blot analysis reveals structural rearrangements and amplification of the SV40 sequences in the choroid plexus tumors, further indicating that overexpression of the SV40 large T antigen is necessary for transforming cells within the choroid plexus.

References

1. Balmain A, Ramsden M, Bowden GT, et al. Activation of the mouse cellular Harvey-ras gene in chemically induced benign skin papillomas. Nature 1984; 307:658–660.
2. Barker D, Wright E, Nguyen K, et al. Gene for von Recklinghausen neurofibromatosis is in the pericentromeric region of chromosome 17. Science 1987; 236:1100–1102.
3. Bigner SH, Mark J, Bullard DE, et al. Chromosomal evolution in malignant human gliomas starts with specific and usually numerical deviations. Cancer Genet Cytogenet 1986; 22:121–135.
4. Bigner SH, Mark J, Burger PC, et al. Specific chromosomal abnormalities in malignant human gliomas. Cancer Res 1988; 48:405–411.
5. Bigner SH, Mark J, Mahaley MS, et al. Patterns of the early,

gross chromosomal changes in malignant human gliomas. *Hereditas* 1984; 101:103–113.

6. Birchmeier C, Birbaum D, Waitches G, et al. Characterization of an activated human *ras* gene. *Mol Cell Biol* 1986; 6:3109–3116.

7. Bishop JM. The molecular genetics of cancer. *Science* 1987; 235:305–311.

8. Bohmann D, Bos TJ, Admon A, et al. Human proto-oncogene c-*jun* encodes a DNA binding protein with structural and functional properties of transcription factor AP-1. *Science* 1987; 238:1386–1392.

9. Bos JL, Fearon ER, Hamilton SR, et al. Prevalence of *ras* gene mutations in human colorectal cancers. *Nature* 1987; 327:293–297.

10. Brodeur GM, Hayes FA, Green AA, et al. Consistent N-*myc* copy number in simultaneous or consecutive neuroblastoma samples from sixty individual patients. *Cancer Res* 1987; 47:4248–4253.

11. Brodeur GM, Seeger RC, Schwab M, et al. Amplification of N-*myc* in untreated human neuroblastomas correlates with advanced disease stage. *Science* 1984; 224:1121–1124.

12. Byrd PJ, Grand RJA, Gallimore PH. Differential transformation of primary human embryo retinal cells by adenovirus E1 regions and combinations of E1A + *ras*. *Oncogene* 1988; 2:477–484.

13. Cavenee WK, Murphree AL, Shull MM, et al. Prediction of familial predisposition to retinoblastoma. *N Engl J Med* 1986; 314:1201–1207.

14. DeCaprio JA, Ludlow JW, Figge JU, et al. SV40 large tumor antigen forms a specific complex with the product of the retinoblastoma susceptibility gene. *Cell* 1988; 54:275–283.

15. Dumanski JP, Carlbom E, Collins VP, et al. Deletion mapping of a locus on human chromosome 22 involved in the oncogenesis of meningioma. *Proc Natl Acad Sci USA* 1987; 84:9275–9279.

16. Forrester K, Almoguera C, Han K, et al. Detection of high incidence of K-*ras* oncogenes during human colon tumorigenesis. *Nature* 1986; 327:298–303.

17. Friend SH, Bernards R, Rogelj S, et al. A human DNA segment with properties of the gene that predisposes to retinoblastoma and osteosarcoma. *Nature* 1986; 323:643–646.

18. Harbour JW, Lai SL, Whang-Peng J, et al. Abnormalities in structure and expression of the human retinoblastoma gene in SCLC. *Science* 1988; 241:353–357.

19. Heldin CH, Westermark B. Growth factors: Mechanism of action and relation to oncogenes. *Cell* 1984; 37:9–20.

20. Hinrichs SH, Nerenberg M, Reynolds RK, et al. A transgenic mouse model for human neurofibromatosis. *Science* 1987; 237:1340–1343.

21. James CD, Carlbom E, Dumanski J, et al. Clonal genomic alterations in glioma malignancy stages. *Cancer Res* 1988; 48:5546–5551.

22. James CD, Carlbom E, Nordenskjold M, et al. Mitotic recombination of a locus on chromosome 17 in astrocytomas. *Proc Natl Acad Sci USA* 1989; 86:2858–2862.

23. Klein G. The approaching era of the tumor suppressor genes. *Science* 1987; 238:1539–1545.

24. Kohl NE, Gee CE, Alt FW. Activated expression of the N-*myc* gene in human neuroblastomas and related tumors. *Science* 1984; 226:1335–1337.

25. Land H, Parada LF, Weinberg RA. Cellular oncogenes and multistep carcinogenesis. *Science* 1983; 222:771–778.

26. Lee W-H, Shew JY, Hong FD, et al. The retinoblastoma susceptibility gene encodes a nuclear phosphoprotein associated with DNA binding activity. *Nature* 1987; 329:642–645.

27. Levine AJ. Oncogenes of DNA tumor viruses. *Cancer Res* 1988; 48:493–496.

28. Lieberman T, Nusbaum HR, Razon N, et al. Amplification, enhanced expression and possible rearrangement of EGF receptor gene in primary human brain tumours of glial origin. *Nature* 1985; 313:144–147.

29. Mapstone TB. Oncogene activity in human CNS tumors. Presented at the 50th Annual Meeting of the American Academy of Neurological Surgery, Cincinnati, Ohio, September 17, 1988.

30. Nowell PC. Molecular events in tumor development. *N Engl J Med* 1988; 319:575–577.

31. Palmiter RD, Chen HY, Messing A, et al. SV40 enhancer and large-T antigen are instrumental in development of choroid plexus tumours in transgenic mice. *Nature* 1985; 316:457–460.

32. Ponder B. Cancer: gene losses in human tumours. *Nature* 1988; 335:400–402.

33. Rauscher FJ III, Cohen D, Curran T, et al. *fos*-associated protein p39 is the product of the *jun* proto-oncogene. *Science* 1988; 240:1010–1016.

34. Rey JA, Bello MJ, de Campos JM, et al. Chromosomal patterns in human astrocytomas. *Cancer Genet Cytogenet* 1987; 29:202–221.

35. Rey JA, Bello MJ, de Campos JM, et al. Chromosomal abnormalities in human brain tumors: an analysis of 52 cases. *Clin Genet* 1985; 27:330–331 (abstr).

36. Ruley HE. Analysis of malignant phenotypes by oncogene complementation. *Adv Viral Oncol* 1987; 6:1–20.

37. Schecter AL, Stern DF, Vaidyanathan L, et al. The *neu* oncogene: an *erb*-B-related gene encoding a 185,000-Mr tumour antigen. *Nature* 1984; 312:513–516.

38. Schmidek HH. The molecular genetics of nervous system tumors. *J Neurosurg* 1987; 67:1–16.

39. Seizinger BR, Martuza RL, Gusella JF. Loss of genes on chromosome 22 in tumorigenesis of human acoustic neuroma. *Nature* 1986; 322:644–647.

40. Seizinger BR, Rouleau GA, Ozelius LJ, et al. Genetic linkage of von Recklinghausen neurofibromatosis to the nerve growth factor receptor gene. *Cell* 1987; 49:589–594.

41. Sinn E, Muller W, Pattengale P, et al. Coexpression of MMTV/v-Ha-*ras* and MMTV/c-*myc* genes in transgenic mice: synergistic action of oncogenes *in vivo*. *Cell* 1987; 49:465–475.

42. Slamon DJ, Clark GM, Wong SG, et al. Human breast cancer: correlation of relapse and survival with amplification of the HER-2/*neu* oncogene. *Science* 1987; 235:177–182.

43. Varmus HE. The molecular genetics of cellular oncogenes. *Annu Rev Genet* 1984; 18:553–612.

44. Weinberg RA. The action of oncogenes in the cytoplasm and nucleus. *Science* 1985; 230:770–776.

45. Whyte P, Buchkovich KJ, Horowitz JM, et al. Association between an oncogene and an anti-oncogene: the adenovirus E1A proteins bind to the retinoblastoma gene product. *Nature* 1988; 334:124–129.

46. Yamada K, Kondo T, Yoshioka M, et al. Cytogenetic studies in twenty human brain tumors: association of no. 22 chromosome abnormalities with tumors of the brain. *Cancer Genet Cytogenet* 1980; 2:293–307.

47. Zang KD. Cytological and cytogenetical studies on human meningioma. *Cancer Genet Cytogenet* 1982; 6:249–274.

24

Risk Factors in the Development of Glioblastoma and Other Brain Tumors

Fred H. Hochberg
Alberto A. Gabbai

The science of epidemiology provides the clinician and investigator with insights into the pathogenesis of brain tumors. Using epidemiologic techniques to study these malignancies, the clinician delineates the population at risk, factors influencing tumor development, and determinants of prognosis. Despite recent advances in our understanding of risk factors for the development of these tumors, most data are gleaned from reports of clustered glioma cases, anecdotes suggesting trauma and occupational exposure as determinants of glioma development, and the studies of glioma induction in animals. These observations await evaluation as part of formalized epidemiologic studies.

MacMahon and Pugh[28] have noted three key steps in the formation of cancer risk or causation hypotheses, as follows:

1. New hypotheses are commonly formed by relating observations from several different fields. Future neuro-oncologic epidemiologists will draw heavily upon recent developments in our understanding of (1) the interface between teratogenesis and carcinogenesis (as in pineal area tumor development, and the dysraphic states); (2) the interrelationship between production of growth factors (of vascular, platelet, or epidermal origin) and oncogene expression; (3) the presence of steroid and peptide receptors within the normal brain and brain tumors; and (4) immune regulation of viral proliferation, tumor cell growth, and vascular neogenesis.
2. Observations of the change in frequency of a disease over time have been very productive of hypotheses. The introduction of noninvasive scanning techniques will allow the screening of large "at risk" populations, providing a better estimate of true glioma incidence. The appearance of

lymphoma of the brain in the sex-linked immunodeficiency syndrome (Duncan's syndrome) provides glimpses into the relationship between nervous system lymphomas and the acquired immunodeficiency syndrome (AIDS), renal transplantation, and Epstein-Barr (EB) viral infections. Similarly related may be the increasing frequency of pineal area tumors in Japan and Taiwan, and clustered infections with the human T-cell leukemia virus.
3. An isolated or unusual case should receive particular attention in the formation of hypotheses. Special attention is drawn to the occurrence of glioma or glioblastoma as a second tumor and to their appearance in association with pregnancy, trauma, progressive multifocal leukoencephalopathy, and AIDS.

In the present chapter, we do not emphasize basic principles in epidemiologic methodology. Instead, we provide an approach to the appropriate literature by which the investigator may plan studies for testing causal hypotheses.

Many of the risk factors that are cited herein have been examined during a recently completed case-control study at our institution involving patients with glioblastoma and controls. Controls consisted of nonrelated best friends of the same sex and within 5 years of the patient's age who lived within 100 mi. A 40-page questionnaire was provided to patients with biopsy-proven glioblastoma and to their controls. Telephone follow-up was used to confirm key information from the self-administered questionnaire. Sixty-seven percent ($N = 160$) of the 237 eligible cases were evaluable, as were 120 matching controls. Cases were similar to controls in educational level, religion, and socioeconomic status (of both the respondent and their parents). We estimated the incidence rate of glioblastoma among persons who were exposed to a specified risk indicator relative to the rate among controls. The analyses from this case-control study that are mentioned below are for unmatched populations (160 glioblastoma patients and 120 controls), there being no difference when similar analyses were done for matched pairs. Subjects were stratified according to potential confounders, and standardized rate ratios (RRs) were estimated by the Mantel-Haenzel procedure.

Definition of Illness (the Sources of Bias)

Population-based studies of intracranial malignancies evaluate the occurrence of "brain tumor" diagnoses on death certificates, union records, or hospital records. Specific tumor histologies (such as oligodendroglioma or glioblastoma) are often not indicated and are rarely, if ever, validated by independent examination of biopsy or autopsy material. Often little effort is taken to establish strict histologic bases for case inclusion. Not uncommonly, the rubric "cancer, brain and other nervous system" is used to report incidence for the population of the United States or a single state such as Connecticut. This retrospective approach accumulates data from death certificates and thus avoids the expensive and laborious procedure of verification of clinical diagnosis and categorization by histology. However, death certificate data are open to sources of error from underreporting as well as imprecision stemming from the dependence on unconfirmed "clinical diagnoses" which may include other, non-neoplastic intracranial lesions, or on "substantiation" by noninvasive computed tomography (CT) or magnetic resonance (MR) scanning techniques rather than histologic confirmation (an approach which carries at least a 10 percent risk of false positive and false negative diagnoses).

In addition, the lack of histologic definition removes the chance of delineating clusters of subcategories of glioblastoma (e.g., glioblastoma with giant cell features). These subcategories are especially important in view of experience with tumor development in other organs (i.e., angiosarcoma of the liver and vinyl chloride exposure, Burkitt's lymphoma and EB viral infection).

As a result of this imprecision, the flaws which exist in the literature include: (1) The lumping of pediatric and adult brain tumors, which produce the common "bimodal" (incidence peaks in early teens and in the sixth decade) age distribution for brain tumors. (2) Uncertainties regarding the true frequencies of selected tumors (e.g., glioblastoma, acoustic neurinoma). With these data, it is impossible to evaluate reports of tumor clusters within certain industries or families. (3) Emphasis on tumor distribution from clinical series to the exclusion of autopsy studies. This emphasis had created underestimates for meningioma and pituitary tumors. For example, Nakasu et al. found 23 patients with "incidental" meningiomas at autopsy in a 32-year period.[33] (4) Paucity of cross-cultural studies with a histologic base. Such studies have been of greater value for other tumors such as those of the gastrointestinal tract and uterus. The recently published pathologic definitions of the World Health Organization will permit better cross-cultural prevalence studies.

The Individual Case

Observation of glial tumors with unique histologic features or among defined populations is the major stimulus for subsequent formal epidemiologic studies. Such observations involve cases clustered among specific populations (e.g., families, workers, veterans), within a certain time interval, or in a certain location. Major advances in our understanding of glioma have stemmed from anecdotal reports of patients with afflicted family members, with a second tumor, with a unique occupation, or with a hereditary abnormality. These neuroepidemiologic advances parallel those in other areas of cancer epidemiology where investigation of a "chance" relationship has led to major advances.

The Relative Frequency of Malignant Glial Tumors

The intracranial malignant glial tumors (glioblastoma, anaplastic astrocytoma, malignant oligodendroglioma, malig-

nant ependymoma) represent between 20 and 30 percent of all intracranial neoplasms and approximately half of all intracranial tumors of glial origin. Disparities in these figures reflect the populations studied and the sources of data. Thus, pediatric clinical series tend to overrepresent posterior fossa or benign tumors,[45] whereas adult series contain more malignant, supratentorial tumors. In autopsy-based series there are overrepresented tumors of metastatic, pituitary, and meningeal origin, reflecting the lack of symptoms associated with some of these lesions during life.

Most authors report frequencies of glioma occurrence that are not significantly different between geographic areas. In published reports from the United States, malignant gliomas account for one quarter of brain growths. Unpublished data from the Japanese Brain Tumor Study Group, European Brain Tumor Study Group, and U.S. Brain Tumor Study Group confirm this figure. Similar data are available from the People's Republic of China and the Republic of China.

Other primary and secondary brain tumors do show geographic clustering. Thus, Sano reported that pineal area tumors account for 8.8 percent of brain tumors among Japanese.[42] This figure is close to that (7.8 percent) recently noted by Mori and Kurisaka in children,[31] but greater than that (2.7 percent) in adults. These rates are not greater than those seen in Australia or Taiwan but are in contrast to the figure of 1 to 2 percent reported from major series elsewhere. The Japanese clustering of pineal tumors is localized to Kyushu.

Incidence data for malignant glial tumors are difficult to determine. Various reports cite the incidence of "brain tumor" as being between 40 and 100 cases per million population. The incidence rate for malignant glial tumors is between 10 and 50 cases per million population, assuming that between one quarter and one half of all brain tumors are of malignant glial origin. These figures compare to the peak figure of 62 per million derived for the population of 60 to 64 years from the Mayo Clinic and Connecticut registries. From the same studies, a peak incidence of 5.5 glioblastoma cases per million was derived for the childhood population at 7 years of age.

Several authors have noted an increase over time in the death rates from malignant neoplasms of the brain and nervous system. Male death rates increased from approximately 50 per million to 75 per million between 1967 and 1974. Certain tumors, such as medulloblastoma, may be becoming increasingly common. Similar sequential increases have been seen for all decades between 1930 and 1960 for men and women of white and nonwhite races, with whites more frequently affected than blacks in one retrospective study. In at least one study the "exposure (or susceptibility) to . . . aetiological factors appears to be higher in males and whites than in females and nonwhites."[55] Bunin noted an increasing occurrence of glioma and medulloblastoma in blacks by time trend analysis.[7] The increased black occurrence of gliomas was especially true for ages 0 to 4 and 10 to 14 years. For medulloblastoma, the male/female ratio differed between whites (1.7) and blacks (1.0). Time and space clusters of glioblastoma have been described (R. A. Morantz, personal communication). These increases are thought to reflect increasingly sophisticated diagnostic techniques and improved ascertainment of occurrence.

The Relationship between Glioblastoma and Age

Although brain tumors are commonly said to have a bimodal age distribution with peaks at 8 and 70 years, this reflects the lumping of tumors of varying histologies. Age-specific data for malignant ependymoma and malignant oligodendroglioma are not available. The median age for glioblastoma occurrence is 50 years, with three quarters of patients being between 40 and 60 years old. Reports exist of isolated cases in neonates and octogenarians. Various authors have noted incidence rates that increase with age; others have indicated that the peak occurrence of malignant brain tumors is from 55 to 64 years.

In general, childhood brain tumors tend toward benign histologies and posterior fossa locations. Before age 20, the most common tumors are low-grade astrocytomas or primitive, differentiated neuroectodermal tumors (PNET). These occur with peak incidence at 3 to 7 and 5 to 15 years, respectively. Childhood midline cerebellar medulloblastomas have a peak occurrence between 8 and 10 years.

Age is a key determinant of tumor biology. Thus, in patients less than 50 years old, survival with glioblastoma is twice that of the more elderly patients having this tumor.

Zülch indicates that at all ages glioblastoma is more common among males than females.[59] At the age of maximal occurrence (55 to 64) there are 18.3 male cases per 100,000 versus 9.8 female cases. A male preponderance exists for all intracranial tumors except meningioma and neurofibroma, where the male/female ratio approaches 6:7 and 1:2, respectively.

Intracranial tumors in either sex seem to be on the rise. Gold[17] (quoting the work of Cutler and Young[11]) refers to male preponderance of all brain tumors since 1937 but notes a diminished frequency among white female children. Kurland et al. noted an increased female risk of glioma since 1950 without an increased male risk or an increase in meningioma occurrence.[25] Annegers et al.[1] and Garfinkel and Sarokhan[15] noted an increasing incidence of "brain cancer" among white and nonwhite females since 1950 (in 1950 the incidence in white females was 2.3 per 100,000, and in nonwhite females was 1.6 per 100,000; in 1976, comparable figures were 3.5 and 2.0, respectively) but also noted similar increases among white and nonwhite males at two time intervals (1950 and 1978).

Recently it has been shown that patients with Klinefelter's syndrome are at high risk for developing cerebral germinoma. No positive association between Klinefelter's syndrome and other primary brain tumors has been found.

Spiers hypothesized hormonal dependence for tumor development.[49] Although these developmental controls remain unknown, they undoubtedly affect the appearance of glioblastoma during pregnancy. The availability of assays for hormone receptors on primary brain tumors will allow for hormonal specification of these tumors.

Familial Glioma

Studies of the occurrence of glioma among families are of three types: (1) those reporting glioma or glioblastoma development as part of a recognized inherited neuroectodermal syndrome, (2) those reporting the occurrence of glioma and glioblastoma among a series of intracranial and extracranial tumors within certain families in which no neuroectodermal syndrome exists, and (3) those presenting data on familial glioma as a consequence of a specific prospective or retrospective investigation. Identification of a putative glioblastoma gene on the short arm of chromosome 17 will aid these studies.

Glioma within Neuroectodermal Syndromes

Neuroectodermal syndromes, especially von Recklinghausen's neurofibromatosis (NF), have been associated with the development of intracranial glial malignancies. For each syndrome, characteristic systemic and intracranial lesions occur coincident with gliomas. The development of central NF-associated brain tumors has been linked to loss of an allele from chromosome 22.

NF and tuberous sclerosis are inherited as autosomal dominant disorders with incomplete penetrance. The classic intracranial tumors which occur in 3 to 5 percent of NF patients include single and multiple meningiomas and neurinomas of cranial nerves (acoustic, trigeminal, and glossopharyngeal). Less common are other intracranial lesions including astrocytoma of the optic nerve which, in youth, may be unique to NF. The frequency of glial tumors is uncertain.

Canale et al. reviewed NF cases and found only three with intracranial nonmalignant astrocytomas.[8] David et al. found three hemispheric and two cerebellar gliomas among 17 cases of central nervous system NF.[12] Van der Weil noted 16 examples of optic glioma in cases of neurofibromatosis reported between 1920 and 1954 in addition to 12 examples of spinal glioma.[54] More striking are his references to 32 previously reported NF cases with intracranial glioma.[54] The malignant changes may include pleomorphism, giant cells, vascular proliferation, and sarcomatous changes, all occurring in fewer than 15 percent of NF tumors and then in a well-localized fashion.

Similarly scanty are data concerning the incidence of NF among large populations of glioma patients. Van der Weil, reviewing an extended glioma family, reported cafe au lait spots in 3 of 38 with glioblastoma multiforme and 5 of 26 with glioma.[54] These cafe au lait marks were present in 767 of 3557 family members versus 7 percent of controls. In our series of 160 brain tumor cases and 120 controls, 0 cases and 3 controls reported having von Recklinghausen's NF. The expected odds ratio (EOR) was 0, and the Taylor series 95 percent upper confidence interval was 1.362.

Tuberous sclerosis is characterized by adenoma sebaceum of the face; renal hamartoma; and tumors of heart, lens, and skin. Brain lesions include both periventricular gliotic growths containing bizarre enlarged glial cells and multiple white matter collections of bizarre enlarged glia and misplaced neuronal cells. These abnormalities may be found among patients without other stigmata of tuberous sclerosis. Thus, forme fruste examples of both diseases may be easily missed in large surveys of neuroectodermal syndromes. Although patients with tuberous sclerosis may harbor well-differentiated glial tumors, rare are the reports of glioblastoma. In our case-control study, no cases and two controls reported having tuberous sclerosis (EOR = 0; 95 percent upper limits = 2.770).

The von Hippel-Lindau syndrome, which is also transmitted as an autosomal dominant trait, is characterized by hemangioblastomas of the retina and cerebellum. Classically, the cerebellar lesion consists of a slowly growing hemangioblastoma with a large cystic component, but there is one example in the literature of a patient with both the von Hippel-Lindau syndrome and an intraventricular neuroblastoma. Reported also are patients with a glioma and an aneurysm of the intracranial circulation and those with a malignant glioma and an intracranial arteriovenous malformation.

Cerebellar hemangioblastoma may also be familial as a forme fruste of von Hippel-Lindau disease. Such familial cases are younger than those with nonfamilial cerebellar hemangioblastoma.

Other Familial Glial Tumors

Considerable interest has been generated in the patterns of inheritance of glial tumors by (1) reports of cancer families harboring an increased risk of the development of cancer of the breast, gastrointestinal tract, and endocrine system, (2) case reports defining glial tumor occurrences in multiple members of a family, and (3) investigations indicating an increased risk of brain and hematologic tumors in family members of known brain tumor patients. Many of these observations have been criticized on methodologic grounds. These reports are often striking and suggest a need for carefully controlled population studies.

There have been many reports of glial tumors in at least two members of a family. Schoenberg et al. cited 52 reports of this occurrence.[44] The majority describe glioblastoma in siblings. Motz et al. emphasized cases of brain tumors in siblings and included five identical twins and parents.[32] Most reports of familial glioma exclude known neuroectodermal disorders, and pathologic examination of these familial gliomas reveals little to suggest that they represent forme fruste NF cases or have unique and characteristic histologic features.

The occurrence of gliomas afflicting more than three members of a single family are unusually interesting and suggest the need for careful chromosome marker evaluations. Younger individuals in the succeeding generations may harbor tumors which appear different from that of the index case. Glioma families may be at increased risk of nonglial brain tumors including meningioma, sarcoma, medulloblastoma, pineal tumor, and ependymoma. Exploration of blood group tumor relationships and HLA markers have been unproductive until now.

Retinoblastoma, a neural neoplasm that is often familial and is sometimes transmitted as an autosomal dominant trait, may also be associated with pinealoma. This association is frequently referred to as trilateral retinoblastoma (affecting both eyes and the pineal). In certain lower animals, the pineal functions as a photoreceptor organ, resembles the retina histologically, and is described as the "third eye." Mutation or loss of the retinoblastoma gene on chromosome 13q14 is related to tumor development.

Bannayan syndrome (macrocephaly, short stature, and mesodermal fatty or vascular hamartomas), when familial, is associated with an increased risk of meningioma. Turcot's syndrome (colonic polyposis) may be associated with malignant astrocytoma. Variants include cases with osteochondrodysplasia or skeletal abnormalities. These cases may merge with those having the cartilage dysplasia and anaplastic astrocytoma of Ollier's disease.

Population-Based Studies

Population-based studies of familial glioma have methodologic deficiencies. Various studies have suggested more frequent familial brain tumors than were noted in controls. However, two studies of Harvald and Hauge noted no greater risk among families with a member with glioblastoma.[19,20]

Van der Weil confirmed 7 gliomas among 1290 relatives of 100 glioma patients.[54] Five additional gliomas were assumed but not confirmed. There were no gliomas among 532 dead relatives of controls. Additionally, there were more frequent occurrences of "dysraphic" states among tumor families versus controls. Cafe au lait spots were present in 27.8 percent of first- and second-degree relatives and in 21.6 percent of all relatives versus between 5.3 percent and 7.0 percent in a variety of control groups.

Although no other populations have been as extensively examined as these, Choi et al., using a case-control approach, found brain tumor attack rates of 57 per 100,000 for family members of brain tumor patients versus 12.4 per 100,000 for family members of controls.[9] In our series, the occurrence of glioblastoma was unrelated to a familial history of CNS malignancies. Seven patients and 10 controls reported at least one parent or sibling with such conditions, a relative risk adjusted for family size of 0.5 (0.2 to 1.4). However, no distinction could be made between primary and metastatic tumors. A variety of factors have been discussed in association with brain tumor inheritance. Each remains interesting but all untested.

Glioma in Children

Gliomas account for 40 percent of childhood intracranial tumors. Astrocytoma accounts for two thirds of these, and glioblastoma for 2 to 10 percent. Cerebellar locations predominate. The peak incidence rate occurs at age 3 (0.65 per 100,000) for glioblastoma. At least one author has noted a sharp drop in incidence for these tumors in girls after the age of 10 versus "a slow fall of incidence for boys."[16] Childhood tumors, except neonatal teratocarcinoma and primitive neuroectodermal malignancies (spongioblastoma, gliosarcoma), have a better prognosis than their adult counterparts.

Available data concerning risk factors in the pathogenesis of childhood brain tumors have been reviewed by Gold.[17] From her data, as well as those from the studies of Choi et al.,[9] several risk factors have been suggested: (1) maternal history of abortion; (2) increased maternal age at index childbirth; (3) tendency to be a first birth (odds ratio [OR] = 1.7); (4) birth weight above 9 lb (OR = 2.6); (5) birth order and weight; (6) unusual delivery history; and (7) maternal diabetes (inverse relationship).

Although extremely rare (Cushing reported one congenital brain tumor among 200 intracranial tumors, and Wollstein and Bartlett[58] noted only nine examples in a pediatric autopsy series of 4562), brain tumors occurring before 1 year of life have been the subject of at least 10 reports of which 3 are comprehensive. Most common among these growths are ependymoma (23 percent) in a periventricular or midline location, as well as hemangioendothelioma, glioblastoma, and sarcoma.

Multiple Tumor Syndromes

Often multiple tumors occur in close temporal or spatial relationship. (We and others have seen the initial resection of a meningioma reveal a glioblastoma in close proximity.) Equally likely, "second" tumor development may reflect intervening therapy. Thus, the second operation for recurrent postirradiation glioblastoma frequently reveals sarcomatous features in the overlying pia arachnoid, or dura. This appearance is distinct from the "multifocal" presentation of gliomas, which include (1) histologically identical glioma or glioblastoma as separate deposits, often in proximity to the ventricles; (2) widespread diffusely abnormal glia in "gliomatosis cerebri"; and (3) closely approximated but histologically separable glial tumors containing features of oligodendroglioma, gemistocytic astrocytoma, and glioblastoma.

The appearance of multifocal or noncontiguous, well-differentiated glial tumors suggests that an uncontrolled normal glial response may merge into malignancy. These multifocal tumors bear striking similarity to those produced in animals in response to an oncogenic viral infection or chemical carcinogen. Although not uniformly present, they may contain giant cells, inclusion bodies, multiple nuclei, or sarcomatous vascular changes. The last may, by rapid growth, develop into a true glioma-sarcoma. This appearance is reminiscent of animal brain tumors produced by RNA tumor viruses (avian, murine, and simian sarcoma viruses) and the DNA papova viruses (bovine papilloma, SA-7, human adeno type 12, and SV-40 viruses). Similar lesions have also been produced in the albino mouse using 20-methyl cholanthrene. In these tumors and in their sporadic human analogue one is left with the impression of sarcoma induction by growth factors produced by glioma cells.

The role of "platelet"-derived growth factor (PDGF) and "epidermal" growth factor (EGF) as modulated by oncogenes (sis, Ros-1, KIT, N-myc, gli) is explored elsewhere. Glioma-specific PDGF- and EFG-receptor mutations and amplifications have been well described and may account for glial tumor cell heterogeneity, gliosarcoma, and mixed astrocytic malignancies.

In addition to multiple brain tumors occurring in individual patients, a variety of systemic malignancies have been reported in brain tumor patients. Miller[30] and Li et al.[26] reported relationships between astrocytoma-glioblastoma and sarcoma (usually osteogenic sarcoma). Hawkins et al. reported an increase in second primary tumors in the brain in patients with hereditary retinoblastoma (see above) or following radiation or chemotherapy of primary tumors not involving the brain.[21] Fontana et al. reported three adolescents whose focal glioma followed years after brain irradiation and intrathecal methotrexate therapy for childhood leukemia.[14] Ingram et al. reported one child whose astrocytoma followed therapy of a non-Hodgkin's lymphoma.[22] We have seen five instances of second tumor in glioblastoma patients including (1) adenocarcinoma of the colon in a 40-year-old man who developed glioblastoma 15 years later; (2) ovarian cancer followed 25 years later by glioblastoma at age 60; (3) carcinoma of the cervix 4 years after nitrosourea chemotherapy for a presumed spinal cord astrocytoma; (4) carcinoma in situ of the cervix in a 25-year-old woman with a grade III astrocytoma diagnosed 4 years before; and (5) fibrosarcoma of the middle fossa eroding into the middle ear 5 years after the irradiation and cure of a glioblastoma.

Clinical Precursors of Malignant Glioma

The Question of Malignant Dedifferentiation

The origin of malignant glioma (glioblastoma) is unknown. A potential precursor cell has been hypothesized, but the role of this cell in tumor development is speculative. Four hypotheses explain glioblastoma development: (1) tumors arise from dormant germ cells; (2) late-life glial inflammation leads to uncontrolled proliferation and neoplasia; (3) hamartomas dedifferentiate into malignant tumors; and (4) the localized expression of a specific growth factor results from, or is responsible for, the activation of a tumor-promoting oncogene. The last appears to be the case for simian sarcoma virus oncogene (V-sis) which modulates the expression of, and in turn may be modulated by, the gene encoding for PDGF as well as for the relation between erbB oncogene and EGF. Such growth factors have been demonstrated in cells of glioma origin and amplification or modulation of their receptors may correlate with neoplastic growth.

As regards glioblastoma, Rubinstein et al. note "most examples of glioblastoma are probably derived from anaplasia from a preexisting astrocytoma of relatively restricted size. . . . their characteristic appearance can be attributed to the rapid progression of anaplastic changes spreading throughout the entire neoplastic area."[40] This concept of dedifferentiation of a well-defined astrocytoma into its more malignant form is based on the work of Kernohan et al.[24] In Kernohan's continuum, benign astrocytoma (grades I and II) might progress to a malignant form (grades III and IV).

Surprisingly, little effort has gone into the confirmation of these concepts. Rubinstein et al., in reviewing 129 glioblastomas, found that 28 "were established as glioblastoma supervening upon a diffuse astrocytoma.''[40] Few other studies exist in the literature. Neuro-oncologic clinicians are well aware of patients whose sequential tumor biopsies exhibit greater malignancy over time. Three possible explanations exist for this antecedent history:

1. A preexistent ''benign'' cause of seizures (hamartoma, glial scar, low-grade glioma) undergoes malignant dedifferentiation with time. Large surgical series of intractable epileptics include at least 30 percent of patients whose seizures are due to low-grade tumors. Brown et al. reported 6 brain tumors in their 25 operated patients[5] and Penfield and Flanigin noted 5 of 68 patients.[36] In the series of Bailey et al. of 25 seizure patients, only 1 had a brain tumor.[3] Additional underlying processes include congenital hamartoma, ''sclerosis,'' or scar formation. Tumor induction from these lesions may be influenced by pregnancy, puberty, and medications, but the precise contribution of such has not been studied.

2. Antiseizure medications may be oncogenic. Barbiturate exposure in the prenatal or early childhood years is associated with an increased risk of brain tumors. Clemmensen and Hjalgrim-Jensen, in a retrospective study of 8078 epileptics treated with phenobarbital or phenobarbital and phenytoin/primidone, found an increased risk of ''brain tumors'' in both sexes below 9 years of age (27 brain tumors were found among boys, in whom 2.13 were expected, and 18 were found among girls, in whom 1.74 were expected).[10] Similar figures for boys 10 to 14 years old were 8/1.32, and for girls of the same age were 5/1.10. In our case-control study, eight of the patients who had received medical treatment for seizures at least 3 years before diagnosis had been treated with both diphenylhydantoin and diazepam, two with phenobarbital alone, and one with diphenylhydantoin alone. Lipson and Bale reported the development of an ependymoblastoma in a 28-month-old whose mother, during pregnancy, had received diphenylhydantoin and methylphenobarbitone.[27]

3. Seizures and gliomas may have a common cause. This cause (possibly neuroectodermal dysplasia, congenital malformation, or a hormonal-nerve growth factor) might produce either coincident seizures and tumors or seizures antedating glioblastomas.

Symptoms may initially be associated with normality or with low absorption areas on CT scans. Within months, repeat CT or MR scans may reveal enhancing masses heralding the histologic diagnosis of malignant glioma. We have seen 20 patients evolve from ''unremarkable'' to an enhancing mass on CT within 4 months of the initial evaluation. This pattern of progression may characterize the emergence of glioblastoma in patients with (1) chronic seizure activity, (2) chronic psychiatric illness, (3) a previously defined low-grade astrocytoma, or (4) a recurrent demyelinating or inflammatory disorder of the nervous system such as multiple sclerosis (MS).

Chronic Seizure Activity

Eighty percent of glioblastoma patients (especially those with temporal lobe tumors) have electroencephalographic slowing that characterizes their tumor. Three quarters of these patients exhibit seizure activity. Surprisingly, these seizures may antedate glioblastoma by 5 years in 30 percent of children and adults. The long duration of seizure symptoms is inconsistent with the growth and doubling time of de novo glioblastoma and implies malignant dedifferentiation of a preexistent benign tumor.

During the last 8 years, 38 of our 650 patients with glioblastoma had seizure activity antedating the tumor by 5 years. Eighteen had seizures for 10 years. The majority of these (75 percent) were of temporal lobe origin. Surgical extirpation of the tumor improved seizure control for 14 of the 36 patients. A similar experience, as seen in 6 of 150 seizure patients and as noted by Spencer and Spencer,[48] has been extended by more frequently obtained CT scans. In our case-control study, 12 cases and no controls had received medical treatment for seizures for at least 3 years prior to diagnosis.

Chronic Psychiatric Illness

We have evaluated 13 patients whose psychiatric illness antedated the development of a glioblastoma by 5 years or more. These patients were without seizure activity until late in the clinical course. Most commonly patients with affective (manic-depressive or unipolar depressive) or psychotic (schizophreniform psychosis) disorders have required hospitalization or chronic medical psychiatric care. In hindsight, many had features suggestive of temporal lobe disorders, but the clinical illnesses did not allow the observer to predict a malignancy. Seizures, usually of temporal lobe appearance, were a late manifestation.

In our case-control study, a number of questions related to psychiatric illness. One item asked, ''Have you been under 'psychologic stress' for most of your life?'' More cases responded affirmatively to this question than controls (EOR = 2.51; 1.4244 to 4.4719). Cases reported a slightly higher occurrence of psychosis than did controls, although this increase was not statistically significant (EOR = 1.06; 0.5559 to 2.0304). With this exception, there was no difference between cases and controls who had ''sought professional help for depression . . . anxiety . . . sleep problems,'' or had a history of treatment for these symptoms.

Dedifferentiation of the Low-Grade Astrocytoma

The modern terms glioblastoma multiforme and anaplastic astrocytoma imply neoplastic tumor formation from ''benign'' astrocytoma. Foci of anaplastic change are common within astrocytomas, and Rubinstein et al. note that ''if the cerebral group (of nonmalignant glioma) alone is assessed, the incidence of some degree of anaplasia amounts to nearly 80 percent.''[40] In a retrospective study, these authors noted some degree of anaplasia in 233 of 243 intracranial gliomas. These figures complement Scherer's[43] finding of anaplastic change in 120 of 125 gliomas. Despite this, he estimated that only 10 percent of astrocytomas become malignant, a figure similar to that of Zülch[59] (7 malignant gliomas among 55 astrocytomas). The discrepancy between data reflects both the size of the specimens examined as well as the major histologic cell type of the glioma.

The appearance of anaplastic changes is best seen over many years. We have seen 11 patients with biopsy-proven glioblastoma, years after operation for grade II astrocytoma. Seven of these exhibited malignant features at least 3 years after their initial operation. One woman had a malignant recurrence of her cerebellar astrocytoma 35 years after the initial diagnosis. Reported cases with malignant recurrence include the progression to malignancy after intervals of 5 years, 8 to $13\frac{1}{2}$ years, and 20 years.

Malignant degeneration is seen in oligodendroglioma. The benign tumor that recurs in this way may develop features suggestive of evolution into a glial fibrillary (glioblastoma) or rosette-forming (medulloblastoma) neoplasm. Rubinstein et al. reported a posterior fossa astrocytoma which presented upon recurrence with features of medulloblastoma and malignant astrocytoma.[41] Rarely, malignant recurrence of an ependymoma develops features of an anaplastic glioma.

The appearance of anaplasia is influenced by therapeutic intervention. Tooth in 1912 noted that "surgical interference, exploration or manipulation . . . is liable to awaken into greater activity a tendency to exuberance. . . ."[53] Similarly confounding are the effects of radiation, chemotherapy, and advancing age, each of which may be associated with malignant histologic changes. Radiation may induce large bizarre forms of tumor cells as well as necrosis and changes in vessel walls.

Preexisting Demyelinating or Inflammatory Lesions and Malignant Glioma

The brain makes a well-defined and limited response to insult. Cerebral trauma incites proliferation and migration of "reactive" glial cells from within the brain parenchyma while attracting macrophages. Aside from head trauma, three other "insults" [i.e., MS, amyotrophic lateral sclerosis (ALS), and progressive multifocal leukoencephalopathy (PML)] have been associated with glioblastoma development. These occurrences are intriguing by virtue of (1) the temporal and spatial linkages between the "benign" inflammatory disorder and tumor development, (2) the implied relationship between putative viral-induced immunopathology (MS, ALS, PML) and tumor development, and (3) the implications of dedifferentiation of reactive glia in the setting of local tumor-promoting factors.

Multiple Sclerosis

At least 20 separate reports have described the coexistence of MS and glioma. Most often afflicted are women, usually about 50 years of age. Clinical evidence of demyelination precedes glioma in most patients, while in the remainder pathologic examination confirms the existence of chronic foci of demyelination populated by reactive glia and macrophages. With the exception of the late age of clinical onset and seeming predominance of subcortical white matter lesions rather than infratentorial lesions, there is little that distinguishes the patient with both demyelination and glioma from the more common nontumorous MS patients seen by neurologists. In five pathologically confirmed cases (four reported and one examined by us), plaques of myelin loss with macrophages and reactive glia merge with anaplastic glia at the border of the lesions. The plaques of demyelination are in contiguity with the anaplastic glioma. In four additional MS-glioma cases, the multicentric gliomas suggested a multifocal relationship to demyelinating plaques.

Amyotrophic Lateral Sclerosis

In our experience, two patients with motor system disease developed unifocal glioblastoma after symptomatic ALS of 3.4 years' duration.

Progressive Multifocal Leukoencephalopathy

PML is a rare cause of multifocal inflammation of white matter in patients with systemic neoplasia (chronic lymphocytic leukemia, Hodgkin's disease, lymphosarcoma), with chronic infections (tuberculosis, sarcoid), or following immunosuppresive medication. The disease is characterized by bizarre and often malignant-appearing giant astrocytic cells with heteroploid nuclei. The causative papovavirus is a DNA tumor virus.

Not surprisingly, other members of the papovavirus group (including polyoma SV-40 virus and the PML-associated strains of JC and BK viruses) have been used to induce meningeal and intracranial tumors (sarcoma, gliosarcoma, ependymoma, choroid plexus papilloma, glioblastoma, and unclassified neuroectodermal tumors) in hamster, rat, rabbit, calf, and primates. Tumor induction has followed viral inoculation by intracerebral, transplacental, and intravenous routes.

Patients have shared PML and glioblastoma. Despite these cases and two patients whose neurologic tumors developed after laboratory exposure to these agents, neuroepidemiologists have been unable to identify the spontaneous human equivalents of animal brain tumors of viral origin, nor have they found viral materials in human brain tumors. The only exceptions are the EB viral related B cell lymphomas in the brain of human beings and the use of SV-40 viral probes for the detection of DNA in a variety of brain tumors including a glioblastoma. In one instance an SV-40-like virus was obtained from a glioblastoma. This tumor had characteristic SV-40 antigen present in 95 percent of the cells tested. Dorriers et al. found no hybridization with JC or SV-40 probes but noted Southern blot hybrids to BkV probes in 11 of 24 tumors.[13] Five of these hybrids occurred in meningiomas, three in neurinomas, and one each in oligodendroglioma, anaplastic astrocytoma, and malignant glioma.

Animal brain tumor models of viral oncogenesis have been extensively reviewed by Bigner and his colleagues.[4,6] Several epidemiologic concerns emerge from this experimental work: (1) In animals, most intracranial gliomas have followed the intracerebral inoculation of papova- or sarcoma viruses into neonates or immunologically compromised (nude or exogenous) mice. (2) Depending on the route of inoculation, the immunologic competency of the animal, the specificity of the virus for the nervous system, and its oncogenic potential, the development of brain tumor may occupy 2 to 40 percent of the animals' expected life span. (3) In general, there is no predictable relationship between the viral inoculum and tumor histology. Thus, the sarcoma-inducing viruses may induce astrocytic tumors, ependymal tumors, sarcomatous tumors, pinealocytoma, and choroid plexus papilloma. (4) Although animal experiments have not provided a convincing basis for the role of oncogenic viruses in human brain tumor, these experiments have led to clinical observations that include the presence of "viral" inclusion bodies within glioblastoma cells, electron microscopic identification of particles similar to C-type RNA viruses in human brain tumors, the negative search for the T antigen associated with polyoma virus in tumor cell lines derived from glial tumor, and the epidemiologic interest in populations with known viral exposure who may be at an increased risk of brain tumor. These populations include Scandinavians whose exposure to the SV-40 virus followed contamination of polio vaccine, Kyushu (Japan) islanders who are at risk for both HTLV infection and pinealoma, and the possible relationship between maternal chicken pox and childhood brain tumors.

Occupational and Environmental Factors

The recent suggestion that petrochemical employees and children of aircraft industry employees are at increased risk of brain tumor has resulted in a resurgence of interest in the relation of occupation to glioma, and the chemical exposures associated with employment.

Occupations at Risk

Six occupations or categories of work-related exposure (rubber worker, petrochemical worker, anatomist, microwave-exposed worker, radiation-exposed worker, and vinyl chloride–exposed worker) have been linked to brain tumor development. With two exceptions, these linkages are unconfirmed by formal studies. Other formal studies have failed to reveal occupational brain tumor linkages.

Rubber Workers

The studies of Mancuso[29] underscore the difficulty in planning and interpreting occupation-based studies. Investigating cancer mortality among Ohio workers, he found elevated death rates from brain and CNS cancer among rubber and plastic workers compared to controls (1.30 versus 0.09 for agricultural industries and 1.30 versus 0.21 for all males 15 years old and over). The excess mortality was restricted to Summit County, the seat of the rubber industry. In a retrospective study (dating cases from 1937), he found an excess of brain tumor deaths among rubber workers (32 observed:23.6 expected) in comparison to nonrubber workers (29 observed:37.4 expected). This difference was especially notable for individuals 25 to 44 years old.

In 1968, social security and union files were used to uncover seven brain tumor cases among production workers employed between 1938 and 1939 in a single large plant.

However, a multicompany cohort study in Ohio in 1974 showed no clustering of brain tumor cases within selected departments across company lines. Later studies confirmed the excess brain tumor mortality among tire building and assembly workers in a single Ohio plant but noted no increased risk for the plant employees. These inconsistent results may reflect (1) differences in the choice of plant and the method of evaluation; (2) imprecision in the categorization of jobs; (3) relative availability of and quality of individual case work histories; (4) changes in job classification with time; and (5) changes in manufacturing techniques, solvents, substrates, exposure, and containment procedures with time within constant job categories. Thus a tire assembler may be exposed to a vast variety of potential toxins as the procedures for manufacture and assembly evolve over years. Small changes in the quality of these data may affect the already small differences in observed versus expected mortalities. Often the search for an excess of brain tumors within industries (such as lead or apparel workers) may thus indicate no increased risk while not evaluating the carcinogenic role of specific carcinogens such as the nitrosoureas or vinyl chloride.

Petrochemical Workers

Equally complex is the question of increased risk of brain tumor among petrochemical workers. The problem reached public attention as the result of the identification by the National Occupational Safety and Health Administration (OSHA) of a Texas petrochemical worker with a brain tumor in November 1978. In a retrospective investigation of brain tumor deaths among former employees in the Texas Gulf Coast petrochemical industry, OSHA investigators compared the risk of brain tumor in former Dow Chemical employees with non-Dow employees. Dow-employed brain tumor deaths accounted for 44 percent of brain tumor deaths in a single county, whereas non-Dow employees accounted for 25 percent [odds ratio (OR) = 2.54]. This initial group of 11 brain tumor deaths in former Dow employees was soon expanded to 25 by inclusion of Dow employees with brain tumors from neighboring counties. These cases resulted from a careful search of company medical records, municipal death files, and "unsolicited leads." Eighty-four percent of these individuals had been hired between 1940 and 1946. Sixty-four percent of these cases were astrocytoma grade III/IV or glioblastoma, but only six had been confirmed by surgical pathology or autopsy examination.

A retrospective evaluation of 5 percent of the work force at the Dow complex is ongoing. However, hourly employees with over 6 months employment did have excess brain cancer development (observed/expected = 10/5.01) as did long-term employees (over threefold for 20-year employees). This study underscores the need for histologic verification of cases. Without this, occupational studies are difficult to evaluate.

Early in 1980, Thomas et al. reported the result of a different approach—the analysis of mortality patterns among members of a single union in Texas oil refineries and petrochemical plants.[51] This study disclosed 25 "brain cancer" deaths in comparison to the 14 expected. For each brain tumor case, three matched (age, year of death, length as a union member) employees were chosen as controls. These controls had succumbed to causes of death other than brain tumor. The results of these studies are pending. Despite these data, epidemiologic evaluations of workers at sites owned by Dupont, Gulf Oil, and Union Carbide have failed to show excess mortality from brain tumor. Similar negative risk data have been reported from Britain.

Anatomists

Stroup et al., evaluating 2317 male anatomists, found standardized mortality ratios of 2.7 [95% confidence limits (CL) = 1.3 to 5.10] (versus white males) and 6.0 (CL = 2.3 to 15.6) (versus psychiatrists).[50] Ten anatomists had glial tumors.

Exposure and Brain Tumor Development

The interest in occupation-linked brain tumor development within the rubber, petrochemical, polymer (vinyl chloride), and pesticide-exposed agriculture industries stems from, and has provided impetus for, studies of the chemical induction of brain tumors in animals. Three groups of chemicals, administered by transplacental, oral, parenteral, or intracerebral routes, have produced neuroectodermal tumors in rodents, dogs, and primates: (1) polycyclic hydrocarbons (by intracerebral or transplacental inoculation), (2) nitroso compounds (following transplacental and intravenous routes), and (3) triazenes. These induction experiments indicate that (1) at least 15 agents can be administered to produce transplacental neuroectodermal tumors; (2) neonatal populations show the highest brain tumor induction rate following carcinogen exposure; (3) chemically induced tumors resemble spontaneous brain malignancies, but each carcinogen is not invariably associated with the same distinct histologic tumor type and a characteristic location; (4) carcinogens tend to induce primitive neuroectodermal tumors, often with sarcomatous elements; and (5) coincident, often multifocal, involvement of white matter, cranial nerves, and spinal nerves is seen following systemic or transplacental induction, whereas neonatal intracerebral carcinogen inoculation often produces a single expanding mass.

There is species specificity for chemical tumor induction. Thus, although in the rodent, nitrosoureas are potent carcinogens, their therapeutic use (BCNU, CCNU) in human beings has not been associated with an increase in tumor risk.

In our case-control study, more controls than cases reported an occupationally related exposure to toxic chemicals (EOR = 0.83; 0.4614, 1.4863) and solvents (EOR = 0.78; −0.448, 1.356). These differences are not statistically significant. Little attempt has been made to evaluate cohorts exposed to known brain carcinogens. The evaluation of vinyl-exposed populations by Waxweiler et al. led to the identification of increased glioblastoma risk, but exposure risk data have not emerged.[56] Austin and Schatter found "no statistically significant differences between the proportion of cases and controls exposed" when evaluating the exposure of glioma cases and controls to five carcinogens (benzene, diethylsulfate, ethylene dichloride, ethylene oxide, and

vinyl chloride) in a single plant.[2] Cases were exposed more frequently than controls to ethylene, isopropanol, vinyl acetate, chlorine, and sodium sulfite—but these are not known to be carcinogens.

Similarly, Johnson et al. found (in evaluating childhood brain tumors) "no significant associations . . . with jobs with exposure to hydrocarbons."[23] Olin et al. in a case-control study (clinical and population controls) of astrocytoma patients (supratentorial) found patients more likely to "live near a petrochemical . . . or municipal sewage treatment plant" or be "working at an airfield."[34] The role of dietary carcinogens is less clear. Preston-Martin et al. found increased odds ratio (2.8; $p < 0.01$) for women with meningiomas who had consumed nitrate-cured bacon, fish, ham, or sausage.[37] The odds ratio for high consumers was 4.8.

Hormones and Estrogen Exposure

There have been sporadic reports which relate diabetes mellitus to diminished brain tumor risk. In addition, clinicians have sought relationships between brain tumors and hormones of endogenous and exogenous origin based on (1) the relationship between exogenous sex hormones and cancer of the breast, endometrium, and uterine cervix (although no linkage between these hormones and glioblastoma has been noted); (2) the frequent clinical appearance of glioblastoma during pregnancy (although this may reflect edema formation, there are no data on the effect of hormonal changes on malignant dedifferentiation); (3) the association of adrenocortical carcinoma with coincidental astrocytoma in two children and with brain malformation in two others; (4) the finding of estrogen receptors within acoustic neurinomas and meningiomas and the role of nerve growth factor in the development of Schwann cell tumors associated with von Recklinghausen's neurofibromatosis; and (5) the unique association between meningioma and breast cancer.

An extensive obstetrical literature has detailed the presentation of brain tumors during pregnancy. Meningioma, optic glioma, oligodendroglioma, and cerebral glioblastoma have all been reported. Most often, these affect primiparous women without prior neurologic difficulties. In the majority, the diagnosis is made in the second or third trimester. Three factors have been considered to explain this relationship: (1) an exacerbation of peritumoral edema or an accumulation of tumor cyst fluid as a consequence of water retention; (2) vasodilatation and edema formation within the tumor; and (3) growth stimulation of the tumor during pregnancy. Ospelt expressed the view that pregnancy produced a noxious influence on the brain tumor.[35] However, Haas et al. in a cohort study found no support for the view that intracranial neoplasms present more often during pregnancy (OR = 0.26 to 0.38).[18]

Radiation Exposure

Radiation has been indentified as a risk factor for brain tumor development (mainly meningioma) as a result of retrospective studies and case-control studies involving patients irradiated for tinea capitis or spondylosis. Early life dental x-ray exposure may predispose to meningiomas in men and women (OR = 3.5 and 4.0). Reports include those of intracranial glioma developing years after therapeutic radiation for benign intracranial tumors and for other tumors of the head and neck. The meningiomas following tinea capitis therapy may have a distinct morphology (giant cells). These are in addition to the rare spinal glioma induced by irradiation.

Experimental induction of intracranial tumors of glial origin follows irradiation from external photon or proton sources as well as from implanted radiation brachytherapy probes. In one study, monkey ependymal tumors were seen (3 of 32 animals exposed to 600 to 800 rad) after an interval of 5 years.

Similar latencies have been observed when malignant glial tumors appear to occur in patients as a result of prior irradiation of head or neck lesions. Controversy exists with respect to induction of glioblastoma in human beings. Two studies have shown that irradiation of children for tinea capitis is associated with an increased risk (3-fold and 1.6-fold, respectively) of malignant head and neck neoplasms, but the occurrence of glioblastoma in this population is uncertain.

Similarly, prenatal x-ray exposure is associated with an increased risk of "neoplasm of the central nervous system" (relative risk, 1.33). However, this risk is less than that (1.42) for all cancers in the same population. No data were presented for glioblastoma occurrence in this population. Irradiation of the spinal cord during treatment of spondylosis is associated with a twofold risk (7.84 versus 4) of tumor development. However, Smith and Doll found no increase in risk of brain tumors among 72 British radiologists receiving an estimated 100 to 500-rad whole body dose between 1940 and 1945.[46]

Similar data are becoming available for radiation-exposed individuals engaged in radar maintenance or experimental detection and transmission research. The latter groups may have had unmeasured microwave or radiation exposure in the period following World War II. Thomas et al. performed a death certificate–based case-control study.[52] The relative risk (RR) for all brain tumors was elevated among men exposed to microwave and other radiofrequency radiation (RR = 1.6; CL = 1.0; 2.4). Those in electronic design, manufacturing, repair, or installation were at greater risk (RR = 2.3). The risk increased with exposure (>20 years) to tenfold. This study did not explore the power source or the significance of coincidental chemical exposure. However, a case-control study at nuclear facilities revealed that the nonoccupational risk factor of epilepsy (OR = 5.7; 95%) strongly associated with brain cancer.

In our case-control series, more controls than cases reported an occupationally related exposure to radiation (EOR = 0.52; 0.1784, 1.4874). Additionally, controls reported a greater overall exposure to x-rays than cases (EOR = 0.27; 0.565, 1.2442). However, cases had slightly more exposure to head x-ray treatment for acne (EOR = 1.62; 0.48, 5.5456) and annual roentgenograms of the chest (EOR = 1.08; 0.601, 1.9526). These differences are not statistically significant.

Head Trauma

Although trauma has been mentioned in the pathogenesis of meningioma, trauma-related glioblastoma has been only rarely noted. Fewer are the cases that satisfy the requirements of Ewing and Zülch: (1) the patient should have been well before the accident; (2) the head trauma must have been adequate (sufficient force to yield brain destruction); (3) the site of tumor formation must correspond to the area receiving the trauma; (4) the time interval between the trauma and the development of the tumor should be adequate (long latency); and (5) the tumor has to be proved histologically. Taking these concerns into account, several reports point to a trauma-glioma linkage. However, in one follow-up study of 2953 head trauma patients followed through 29,859 person years, no excess was observed in brain tumor occurrence.

In our case-control study, we observed a positive association between head trauma and glioblastoma. The overall EOR for a positive history of head trauma was 2.1 (1.1 to 4.0). The EOR varied with the severity of trauma: EOR was 1.5 for mild trauma (0.7 to 3.3) and was 3.8 for severe trauma (1.3 to 11.0). Preston-Martin and associates found increased odds ratios (case/neighbor) of meningioma in men who had boxed (OR = 2.0) or had had head injury (OR = 1.9) and in women who had had head trauma (OR = 2.0).[37,38] In a similar case-control study of "brain cancer" patients, the role of prior trauma was not upheld (OR = 0.9, 95%).

Predisposition and Risk Factors for the Development of non-Hodgkin's Lymphoma of the CNS (Primary Brain Lymphoma)

The present annual incidence of primary brain lymphoma [non-Hodgkin's lymphoma of the CNS (NHL-CNS)] is about 240 cases per year in the United States. The occurrence of NHL-CNS has slowly increased since 1960, but in the 5-year interval between 1980 and 1984, the incidence has trebled in comparison to any previous 5-year interval. The above-mentioned figures include all patients, with or without increased risk factors for the development of NHL-CNS. As a matter of fact, the majority of NHL-CNS cases do not fall into any of the categories mentioned below.

Three populations are at increased risk of developing NHL-CNS: transplant recipients, patients with AIDS, and patients with a congenital immunodeficiency syndrome. In reports from several medical centers, as many as 30 percent of patients with NHL-CNS have been those with a renal or cardiac transplant. For kidney recipients, the risk of systemic lymphoma is 2.2 cases per 1000 transplant recipients per year—a figure that is 350-fold greater than that for the population at large. The risk for NHL-CNS in these patients, although smaller, is still substantial because half of all these lymphomas are NHL-CNS. The risk of NHL-CNS for heart transplant recipients may be slightly higher. Weintraub and Warnke reported 3 cases per 182 recipients.[57] For both groups, the risk accrues as a result of the extent and duration of the immunosuppression. A median interval of 9 months elapsed from transplantation to tumor development in the reported cases of NHL-CNS arising in transplant recipients, with a range of 5.5 to 46 months. Data do not exist on the particular risk associated with antithymocyte globulin or as a consequence of HLA dyscompatibility.

Drug- or disease-induced immunosuppression has been associated with the development of NHL-CNS. There are reports of NHL-CNS accompanying sarcoidosis, systemic lupus erythematosus, Sjogren's syndrome, vasculitis, rheumatoid arthritis, and idiopathic thrombocytopenic purpura. Cases of NHL-CNS have been reported in association with PML, generally in settings of immunosuppression predisposing to both diseases. These cases include one in which the immunosuppression was associated with renal transplantation and one in which the patient had leukemia. Additional cases of coexisting PML and NHL-CNS have occurred in patients with AIDS.

Other acquired illnesses may be associated with NHL-CNS, even in the absence of overt immunosuppression or immunosuppressive medications. These illnesses include tuberculosis, multiple sclerosis, colon carcinoma, and glioblastoma. One case was reported in association with PML with no other proven immunosuppression disorder.

Primary brain lymphoma of the CNS has been reported in approximately 3 percent of patients with AIDS. This tumor occurring in individuals otherwise considered to be at "high risk" for AIDS but as yet lacking the specific diagnosis is considered by many to be indicative of the diagnosis. Based on the current rate of development of NHL-CNS in AIDS patients, we would expect 600 new cases to emerge from the American population of (currently) approximately 20,000 patients with AIDS. Using a polynomial mathematical model to predict the number of AIDS cases by the year 1991 and taking into account their own experience, Rosenblum et al. predicted the number of AIDS-related NHL-CNS cases to be 1848 by 1991.[39] Those already reported affect male patients who are younger (median age, 39 years) than the usual NHL-CNS population. These patients often have other peripheral and CNS stigmata of AIDS, including cytomegalovirus or EB virus infections of the brain as well as PML and toxoplasmosis, either alone or in combination. However, the CNS lymphoma may precede the appearance of AIDS-related opportunistic infections. In a report of 20 patients with NHL-CNS, So et al. noted no common antecedent systemic or brain lesions.[47]

CNS lymphomas have been reported to make up 4 percent of malignancies seen in patients with congenital immunodeficiency syndromes. Two disorders, the Wiskott-Aldrich syndrome (WAS) and severe combined immunodeficiency, predispose patients to NHL-CNS. Less common congenital immunoregulatory abnormalities have also been associated with such tumors. These include immunoglobulin (Ig)A deficiency and increased IgE. These disorders share inherited abnormalities of immunoglobulin production, deficiencies or absence of normal T-cell function, and a predisposition to infection. NHL-CNS represented 17.9

percent of the 78 cases of cancer in patients with WAS reported to the Immunodeficiency Cancer Registry (ICR) and 24 percent of the 59 lymphomas occurring in these WAS patients. Interestingly, although another similar congenital syndrome, ataxia telangiectasia, is clearly associated with systemic lymphoma, there are no cases of NHL-CNS reported to the ICR among the 152 tumors associated with ataxia telangiectasia, including 67 systemic lymphomas.

Duncan's syndrome, or x-linked lymphoproliferative syndrome, provides a link between the inability to control infection with a specific agent, the EB virus, and NHL-CNS. This work complements other reports suggesting a role for EB virus or papovaviruses in NHL-CNS and systemic lymphoma. This relationship is not easily established from serologic data. Reviewing serum samples from 20 patients with NHL-CNS, we were able to find evidence of persistent or reactivated EB virus infection (EB virus–nuclear antigen titer in excess of 1:40) in only six patients. However, the demonstration by Southern blot hybridization of EB virus genomic material within tumor tissue from four patients with NHL-CNS suggests a causative role for this virus. Alternatively, EB virus may preferentially infect certain malignant B cells; EB virus infection of selected subpopulations of B cells has been described. More recently, in situ hybridization studies have revealed positive EB virus genomic material in four cases of NHL-CNS in AIDS patients (Bashir RM, Hochberg FH, unpublished data).

References

1. Annegers JF, Schoenberg BS, Okazaki H, et al. Primary intracranial neoplasms in Rochester, Minnesota 1937–1977. In: Rose FC (ed.), *Clinical Neuroepidemiology*. Kent: Pittman Medical 1980:366–371.
2. Austin SG, Schnatter AR. A cohort mortality study of petrochemical workers. *J Occup Med* 1983; 25:304–312.
3. Bailey P, Green JR, Amador L, et al. Treatment of psychomotor states by anterior temporal lobectomy. *Arch Res Neurol Ment Dis* 1953; 31:341–345.
4. Bigner DD, Pegram CN. Virus-induced experimental brain tumors and putative associations of viruses and human brain tumors: a review. *Adv Neurol* 1976; 15:57–83.
5. Brown IA, French LA, Ogle WS, et al. Temporal lobe epilepsy: its clinical manifestations and surgical treatment. *Medicine* 1956; 35:425–459.
6. Bullard DE, Bigner DD. Animal models and virus induction of tumours. In: Thomas DGT, Graham D (eds.), *Brain Tumours*. London: Blackwells, 1980:51–84.
7. Bunin G. Racial patterns of childhood brain cancer by histologic type. *J Natl Cancer Inst* 1987; 78:875–880.
8. Canale D, Bebin J, Knighton RS. Neurologic manifestations of von Recklinghausen's disease of the nervous system. *Confin Neurol (Basel)* 1964; 24:359–403.
9. Choi NW, Schuman LM, Gullen WH. Epidemiology of primary central nervous system neoplasms. II: Case-control study. *Am J Epidemiol* 1970; 91:467–484.
10. Clemmensen J, Hjalgrim-Jensen S. Brain tumors in children exposed to barbiturates. *J Natl Cancer Inst* 1981; 66:215.
11. Cutler SJ, Young JL (eds.), *Third National Cancer Survey Incidence Data*. Publication No. (NIH) 75-787-NCI. Bethesda, MD: National Institutes of Health, 1975.

12. David M, Hecaen H, Bonis A. Tumeurs de système nerveaux central et maladie de Recklinghausen. *Semaine Hop Paris Ann Chir* 1956; 32:C335–384.

13. Dörries K, Loeber G, Meixensberger J. Association of polyomaviruses JC, SV40, and BK with human brain tumors. *Virology* 1987; 160:268–270.

14. Fontana M, Stanton C, Pompili A, et al. Late multifocal gliomas in adolescents previously treated for acute lymphoblastic leukemia. *Cancer* 1987; 60:1510–1518.

15. Garfinkel L, Sarokhan B. Trends in brain cancer mortality and morbidity in the U.S. *Ann NY Acad Sci* 1982; 381:1–5.

16. Gol A. Cerebellar astrocytomas in children. *Am J Dis Child* 1963; 106:21–24.

17. Gold EB. Epidemiology of brain tumors. In: Lilienfeld AM (ed.), *Reviews in Cancer Epidemiology*, Vol I. New York: Elsevier-North Holland, 1980:245–292.

18. Haas JF, Jänisch W, Staneczek W. Newly diagnosed primary intracranial neoplasms in pregnant woman: a population-based assessment. *J Neurol Neurosurg Psychiatry* 1986; 49:874–880.

19. Harvald B, Hauge M. On the heredity of glioblastoma. *J Natl Cancer Inst* 1956; 17:289–296.

20. Hauge M, Harvald B. Genetics in intracranial tumours. *Acta Genet* 1957; 7:573–591.

21. Hawkins MM, Draper GJ, Kingston JE. Incidence of second primary tumours among childhood cancer survivors. *Br J Cancer* 1987; 56:339–347.

22. Ingram L, Mott MG, Mann JR, et al. Second malignancies in children treated for non-Hodgkin's lymphoma and T-cell leukaemia with the UKCCSG regimens. *Br J Cancer* 1987; 55:463–466.

23. Johnson CC, Annegers JF, Frankowski RF, et al. Childhood nervous system tumors–an evaluation of the association with paternal occupational exposure to hydrocarbons. *Am J Epidemiol* 1987; 126:605–613.

24. Kernohan JW, Mabon RF, Svien HJ, et al. A simplified classification of the gliomas. *Proc Staff Meet Mayo Clinic* 1949; 24:71–75.

25. Kurland LT, Schoenberg BS, Annegers JF, et al. The incidence of primary intracranial neoplasms in Rochester, Minnesota, 1935–1977. *Ann NY Acad Sci* 1982; 381:6–16.

26. Li FP, McIntosh S, Peng-Whang J. Double primary cancers in 2 young sibs, leukemia in another, and dextrocardia in a fourth. *Cancer* 1977; 39:2633–2636.

27. Lipson A, Bale P. Ependymoblastoma associated with prenatal exposure to diphenylhydantoin and methylphenobarbitone. *Cancer* 1985; 55:1859–1862.

28. MacMahon B, Pugh TF. *Epidemiology; Principles and Methods.* Boston:Little, Brown, 1970.

29. Mancuso TF. Cited by RR Monson. *Occupational Epidemiology.* Boca Raton, FL: CRC Press, 1980.

30. Miller RW. Death from childhood leukemia and solid tumors among twins and other sibs in the United States, 1960–67. *J Natl Cancer Inst* 1971; 46:203–209.

31. Mori K, Kurisaka M. Brain tumors in childhood: statistical analysis of cases from the Brain Tumor Registry of Japan. *Childs Nerv Syst* 1986; 2:233–237.

32. Motz IP, Bots GTAM, Endtz LJ. Astrocytoma in three sisters. *Neurology* 1977; 27:1038–1041.

33. Nakasu S, Hirano A, Shimura T, et al. Incidental meningiomas in autopsy study. *Surg Neurol* 1987; 27: 319–322.

34. Olin RG, Ahlbom A, Lingberg-Navier I, et al. Occupational factors associated with astrocytomas: a case-control study. *Am J Ind Med* 1987; 11:615–625.

35. Ospelt M. Glioma cerebri und Schwangerschaft. *Zentralbl Gynäk* 1939; 63:1401–1405.

36. Penfield W, Flanigin H. Surgical therapy of temporal lobe seizures. *Arch Neurol Psychiatry* 1950; 64:491–500.

37. Preston-Martin S, Paganini-Hill A, Henderson BE, et al. Case-control study of intracranial meningiomas in women in Los Angeles County, California. *J Natl Cancer Inst* 1980; 65:67–73.

38. Preston-Martin S, Yu MC, Henderson BE, et al. Risk factors for meningiomas in men in Los Angeles County. *J Natl Cancer Inst* 1983; 70:863–866.

39. Rosenblum ML, Levy RM, Bredesen DE. Overview of AIDS and the nervous system. In: Rosenblum ML, Levy RM, Bredesen DE (eds.), *AIDS and the Nervous System.* New York: Raven Press, 1988:1–12.

40. Rubinstein LJ. *Tumors of the Central Nervous System.* Washington, DC: Armed Forces Institute of Pathology, 1972.

41. Rubinstein LJ, Herman MM, Hanbery JW. The relationship between differentiating medulloblastoma and dedifferentiating diffuse cerebellar astrocytoma. *Cancer* 1974; 33:675–698.

42. Sano K. Statistics on brain tumors and glioma. *Brain Nerve (Tokyo)* 1969; 21:463–465.

43. Scherer HJ. Cerebral astrocytomas and their derivatives. *Am J Cancer* 1940; 40:159–198.

44. Schoenberg BS, Glista GG, Reagan TJ. The familial occurrence of glioma. *Surg Neurol* 1975; 3:139–145.

45. Schoenberg BS, Schoenberg DG, Christine BW, et al. The epidemiology of primary intracranial neoplasms of childhood: a population study. *Mayo Clin Proc* 1976; 51:51–56.

46. Smith PG, Doll R. Mortality from cancer and all causes among British radiologists. *Br J Radiol* 1981; 54:187–194.

47. So YT, Beckstead JM, Davis RL. Primary central nervous system lymphoma in acquired immune deficiency syndrome: a clinical and pathological study. *Ann Neurol* 1986; 20:566–572.

48. Spencer DD, Spencer SS, Mattson RH, et al. Intracerebral masses in patients with intractable partial epilepsy. *Neurology* 1984; 34:432–436.

49. Spiers PS. Sex ratio by age in childhood malignancies. *J Chronic Dis* 1971; 23:907–911.

50. Stroup NE, Blair A, Erikson GE. Brain cancer and other causes of death in anatomists. *J Natl Cancer Inst* 1986; 77:1217–1224.

51. Thomas TL, Decoufle P, Moure-Eraso R. Mortality among workers employed in petroleum refining and petrochemical plants. *J Occup Med* 1980; 22:97–103.

52. Thomas TL, Stolley PD, Stemhagen A, et al. Brain tumor mortality risk among men with electrical and electronics jobs: a case-control study. *J Natl Cancer Inst* 1987; 79:233–238.

53. Tooth HH. Some observations on the growth and survival period of intracranial tumours, based on the records of 500 cases, with special reference to the pathology of the gliomata. *Brain* 1912; 35:61–108.

54. Van der Wiel HJ. *Inheritance of Glioma.* Amsterdam: Elsevier, 1959.

55. Velema JP, Walker AM. The age curve of nervous system tumour incidence in adults: common shape but changing levels by sex, race, and geographical location. *Int J Epidemiol* 1987; 16:177–183.

56. Waxweiler RJ, Stringer W, Wagoner JK, et al. Neoplastic risk among workers exposed to vinyl chloride. *Ann NY Acad Sci* 1976; 271:40–48.

57. Weintraub J, Warnke RA. Lymphoma in cardiac allotransplant recipients. Clinical and histological features and immunological phenotype. *Transplantation* 1982; 33:347–351.

58. Wollstein M, Bartlett FH. Brain tumors in young children: a clinical and pathologic study. *Am J Dis Child* 1923; 25:257–283.

59. Zülch KJ. *Brain Tumors; Their Biology and Pathology.* 2d ed. New York: Springer, 1965.

25

Controversial Issues in the Management of Low-Grade Astrocytomas

Robert A. Morantz

Recent advances in neurodiagnostic technology have caused a resurgence of interest in the question of what constitutes the optimal treatment of the cerebral astrocytoma. When isotope brain scans and cerebral angiography were the mainstays of brain tumor detection, the majority of patients were diagnosed late in the course of their disease and presented with large, high-grade lesions. The treatment of anaplastic gliomas and glioblastoma multiforme has consequently received most attention during the past several decades. With the advent of computed tomography (CT) and magnetic resonance imaging (MRI), however, we are now detecting smaller, less malignant lesions in younger patients. By the use of new techniques such as stereotactic biopsy, we have been able to obtain pathologic confirmation of tumor foci in many more instances then was previously possible. When the pathologic analysis indicates that a low-grade astrocytoma is present, the question arises as to what constitutes the best available therapy. By this, we mean that therapy which offers the longest and best quality of survival with the lowest risk of side effects. The latter issue is especially important, since these tumors affect patients who are relatively young and thus who can be expected to have a fairly long survival. In this chapter, I shall first discuss briefly what is known about the behavior of the low-grade astrocytoma and then review the main areas of controversy in the treatment of this ever more important neoplasm.

Nomenclature

The tumors that we shall be concerned with in this chapter are those that arise from the supporting cells of the central nervous system. These tumors have been called astrocytomas in the recent three-tier World Health Organization clas-

sification. They correspond to the grade I and grade II astrocytomas of the Kernohan classification, or what have been called "low-grade" astrocytomas in the past. This group includes lesions that previously were classified descriptively by such terms as *fibrillary* and *protoplasmic*. Some types of astrocytomas would appear to have a well-defined prognosis that is unique unto themselves and therefore will not be included in this review. Specifically, the "gemistocytic" astrocytoma seems to have a high incidence of conversion into more malignant forms and thus a worse prognosis than the other low-grade astrocytomas; conversely, the "pilocytic" astrocytoma appears to have an excellent prognosis no matter how radical the surgical resection or the type of postoperative adjuvant therapy.[3,18] Finally, this chapter specifically excludes tumors with a pathologic diagnosis of malignant glioma, anaplastic astrocytoma, astrocytoma grade III or grade IV, and glioblastoma multiforme. While certain of the conclusions of the chapter might also apply to low-grade oligodendroglioma and mixed oligodendroglioma-astrocytoma, there is little agreement as to how such lesions should be graded and few studies in the literature as to their optimal treatment. Thus, this chapter will focus on the low-grade astrocytomas rather than low-grade gliomas.

Epidemiology, Clinical Presentations, and Diagnostic Workup

Supratentorial astrocytomas account for between 10 and 15 percent of all brain tumors and constitute between 25 and 35 percent of all gliomas. They occur predominantly in middle age, with the peak incidence falling between 35 and 45 years. They arise predominantly within the convexity of the brain. The frontal lobe is the most common location, followed by the temporal lobe. On gross examination, they are often firm, whitish tumors. When growth occurs deep within the brain, formation of small and large cysts will often occur.[29]

The most common presenting symptom is epilepsy; other common ones are headache, mental changes, or focal neurologic deficit. In the past, the neuroradiologic procedures used to diagnose the lesion included isotope brain scanning and cerebral angiography. The isotope brain scan might or might not demonstrate the lesion; the angiogram would usually demonstrate a mass lesion without evidence of abnormal vascularity. In recent years, the diagnostic procedures of choice have become CT and/or MR imaging. Whether or not enhancement of the lesion on the CT scan is correlated with a poorer prognosis in patients with low-grade astrocytomas is controversial. Silverman and Marks reported that contrast enhancement had no prognostic value in patients with these tumors.[25] But Piepmeier, in a larger series, concluded that those patients whose tumors enhanced on CT scanning had a poorer prognosis than those whose lesions did not enhance after the administration of an intravenous contrast agent.[19] This poorer prognosis was evident even when adjustment was made for the age of the patient, which is the strongest of all prognosticators.

CT scanning in a typical case reveals a nonenhancing lesion whose density is lower than that of the surrounding brain. A mass effect upon surrounding ventricular structures is common. When enhancement does occur, it is generally faint and homogeneous. On the MR images, the lesion typically presents as a low-intensity area on the T1 images, whereas there is almost always an increase in signal intensity corresponding with an increase in relaxation time on T2-weighted (SE2500/40–80 ms) images. The area of increased signal is usually homogeneous and well circumscribed, with no evidence of hemorrhage or necrosis.[4] In many cases, it is difficult to differentiate on MR scans the tumor itself from surrounding areas of edema. Recent studies employing serial stereotactic biopsies of various regions of CT- and MR-defined abnormalities in patients with gliomas have indicated that there is infiltration of tumor cells into areas that were previously thought to represent only edematous white matter.[10]

Prognostic Factors

A great deal of effort has been expended to determine which factors might be of significance in determining the prognosis in a particular patient. All of the recent studies seem to agree that a young age at the time of diagnosis is by far the most important factor that correlates with a prolonged survival. Laws et al. found that other factors correlating with a prolonged survival were gross total surgical removal, lack of a major preoperative neurologic deficit, long duration of symptoms prior to surgery, seizures as a presenting symptom, lack of a major postoperative neurologic deficit, and having had surgery performed within recent decades.[11] There has not been agreement, however, as to the positive prognostic impact of some of these latter factors; for instance, neither Weir and Grace[28] nor Piepmeier[19] found that the extent of surgical resection was significantly correlated with length of survival. Most previous studies did indicate, however, that patients who received biopsy only had a poorer prognosis than those who received gross total resection.[7] The issue of whether there is an advantage to attempting a gross total removal as compared to a subtotal resection has not been answered.

The Question of Sampling and Dedifferentiation

Scherer was one of the first to emphasize that great care must be taken to examine all areas of a lesion before deciding that anaplastic foci are not present.[22] In his classic study, he made careful sections of the cerebral hemispheres of 18 patients with astrocytomas and found foci of anaplasia in 13. In a similar manner, Russell and Rubenstein examined 55 autopsy specimens of patients who had been diagnosed clinically as having an astrocytoma.[20] In more than 50 percent of these cases, areas of anaplastic change were found. Looked at from another perspective, Russell and Rubenstein analyzed a series of 129 autopsied cases of glioblastoma multiforme and concluded that approximately 28 percent could be considered to have arisen from a preexisting astrocytoma.

This issue has been studied recently by several authors. Müller and associates examined 72 patients whose pathologic diagnosis at the time of initial operation was astrocytoma.[17] At the time of recurrence, 14 percent of the tumors were unchanged pathologically, but 55 percent were now classified as anaplastic astrocytoma, and 30 percent were now classified as glioblastoma multiforme. The time between the initial pathologic diagnosis and the second operation averaged 31 months. The authors concluded that, in approximately two-thirds of all astrocytomas (i.e., including both the astrocytomas and the anaplastic astrocytomas), one can expect an increase in malignancy (i.e., dedifferentiation). In 79 patients with recurrent tumor growth documented either at subsequent surgery or at autopsy, Laws et al. found that a change to astrocytoma grade III or grade IV had occurred approximately 50 percent of the time.[11] More recently, however, Piepmeier found that malignant transformation was seen in only 13 percent of patients at the time of second operation or autopsy.[19] This number is almost certainly low, however, because the patient population reviewed in his study had a mean follow-up of only 5 years, and such malignant dedifferentiation will undoubtedly occur in more patients as the follow-up period increases.

Although this is still a subject of some debate and no definite answer can be given, it is probably fair to suggest that the presence of anaplastic areas at the time of a second resection or biopsy in a patient with a previously diagnosed low-grade astrocytoma is not necessarily due to an initial sampling error. Rather, in up to one-half of the cases, dedifferentiation of the low-grade astrocytoma to a more malignant form occurs. Thus, the clinical problem of most concern is whether radiation therapy can retard the occurrence of dedifferentiation to a more anaplastic state, or possibly whether radiation therapy can destroy small anaplastic foci that are already present in the astrocytoma, as has been suggested in a recent pathologic study.[23]

Optimal Methods of Therapy

Time of Operation

It is a general rule of surgical oncology that surgery should be carried out as early in the course of malignancy as possible. However, it has never been proved that earlier treatment of a low-grade astrocytoma produces an increase in life-span as measured from the time of diagnosis. Furthermore, because more and more patients are having their tumors detected while they are neurologically intact and because operative intervention in some locations will carry a significant risk of postoperative morbidity, some have made the case that surgery should be delayed in lesions that do not show a change in appearance on sequential radiologic studies. Unfortunately, however, since it is still almost impossible to make a precise pathologic diagnosis in a particular patient by neuroradiologic procedures alone, this consideration would appear to be outweighed in most instances by the necessity of obtaining pathologic confirmation of the exact nature of the lesion demonstrated.

Type of Surgery

Most, but certainly not all, of the retrospective studies that have been carried out have indicated that patients who underwent a "gross total" removal of their lesion experienced a longer survival than those who did not. We must be quite careful in evaluating such data, however, since it is quite likely that the patients in these two groups were not comparable—i.e., in those patients whose tumors were widely infiltrating into vital areas, surgical judgment was at variance with an attempt at "gross total" removal. However, given the general oncologic principle that one should try to obtain the maximum reduction of tumor burden possible and the known propensity of residual cells to undergo malignant dedifferentiation, it would appear prudent to attempt a "gross total" removal in those lesions where this can be done without producing a postoperative neurologic deficit.

The Role of Postoperative Adjuvant Radiation Therapy

Perhaps the most controversial area in the treatment of low-grade astrocytomas is the question of whether postoperative radiation therapy should be used as an adjunctive form of therapy.[16,24] The answer to this question should be relatively easy to come by. Ideally, such an answer would be forthcoming from what is probably our most powerful tool for scientifically answering clinical questions such as this one—the randomized, controlled, prospective clinical trial. In this case, one would have to carry out a multigroup, long-term (perhaps as long as 10-year) study in which two large groups of patients (containing individuals who are balanced with respect to important variables such as age, tumor location, histologic classification, etc.) were treated identically in every respect (i.e., extent of operation, use of steroids, etc.) except that one group received an exactly specified course of radiation therapy and the other group did not. Whether there was a statistically significant difference in the length and/or quality of survival between these two groups could then be determined. Such a study has never been completed, although at the present time such cooperative studies are being planned in the United States by the Brain Tumor Cooperative Group and are presently being carried out in Europe. Unfortunately, the results of these studies will not be available for many years to come.

Because no single neurosurgeon's experience is adequate to answer properly how patients with a low-grade astrocytoma should be optimally treated postoperatively, and the results of present cooperative trials will not be available for many years, we are faced with the question of how to presently manage this group of patients. The imperfect present-day solution would seem to be a review of the major studies in this area to see whether they can furnish any guidance.

What is immediately apparent in carrying out such a review, however, is that the reports previously published have almost universally not satisfied even the minimal criteria that could be set forth for a study that could properly answer this question (Table 25-1). More specifically, the previous studies have been retrospective analyses in which the irradi-

TABLE 25-1 Difficulties with Previous Studies of the Role of Radiation Therapy in the Treatment of Astrocytoma

No uniformity of patient selection
No uniformity in the varying neurologic status of the patients (e.g., Karnofsky scale)
No uniform system of pathologic classification
No uniformity of radiation therapy dosage and field size
No uniformity in the extent of surgical removal of the tumor (i.e., gross total removal vs. biopsy)
No uniformity in the location of the lesion (i.e., cerebrum vs. cerebellum vs. brain stem)
No simultaneous control group of patients who are not treated with radiation therapy

ated and nonirradiated groups of patients have not been similar in important characteristics (e.g., age, Karnofsky rating, etc.). The pathologic classification of the lesions has been different (e.g., varying numbers of grade I and grade II tumors). The location and size of the tumors have been different, and the extent of operation has not been uniform (e.g., biopsy versus complete resection). Finally, the parameters of the treatment being tested (i.e., radiation therapy) have not been standardized with respect to total dose, duration of therapy, field size, etc. With these objections in mind, let us review the previous literature, such as it is, in an attempt to discover whether there is any trend that can provide us with at least some general guidelines.

One of the earliest reports was that of Levy and Elvidge, who reviewed 176 cases that were treated at the Montreal Neurological Institute between 1940 and 1949.[13] These authors found what has been confirmed subsequently by many other authors—that the "gemistocytic" type of astrocytoma has a poorer prognosis than that of other variants and that patients with cerebellar astrocytomas did better than those with cerebral lesions, even in the face of incomplete removal. Several years later, Bouchard and Peirce reviewed all patients seen at this same institution over a much longer period and compared the survival of 81 low-grade astrocytoma patients who had received radiation therapy with a group of 71 patients who had not.[2] They found that, although the 3-year survival rate was virtually identical (i.e., 62 versus 59 percent), the 5-year survival statistics showed an increased longevity in those who had received radiation therapy (i.e., 49 versus 38 percent). From these data, they concluded that ionizing radiation should play a major role in the treatment of such patients.

Gol in 1961 reviewed 194 cases of cerebral astrocytoma seen at the Baylor University College of Medicine.[7] Two-thirds of the postoperative patients were given radiation therapy. He found that, irrespective of whether biopsy or resection was the surgical procedure used, the addition of radiation therapy caused an increase in survival (biopsy, 10 versus 2 months; resection, 32 versus 23 months). In addition, this study was the first indicating that patients whose tumor was resected rather than just biopsied did better no matter what other therapy was utilized.

Uihlein et al. published the first of three major studies utilizing the clinical material of the Mayo Clinic.[27] In this report, they reviewed 83 patients with astrocytoma treated between 1955 and 1959. Thirty-three of their patients underwent operation alone, and 50 were treated with operation followed by radiation therapy. They found that 65 percent of those treated with operation alone were alive at 5 years and only 54 percent of those treated by operation and radiation therapy were alive at 5 years. If anything, this indicated a decreased survival after the addition of radiation therapy. However, when they separated the irradiated cases into those that had received 3500 rad or more and those that had received a lower dosage, the 5-year survival rates were 63 and 42 percent. From this analysis, they concluded that there is a "suggestion" that irradiation may be helpful in the treatment of the low-grade astrocytoma.

In 1974, Stage and Stein reviewed the University of California, Los Angeles, experience with supratentorial brain tumors and found six patients with grade I lesions and 45 patients with grade II lesions.[26] An analysis of their survival curves indicated a 40 percent 5-year survival for those treated with resection and radiation therapy compared to a 20 percent 5-year survival for those treated with operation alone.

Marsa and coworkers reviewed the survival data for all patients treated with radiation therapy at Stanford University between 1957 and 1973.[15] They found a 5-year survival rate of approximately 41 percent and a 10-year survival rate of approximately 22 percent. In addition, they confirmed that dedifferentiation to a higher degree of malignancy seemed to occur in a substantial proportion of patients in whom the surgical diagnosis was compared to that found at subsequent autopsy.

In 1975, Leibel et al. reviewed the experience at the University of California, San Francisco, in the treatment of astrocytoma.[12] They found 147 patients who were treated at their institution between 1942 and 1967. If the patients who had complete resection of their lesion were excluded from the analysis, there was a clear-cut increased survival in the group undergoing radiation therapy (i.e., 5-year survival of 46 versus 19 percent; 10-year survival of 35 versus 11 percent). Based on their analysis, patients with complete removal of their tumor did well even if they did not receive radiation therapy, and patients with cerebellar lesions also did well irrespective of whether radiation therapy was given. Finally, they indicated that the quality of life was acceptable in long-term survivors and that there were no instances of radiation damage in those who experienced long-term survival.

Weir and Grace in 1976 studied 107 patients with a grade I or grade II supratentorial astrocytoma treated in the Province of Alberta, Canada, between 1960 and 1970.[28] They analyzed the patients with respect to prognostic factors that might be related to survival and found that young age, lower grade at operation (i.e., grade I > grade II), and the addition of radiation therapy were correlated with an increased survival. Fazekas in 1977 reviewed 68 patients with grade I or grade II lesions treated at the Geisinger Clinic between 1958 and 1974.[5] He concluded that completely excised lesions and those in the cerebellum did well whether or not radiation was given. For those with incomplete resection, radiation increased the 5-year survival from 32 to 54 percent, although by 10 years this difference was thought not to be significant (i.e., 26 versus 32 percent).

Scanlon and Taylor in 1979 published a second report from the Mayo Clinic in which they reviewed 134 cases of low-grade glioma treated between 1960 and 1969.[21] Specifically eliminated were cases with complete resection of the lesion because they were not referred for radiation therapy. After analyzing their data, they concluded that young age and location in the cerebellum were important positive prognostic factors. In contrast to previous findings, they were able to show no advantage of subtotal resection over biopsy. In addition, they found that patients receiving less than 1400 ret did just as well as those receiving a larger dose and that there was a worsening of survival when whole brain rather than localized radiation therapy was given.

In 1982, Bloom reviewed the experience at the Royal Marsden Hospital in treating brain tumors with radiation therapy.[1] His treatment group consisted of 120 patients with grade I or grade II lesions. Although survival data are given only for those treated with operation and radiation therapy (grade I, 5-year survival of 33 percent; 10-year survival, 16 percent; grade II, 5-year survival, 21 percent; 10-year survival, 6 percent), he concluded that "delay of recurrence and greater survival can be expected following postoperative radiotherapy than after surgery alone."[1]

In 1984, Laws et al. again used the patient population at the Mayo Clinic to review 461 astrocytoma patients treated between 1915 and 1975.[11] These cases were selected from a much larger group of patients and represented only those with supratentorial tumors who survived at least 30 days postoperatively and for whom follow-up data were available. Multiple prognostic factors were analyzed for possible correlation with an increase in survival. The authors found that the age of the patient was the most important variable and surpassed all others in its positive correlation with long-term survival. In addition, they interpreted the data as supporting radical operation and a beneficial effect of radiation therapy only in those patients with poor prognostic factors (e.g., older age).

In 1985, Garcia and coworkers reported a retrospective study of 86 adults treated at Washington University between 1950 and 1979.[6] Although the number of patients with well-differentiated astrocytomas was small, they found that those with a juvenile pilocytic type of astrocytoma did well regardless of treatment and did not require radiation therapy, a conclusion that has been confirmed in other recent studies.

Piepmeier reviewed the records of 60 patients with low-grade astrocytomas seen at the Yale–New Haven Hospital between 1975 and 1985.[19] In this retrospective review, there was no significant difference found in survival between those patients who received radiation therapy in addition to surgery and those who did not. What is important in this study is that all patients who were irradiated received between 50 and 60 Gy delivered over 5 to 6 weeks to fields that were constructed by using CT scanning to include the tumor plus a wide margin of surrounding brain. One caveat expressed by the author, however, was that since the patient population reviewed in this paper was treated over the last decade, the mean follow-up time was slightly less than 5 years and thus this may have been insufficient time to allow a potential effect of radiation to become evident. However, it should also be noted that most previous studies which did indicate a beneficial effect of radiation therapy did so mainly

TABLE 25-2 Treatment of Cerebral Astrocytoma

Authors and Year Reported	Years of Study	Patients Included	No. of Cases	Radiation Dose	Survival 3 Years		Survival 5 Years		Survival 10 Years	
					Surgery	Surgery and Radiation	Surgery	Surgery and Radiation	Surgery	Surgery and Radiation
Levy and Elvidge, 1956	1940–49	Astrocytomas, grades I and II	176	?	52%	62%	26%	36%		
Bouchard and Peirce, 1960	1939–58	Astrocytomas	126	5000–6000 rad	59%	61.7%	38%	49%		35.8%
Gol, 1961	?	Astrocytomas, grades I and II	194	?	Median survival		Biopsy alone: 2 months; Biopsy and radiation: 10 months		Resection alone: 23 months; Resection and radiation: 32 months	
Uihlein et al., 1966	1955–59	Astrocytomas, grades I and II	83	2000–6000 rad	63.6%	64%	65%	54%		
Stage and Stein, 1974	1956–70	Cerebral astrocytomas, grade II	45	3500–6500 rad	—	—	20%	42%		
Marsa et al., 1975	1957–73	Astrocytomas	40	4900–6650 rad	—	62%		~41%		~22%
Leibel et al., 1975	1942–67	Astrocytomas, grades I and II	147	3500–5000 rad	27%	59%	19%	46%	11%	35%
Weir and Grace, 1976	1960–70	Astrocytomas, grades I and II	107	—	Average survival		Surgery: 28 months; Surgery and radiation: 35 months			
Fazekas, 1977	1958–74	Astrocytomas, grades I and II	68	850–1400 ret	—	—	32%	54%	26%	32%
Scanlon and Taylor, 1979	1960–69	Astrocytomas, grades I and II	134	~1400 ret	—	—	64%			
Bloom, 1982	1952–70	Astrocytomas, grades I and II	120 (adults)	?	—	—		Grade I: 33% Grade II: 21%		Grade I: 16% Grade II: 6%
Laws et al., 1984	1915–75	Astrocytomas, low-grade	461	4000–7900 rad	—	—	~35%	~50%	~10%	~15%
Garcia et al., 1985	1950–79	Astrocytomas, grades I, II, and III	86	3500–6100 rad	35%	61%	22%	40%	9%	9%
Piepmeier, 1987	1975–85	Astrocytomas, low-grade	60	5000–6000 rad	Mean survival		Biopsy alone: 6.67 yr; Biopsy + radiation: 6.01 yr		Subtotal alone: 9.58 yr; Subtotal + radiation: 6.34 yr	

Total alone: 5.10 yr
Total + radiation: 7.65 yr

at 5 years, with such beneficial effect decreasing at 10 years and longer.

As indicated in the literature review above, the majority of the major English-language studies have found that radiation therapy is beneficial when added to surgery in the treatment of cerebral astrocytoma (Table 25-2). One must, however, be extremely cautious in interpreting the retrospective data from these reports. As we have indicated previously, it is mandatory to take into account the various prognostic factors that may be present to differing degrees in the two groups of patients that are being compared. Age, functional status of the patient, extent of surgical removal, and pathologic grade (i.e., grade I or grade II) are at least some of the important variables that must be known. In almost none of the studies reviewed is this information readily available. In addition, all of these studies suffer from being retrospective analyses in which the two groups are not strictly comparable with respect to various selection factors or even the treatment given. Consequently, any conclusions reached must be considered only tentative until the proper studies are carried out.

It is possible that future advances in technology will allow us to select a subgroup of patients with low-grade astrocytomas who should receive postoperative radiation therapy. Procedures that are just now being perfected allow us to directly measure the proliferative potential of low-grade astrocytomas[9] using immunohistochemical techniques such as in situ labeling with bromodeoxyuridine. Preliminary data would appear to correlate a poor prognosis with an increase in proliferative potential. If this is confirmed, then perhaps only patients whose tumors have a labeling index above a certain level should receive radiation therapy.

The issue of whether radiation therapy should be utilized in these patients is not one that can be taken lightly. In patients with anaplastic astrocytoma or glioblastoma multiforme, it is quite probable that the relatively short survival time prevents the long-term deleterious effects of radiation therapy from becoming evident. This would not be the case in the group of patients with grade I or grade II astrocytoma, who have a 5-year survival rate of approximately 40 percent and a 10-year survival rate of perhaps 20 percent. Although the reported incidence of radiation necrosis varies widely, a recent study indicated its presence in 9 percent of a series of 76 patients treated with whole brain irradiation for various intrinsic brain tumors.[8] In this regard, it is of interest that a recent review of 371 irradiated brain tumor patients by Marks and Wong found the incidence of radiation necrosis to be 1.5 percent at 5500 rad and 4 percent at 6000 rad and to increase substantially for higher doses.[14] It is also generally accepted that the risk of untoward sequelae from radiation therapy is greater after whole brain radiation therapy than after more localized treatment.

Conclusions

Because the proper prospective, randomized study has not yet been done, the optimal treatment of the low-grade astrocytoma remains controversial, and thus dogmatic statements as to optimal treatment should be avoided. Nevertheless,

until more definitive data become available, we may draw certain tentative conclusions:

1. An attempt should be made to obtain pathologic confirmation of the nature of a supratentorial lesion that is seen on CT or MR scans and has at least some of the features of an intrinsic brain tumor.
2. Consistent with sound neurosurgical judgment as to postoperative sequelae, an attempt should be made to carry out gross total removal of a hemispheric astrocytoma or to remove as much tumor as possible.
3. In the case of such a gross total surgical removal, radiation therapy can be withheld and the patient carefully followed with periodic CT and/or MR scans. If the lesion does not show definite evidence of recurrence, then radiation therapy should be withheld.
4. In cases where total removal cannot be accomplished, postoperative radiation therapy seems warranted.
5. Such radiation therapy should be given in a conventional fractionation schedule to a dose not exceeding 5500 rad. This radiation therapy should be given to a limited volume as determined by the CT and MR scans rather than to the whole brain.
6. Such a treatment regimen may be expected to yield a 5-year survival of approximately 40 percent and a 10-year survival of up to 20 percent, although a more precise estimate of survival time can be made if the particular prognostic variables (especially age) of the individual patient are known.
7. The results of several multigroup, long-term, prospective, randomized studies of this important question are eagerly awaited.

References

1. Bloom HJG. Intracranial tumors: response and resistance to therapeutic endeavors, 1970–1980. *Int J Radiat Oncol Biol Phys* 1982; 8:1083–1113.
2. Bouchard J, Peirce CB. Radiation therapy in the management of neoplasms of the central nervous system, with a special note in regard to children: twenty years' experience, 1939–1958. *AJR* 1960; 84:610–628.
3. Clark GB, Henry JM, McKeever PE. Cerebral pilocytic astrocytoma. *Cancer* 1985; 56:1128–1133.
4. Drayer BP, Johnson PC, Bird CR. Magnetic resonance imaging and glioma. *BNI Quart* 1987; 3:44–55.
5. Fazekas JT. Treatment of grades I and II brain astrocytomas: the role of radiotherapy. *Int J Radiat Oncol Biol Phys* 1977; 2:661–666.
6. Garcia DM, Fulling KH, Marks JE. The value of radiation therapy in addition to surgery for astrocytomas of the adult cerebrum. *Cancer* 1985; 55:919–927.
7. Gol A. The relatively benign astrocytomas of the cerebrum: a clinical study of 194 verified cases. *J Neurosurg* 1961; 18: 501–506.
8. Hohwieler ML, Lo TCM, Silverman ML, et al. Brain necrosis after radiotherapy for primary intracerebral tumor. *Neurosurgery* 1986; 18:67–74.
9. Hoshino T. A commentary on the biology and growth kinetics of low-grade and high-grade gliomas. *J Neurosurg* 1984; 61:895–900.
10. Kelly PJ, Daumas-Duport C, Scheithauer BW, et al. Stereotac-

tic histologic correlations of computed tomography and magnetic resonance imaging-defined abnormalities in patients with glial neoplasms. *Mayo Clin Proc* 1987; 62:450–459.

11. Laws ER Jr, Taylor WF, Clifton MB, et al. Neurosurgical management of low-grade astrocytomas of the cerebral hemispheres. *J Neurosurg* 1984; 61:665–673.

12. Leibel SA, Sheline GE, Wara WM, et al. The role of radiation therapy in the treatment of astrocytomas. *Cancer* 1975; 35:1551–1557.

13. Levy LF, Elvidge AR. Astrocytoma of the brain and spinal cord: a review of 176 cases, 1940–1949. *J Neurosurg* 1956; 13:413–443.

14. Marks JE, Wong I. The risk of cerebral radionecrosis in relation to dose, time and fractionation: a follow-up study. *Prog Exp Tumor Res* 1985; 29:210–218.

15. Marsa GW, Goffinet DR, Rubenstein LJ, et al. Megavoltage irradiation in the treatment of gliomas of the brain and spinal cord. *Cancer* 1975; 36:1681–1689.

16. Morantz RA. Radiation therapy in the treatment of cerebral astrocytoma. *Neurosurgery* 1987; 20:975–982.

17. Müller W, Áfra D, Schröder R. Supratentorial recurrences of gliomas: morphological studies in relation to time intervals with astrocytomas. *Acta Neurochir (Wien)* 1977; 37:75–91.

18. Palma L, Guidetti B. Cystic pilocytic astrocytomas of the cerebral hemispheres: surgical experience with 51 cases and long-term results. *J Neurosurg* 1985; 62:811–815.

19. Piepmeier JM. Observations on the current treatment of low-grade astrocytic tumors of the cerebral hemispheres. *J Neurosurg* 1987; 67:177–181.

20. Russell DS, Rubenstein LJ. *Pathology of Tumors of the Nervous System*, 3d ed. Baltimore: Williams & Wilkins, 1971:126, 169.

21. Scanlon PW, Taylor WF. Radiotherapy of intracranial astrocytomas: analysis of 417 cases treated from 1960 through 1969. *Neurosurgery* 1979; 5:301–308.

22. Scherer JH. Cerebral astrocytomas and their derivatives. *Am J Cancer* 1940; 40:159–198.

23. Schiffer D, Giordana MT, Sofietti R, et al. Effects of radiotherapy on the astrocytomatous areas of malignant gliomas. *J Neurooncol* 1984; 2:167–175.

24. Sheline GE. The role of radiation therapy in the treatment of low-grade gliomas. *Clin Neurosurg* 1986; 33:563–574.

25. Silverman C, Marks JE. Prognostic significance of contrast enhancement in low-grade astrocytomas of the adult cerebrum. *Radiology* 1981; 139:211–213.

26. Stage WS, Stein JJ. Treatment of malignant astrocytomas. *AJR* 1974; 120:7–18.

27. Uihlein A, Colby MY Jr, Layton DD, et al. Comparison of surgery and surgery plus irradiation in the treatment of supratentorial gliomas. *Acta Radiol* 1966; 5:67–78.

28. Weir B, Grace M. The relative significance of factors affecting postoperative survival in astrocytomas, grades one and two. *Can J Neurol Sci* 1976; 3:47–50.

29. Zülch KJ. *Brain Tumors: Their Biology and Pathology*, 3d ed. Berlin: Springer-Verlag, 1986:210–213.

26

Monoclonal Antibodies: Their Applications in the Diagnosis and Management of Brain Tumors

Herbert E. Fuchs
Michael R. Zalutsky
Sandra H. Bigner
Darell D. Bigner

The use of antibodies to deliver chemotherapeutic agents was first proposed by Paul Ehrlich in 1906.[16] The potential for antibodies to specifically diagnose and treat human tumors has been the subject of active investigation ever since. The identification of tumor-associated antigens on human brain tumors[2,10,13,54] has paved the way for the application of antibodies in neuro-oncology.

In 1965, Mahaley and Day first reported a rabbit antihuman glioma antiserum, which could, after extensive absorption and fractionation, preferentially localize in human glioma tissue after intra-arterial injection.[29,30] Coakham described a rabbit antiglioma antiserum against human astrocytoma antigens, although this serum was not shown to be definitely HLA-nonreactive.[11,13] Both Miyake et al.[33] and Sato et al.[44] produced rabbit antisera against human glioma cells, although neither preparation underwent adequate absorption with normal brain, and neither antiserum was usable as a glioma-specific probe. In none of these reports has a specific response to a tumor-associated antigen been well defined using polyclonal antisera.[52,53] More recent results suggest that this failure is due to the limitations of the polyclonal antisera which were not made by immunizing with purified tumor-associated antigens.

The Development of Monoclonal Antibodies

The immunologic response of an organism to a foreign substance is heterogeneous. If the foreign substance contains only a single antigenic determinant, the heterogeneity of the response lies in the variable affinities, and often the immunoglobulin class (IgG subtypes versus IgM) of the multiple antibodies produced against this single determinant. Most immunogens have multiple antigenic determinants, resulting in heterogeneity in antibody specificity to the various determinants as well as varying antibody affinity for each determinant.

There are several methods to reduce the heterogeneity of the immune response. Serial immunization tends to increase the affinity of the antiserum for the immunogen. The antiserum produced by serial immunization is still very heterogeneous, with as much as 90 percent of the immunoglobulin in the antiserum having little or no avidity for the immunogen. Serial absorption of the antiserum reduces both the heterogeneity and the ultimate yield of antiserum, requiring a number of animals to produce usable quantities of antiserum.

A tremendous technological advance occurred in 1975, with the development of monoclonal antibodies (MAbs) by Köhler and Milstein.[24] Hybridomas are cell lines produced by the fusion of a B lymphocyte, which secretes a single antibody, with a nonimmunoglobulin-secreting, immortal myeloma cell. The vast majority of hybridomas produced to date are derived from murine cell lines. Following immunization of a mouse with the desired immunogen, spleen cells are fused using polyethylene glycol or Sendai virus, with a murine myeloma cell line which does not secrete immunoglobulin but is capable of indefinite proliferation in cell culture. The myeloma cell line is also deficient in one of the enzymes essential for nucleic acid salvage pathways. Following fusion, cells are plated at dilutions allowing, on the average, less than one hybridoma cell per well, in hypoxanthine, aminopterin, and thymidine (HAT) media, which allows only hybrid cells, and not the parent cells, to grow. Supernatants from the wells are screened for antibody to the original immunogen. Since the hybridoma cell line is produced from a single antibody-producing cell, all molecules of antibody produced are identical, and are directed against a single antigenic determinant. These cloned hybridoma cell lines may be propagated indefinitely, producing vast quantities of pure, monospecific monoclonal antibodies. This represents a significant improvement over polyclonal antisera, which are heterogeneous in composition, which vary from animal to animal, and which are limited in production by the mortality of the animal. Once sufficient quantities of MAb are available, the MAb can be characterized as to immunoglobulin class and subclass, affinity for the immunogen, and potential cross-reactivity with related antigens or tissues.

Murine MAbs have several potential limitations in their clinical use. Murine MAbs have been unable to detect certain major histocompatibility complex (HLA) antigens readily detected by conventional human polyclonal antisera, suggesting a reduced interspecies response.[23] Also, exact duplication of the unique autochthonous human immune responses which occur in regional draining lymph nodes or intratumoral lymphocytes is not possible with murine MAbs.[38,39,43] There is also the potential for interspecies reaction with marine MAbs in human clinical use. Hybridomas producing human antibodies would be able to circumvent these difficulties. To date, however, efforts to fuse human B lymphocytes with murine myeloma cells have resulted in unstable mixed hybrids which shed chromosomes. Efforts are currently under way to identify a more effective human tumor cell line to produce human hybridomas. Recently, genetic engineering has allowed cloning of murine hybridoma immunoglobulin genes, including the antigen-specific portion of the molecule, into human hybridoma cells, allowing the production of chimeric antibodies predominantly human in composition.[48]

It has been suggested that the specificity of MAbs may limit their usefulness with malignant gliomas, which may demonstrate tremendous genotypic and phenotypic heterogeneity.[2] For this reason, a single MAb may not demonstrate reactivity with all tumors. This may be overcome by using a MAb directed at basic tumor functions, such as vital membrane transport mechanisms, or tumor-induced neovascularization, or through the use of a panel of MAbs, each with a unique specificity.

Monoclonal Antibodies in Vitro

Monoclonal antibodies are valuable tools in the purification and characterization of antigens. Making monospecific polyclonal antisera requires a purified antigen preparation for immunization. MAbs, however, may be produced using complex mixtures of antigens, even intact cells for immunization. After hybridoma production, MAbs may be selected for the desired specificity. Affinity chromatography techniques with MAbs may then be used to purify the antigen for further characterization. In this manner, previously described antigens may be better defined, and new antigens may be discovered.

Monoclonal antibodies have been developed against a wide variety of antigens, including receptor molecules, hormones, extracellular matrix proteins, neuroectodermal tumor–associated antigens and normal CNS-associated antigens.

Well-characterized MAbs directed against a variety of antigenic specificities can be utilized as diagnostic tools with immunohistochemistry. The presence of antigen at either the cellular or subcellular level can be precisely defined using horseradish peroxidase, immunofluorescence, enzyme-linked immunosorbent assay (ELISA), or radioimmunoassay. The use of MAbs in these techniques allows a reproducibility and standardization which was not possible with polyclonal antisera. MAbs have been used to define the expression of antigens on cells of the CNS. With antigens as markers for the different cell components of the CNS, the development of the normal CNS may be studied, and specific tumor-associated antigens may be described. The neuroectodermal tumor-associated antigens defined by MAbs

may be classified as biochemically defined markers, shared nervous system–lymphoid cell markers, shared neuroectodermal–oncofetal markers, and restricted tumor markers.[6]

The best characterized, biochemically defined marker in the CNS is glial fibrillary acidic protein (GFAP), an intracellular intermediate filament protein which was originally isolated from multiple sclerosis plaques and is expressed specifically by astroglial cells. GFAP has been demonstrated in normal astroglial cells and in virtually all astroglial-derived tumors, including ependymomas, oligodendroglioma-astrocytomas, gliosarcomas, angiogliomas, astroblastomas, and in the more differentiated regions of glioblastomas, but not in ganglion cells or in mesenchymal tumors. The problem of questionable specificity of early polyclonal anti-GFAP antisera has been resolved with anti-GFAP MAbs, and these MAbs are now in use both in the diagnosis of neurosurgical tumor biopsies as well as in experimental neuro-oncology.

Neurofilaments have proven to be reliable markers for neurons. Using MAbs, neurofilaments have been identified in both peripheral and CNS tumors including neuroblastomas, ganglioneuroblastomas, ganglioneuromas, pheochromocytomas, pineoblastomas, ganglion cells of gangliogliomas, and some medulloblastomas. As was the case with GFAP, neurofilaments appear to be differentiation markers, as they are found in much higher levels in the more differentiated regions of such tumors.

Recently, synaptophysin, an M_r 38,000 integral membrane glycoprotein of neurotransmitter vesicles, has been identified in normal neurons, and a variety of neuroendocrine tumors, including medulloblastomas, neuroblastomas, ganglioneuroblastomas, ganglioneuromas, pheochromocytomas, paragangliomas, medullary thyroid carcinomas, and pancreatic islet cell neoplasms, but not melanomas, gliomas, or non-neuroendocrine carcinomas.[20,50] Immunocytochemical techniques using the MAb SY38 have documented the presence of synaptophysin in both primary tumors and metastases of these neuroendocrine tumors, and this technique may potentially be useful for diagnosis using both CSF and needle-aspiration biopsies.[51]

The soluble protein S-100 was originally reported as a CNS marker to distinguish schwannomas from histologically similar tissues. More recent studies have demonstrated S-100 also in neural crest–derived tumors, and varying levels of S-100 in glioblastomas, anaplastic astrocytomas, oligodendrogliomas, and acoustic neuromas. Although the levels of S-100 have not been demonstrated to be useful in either diagnostic studies or as prognostic indicators, S-100 is highly useful in antibody panels for malignant melanoma, including CSF cytology and fine-needle stereotactic brain biopsies.[47]

Neural crest–derived melanoma cells have been used to produce MAbs which also recognize antigens on neuroectodermal tumors. These antigens have been identified as gangliosides, including GD2, GD3, and GM3.[18,31] These gangliosides are generally found in fetal brain but are also present in normal brain, retina, and kidney.[37,41] The identification of novel tumor-associated gangliosides such as 3′-iso-LM1, a ganglioside specific for human malignant gliomas,[19] and the production of MAbs directed against them is

TABLE 26-1 MAb Reactivity with CNS Tumors*

Diagnosis	No. Cases	FD19	UJ13A	UJ127.11	UJ181.4	LE61	2D1	A$_2$B$_5$
Malignant glioma	31	+	+	1	5	−	−	+
Astrocytoma	18	+	+	−	−	−	−	+
Oligodendroglioma	6	+	+	−	3	−	−	+
Ependymoma	14	+	+	−	−	−	−	+
Schwannoma	10	−	+	+	−	−	−	+
Meningioma	14	−	+	−	−	−	−	+
Medulloblastoma	10	+	+	8	+	−	−	+
Neuroblastoma	2	−	+	+	+	−	−	+
Primitive neuroectodermal tumor	3	−	+	−	−	−	−	+
Choroid plexus tumor	3	−	−	−	−	+	−	−
Metastatic carcinoma	41	−	5	−	1	36	−	26
Primary brain lymphoma	9	−	−	−	−	−	+	−
Spinal extradural lymphoma	3	−	−	−	−	−	+	−
Total	164							

*From Coakham et al.[12]

a promising area of current research, with potential future in vitro and in vivo applications.

Shared nervous system–lymphoid cell markers were first described in 1964 by Reif and Allen using a polyclonal antiserum which detected an antigen present on murine lymphocytes and brain cells, Thy 1.[42] This and other similar antigens have been reported on B and T cells from a variety of animal species and humans, as well as on human brain, glioma, melanoma, endometrial carcinoma, and osteosarcoma. These antigens have been demonstrated using MAbs originally prepared against either lymphoid or neuroectodermal tumor cells. Seeger et al. reported an anti-Thy-1 MAb, prepared using fetal brain as an immunogen, which reacts with glioma, neuroblastoma, rhabdomyosarcoma, leiomyosarcoma, and teratoma cell lines, but not medulloblastoma, melanoma, or carcinoma cell lines.[45] It appears that the anti-Thy-1 reactivity of these cells may be due to homology between the Thy 1.2 protein and actin. Another MAb, PI 153/3 recognizes an antigen present on glioma, neuroblastoma, retinoblastoma, null, B cell ALL, and B cell CLL cells. This antigen appears to be present on fetal brain and B lymphocytes.

A number of tumor-associated antigens have been described which are shared by human neuroectodermal tumors and oncofetal tissue, including both fetal CNS and lymphoid tissues. The MAbs defining these antigens have been produced using melanoma or glioma cell lines, or fetal brain as immunogens. These MAbs generally have a restricted reactivity pattern, including gliomas, neuroblastomas, and melanomas.

Using MAbs of varying specificities, a panel of MAbs may be constructed to aid in the diagnosis of CNS tumors. Coakham et al. reported 164 cases of CNS tumors in which immunohistochemistry was performed using a panel of seven MAbs.[12] The panel was most useful in the diagnosis of small round cell tumors, such as lymphoma or neuroblastoma, but most other CNS tumors were also accurately characterized (Table 26-1). UJ13A is an MAb produced using fetal brain as an immunogen and which recognizes a membrane protein on normal and neoplastic neuroectoderm. UJ127.11 was also produced with fetal brain as an immuno-

gen and recognizes a membrane glycoprotein present on neuroblastic tissues and tumors, and schwannomas. UJ181.4 was produced using fetal brain as an immunogen and recognizes a membrane protein on neuroblastic tumors. FD19 is an anti-GFAP MAb, produced using an astrocytoma as immunogen. LE61 recognizes a cytoplasmic cytokeratin on simple epithelium and carcinomas. 2D1 recognizes a membrane protein on leukocytes and lymphomas. A$_2$B$_5$ recognizes an epitope which is broadly distributed on gangliosides.

More recently, a panel of MAbs has been utilized in the evaluation of CSF cytology specimens to accurately differentiate between primary brain tumors, metastases, leukemias, and lymphomas (Table 26-2).[49] The antibodies utilized included UJ13A and 2D1 as discussed above, along with a panel of three anti-GFAP MAbs, and B72.3, which recognizes a carcinoma-distinctive tumor-associated glycoprotein complex. The use of such panels of MAbs in both immunohistochemistry and immunocytochemistry may serve to supplement conventional histologic and cytologic techniques in the diagnosis of CNS tumors. A similar approach has been taken for the diagnosis of malignant melanoma in cytologic preparations from a variety of body sites including CSF. Most melanomas stain with Mel-14, antisera against S-100

TABLE 26-2 MAb Reactivity Patterns in Cytologic Analysis*

	UJ13A	α-GFAP	B72.3	2D1
Glioma	+	+	−	±
Normal brain	+	+	−	−
Nonglial primary CNS tumors	+	−	−	−
Small-cell undifferentiated carcinoma and embryonal rhabdomyosarcoma	+	−	−	−
Non–small cell carcinoma	−	−	+	−
Melanoma	−	−	−	−
Lymphoma-leukemia	−	−	−	+
Inflammation	−	−	−	+

*From Vick et al.[49]

protein, or both, while these tumors are usually negative for expression of cytokeratin, B72.3, and 2D-1 (Fig. 26-1).[47] This pattern allows their distinction from metastatic carcinoma and lymphoma conditions, which frequently present a problem in differential diagnosis. Although many primary CNS tumors exhibit the same pattern of staining as melanoma with these antibodies, they can readily be differentiated using UJ13A and GFAP, which are consistently negative in melanomas.[49] Currently, however, there are no MAbs available which will distinguish the tissue of origin of the most frequent sources of metastasis, which include lung, breast, and stomach. Furthermore, reagents are not yet available which will consistently distinguish reactive astrocytes from astrocytoma, or distinguish between glial tumors of astrocytic, oligodendroglial, or ependymal origin.

Panels of MAbs and monospecific antisera may be used to detect phenotypic differences between tumor cell lines. He et al. were able to distinguish two patterns of antigen expression among four medulloblastoma cell lines.[22] The two "glial" medulloblastoma cell lines expressed HLA antigens, epidermal growth factor (EGF) receptor, and tenascin but not neurofilament protein, whereas the "neuronal" medulloblastoma cell lines expressed neurofilament protein but not HLA antigens, tenascin, or EGF receptor. Phenotypic differences, such as these, may provide a basis for the

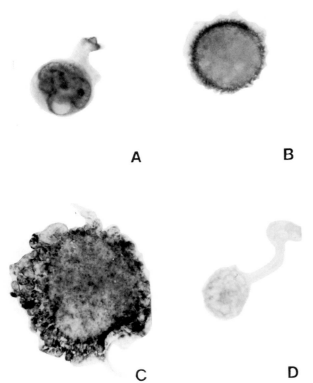

A   B

C   D

Figure 26-1. Metastatic melanoma in CSF. *A.* Cytocentrifuged preparation stained with Papanicolaou's stain shows large malignant tumor cells (×1000). *B.* Immunocytochemistry with Mel-14 demonstrates intensive cytoplasmic staining (×1000). *C.* Immunocytochemistry with a polyclonal S-100 antiserum is also positive (×1000). *D.* Anticarcinoma antibody B72.3 fails to react with these cells in immunocytochemistry (×1000).

investigation of differences in biologic behavior among medulloblastomas, and may be of diagnostic and prognostic value in histologic and cytologic diagnosis and antibody-mediated imaging and therapy.

Another application of MAb technology to CNS tumors is the evaluation of the proliferative potential of tumors. This determination is usually based on histologic criteria, including nuclear cytologic appearance, vascular proliferation, necrosis, and mitotic index, although mitoses are frequently not observed, even in most malignant tumors. More recent autoradiographic techniques utilize tritiated thymidine, either infused preoperatively, or incubated with a tumor biopsy. Immunohistochemical techniques have been developed for the detection of bromodeoxyuridine, a thymidine analog, which is infused preoperatively. These methods are somewhat cumbersome, requiring prior patient selection and diffusion of isotope or thymidine analog into the tumor.

Several nuclear antigens specific for proliferating cells have been described. Ki-67 is an MAb which recognizes a nuclear protein expressed in the G_1, S, G_2, and M phases of the cell cycle. Immunohistochemical techniques utilizing frozen sections have been developed with Ki-67 to demonstrate proliferating cells in CNS neoplasms. The percentage of Ki-67 positive cells was generally in good agreement with histologic grade and the known biologic behavior of various tumors, ranging from less than 1 percent in meningiomas and schwannomas, to 0 to 4.5 percent in low-grade astrocytomas, to 0.7 to 7.4 percent in anaplastic astrocytomas, to 1.7 to 32.2 percent in glioblastoma multiforme, to 57 percent in metastatic carcinomas.[9,61] The potential prognostic significance of this technique is currently under evaluation.

Monoclonal Antibodies in Vivo

The technique of delivering antibodies to tissue in vivo, immunolocalization, was developed by Pressman et al.[40] and Bale and Spar.[1] These studies demonstrated the potential of antibodies to localize in tumors and to alter tumor growth. With the development of MAbs, many of the limitations of immunolocalization with polyclonal antisera were overcome. There remain, however, several obstacles to the in vivo use of MAbs in the diagnosis and treatment of CNS tumors, and an antigen affinity-purified polyclonal serum may provide at least equivalent results to those obtained with a low-affinity MAb.

Human neuroectodermal tumors exhibit a marked phenotypic and genotypic heterogeneity, as evidenced by gliomas, which commonly demonstrate intratumoral variation in both blood-brain barrier permeability and antigen expression.[32,54] The heterogeneity in antigen expression may be cell-cycle dependent, and certain antigens may be temporarily or even permanently lost. This variability may be overcome by using a panel of MAbs, each with differing specificities, in the diagnosis and treatment of CNS tumors.

The specific localization of MAbs within tumors is dependent on the affinity of antibody for antigen, antigen density in the tumor, and the kinetics of transport of MAb within the various biologic compartments. The degree of localization may also be adversely affected by antigen shedding and modulation, as seen with soluble or secreted antigens such as carcinoembryonic antigen. Cross-reactivity of MAbs with shared antigens on normal tissues such as bone marrow also interferes with tumor localization and more importantly could potentially increase toxicity.

The delivery of MAbs to tumors is also influenced by the vascularity of the tumor, vascular permeability, blood flow, and extracellular fluid dynamics within the tumor. The presence of the blood-brain barrier may provide a further hindrance to the delivery of MAbs to CNS tumors, although the limited human data available in general show that the percent localized dose in intracranial tumors is comparable to that in tumors in extracranial sites. The blood-brain barrier exists anatomically at the level of the tight junctions between endothelial cells in cerebral capillaries, restricting the passage of low molecular weight, ionic compounds, as well as higher-molecular-weight molecules, such as proteins, from the blood to the brain. The blood-brain barrier has been shown to be heterogeneous in both human gliomas and in experimental animal tumors, due to the presence of abnormal blood vessels in gliomas, intratumoral variation in vascular permeability, and altered intratumoral blood flow.[21]

The role of delivery to CNS tumors of both MAbs and chemotherapeutic agents has been extensively studied, including such factors as route of delivery (intracarotid, intravenous, intrathecal, and intratumoral), the use of smaller and thus more freely diffusable Fab or F(ab')$_2$ fragments, and transient blood-brain barrier disruption. Direct intracarotid injection offers two potential advantages over the intravenous route: higher levels in tumor and lower systemic toxicity due to the potential for lower doses to achieve equivalent brain levels. Small, lipid-soluble molecules, such as 1,3,-bis-(2-chloroethyl)-1-nitrosourea (BCNU) demonstrate the greatest advantage.[7,17] In rats with a highly permeable experimental human glioma xenograft, even higher-molecular-weight MAbs demonstrated a 20 percent increase in delivery to intracranial tumor with intracarotid versus intravenous administration.[27] However, recent human studies with paired-label intracarotid and intravenous injection in anaplastic glioma patients have shown no intracarotid advantage for the delivery of either IgG or F(ab')$_2$ fragments to tumor.[35] Hyperosmotic blood-brain barrier disruption by intracarotid infusion of mannitol, arabinose, or urea has been shown to increase delivery to normal brain of diverse molecules ranging from methotrexate and adriamycin to proteins such as albumin and immunoglobulin. The effect of blood-brain barrier disruption on tumor permeability is controversial. Neuwelt et al. reported increased delivery of methotrexate to an intracranial xenograft of a human small cell lung carcinoma,[36] but other reports indicate only a modest increase in methotrexate delivery to intracranial tumors, at the expense of 10- to 25-fold higher levels in normal brain.[46] Since many of the chemotherapeutic agents are neurotoxic, the nonspecific increase in drug delivery to the normal CNS may be harmful. MAbs which bind specifically to tumor antigens have a potential advantage over nonspecific chemotherapeutic agents. Hyperosmolar blood-brain barrier disruption has been shown to dramatically increase the delivery of MAb to normal brain.[8] The potential for blood-brain barrier disruption to increase delivery of MAbs to

CNS tumors remains to be determined. Other methods of circumventing the blood-brain barrier include intrathecal administration, especially for neoplastic meningitis (both from primary CNS tumors such as medulloblastoma and pineoblastoma and from carcinomas or lymphoid neoplasms), and direct intratumoral injection.

MAb administration alone has been shown to have therapeutic benefit in both animal models and patients. These responses appear to require the Fc portion of the immunoglobulin, with complement-mediated cytolysis resulting in tumor cell necrosis without inflammatory infiltrates or as an antibody-dependent cell-mediated cytotoxicity. The efficacy of these mechanisms varies with immunoglobulin isotype, and careful MAb selection may be required to demonstrate therapeutic efficacy of passive serotherapy in patients.

Once the issues of delivery and specific localization are resolved, MAbs hold tremendous potential as carriers of radionuclides or drugs for diagnosis and treatment of brain tumors. For purposes of localization, imaging, and treatment, MAbs have been successfully conjugated to a variety of toxins such as the plant toxins ricin and abrin and bacterial toxins such as diphtheria toxin A and the toxin of *Pseudomonas aeruginosa*; to drugs such as methotrexate and chlorambucil; and to both halogen and metallic radionuclides, including ^{123}I, ^{131}I, and ^{111}In. In addition, MAbs have also been shown to have direct toxicity through antibody-mediated immunologic mechanisms.

Immunotoxins are cytotoxic reagents composed of an MAb linked to a protein toxin. The plant toxins ricin and abrin have served as model agents, being composed of A chains which catalytically inhibit protein synthesis and a B chain which binds the toxin nonselectively to cell-surface receptors and facilitates the entry of the A chain into the cell. Either the A chain alone or that intact toxin may be coupled to the MAb. A variety of animal and human tumor model systems have been used, with demonstrated efficacy using MAbs directed at antigens such as Thy-1 or the transferrin receptor.[57,60] The A-chain conjugate demonstrates greater cell specificity than the whole toxin conjugate but also decreased toxicity, rendering the A-chain conjugate effective only against smaller tumors. The bacterial toxins of *Corynebacterium diphtheriae* and *Pseudomonas aeruginosa* are similar to the plant toxins discussed above but differ in their site of toxicity from ricin in enzymatically inactivating the eukaryotic ribosomal elongation factor EF-2. There are two main disadvantages to their potential clinical use: (1) they are more difficult to obtain than plant toxins, and (2) a significant percentage of the population has been actively immunized against diphtheria.

Chemotherapeutic agents may also be coupled to MAbs, to increase the specificity of drug delivery to tumor and maintain therapeutic levels in tumor with decreased systemic toxicity. MAb-drug conjugates have been studied in a variety of model tumor systems, utilizing such agents as methotrexate, chlorambucil, and melphalan,[3] but the most encouraging results were obtained in a rat mammary carcinoma in which an MAb-adriamycin conjugate significantly delayed tumor growth and prolonged survival in tumor-bearing animals, with a fivefold lower dose than with adriamycin alone.

Radionuclides coupled to MAbs offer several advantages

over the agents discussed above. The pharmacokinetics and dosimetry of radionuclides can be more easily monitored and quantitated in vivo through the use of direct tissue counting, radioscintigraphy, and quantitative autoradiography. Furthermore, for alpha and beta emitters, the radionuclide does not have to enter the cell to exert its tumoricidal effect, because these radiations are effective over distances between several cell diameters (alphas) and hundreds of cell diameters (betas). This is also a disadvantage, particularly for beta emitters, because normal tissue is also exposed to ionizing radiation. The goal of MAb-radionuclide therapy is to target rapidly as much radionuclide as possible to tumor while minimizing exposure of normal tissues.

Several MAbs have been shown to specifically localize in subcutaneous and intracranial human glioma xenografts in athymic mice and rats.[55] Of these, the MAb 81C6 is the best studied. 81C6 recognizes a 220,000-MW glioma-mesenchymal matrix protein present on gliomas and melanoma. In paired-label studies, higher levels of ^{125}I-81C6, compared to a nonspecific control antibody, were localized in intracranial and subcutaneous human glioma xenografts in athymic mice by 24 to 48 h, with tumor uptake persisting for 5 to 7 days.[4] The specific localization of 81C6 allowed imaging of intracranial human glioma xenografts as small as 20 mg in athymic rats. Only tumors greater than 300 mg could be imaged with nonspecific control antibody.[5] Treatment studies with ^{131}I-81C6 in subcutaneous human glioma xenografts in athymic mice demonstrated significant tumor growth delays with 500 to 1000 μCi doses.[28] Similarly, significant survival benefits were seen with ^{131}I-81C6 in intracranial human glioma xenografts in athymic rats, using doses up to 2.5 mCi, with several cures.[26] In both studies, the smaller or absent response following ^{131}I-control antibody administration demonstrated the specificity of the therapeutic effects.

Immunoglobulin fragments, such as Fab and F(ab')$_2$, offer many potential advantages over intact immunoglobulin as carriers of radionuclides. The fragments are more rapidly cleared from tissues and from plasma, resulting in lower background for imaging studies, and lower normal tissue radiation exposure. Also, the smaller fragments may more easily penetrate the blood-brain barrier to gain access to tumor. The absence of the Fc portion of the molecule may reduce the immunogenicity of the murine protein administered to humans and may also result in decreased nonspecific Fc-mediated binding, especially limiting nonspecific binding to bone marrow and other cells of the reticuloendothelial system.

The Fab fragment of 81C6 is a low-affinity fragment with a single antigen recognition site. It undergoes rapid plasma clearance (7.1 h versus 2.1 days for intact 81C6) and localizes in both subcutaneous and intracranial human glioma xenografts in athymic mice but at lower levels than intact 81C6.[14] Dosimetry calculations suggest the rapid plasma clearance could yield improved tumor-to-tissue radiation dose ratios with short-lived nuclides, such as the alpha emitters like ^{211}At or ^{212}Bi.

A higher-affinity divalent F(ab')$_2$ fragment cannot be generated from 81C6 because it is of the IgG$_{2b}$ subclass. Mel-14 is in IgG2a, which can yield F(ab')$_2$ fragments. Mel-14 recognizes a membrane chondroitin sulfate proteoglycan present in melanomas, gliomas, and some medulloblasto-

mas. Using the athymic mouse-human glioma xenograft model described above, the Mel-14 F(ab')$_2$ fragment was shown to rapidly localize in subcutaneous or intracranial tumor as early as 6 to 8 h, with more favorable tumor to normal tissue radiation dose ratios than intact Mel-14.[15]

Based on the encouraging results of these animal studies, phase I imaging of patients with gliomas has been performed with several MAbs, including 81C6 and Mel-14 F(ab')$_2$. Paired-label investigations have compared the pharmacokinetics of ^{131}I-81C6 and isotype-matched control antibody 45.6 labeled with ^{125}I. Examination of tissue obtained at craniotomy revealed localization indices for 81C6 as high as five for tumor, while values of about one were obtained for normal brain.[34] These data demonstrate that uptake and retention of 81C6 in tumor are related to its specificity and are not simply the result of nonspecific accumulation due to alteration in blood-brain barrier by tumor. No toxicity has been observed in patients receiving as much as 50 mg of 81C6 MAb.

One promising application of MAb-targeted radiotherapy is in patients with carcinomatous meningitis. Lashford et al. reported the treatment of a group of five patients with leptomeningeal spread of tumors such as lymphoma, melanoma, and ependymoma with 11 to 40 mCi ^{131}I-coupled to MAbs.[25] Imaging studies were performed to document the distribution and retention of radioactivity within the CNS (Fig. 26-2). Four of five demonstrated an objective improvement in response to treatment, lasting from 7 months to 2 years. No clinical signs of chronic toxicity have been observed in follow-up up to 2 years after therapy.

The potential of radiolabeled monoclonal antibodies for improving the diagnosis and treatment of brain tumors has only begun to be explored. Second- and third-generation antibodies of higher affinity for tumors with less reactivity with normal tissues are already under development. With

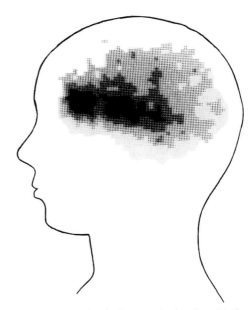

Figure 26-2. Lateral scintigram obtained at 14 days after intrathecal injection of ^{131}I-UJ181.4 showing basal uptake in a patient with neoplastic meningitis from a pineal tumor. (From Lashford et al.[25])

regard to the nuclide, most studies to date with MAb and brain tumors have used ^{131}I as the label. A significant problem with the use of radiohalogenated MAb is that they are often extensively dehalogenated in vivo, resulting in a decreased cumulative radiation dose to tumor. Recently, a new antibody radioiodination method has been reported which has decreased the loss of ^{131}I from MAb in vivo and also has increased the retention of antibody affinity after labeling.[59] These two factors have increased the cumulative radiation dose to tumors by as much as sixfold compared to conventional iodination methods.

Other nuclides with physical properties different from ^{131}I will be more optimal for some applications of labeled MAb. Preliminary studies using 81C6 labeled with ^{123}I have shown the advantages of single-photon computed tomography for imaging gliomas. For radiotherapy, alpha emitters such as the 7.2-h radiohalogen [211]At offer certain advantages. Compared to the beta particles of ^{131}I, they have a higher radiobiologic effectiveness, and their cytotoxic effects are nearly oxygen-independent, offering the possibility of treating hypoxic areas of tumor. The range of alpha particles is only a few cell diameters, making them ideal for the treatment of leptomeningeal disease because of its surface nature and the proximity of radiation-sensitive normal CNS tissues. Recently, a new method for labeling MAb with [211]At without loss of immunoreactivity has been reported.[58] Another possibility for antibodies which are rapidly internalized by tumor cells is to use extremely low energy Auger electron emitters which are highly radiotoxic if localized in close proximity to DNA. This approach is being investigated by the Wistar group using an anti-EGF receptor MAb labeled with [125]I.[56]

In summary, better antibodies, improved labeling methods, more optimal radionuclides, and more favorable routes of delivery are all under investigation. Advances in these areas have the potential to transform the labeled antibody approach from a research tool to a clinically useful technique for the diagnosis and treatment of brain tumors.

References

1. Bale WF, Spar IL. Studies directed toward the use of antibodies as carriers of radioactivity for therapy. *Adv Biol Med Phys* 1957; 5:285–356.
2. Bigner DD. Biology of gliomas: potential clinical implications of glioma cellular heterogeneity. *Neurosurgery* 1981; 9:320–326.
3. Bourdon MA, Coleman RE, Bigner, DD. The potential of monoclonal antibodies as carriers of radiation and drugs for immunodetection and therapy of brain tumors. *Prog Exp Tumor Res* 1984; 28:79–101.
4. Bourdon MA, Wikstrand CJ, Furthmayr H, et al. Human glioma-mesenchymal extracellular matrix antigen defined by monoclonal antibody. *Cancer Res* 1983; 43:2796–2805.
5. Bullard DE, Adams CJ, Coleman RE, et al. In vivo imaging of intracranial human glioma xenografts comparing specific with nonspecific radiolabeled monoclonal antibodies. *J Neurosurg* 1986; 64:257–262.
6. Bullard DE, Bigner DD. Applications of monoclonal antibodies in the diagnosis and treatment of primary brain tumors. *J Neurosurg* 1985; 63:2–16.
7. Bullard DE, Bigner SH, Bigner DD. Comparison of intrave-

nous versus intracarotid therapy with 1,3-bis (2-chloroethyl)-1-nitrosourea in a rat brain tumor model. *Cancer Res* 1985; 45:5240–5245.
8. Bullard DE, Bourdon M, Bigner DD. Comparison of various methods for delivering radiolabeled monoclonal antibody to normal rat brain. *J Neurosurg* 1984; 61:901–911.
9. Burger PC, Shibata T, Kleihues P. The use of the monoclonal antibody Ki-67 in the identification of proliferating cells: application to surgical neuropathology. *Am J Surg Pathol* 1986; 10:611–617.
10. Carrel S, deTribolet N, Mach JP. Expression of neuroectodermal antigens common to melanomas, gliomas, and neuroblastomas: I. Identification by monoclonal anti-melanoma and anti-glioma antibodies. *Acta Neuropathol (Berl)* 1982; 57:158–164.
11. Coakham H. Surface antigen(s) common to human astrocytoma cells. *Nature* 1974; 250:328–330.
12. Coakham HB, Garson JA, Allan PA, et al. Immunohistological diagnosis of central nervous system tumours using a monoclonal antibody panel. *J Clin Pathol* 1985; 38:165–173.
13. Coakham HB, Lakshmi MS. Tumour-associated surface antigen(s) in human astrocytomas. *Oncology* 1975; 31:233–243.
14. Colapinto EV, Humphrey PA, Zalutsky MR, et al. Comparative localization of murine monoclonal antibody Mel-14 F(ab′)$_2$ fragment and whole IgG2a in human glioma xenografts. *Cancer Res* 1988; 48:5701–5707.
15. Colapinto EV, Lee YS, Humphrey PA, et al. The localization of radiolabeled murine monoclonal antibody 81C6 and its Fab fragment in human glioma xenografts in athymic mice. *Br J Neurosurg* 1988; 2:179–191.
16. Ehrlich P. *Collected Studies on Immunity*. New York: Wiley, 1906.
17. Fenstermacher J, Cowles AL. Theoretical limitations of intracarotid infusions in brain tumor chemotherapy. *Cancer Treat Rep* 1977; 61:519–526.
18. Fredman P, von Holst H, Collins VP, et al. Potential ganglioside antigens associated with human gliomas. *Neurol Res* 1986; 8:123–126.
19. Fredman P, von Holst H, Collins VP, et al. Sialyllactotetraosylceramide, a ganglioside marker for human malignant gliomas. *J Neurochem* 1988; 50:912–919.
20. Gould VE, Wiedenmann B, Lee I, et al. Synaptophysin expression in neuroendocrine neoplasms as determined by immunocytochemistry *Am J Pathol* 1987; 126:243–257.
21. Groothuis DR, Molnar P, Blasberg RG. Regional blood flow and blood to tissue transport in five brain tumor models. *Prog Exp Tumor Res* 1984; 27:132–153.
22. He X, Skapek SX, Wikstrand CJ, et al. Phenotypic analysis of four human medulloblastoma cell lines and transplantable xenografts. *J Neuropathol Exp Neurol* 1989; 48:48–68.
23. Iglehart JD, Weinhold KJ, Ward EC, et al. Prospects for the immunological management of lethal tumors. *Cancer Invest* 1983; 1:409–421.
24. Köhler G, Milstein C. Continuous cultures of fused cells secreting antibody of predefined specificity. *Nature* 1975; 256:495–497.
25. Lashford LS, Davies AG, Richardson RB, et al. A pilot study of ^{131}I monoclonal antibodies in the therapy of leptomeningeal tumors. *Cancer* 1988; 61:857–868.
26. Lee YS, Bullard DE, Humphrey PA, et al. Treatment of intracranial human glioma xenografts with ^{131}I-labeled anti-tenascin monoclonal antibody 81C6. *Cancer Res* 1988; 48:2904–2910.
27. Lee YS, Bullard DE, Wikstrand CJ, et al. Comparison of monoclonal antibody delivery to intracranial glioma xenografts by intravenous and intracarotid administration. *Cancer Res* 1987; 47:1941–1946.
28. Lee YS, Bullard DE, Zalutsky MR, et al. Therapeutic efficacy of antiglioma mesenchymal extracellular matrix ^{131}I-radiola-

beled murine monoclonal antibody in a human glioma xenograft model. *Cancer Res* 1988; 48:559–566.

29. Mahaley MS Jr. Experiences with antibody production from human glioma tissue. *Prog Exp Tumor Res* 1972; 17:31–39.

30. Mahaley MS Jr, Day ED: Immunological studies of human gliomas. *J Neurosurg* 1965; 23:363–370.

31. Månsson JE, Fredman P, Bigner DD, et al. Characterization of new gangliosides of the lactotetraose series in murine xenografts of a human glioma cell line. *FEBS Lett* 1986; 201:109–113.

32. McComb RD, Bigner DD. The biology of malignant gliomas: a comprehensive survey. *Clin Neuropathol* 1984; 3:93–106.

33. Miyake E, Kitamura K, Nomoto K, et al. An attempt to detect cell surface antigens in cultured human brain tumors by mixed hemadsorption test: first report. *Acta Neuropathol (Berl)* 1977; 37:27–29.

34. Moseley R, Zalutsky MR, Coakham HB, et al. Distribution of I-131 81C6 monoclonal antibody (Mab) administered via carotid artery in patients with glioma (G). *J Nucl Med* 1987; 28:603–604 (abstr).

35. Moseley R, Zalutsky MR, Coakham HB, et al. Monoclonal antibody imaging of gliomas: comparison of intracarotid and intravenous administration in patients. *J Nucl Med* 1988; 29:897 (abstr).

36. Neuwelt EA, Frenkel EP, D'Agostino AN, et al. Growth of human lung tumor in the brain of the nude rat as a model to evaluate antitumor agent delivery across the blood-brain barrier. *Cancer Res* 1985; 45:2827–2833.

37. Nudelman E, Hakomori S, Kannagi R, et al. Characterization of a human melanoma-associated ganglioside antigen defined by a monoclonal antibody, 4.2. *J Biol Chem* 1982; 257:12,752–12,756.

38. Palma L, DiLorenzo N, Guidetti B. Lymphocytic infiltrates in primary glioblastomas and recidivous gliomas: incidence, fate, and relevance to prognosis in 228 operated cases. *J Neurosurg* 1978; 49:854–861.

39. Phillips J, Alderson T, Sikora K, et al. Localization of malignant glioma by a radiolabelled human monoclonal antibody. *J Neurol Neurosurg Psychiatry* 1983; 46:388–392.

40. Pressman D, Day ED, Blau M. The use of paired labeling in the determination of tumor-localizing antibodies. *Cancer Res* 1957; 17:845–850.

41. Pukel CS, Lloyd KO, Travassos LR, et al. GD$_3$, a prominent ganglioside of human melanoma: detection and characterization by mouse monoclonal antibody. *J Exp Med* 1982; 155:1133–1147.

42. Reif AE, Allen JMV. The AKR thymic antigen and its distribution in leukemias and nervous tissues. *J Exp Med* 1964; 120:413–433.

43. Ridley A, Cavanagh JB. Lymphocytic infiltration in gliomas: evidence of possible host resistance. *Brain* 1971; 94:117–124.

44. Sato K, Raimondi AJ, Dray S, et al. Comparison of tumor-associated surface antigens on cells from medulloblastomas and from other neoplasms of the human nervous system. *Childs Brain* 1978; 4:83–94.

45. Seeger RC, Danon YL, Rayner SA, et al. Definition of a Thy-1 determinant on human neuroblastoma, glioma, sarcoma, and

teratoma cells with a monoclonal antibody. *J Immunol* 1982; 128:983–989.

46. Shapiro WR, Voorhies RM, Hiesiger EM, et al. Pharmacokinetics of tumor cell exposure to [^{14}C] methotrexate after intracarotid administration without and with hyperosmotic opening of the blood-brain and blood-tumor barriers in rat brain tumors: a quantitative autoradiographic study. *Cancer Res* 1988; 48:694–701.

47. Shoup SA, Tello JW, Seigler HF, et al. The immunocytochemical diagnosis of metastatic melanoma in cytologic specimens. *Acta Cytol* (in press).

48. Verhoeyen M, Milstein C, Winter G. Reshaping human antibodies: grafting an antilysozyme activity. *Science* 1988; 239:1534–1536.

49. Vick WW, Wikstrand CJ, Bullard DE, et al. The use of a panel of monoclonal antibodies in the evaluation of cytologic specimens from the central nervous system. *Acta Cytol* 1987; 31:815–824.

50. Wiedenmann B, Franke WW, Kuhn C, et al. Synaptophysin: a marker protein for neuroendocrine cells and neoplasms. *Proc Natl Acad Sci USA* 1986; 83:3500–3504.

51. Wiedenmann B, Kuhn C, Schwechheimer K, et al. Synaptophysin identified in metastases of neuroendocrine tumors by immunocytochemistry and immunoblotting. *Am J Clin Pathol* 1987; 88:560–569.

52. Wikstrand CJ, Bigner DD. Immunobiologic aspects of the brain and human gliomas. *Am J Pathol* 1980; 98:515–568.

53. Wikstrand CJ, Bigner DD. Expression of human fetal brain antigens by human tumors of neuroectodermal origin as defined by monoclonal antibodies. *Cancer Res* 1982; 42:267–275.

54. Wikstrand CJ, Bigner SH, Bigner DD. Demonstration of complex antigenic heterogeneity in a human glioma cell line and eight derived clones by specific monoclonal antibodies. *Cancer Res* 1983; 43:3327–3334.

55. Wikstrand CJ, McLendon RE, Carrel S, et al. Comparative localization of glioma-reactive monoclonal antibodies in vivo in an athymic mouse human glioma xenograft model. *J Neuroimmunol* 1987; 15:37–56.

56. Woo DV, Brady LW, Karlsson U, et al. Radioimmunotherapy of human gliomas using I-125 labeled monoclonal antibody to epidermal growth factor receptor. *J Nucl Med* 1988; 29:847 (abstr).

57. Youle RJ, Neville DM Jr. Kinetics of protein synthesis inactivation by ricin-anti-Thy 1.1 monoclonal antibody hybrids: role of the ricin B subunit demonstrated by reconstitution. *J Biol Chem* 1982; 257:1598–1601.

58. Zalutsky MR, Garg PK, Narula AS. Labeling monoclonal antibodies with halogen nuclides. *Acta Radiol* (in press).

59. Zalutsky MR, Narula AS. Radiohalogenation of a monoclonal antibody using an N-succinimidyl 3-(tri-n-butylstannyl) benzoate intermediate. *Cancer Res* 1988; 48:1446–1450.

60. Zovickian J, Youle RJ. Efficacy of intrathecal immunotoxin therapy in an animal model of leptomeningeal neoplasia. *J Neurosurg* 1988; 68:767–774.

61. Zuber P, Hamou M-F, deTribolet N. Identification of proliferating cells in human gliomas using the monoclonal antibody Ki-67. *Neurosurgery* 1988; 22:364–368.

27

Photoradiation Therapy for Malignant Gliomas

Edward R. Laws, Jr.
Robert E. Wharen, Jr.
Robert E. Anderson

The concept of photoradiation therapy (PRT) is based upon the ability of certain substances known as photosensitizers to concentrate preferentially in malignant tissue. These photosensitizers then have the capability for the selective destruction of malignant tissue when activated by light of the appropriate wavelength and intensity in the presence of oxygen. Phototherapy, photodynamic therapy, and photochemotherapy are all terms for this phenomenon of photoradiation therapy.

The action of a photosensitizer is produced by the absorption of photons of a wavelength sufficient to promote electrons within the sensitizer to an excited triplet state. This excited molecule may then interact either directly with substrates within a cell or indirectly with those substrates through the production of singlet oxygen ($^1O_2$). The various photochemical reactions that are excited by light are subsequently capable of killing cells through multiple interactions with the cell membrane, cytoplasm, nuclear membrane, and nucleus.

An ideal photosensitizer should (1) be nontoxic to normal tissues, (2) be selectively absorbed or retained by all neoplastic or dysplastic cells, (3) have some characteristic such as fluorescence that makes it easily detectable, and (4) be efficient in killing malignant tissue following the application of light at a wavelength capable of significant tissue penetration.

The search for an ideal photosensitizer is currently being pursued. Although far from ideal, the photosensitizer which has received the most extensive investigation both in the laboratory and clinically is hematoporphyrin derivative (HpD).

History of Photoradiation Therapy

The first application of HpD to the management of brain tumors took place in the 1950s at The Johns Hopkins Hospital.[29,35] At that time, a series of experiments were performed to evaluate HpD fluorescence in the detection of brain tumors at the time of surgery. These experiments demonstrated that detectable levels of HpD would concentrate in brain tumors and that HpD was effectively excluded by an intact blood-brain barrier.

The first studies that suggested that photoactivation of HpD might be cytotoxic to brain tumors were performed in 1975.[15] In a tumor model system, cell death was produced by exposure of the tumor containing HpD to light. Interest in this phenomenon was rekindled in Italy,[26,27] Australia,[13] and the United States[21] in 1980–1981 when several groups reported the initial results of photodynamic therapy (PDT) directed toward brain tumors in humans.

The application of PRT in neurosurgery was initially very encouraging. A number of investigators have reported the capability of HpD to kill glioma cells both in vitro and in vivo.[2,4–6,11,14,31,34] More recent reports have described additional attempts at the use of PRT for the treatment of malignant brain tumors,[10,17,20,22–25,28,32,33] and although the results are equivocal, it is evident that despite major differences in the protocols by various investigators, HpD phototherapy is capable of tumor cell destruction in humans. Hematoporphyrin is not entirely contained within neoplastic tissue, and some HpD accumulates in brain tissue. This small amount of HpD within normal brain tissue can produce significant morbidity and mortality in experimental animals upon application of a sufficient dose of light.[7]

Efforts to quantitate the uptake of hematoporphyrin within tumors and normal tissue have been performed,[12,18,30] and Wharen et al. have quantitated the amount of HpD achieved in human gliomas and normal brain tissue 24 to 48 h after the administration of 5 mg/kg HpD.[31] The uniformity of brain tumor uptake was assessed by Boggan et al.,[6] who found considerable heterogeneity of uptake in their tumor model and attributed cell death in such tumors as much to an effect on the vasculature[3] as to direct toxicity to tumor cells.

Current efforts are being directed toward an understanding of the fundamental principles and the scientific application of this modality of PRT. This has been stimulated by the desire to develop a treatment which may open new possibilities for therapy of malignant tumors where surgery, radiotherapy, and chemotherapy are inadequate.

Current Status of Photoradiation Therapy

Analysis of the Photoactive Drug

In parallel with our initial clinical investigations,[21] a number of laboratory experiments were performed. These utilized cell culture models of human and experimental brain tumors and an animal model of malignant ethylnitrosourea (ENU)–induced brain tumors in rats.[31,35] These experiments have confirmed HpD photodynamic cytotoxicity for brain tumor cells at practical concentrations of HpD and achievable doses of light. They also provided information relative to the time course and quantitative aspects of HpD concentration within the tumor cells. Several aspects of PDT were elucidated by these studies. First, a dose of 5 mg/kg of HpD seemed adequate. Second, a delay of 4 to 24 h resulted in satisfactory concentrations of HpD in the tumor cells and optimal tumor/brain ratios. Third, the exclusion of HpD by an intact blood-brain barrier was again confirmed. Fourth, the superiority of violet light (405 nm) activation to red light activation was confirmed. Fifth, the superiority of red light (633 nm) to violet light penetration of brain and brain tumor was confirmed. More recent experiments have suggested that the postulated cytotoxic mechanisms are dependent upon production of singlet oxygen in these experimental brain tumors.[10,16]

The optimum time to administer photoradiation therapy after drug administration would be when the HpD concentration in tumor is maximum, as compared to normal brain, provided that the absolute amount in normal brain is low enough to be nontoxic. Although Wharen et al. noted a ratio approximately twofold higher at 4 h compared to 24 h after drug administration,[31] Boggan et al. found maximal ratios at 24 h.[4] This ratio will also be dependent upon the HpD preparation, and further development is necessary before the timing of photoradiation therapy after drug administration can be optimized. Efforts to use subfractions of HpD (Hp, porphyrin C) or other photoactive compounds such as phthalocyanines, are also being investigated.

The toxicity of HpD in clinical applications has thus far been limited primarily to skin sensitization. Patients must remain out of bright sunlight for approximately 4 weeks after drug administration. McCulloch et al. have also reported one patient who developed cerebral edema following the administration of 150 J/cm^2 of red light 48 h after the injection of 5 mg/kg of HpD.[24] As suggested by El-Far and Pimstone[12] and Dougherty,[10] the use of a more pure preparation of HpD or a different porphyrin such as uroporphyrin-I may limit or eventually eliminate skin toxicity.

Analysis of the Drug-Light Interaction

The action mechanism in PRT and in dye-sensitized photooxidation reactions for both in vitro and in vivo systems has been an area of avid research from which some understanding of the basic processes involved has developed.

With few exceptions, photosensitized oxidations proceed by way of a triplet sensitizer. The excited triplet state (^3S) of the sensitizer (S) is produced by the absorption of a photon of light with an energy sufficient to raise the sensitizer to an excited singlet state (^1S). Subsequent intersystem crossing results in the transformation of an excited singlet state (^1S) to an excited triplet state (^3S), because the direct excitation of the triplet state (^3S) from the ground state (S) is a forbidden process.

The excited triplet state (^3S) can then react with biologic substrates by two major mechanisms: either directly with the substrate (type I) by electron or hydrogen-ion transfer, or indirectly with the substrate (type II) through the production of singlet molecular oxygen.

The efficiency of each path is dependent upon the relative concentrations of oxygen (O_2) and substrate available for the sensitizer (^3S) to react, and the relative rate constants for each reaction (K_{O_2} and K_S) and for the rate of triplet decay (K_d). The overall process is limited by the quantum yield of triplet sensitizer formation. The rate constants will be dependent upon such factors as the chemical structure of the sensitizer (^3S), the aggregation state of the porphyrin, and the nature of the reaction medium.

The transfer of energy from the excited triplet state of the sensitizer (^3S) to oxygen proceeds by a process of electronic or resonance energy transfer, which is a diffusion-controlled process. The $^1O_2$-producing ability of photoexcited porphyrins and hence their photosensitizing efficiency is directly related to the lifetime or the decay rate of the porphyrin triplet state.

Dougherty et al. proposed in 1976 that singlet oxygen ($^1O_2$) was the cytotoxic agent responsible for the in vitro inactivation of TA-3 mouse mammary carcinoma cells exposed to HpD photoradiation using red light therapy.[11] $^1O_2$ was produced by the transfer of energy from an excited triplet state of hematoporphyrin to oxygen with a quantum yield for $^1O_2$ of 0.16 within the TA-3 cells. Further work has demonstrated that although most porphyrin-sensitized reactions occur via a type II mechanism involving $^1O_2$, other type I mechanisms involving electron transfer may be important. It has been documented that HpD (photofrin I and II) which consists of porphyrin aggregates produces $^1O_2$ with significantly smaller yields than Hp. Thus, although the use of $^1O_2$ quenchers such as β-carotene, ascorbic acid, and N_3 along with the enhancing effect of D_2O on the production of $^1O_2$ have clearly demonstrated the participation of $^1O_2$ in reactions in vivo, no photodynamic action so far investigated in vivo is solely explained by the $^1O_2$ mechanism.

The mechanisms responsible for the loss of cell viability in photoradiation therapy are difficult to characterize because of the multiplicity of damaging reactions that occur. Photoradiation of porphyrin-loaded cells results in inhibition of membrane transport functions and membrane damage; effects which may occur from photodynamic cross-linking of membrane proteins. Photodynamic damage to DNA and to lysosomes also occurs.[16]

Proteins, nucleic acids, unsaturated lipids, NADH, NADPH, hyaluronic acid, and other biomolecules are photo-oxidized with porphyrins as sensitizers. The predominant susceptible sites on proteins are the unprotonated thiol group of cysteine, the unprotonated imidazole ring of histidine, the thio-ether group of methionine, the indole ring of tryptophan, and the phenolate anion of tyrosine. Photo-oxidation of these sites on proteins results in the loss of enzymatic and hormonal activity, loss of toxic properties of snake venoms and bacterial toxins, loss of antigenic properties, and loss of antibody reactivity. Unsaturated lipids and cholesterol are converted to hydroperoxides. Nucleic acids are photo-oxidized by porphyrins predominately at guanine residues, and both single and double strand breaks can be produced in DNA.

Inactivation of cells by photoradiation can be classified into three major modes of action. First the porphyrin remains either outside the cell or within the cell membrane. In this case, the cell membrane would be expected to be the major site of photodamage. Membrane damage would result from the photo-oxidation of membrane lipids, structural proteins, and enzymes with resultant inhibition of transport processes, alterations of receptors, changes in permeability, or cross-linking of proteins in the membrane. Second, the porphyrin penetrates into the cytoplasm resulting in damage to mitochondria, lysosomes, ribosomes, and proteins. Cell death would then occur from uncoupling or inhibition of oxidative phosphorylation, leakage of hydrolases from lysosomes into the cytoplasm, and inhibition of microsomal activity. Third, the porphyrin penetrates the nucleus to sensitize the nucleic acids and chromosomes, with resulting chromosomal breaks. As yet, no chromosomal breaks have been demonstrated in mammalian cells. Currently, the modes of action of porphyrin photosensitized reactions are considered to be multifactorial involving predominately the cell membrane and cytoplasm.

Optimization of the parameters of photoradiation therapy involves not only considerations of the uptake, distribution, and action mechanisms of the dye but also considerations of the wavelength, quantity, and energy density of light necessary to achieve cell kill. The action spectrum for porphyrin-sensitized cytotoxicity corresponds closely to the absorption spectrum of the porphyrin. Kinsey et al. found that the cytotoxic action of HpD was directly proportional to the number of light quanta absorbed by HpD in the cell.[19] For thin layers of cells, the Soret band at 405 nm had 12 to 30 times the cytotoxicity of red light.

Anderson et al. investigated the effect of optical spectrum, power density, HpD concentration, and HpD preparation on the HpD tumor cell killing efficiency of MEWO cells in culture.[2] Using a trypan blue exclusion assay, cell survival curves were obtained following irradiation with violet (405 nm), red (630 nm), and white (340 to 680 nm) light at energies of 0 to 320 J and at power densities of 20 to 160 mW/cm^2 for cells exposed for 6 h to HpD concentrations of 0 to 25 μg/ml.

Not only the wavelength and power density but also the type of light appears to affect the cellular killing efficiency of HpD-photoradiation therapy. Cowled et al. observed no difference in the HpD cell killing efficiency of a continuous-wave argon-pumped dye laser using rhodamine B with a wavelength of 625 to 635 nm when compared to a pulsed-wave gold vapor laser at a pulse frequency of 10 to 14 kHz having a wavelength of 627.8 nm.[8] Wharen et al. found a markedly decreased cellular killing efficiency for pulsed red light (625 to 645 nm) produced from a tunable flash-pumped dye laser at a repetition rate of one to six per second compared to continuous-wave red light (625 to 635 nm) from a filtered xenon arc lamp.[33] In addition, it has been reported that pulsed light from a nitrogen laser with a wavelength of 332 nm and a repetition rate of 30 Hz had a HpD cellular killing efficiency greater than that of a continuous

light from an argon ion laser with a wavelength of 334 nm. This was attributed to a mechanism of two-photon absorption and production of cytotoxic radicals of HpD. It appears that not only the wavelength of light but also the form of the light (pulsed versus continuous) and the repetition rate, pulse width, and peak pulse power are all important variables in need of further study.

After all the drug and light parameters have been maximized in HpD photoradiation therapy, the limiting factor in its clinical application may remain the penetration of light through brain and tumor tissue. Light penetration into tissue is determined by the optical characteristics of the tissue, the wavelength of the light, and the concentration of the photosensitizer that has been used. Photons are either absorbed or scattered, and the ultimate penetration of light is both wavelength- and tissue-dependent in an exponential manner.

The relative penetration of light through in vivo cat brain as a function of wavelength has been measured and demonstrates the significantly greater depth of penetration of red light (630 nm) compared to violet light (405 nm). Dougherty, however, has recently stated that the useful penetration of visible light in adult brain at 630 nm is on the order of 1 to 1.5 mm.[10] If that is the case, then the depth of penetration of light at 630 nm represents a significant limiting factor for the use of photoradiation therapy for brain tumors. It is known, however, that the penetration of light through tissue continues to improve by several orders of magnitude as the wavelength increases from approximately 600 nm to 1.1 m. Thus, the possibility exists that photoradiation therapy at these wavelengths might provide a more effective depth of tissue penetration.

Clinical Studies

Clinical experience (Table 27-1) has expanded slowly. The majority of patients have had recurrent malignant tumors and have failed prior attempts at therapy. The mean survival for those patients who died after surgery was 11.6 months.

At present, a number of modalities of PDT for malignant brain tumors are suggested. For inoperable deep tumors, the stereotactic implantation of one or more quartz fibers to provide argon-dye laser photoradiation (500 to 1000 J) has been utilized, in conjunction with prior intravenous administration of HpD. For recurrent tumors which can be resected, PDT of the tumor bed has been utilized after intravenous and, in some cases, additional topical administration of HpD. The light delivery system has consisted of a filtered high-intensity xenon-arc lamp and a fiberoptic cable with a Lucite (E.I. du Pont de Nemours & Co., Wilmington, DE) tip. The latter is inserted into a diffusion medium (0.1% Liposol in saline) which fills the tumor bed and also may be used to cool the operative field. A dose of 150 to 200 J is employed. A third mechanism of PDT is employed for cystic or cavitary lesions. After intravenous and/or topical administration of HpD, the cyst or cavity is filled with a diffusion medium and illuminated either with the laser-quartz fiber system or the high-intensity xenon-arc lamp fiberoptic system.

TABLE 27-1 Brain Tumor Patients Treated by HpD-Photodynamic Therapy*

Tumor	Location	HpD	Light	Result
Malignant astrocytoma	Right frontal	5 mg/kg IV, 48 h	Laser—630 nm	Alive, 6 months
Malignant astrocytoma	Left frontal	5 mg/kg IV, 72 h	Laser—630 nm	Dead, 5 months
Malignant astrocytoma, cystic	Left temporal	5 mg/kg IV, 48 h	Laser—630 nm	Dead, 37 months
Malignant astrocytoma	Right frontal	5 mg/kg IV, 48 h	Laser—630 nm	Dead, 4 months
Malignant astrocytoma	Left temporal	5 mg/kg IV, 36 h	Postresection, xenon lamp—450 + 630 nm	Dead, 7 months
Malignant astrocytoma	Left parietal	5 mg/kg IV, 24 h	Postresection, xenon lamp—white	Dead, 9 months
Malignant astrocytoma	Right frontal	5 mg/kg IV, 24 h	Postresection, xenon arc—white	Dead, 26 months
Malignant astrocytoma	Right thalamus	5 mg/kg IV, 24 h	Postresection, xenon arc—white	Alive, 33 months
Malignant astrocytoma	Right thalamus	5 mg/kg IV, 6 h	Postresection, xenon arc—630 nm	No follow-up
Malignant astrocytoma	Left frontal	5 mg/kg IV, 6 h	Postresection, xenon arc—630 nm, diffusion medium	Dead, 2 months
Malignant astrocytoma	Left frontal	5 mg/kg IV, 8 h	Postresection, xenon arc—630 nm, diffusion medium	Dead, 2 months
Malignant astrocytoma	Left frontal	5 mg/kg IV, 8 h	Postresection, xenon arc—630 nm, diffusion medium	Alive, with recurrence, 13 months
Malignant oligodendroglioma	Right frontal	5 mg/kg IV, 48 h	Postresection, xenon arc—405 + 630 nm	Dead, 3 months
Malignant small cell neoplasm (probably metastatic)	Right frontal	5 mg/kg IV, 48 h	Laser—630 nm	Dead, 1 month, infection
Malignant small cell neoplasm (probably metastatic)	Right frontal	5 mg/kg IV, 48 h	Laser—630 nm	Alive, 6 months
Medulloblastoma	Cerebellum	5 mg/kg IV, 6 h	Postresection xenon arc—white	Alive, 31 months
Medulloblastoma	Cerebellum	5 mg/kg IV, 6 h	Postresection xenon arc—630 nm, diffusion medium	Alive, 13 months
Ependymoma	Cerebellum	5 mg/kg IV, 4 h	Postresection, xenon arc—405 nm	Dead, postoperative, DIC
Ependymoma	Cerebellum	5 mg/kg IV, + topical, 6 h	Postresection, xenon arc—630 nm, diffusion medium	Alive, 8 months
Metastatic carcinoma (pulmonary)	Left parietal	5 mg/kg IV, 6 h	Postresection, xenon arc—630 nm, diffusion medium	Alive, with recurrence, 11 months
Metastatic melanoma	Left frontal	5 mg/kg IV, 10 h	Postresection, xenon arc—620 nm, diffusion medium	Alive, 9 months
Rhabdomyosarcoma	Left orbit	5 mg/kg IV, 24–72 h	Xenon arc—405 + 630 nm	Dead, 2 months
Craniopharyngioma	Sella turcica	Topical 5 mg/cc, 15 min	Xenon arc—630 nm	Dead, pulmonary embolus, 4 months

*Modified from Laws et al.[23]

The technical aspects of these clinical trials in brain tumor patients have been quite satisfactory. There have been no adverse effects related to either intravenous or topical administration of HpD.

The light delivery systems have functioned well, but the importance of temperature monitoring should be emphasized. Power densities greater than 200 mW of red light through a 0.6-mm quartz fiber will produce significant heat-ing of tissue. There is less significant heating when light is delivered through a large diameter (>5.0-mm) fiberoptic system. Because hyperthermia has its own cytotoxic effects, and because heat interferes with the photodynamic effect, it is essential to monitor this parameter and to avoid any significant thermal effects while delivering photoradiation.

If tissue heating is avoided, we have not recognized any significant degree of post-therapy cerebral edema in any of these patients, all of whom had CT scans within 48 h of treatment. Two patients had new neurologic signs related to either surgery or PDT, but they were transient in both. All patients were managed with pre- and postoperative corticosteroid therapy. Two patients developed postoperative wound infections, which is not surprising in light of the extensive prior therapy both had received. Both responded to antibiotic therapy. One patient died postoperatively of disseminated intravascular coagulopathy (DIC), and one late death occurred at 4 months from a pulmonary embolus. Two patients developed symptoms and signs of cutaneous photosensitivity as a result of disregarding advice to protect themselves from direct sunlight.

As mentioned earlier, the analysis of this series of brain tumor patients treated by PDT with HpD does not yet permit any conclusions as to the effectiveness of the method. The results, however, are encouraging for several reasons. The theoretical basis of PDT for brain tumors still appears to be sound. The administration of effective amounts of HpD is relatively well tolerated by these patients. The light delivery systems are practical in use. At least some of these patients appear to have derived some benefit from PDT. These conclusions have been supported by the work of others.[28]

As basic knowledge with regard to PDT and malignant brain tumors increases and further laboratory work in cell culture and animal model systems progresses, it should be possible to improve the efficiency and the efficacy of PDT. Clinical indications may expand as well, to include the treatment of nonmalignant but invasive brain tumors such as meningiomas, pituitary adenomas, and craniopharyngiomas and the treatment of some forms of brain abscesses or parasitic infestations. Other prospects for the future include the following: new light-drug combinations[1] of higher efficiency, less toxicity, and deeper penetration of tumor tissue; new light delivery systems, such as multiple fiber lasers, for more complete photoradiation of tumor tissue; the development of methods (systemic or topical) to improve dye uptake by tumor cells; the use of metabolic enhancers of the cytotoxic effect in tumor tissue[9] and quenchers of the photodynamic effect in normal tissue; and combination of PDT with other methods (stereotactic CO_2 laser resection, interstitial and conventional chemotherapy, radiation therapy,[20] hyperthermia, immunotherapy) in an effort to achieve ultimate control of these devastating tumors.

References

1. Abernathey CD, Anderson RE, Kooistra KL, et al. Activity of phthalocyanine photosensitizers against human glioblastoma in vitro. *Neurosurgery* 1987; 21:468–473.
2. Anderson RE, Wharen RE Jr, Jones CA, et al. Parameters of hematoporphyrin derivative tumor cell killing efficiency: decomposition of hematoporphyrin derivative at high power densities. In: Doiron DR, Gomer CJ (eds.), *Porphyrin Localization and Treatment of Tumors.* New York: Liss, 1984:483–500.
3. Berenbaum MC, Hall GW, Hoyes AD. Cerebral photosensitization by haematoporphyrin derivative: evidence for an endothelial site of action. *Br J Cancer* 1986; 53:81–89.
4. Boggan JE, Berns M, Edwards M. Uptake, distribution, and retention of hematoporphyrin derivative in metastic and intrinsic rat tumor models. Presented at the Clayton Foundation Symposium on Porphyrin Localization and Treatment of Tumors, Santa Barbara, California, 1983.
5. Boggan JE, Bolger C, Edwards MSB. Effect of hematoporphyrin derivative photoradiation therapy on survival in the rat 9L gliosarcoma brain-tumor model. *J Neurosurg* 1985; 63:917–921.
6. Boggan JE, Walter R, Edwards MSB, et al. Distribution of hematoporphyrin derivative in the rat 9L gliosarcoma brain tumor analyzed by digital video fluorescence microscopy. *J Neurosurg* 1984; 61:1113–1119.
7. Cheng MK, McKean J, Boisvert D, et al. Effects of photoradiation therapy on normal rat brain. *Neurosurgery* 1984; 15:804–810.
8. Cowled PA, Grace JR, Forbes IJ. Comparison of the efficacy of pulsed and continuous-wave red laser light in induction of phototoxicity by hematoporphyrin derivative. *Photochem Photobiol* 1984; 39:115–117.
9. Cowled PA, MacKenzie L, Forbes IJ. Potentiation of photodynamic therapy with haematoporphyrin derivatives by glucocorticoids. *Cancer Lett* 1985; 29:107–114.
10. Dougherty TJ. Photodynamic therapy (PDT) of malignant tumors. *CRC Crit Rev Oncol Hematol* 1984; 2:83–116.
11. Dougherty TJ, Gomer CJ, Weishaupt KR. Energetics and efficiency of photoinactivation of murine tumor cells containing hematoporphyrin. *Cancer Res* 1976; 36:2330–2333.
12. El-Far MA, Pimstone NR. Selective in vivo tumor localization of uroporphyrin isomer I in mouse mammary carcinoma: superiority over other porphyrins in a comparative study. *Cancer Res* 1986; 46:4390–4394.
13. Forbes IJ, Cowled PA, Leong AS, et al. Phototherapy of human tumours using haematoporphyrin derivative. *Med J Aust* 1980; 2:489–493.
14. Gomer CJ, Doiron DR, Bucker N, et al. Examination of action spectrum, dose rate and mutagenic properties of haematoporphyrin derivative photoradiation therapy. In: Doiron DR, Gomer CJ (eds.), *Porphyrin Localization and Treatment of Tumors.* New York: Liss, 1984:459–469.
15. Granelli SG, Diamond I, McDonagh AF, et al. Photochemotherapy of glioma cells by visible light and hematoporphyrin. *Cancer Res* 1975; 35:2567–2570.
16. Grossweiner LI, Patel AS, Grossweiner JB. Type I and type II mechanisms in the photosensitized lysis of phosphatidylcholine liposomes by hematoporphyrin. *Photochem Photobiol* 1982; 36:159–167.
17. Kaye AH, Morstyn G, Brownbill D. Adjuvant high-dose photoradiation therapy in the treatment of cerebral glioma: a phase 1-2 study. *J Neurosurg* 1987; 67:500–505.
18. Kessel D. Components of hematoporphyrin derivatives and their tumor-localizing capacity. *Cancer Res* 1982; 42:1703–1706.
19. Kinsey JH, Cortese DA, Moses HL, et al. Photodynamic effect of hematoporphyrin derivative as a function of optical spectrum and incident energy density. *Cancer Res* 1981; 41:5020–5026.
20. Kostron H, Weiser G, Fritsch E, et al. Photodynamic therapy of malignant brain tumors: clinical and neuropathological results. *Photochem Photobiol* 1987; 46:937–943.
21. Laws ER Jr, Cortese DA, Kinsey JH, et al. Photoradiation therapy in the treatment of malignant brain tumors: a phase I (feasibility) study. *Neurosurgery* 1981; 9:672–678.
22. Laws ER Jr, Wharen RE, Anderson RE. Photodynamic therapy of brain tumors. In: Jori G, Perria C (eds.), *Photodynamic Therapy of Tumors and Other Diseases.* Padova: Libreria Progetto, 1985:311–316.
23. Laws ER Jr, Wharen RE Jr, Anderson RE. The treatment of

brain tumors by photoradiation. In: Pluchino F, Broggi G (eds.), *Advanced Technology in Neurosurgery*. Berlin: Springer-Verlag, 1988:46–60.

24. McCulloch GAJ, Forbes IJ, See KL, et al. Phototherapy in malignant brain tumors. In: Doiron DR, Gomer CJ (eds.), *Porphyrin Localization and Treatment of Tumors*. New York: Liss, 1984:709–717.

25. Muller PJ, Wilson BC. Photodynamic therapy of malignant primary brain tumors: clinical effects, postoperative ICP, and light penetration of the brain. *Photochem Photobiol* 1987; 46:929–935.

26. Perria C. Photodynamic therapy of human gliomas by hematoporphyrin and He-Ne laser. *IRCS Med Sci (Cancer)* 1981; 9:57–58.

27. Perria C, Capuzzo T, Cavagnaro G, et al. First attempts at the photodynamic treatment of human gliomas. *J Neurosurg Sci* 1980; 24:119–129.

28. Perria C, Carai M, Falzoi A, et al. Photodynamic therapy of malignant brain tumors: clinical results of, difficulties with, questions about, and future prospects for the neurosurgical applications. *Neurosurgery* 1988; 23:557–563.

29. Rasmussen-Taxdal DS, Ward GE, Figge FHJ. Fluorescence of human lymphatic and cancer tissues following high doses of intravenous hematoporphyrin. *Cancer* 1955; 8:78–81.

30. Rounds DE, Jacques S, Shelden CH, et al. Development of a protocol for photoradiation therapy of malignant brain tumors: Part I. Photosensitization of normal brain tissue with hematoporphyrin derivative. *Neurosurgery* 1982; 11:500–505.

31. Wharen RE Jr, Anderson RE, Laws ER Jr. Quantitation of hematoporphyrin derivative in human gliomas, experimental central nervous system tumors, and normal tissues. *Neurosurgery* 1983; 12:446–450.

32. Wharen RE Jr, Anderson RE, Laws ER Jr. Photoradiation therapy with hematoporphyrin derivative in the management of brain tumors. In: Fasano VA (ed.), *Advanced Intraoperative Technologies in Neurosurgery*. Vienna: Springer-Verlag, 1987:211–227.

33. Wharen RE Jr, Anderson RE, Laws ER Jr. Photoradiation therapy of malignant brain tumors. In: Cerullo LJ (ed.), *Application of Lasers in Neurosurgery*. Chicago: Year Book Medical Publishers, 1988:156–171.

34. Wharen RE Jr, So S, Anderson RE, et al. Hematoporhyrin derivative photocytotoxicity of human glioblastoma in cell culture. *Neurosurgery* 1986; 19:495–501.

35. Wise BL, Taxdal DR. Studies of the blood-brain barrier utilizing hematoporphyrin. *Brain Res* 1957; 4:387–389.

28

Surgical Approaches to Tumors of the Skull Base: An Overview

Don M. Long

Tumors of the skull base have been terra incognita for neurosurgeons.[11] Most were approached by craniotomy for biopsy or unsatisfactory attempts at removal followed by radiation.[12,44] Those which are largely intracranial with a minor skull base component such as the usual subfrontal or sphenoid wing meningioma have been removed successfully.[15] Even with these tumors, the recurrence rate is high.[9] The only skull base tumors to be managed in a truly satisfactory fashion are pituitary and acoustic tumors.[39] There have been a few pioneers who have attempted to improve the approaches to both common and unusual tumors of the skull base. Fisch has been chief among these, writing for a decade about extracranial approaches to intracranial tumors.[13,19] A number of others have described individual approaches. In the recent past, there has been a considerable increase in the interest in these previously untreatable tumors. A number of individual physicians and a few specialized centers interested in these tumors have appeared.[22,24,25,42]

This surgery is difficult and time-consuming and requires a number of skills which are not commonly taught in neurosurgical training. Most are in evolution. Nevertheless, it is important for neurosurgeons to know that the work is being done and that some procedures exist which offer benefit to these unfortunate patients. Over the next few years it is probable that nearly all these procedures can be incorporated into standard neurosurgical practice.

Tumors of the Anterior Fossa

Midline Nasopharyngeal Tumors

The most common skull base lesions which require more than conventional craniotomy are malignancies of the para-nasal sinuses and nasopharynx. These tumors can be approached by a combined operation in which the intracranial portion of the tumor is managed by craniotomy and the nasopharyngeal portion of the tumor by the en bloc dissections of the head and neck surgeon. Current magnetic resonance (MR) and computed tomography (CT) imaging, particularly three-dimensional CT imaging, provide an accurate assessment of these tumors, their relationships, and extent. Resectability can be determined in advance. At one time it was thought that any intracranial extension made these tumors inoperable. This is no longer the case, and wide resections including dura are possible for palliation and even cure.[11]

Operative Technique The neurosurgical portion of the operation is carried out with the patient in the supine position. Arrangements must be made for a bicoronal skin incision and bifrontal craniotomy to be followed by the head and neck procedure. The neurosurgical portion of the operation is done first. A standard coronal incision and bifrontal craniotomy carried as low as possible without regard for the frontal sinuses are the first steps. The pericranium must be preserved as a sheet for later reconstruction of the skull base. The pericranium must be lifted from the frontal bone without perforation and left attached to the supraorbital rim. If any perforation occurs, it must be closed at the time it is noticed, for it will be extremely difficult to find at the end of a long procedure. An extradural elevation of the frontal lobes is then performed. In most instances surgery is undertaken when there is no dural involvement. At one time it was thought that dural involvement precluded definitive operation. However, advances in technique now make it possible to widely excise the dura, lift the frontal lobe off the tumor mass, and then repair the dura with a graft after en bloc resection of the tumor from below. More commonly, the frontal lobes are elevated in an extradural fashion, and the dura remains intact to prevent a CSF leak. With the frontal fossa exposed, the location of the optic nerves is estimated and a high speed drill or chisel used to cut through the frontal bone at the lateral margins of the ethmoid sinuses and the roof of the sphenoid sinus, leaving the orbits and optic canals intact. A cut is made through the cribriform plate anteriorly, and the entire mass is then freed from the intracranial contents. This allows the head and neck surgeon to carry out definitive resection from below and remove the skull base as a part of the tumor specimen. When the tumor is removed, the pericranial flap is then swung into the field and placed over the skull defect, and the frontal lobes allowed to return to their normal location. The double layer of pericranium and dura has been sufficient to prevent herniation of the brain through the bony defect. Reconstitution of the skull base with other materials has not been necessary. The results of this aggressive approach to these tumors are not yet documented by long-term follow-up, but it appears that cure is possible and may occur in 30 to 50 percent.

Meningiomas and Other Tumors of the Sphenoid Bone, Lateral and Posterior Orbit

The most common tumor to occur in the region of the sphenoid bone is the meningioma (Fig. 28-1).[10,23,28,33] Meningi-

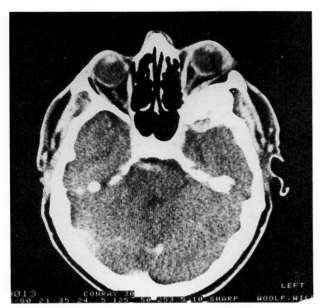

Figure 28-1 Hyperostosis of the sphenoid bone with a small tumor producing proptosis and mechanical limitation of vision. This tumor and bony abnormality are ideal for an extradural lateral approach.

omas of the optic sheath and sphenoid bone with major intracranial extensions are best managed by craniotomy. However, there are a significant number of these tumors arising within the sphenoid bone which cause hyperostosis, restriction of eye mobility, pain, and eventually, loss of vision.[10,23,26,28] These tumors may be approached by a standard craniotomy, but a lateral extradural approach is often superior and safer for the patient. This is the procedure of choice when there is little intracranial extension of the tumor.[45]

Operative Technique The operation is carried out with the patient under general anesthesia and prepared in the lateral position. A skin incision is made just behind the temporal hairline from above the level of insertion of the temporalis muscle down to the zygoma. It then turns posteriorly to parallel the zygoma to the tragus and then angles down behind the jaw in a convenient skin fold. If there is a large extension of the tumor into the pterygoid fossa, the incision can be carried down parallel to the anterior border of the sternocleidomastoid muscle. For tumors associated only with the orbit and sphenoid bone, this is not necessary. The temporalis muscle is cut from its attachments, leaving a small rim of muscle for resuturing, and is reflected down over the zygoma. If the tumor is large, it is probably wise to cut the zygoma at both extremities and then resuture it in place when the surgery is finished. The goal of surgery is to remove the abnormal tumor-bearing or hyperostotic sphenoid bone and the entire lateral orbit, most of its roof, and most of its floor in order to provide access to the posterior orbit and canal. This is done with a high speed drill. The drill is used to remove sphenoid bone medially until the anterior clinoid and orbital sheath are encountered. The clin-

oid can be removed and the orbital sheath skeletonized. It is possible to remove the orbital roof virtually to the midline. The floor can be removed extensively, and the entire sphenoid bone down to the superior orbital fissure is drilled away. When the tumor is exclusively in the sphenoid bone or when the problem is hyperostotic reaction to a small meningioma, the bony removal is all that is required. Small intracranial extensions are removed without opening the dura. The tumor is identified where it penetrates the dura and removed using standard techniques. If there is a sizable intracranial extension, it probably is wiser to open the dura, identify the mass, and be certain that there are no intimate connections with important structures before extradural removal is attempted. Those tumors which penetrate the orbit usually leave the periorbita intact and can be removed as soon as the bone is drilled away. If the periorbita is penetrated, the tumor must be dissected free from the orbital contents. The major risks of the procedure are entering the carotid artery near the clinoid, entering the superior orbital fissure, and injuring the optic nerve near the orbital apex or in the canal.

There are several factors which mandate the use of a combined intradural-extradural approach for tumors of this location. If the mass appears to involve the chiasm, it is better to remove the portion which surrounds the intracranial optic apparatus directly and then continue the extradural dissection. If the carotid artery and cavernous sinus are involved, as they often are with these tumors, it is better to explore intracranially first to identify cranial nerves and the carotid artery. These can be followed into a tumor mass much more easily from their normal intracranial components than trying to identify them within the cavernous sinus and posterior orbit in the tumor mass. These tumors often surround the cranial nerves and vessels, making it impossible to remove the tumor from the extracranial approach alone.

When the procedure is completed, the large bony defect which is left is filled with a fat graft harvested from the abdomen. Even if the dura is open, no closure is required.

The results of surgery of this kind are excellent. In 32 operations in which varying combinations of this intracranial-extracranial approach were utilized, there has been no mortality and no increased visual loss. The only morbidity has been the development of a sixth nerve palsy in two patients. Both have been corrected, though one requires further revision of the muscle-shortening operation.

Tumors of the Medial Middle Fossa and Gasserian Ganglion

The Lateral Temporal Approach

The most common tumors to occur in the medial middle fossa which require more than a traditional craniotomy are meningiomas with large extensions through the skull base into the pterygoid fossa, and schwannomas of the gasserian ganglion.[13] Both present with facial pain and sensory loss, trigeminal motor deficits, and abnormalities of extraocular function. Although the two tumors and the rare neurofibroma of the trigeminal system cannot be differentiated with certainty with imaging studies, it is possible to identify the anatomic configuration of the tumor and surrounding structures with accuracy.[29] Angiography should be employed if it appears that the tumor involves the carotid artery. Schwannomas are usually circumscribed ovoid tumors, whereas meningiomas are more invasive and conform more to the anatomic configuration of the structures at the skull base. The approach to both is the same.[20]

Operative Technique The operation utilized is virtually identical to that for the lateral approach to the orbit. The procedure is performed under general anesthesia with the head turned and the patient turned so that the zygoma is parallel with the floor. The same skin incision is made. The temporalis muscle is removed and the zygoma is resected. If there is a significant pterygoid extension, it may be necessary to dislocate the mandible or to section the mandible and reflect it forward. The squamous portion of the temporal bone and the base of the middle fossa are exposed by these maneuvers, and a high speed drill is utilized to drill away the floor of the middle fossa. It is not necessary to remove much bone over the lateral surface of the temporal lobe. The drilling is continued until the foramen ovale is skeletonized. The middle meningeal artery will be encountered and can be coagulated easily after the bone around it is totally removed. It must be divided. The drilling continues until the second division of the trigeminal nerve is also isolated. At this point it will be possible to palpate the tumor through the dura. If a schwannoma is expected, it will not be necessary to open into the subtemporal subarachnoid space. The junction of temporal dura with the dural covering of Meckel's cave is identified and opened. The tumor becomes immediately apparent. These tumors are soft and easily removable with an ultrasonic dissector or powerful suction. Often many fascicles of the trigeminal nerve can be saved. The same techniques which are employed for removal of large acoustic tumors will be satisfactory here. The capsule of the tumor is opened, its soft contents are evacuated, and then the capsule is gradually stripped from the surrounding dura and the remaining fascicles of the trigeminal nerve. Anteriorly and medially, the tumor will usually surround the carotid artery, and it may invade the cavernous sinus. However, the capsule is usually such that the cranial nerves in the cavernous sinus are simply adherent, and they can be dissected away. Venous bleeding can be packed with thrombin-soaked Gelfoam. If the tumor extends out along one of the branches or posteriorly into the canal, it may be necessary to extend the dural incisions appropriately.

If there is a significant mass of tumor in the posterior fossa, it is better to remove this through a more conventional dural opening. In such a situation, the tumor in the middle fossa is completely evacuated. The temporal lobe is allowed to return to normal position after hemostasis, and the temporal dura is opened at any convenient point along the base where it will be easy to close. The temporal lobe is then elevated to the free edge of the tentorium, and the tumor is identified. It can be removed using conventional intracranial techniques. The dural incision is then closed in a watertight fashion. It is not necessary to close the gasserian dura. Closure includes replacement of the zygoma which is wired in

place, reattachment of the temporalis muscle to bone, and routine skin closure.

For meningiomas the techniques differ somewhat. In general, if the tumor is completely extradural, the approach can be as described. However, when the tumor is both intra- and extradural, it is necessary to add a standard craniotomy approach. This can be very difficult to tell from imaging studies. Therefore, for a meningioma, the procedure should include a larger temporal craniectomy that will allow the lateral temporal dura to be opened and the temporal lobe elevated to expose the medial middle fossa and the region of the tumor. It is then possible to judge what can be done extradurally and what must be performed intradurally. It is usually easier to remove the intradural portion of the tumor first. Standard techniques are employed. There are some differences, however. It is possible to carry out radical tumor removal for extensions within the cavernous sinus. In order to do so, the cranial nerves entering the sinus should be isolated and followed until they enter the tumor. The tumor is then carefully peeled away, following the nerves through the sinus and only removing the tumor after the courses of all of the nerves are identified. Once the intracranial portion of the tumor is removed, the extracranial portion is then approached by the same technique described for trigeminal schwannomas. Meningiomas are much more difficult because they do not dissect as easily. The laser is an ideal tool in this location. It is easier to skeletonize the carotid artery from the extradural approach, but the surgeon may have to go back and forth between intradural and extradural exposures in order to verify the location of cranial nerves and the carotid artery to make tumor removal safe.

Meningiomas of the Cavernous Sinus

Most of these tumors which require surgery have posterior fossa extensions with brain stem compression, or they compress the visual apparatus.[27,51] They are best approached by pterional craniotomy. Once the tumor is exposed by traditional methods, the surgical techniques vary. It is usually better to remove the soft portions which are intradural before approaching the intra- and extradural portions in the sinus. This means dissection of the tumor free from the visual apparatus and removal of all possible tumor in that location. Then the tumor compressing the brain stem is removed in the same way. The dissection of the visual apparatus, while delicate, is much easier than the removal of the posterior fossa tumor because these lesions which are under the tentorium have virtually always involved the third, fourth, and sixth cranial nerves. The optic nerve and the trigeminal nerve which are also involved are larger structures and easier to dissect. The tumor must be exposed so that its posterior and medial borders are seen as well as its superior surface. The cranial nerves should be identified before they enter the tumor. This is usually possible with the fourth and sometimes with the third, but the sixth is almost always obscured by the tumor mass. A nerve-free segment of the tumor is thus identified and the tumor debulked using either ultrasonic dissection or a laser. The individual cranial nerves are then identified and dissected through the tumor mass. The additional tumor removal can continue only after the nerve has been dissected free. The small fourth and sixth nerves are extremely difficult to dissect through these invasive tumors. Sometimes it is simply impossible to do so. Fortunately, these nerves are usually redundant and can be sutured should they be divided during the dissection. The dissection can be carried into the sinus and tumor removed from within the sinus. There is usually enough medial reaction that venous bleeding is not a problem. However, if it should occur, packing with hemostatic agents, muscle, or fat will suffice to stop the bleeding. The risks of bleeding from the sinus have been overestimated, but lesions in this region can be approached only by those with a thorough understanding of the anatomy and the techniques involved. The carotid artery also requires a delicate dissection. Sometimes the tumor has actually invaded the wall of the carotid. The preoperative angiogram will have demonstrated compromise of the carotid lumen, which usually suggests direct invasion of the wall. Total removal is sometimes possible but may not be feasible without neurologic deficit. In such situations, postoperative radiation is used to reduce the risk of recurrence.

There may be an occasional patient who should be treated by a radical operation with resection of the whole area including the carotid artery. These are benign tumors, and such a radical course is rarely indicated. It should be reserved for those tumors which have recurred in spite of adequate surgery and maximal adjunctive treatment. The risks of this aggressive approach are great enough that it should be employed only for life-threatening lesions.[51]

Tumors of the Clivus

Midline Tumors of the Upper Third of the Clivus

Tumors in the upper third of the clivus are usually chordomas. An occasional unusual pituitary tumor may present in this way, and meningiomas are uncommon but occur with enough frequency that they must be considered in the differential diagnosis.[8] All other tumors are exceedingly rare. The critical factor is whether the tumor appears to have a significant intradural extension. This differentiation can be difficult, but it is crucial. If the tumor has a large intradural extension, then a staged operation is required. In such a situation the intracranial portion of the tumor is removed first and the dura reconstituted with a graft. Then one of the anterior midline approaches is employed. If the tumor appears to be intraosseous and extradural, the midline approaches can be utilized.[2,22,32] (See Fig. 28-2.)

Midline Approaches to the Upper Clivus

Trans-sphenoidal Approach

Tumors which involve only the clival bone and the sphenoid sinus without major extensions can be approached by a simple trans-sphenoidal route. This may also be utilized to biopsy tumors. These large tumors that are within the sinus can be easily biopsied by endoscopic techniques, so a full-scale operation is rarely required for diagnosis alone. The trans-sphenoidal approach allows a tumor within the sinus to be removed, and a tumor which is within the upper third of the clivus but not extending laterally or posteriorly can also be approached in this way.

The Transpalatal Approach

Tumors which do not involve the sinus but are confined to the body of the clivus extending down as far as the upper cervical region may be approached by a simple transpalatal procedure. Significant lateral extensions cannot be easily removed, and large tumors require a greater exposure.

Again, the critical factor is intradural extension. MRI and three-dimensional CT scanning will usually settle this question. Angiography should be utilized if there is any suggestion that the basilar artery system may be involved.

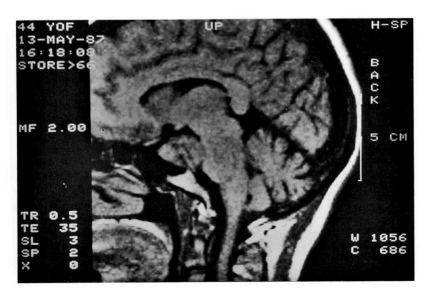

Figure 28-2 MRI reveals a small tumor in the upper clivus which encroaches on the brain stem and has a significant extension into the sphenoid sinus. The tumor can be approached via the pterional or trans-sphenoidal route.

Operative Technique These operations are carried out under general anesthesia with the patient in the supine position. Oral intubation is required, and a special tongue retractor which accommodates the tube is mandatory. The incision splits the uvula and soft palate. A portion of the hard palate can easily be removed without problem if necessary to get higher exposure on the clivus. The incision is then carried through the posterior pharyngeal wall, and the whole clivus, arch of C1, odontoid, and body of C2 can be exposed. The tumor is entered and debulked using standard techniques. Soft gelatinous tumors such as chordomas can easily be removed entirely. Meningiomas are much more difficult and could not be approached effectively before lasers and ultrasonic dissectors became available. It is very important not to enter the subarachnoid space. Leaks are very hard to control with this exposure and should be avoided.

The Transmandibular-Glossopharyngeal-Clival Approach

Large tumors involving the body of the clivus with extensive invasion of the skull base cannot be exposed adequately through the limited transpalatal approach. In order to deal with these tumors, it is necessary to split the mandible and divide the tongue and palate. This affords broad exposure to the entire skull base. It is our practice for these procedures to be carried out by a team of surgeons. The otolaryngologist/head and neck surgeon is responsible for the approach, the neurosurgeon removes the tumor, and closure is carried out by the head and neck surgeon.

Operative Technique The procedure is done under general anesthesia with a tracheostomy. The tracheostomy is carried out as the first step of the procedure. A midline incision is made through the lower lip exposing the mandible in the midline. The mandible is divided with a small step to allow perfect reapproximation. Preformed bite blocks allow perfect occlusion at the end of the procedure, but are not absolutely necessary. The tongue is split in the midline to and including its base. This opens the entire pharyngeal area widely. The pharynx is opened in the midline after division of the soft palate. Much of the hard palate can be removed if necessary for exposure. The clival bone, C1, and C2 can be broadly exposed by this route. The tumors are removed in the conventional way. The ultrasonic dissector and laser are extremely important adjuncts. Chordomas, being soft, can usually be removed entirely, leaving the dura more or less intact. Other types of bony tumors of the clivus can usually be removed with an intact dura. Meningiomas are most likely to have involved the dura, and total removal may not be possible. The mass can be reduced in bulk, providing brain stem decompression and making radiotherapy feasible. Tumors can be removed laterally. The principal limiting factors are the carotid and vertebral arteries and the twelfth nerves. A bilateral twelfth nerve paralysis is a catastrophe and must be avoided. Following tumor excision, the whole defect can be filled with fat taken from the abdomen. This provides a good CSF seal and eliminates the dead space which otherwise would exist in the bony defect. Reconstruc-

tion of the pharyngeal, glossal, and mandibular incisions is critical for a functional jaw. Restoration of proper occlusion is another important factor.

Midface Degloving

There are some tumors which are too widespread to be approached by simple trans-sphenoidal surgery but which can be reached by the so-called midface degloving operation. The goal is a radical sphenoidectomy. Any clival tumor that has a major lateral extension on one or both sides can be managed by this approach.

Operative Technique The operation is carried out under general anesthesia with the patient in the supine position. An oral endotracheal tube is used. The initial skin incision is made beneath the lip but is extended much more laterally than is necessary for transnasal trans-sphenoidal surgery. The skin of the face is then dissected up to the infraorbital nerves, and the skin of the nose lifted from the cartilaginous and bony nose. This allows the skin of the face to be elevated, exposing the entire anterior surface of the maxillary sinuses bilaterally to the level of the inferior rim of the orbit. One or both maxillary sinuses are entered and removed. Through the medial walls of one or both sinuses, the sphenoid sinus is opened and removed. The surgeon may work from either side. This approach gives a broad view of the upper clivus and allows far lateral dissection. It is most appropriate for tumors of the posterior sphenoid and clivus that have lateral extensions. It is particularly important not to enter the subarachnoid space from this approach because there is nothing left to pack to control a CSF fistula. This approach has been most useful for extraordinarily large pituitary tumors, asymmetric chordomas, and sinus carcinomas. Meningiomas may be palliated in this way, but total removal is unlikely.

Tumors Primarily in the Posterior Fossa

Petroclinoclival Meningiomas

Meningiomas which arise from the posterior clinoid and the petrous apex are particularly difficult surgical challenges.[30] They tend to grow to enormous size without causing symptoms (Figs. 28-3 and 28-4). They distort the brain stem and involve the basilar artery and its branches. They involve cranial nerves III through XII routinely. They may extend anteriorly and involve the optic apparatus and pituitary as well.[49] Their total removal is a formidable undertaking. Most of these tumors displace the neural and vascular structures and so are amenable to radical treatment. Another group, approximately 25 percent in our experience, so invest the blood vessels, particularly the basilar artery, that total removal is impossible. The bulk of these tumors can often be removed by the transoral route as long as significant extension into the subarachnoid space does not occur. They can also be debulked by a more traditional subtemporal approach, as well as through the posterior fossa.[2]

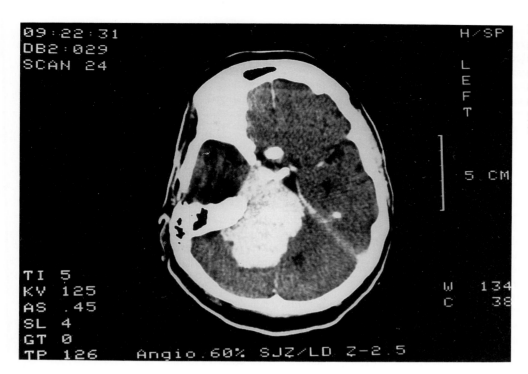

Figure 28-3 This enormous clival meningioma arises from the region of the posterior clinoid and upper clivus. It was approached through the posterior fossa and a total removal obtained.

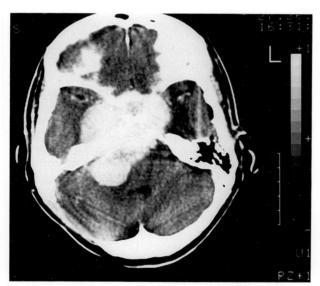

Figure 28-4 This enormous clival meningioma involves all four compartments. A lesion of this kind is beyond surgical cure at the moment. The patient was treated with removal of the posterior fossa component of the tumor which was causing brain stem compression. She has remained without neurologic deficit, so no further treatment has been undertaken.

The Posterior Fossa Approach to Petroclival Tumors

The traditional approach to petroclival tumors has been beneath the temporal lobe.[21] However, the amount of brain retraction required puts the temporal lobe at risk, and the potential for cranial nerve injury is much greater than through the posterior fossa. This is now the favored route by which these tumors can be partially or totally removed.[46]

Operative Technique The operations are done under general anesthesia with the patient placed in the lateral position with the head parallel to the floor. A unilateral posterior fossa incision suffices. Removal of one half of the occipital bone should be carried as far superiorly and laterally as possible without entering the venous sinuses. A rare tumor may require a combined supratentorial and infratentorial approach. Therefore, it is wise to prepare the occipitoparietal area for extension of the incision and a supratentorial craniotomy flap. The approach is identical to that used for large tumors of the cerebellopontine angle. CSF is drained from the cisterna magna until the cerebellum falls away and the operation can be carried out virtually without retraction once CSF is drained. The tumor itself displaces the brain stem posteriorly, and it is rarely necessary to put retractors on the brain stem until the final stages of removal of tumor from the basilar artery and its branches. The first step is to identify all of the cranial nerves possible. It is not unusual for these tumors to involve cranial nerves II through XII. Access to them will generally be between cranial nerve V and the VII-VIII complex or between VII-VIII and IX-X-XI. These structures should be identified first. As they are dissected from the posterior aspect of the tumor, a nerve-free area can be defined and entered. Internal debulking is the key to successful surgery. The ultrasonic aspirator or laser makes this task possible even with the extremely firm tumors which are so common in this location. These tumors share the twin characteristics of firmness and high vascularity. Preoperative angiography and embolization can be an invaluable adjunct. As these tumors are debulked along the base, the cranial nerves become more obvious and the brain stem will begin to sag into the field. The portions adherent to the brain stem and basilar arteries should be removed last to minimize the need for brain stem retraction. The tumor should be allowed to do this work as long as possible. As the tumor shrinks, it should be possible to define cranial nerves IV and XII. The sixth cranial nerve is most likely to be lost during surgery because of the fact that these tumors often arise from the area of Dorello's canal. Tumors of this type have frequently enlarged the incisura of the tentorium so much that it is a simple matter to go up into the middle fossa and strip them from the carotid artery and even from the underside of the optic nerve and chiasm. The last step should be removal from the brain stem and dissection from the basilar artery. Sometimes the tumor is so adherent to the basilar artery that it is not safe to attempt removal.

The base of the tumor in bone is then vaporized with the laser and any tumor-bearing bone is drilled away. Total removal even of extremely large tumors is frequently possible, and the outcome is excellent.

Lateral and Posterior Fossa Approaches to the Skull Base

Asymmetrical tumors involving the petrous bone and the skull base laterally around the exit foramina of the cranial nerves are best approached from a lateral exposure. The most common lesion in this location is the glomus tumor (Fig. 28-5).[5,6,17] Meningiomas are relatively frequent; chordomas occur in this location as do chondromas and chondro-

sarcomas. Occasionally a schwannoma or neurofibroma of a cranial nerve other than the VIIIth occurs here. Large cholesteatomas may also be encountered.

There are two ways to approach these lesions. One is by a single-stage operation designed for cure, and the other is by a two-stage operation for the same purpose. There are no definitive data that indicate that one technique is superior to the other, so both will be described.[1]

Two-Stage Operation for Skull Base Tumors

The goal of a two-stage operation is to prevent CSF fistula and to provide the greatest protection of the intracranial structures during surgery. When the two-stage operation is contemplated, the first approach is a standard unilateral suboccipital craniectomy carried out in the same fashion as for a large acoustic schwannoma. No attempt is made to remove glomus tumors on the first stage. However, other tumors may be debulked intracranially. The major goal is not tumor removal but to isolate cranial nerves and vessels from the tumor. A dural graft is then interposed between these structures and the tumor. Fascia lata or the newer human dural substitutes may be interposed. Artificial substances are not effective in providing the desired CSF barrier. At a second stage, radical resection of the petrous bone and skull base from the lateral approach is undertaken with the brain protected behind a thick layer of artificial dura. In our series of 13 such patients, no CSF leak has been encountered.

The only differences required over standard surgery relate to the skin incision. A curvilinear incision is made behind the ear. It is not carried down to the posterior cervical region but is swung forward toward the angle of the jaw so that it can be continued down into the neck to provide access to the major vessels. This is mandatory for glomus tumors where control of both carotid artery and jugular vein must be obtained. It is desirable for all tumors in the base so that proximal control of both carotid and jugular are obtained.

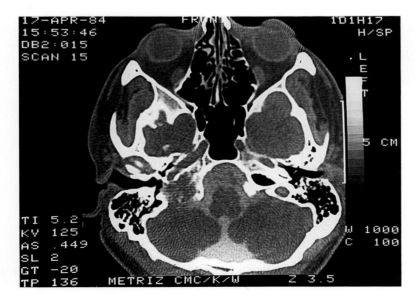

Figure 28-5 A tumor of the glomus jugulare has enlarged the jugular foramen and resulted in significant bone destruction. There is no intracranial extension. Such a tumor can be approached by either a one- or a two-stage procedure.

This means that the cervical musculature is reflected medially off the occipital bone rather than being divided.

Single-Stage Operation for Petrous and Skull Base Tumors

The same operation can be carried out in a single stage. When the tumor is principally involving the petrous bone and is extradural in location, there is no need to consider a two-stage procedure. In such a circumstance a curvilinear incision is made behind the ear, approximating that employed for an acoustic tumor but more laterally placed. The lower end of the incision curves to the angle of the jaw and is extended down the neck to expose the carotid artery and jugular vein. These structures are followed up to either the skull base or tumor, whichever is encountered first. The cervical musculature is detached from the skull base and from the occipital bone. A drill is then utilized to drill away the structures of the bone of the skull base. This technique is not a usual neurosurgical skill. In our institution these operations are shared between otolaryngology/head and neck surgery and neurosurgery. It is quite reasonable for neurosurgeons to do them, but it will require practice and anatomic knowledge not usual in neurosurgical training. The surgeon must learn to spare the structures of the inner ear when necessary, to reroute the VIIth nerve, and to skeletonize the jugular bulb and sigmoid sinus. The extent of destruction of these structures relates entirely to the extent of the tumor. In most instances, hearing is already destroyed, so preservation of the inner ear is not important. However, the VIIth nerve must be preserved in all cases.

It is possible to go all the way to the petrous apex by this approach. The extent of the exposure can be from the petrous apex to the foramen magnum and below if indicated. Extensions upward into the middle fossa can be followed. This lateral posterior fossa approach is the most unfamiliar of all of the extracranial skull base approaches for the neurosurgeon. No one should undertake it without thorough familiarity with the techniques. There are a number of specialized publications available for reference which detail the surgical procedures.

Tumors of the Inferior Third of the Clivus and Upper Cervical Area

The most common tumor in the inferior third of the clivus and the upper cervical area is meningioma.[8] Chordomas may occur here, and an occasional lymphoma of the bone is encountered. If there is no intradural extension expected, the simple transoral route is the most effective way to remove these tumors. Fusion when undertaken through the mouth has a high incidence of infection, and therefore, this approach can be utilized only when there is posterior stability so that fusion will not be necessary. If anterior fusion is contemplated, it is better to use the lateral superior cervical approach.

Operative Technique The patient is intubated in the usual fashion in the supine position. The head is then turned to the side opposite the incision. It is easier for a right-handed surgeon to work on the left. A transverse incision in a convenient skin fold just below the mandible is made, and an approach anterior to the sternocleidomastoid similar to that employed for anterior cervical fusion at a lower level is performed. The jugular vein and carotid artery are reflected laterally with the sternomastoid. The digastric must be cut, and the laryngeal structures are reflected medially. It is usually necessary to cut some or all of the insertion of the sternocleidomastoid on the skull base. This should be done through the tendinous portion so it can be resutured upon closure. This approach brings the surgeon to the retropharyngeal space at the C1-2 level. By dissecting upward it is possible to isolate the lower third of the clivus; C1, the odontoid, and the body of C2 are already exposed. Resection of the tumor is undertaken by standard techniques. A fibular or iliac graft is taken, molded to fit from the lower portion of the intact clivus into the body of C2, and firmly keyed into position. The patient should be stabilized in a halo postoperatively. It is critical not to enter the subarachnoid space by this route.

For tumors with large intradural extensions in this location, a modified lateral approach is preferred. The typical posterior fossa craniectomy is carried out, but the incision is extended farther down the neck to allow the arch of C1 and the spine and the lamina of C2 to be exposed. Cervical laminectomy is added to the craniectomy. The tumor usually has displaced the brain stem and upper cervical cord posteriorly, so that there is room to work in front of the cord and brain stem without retraction. The principles of working between cranial and spinal nerves, debulking the tumor near the base, and gradual extraction of the remaining capsule from beneath the brain stem and cord are the same for all clival tumors. The tumor can be devascularized by drilling away its bony base early in the course of the surgery. This requires careful preservation of the cranial nerves by skeletonizing the jugular foramen. The critical feature in total removal is likely to be the penetration of the tumor by the vertebral artery. The tumor must be dissected from the vertebral and the posterior inferior cerebellar artery. Skeletonization of the vertebral at the skull base in the tumor mass can be difficult.

The Posterior Fossa Approach to the Cerebellopontine Angle

Most tumors in the cerebellopontine angle are acoustic schwannomas (Fig. 28-6).[7,31,34,43] Meningiomas occur less commonly (Fig. 28-7), and other lesions such as cholesteatomas are unusual.[3,37,48,50] There are three basic approaches to these tumors: a posterior fossa craniectomy, a translabyrinthine approach, and middle fossa exposure. Much is written about the utility of these approaches. My own preference is to use the posterior fossa approach whenever the tumor is large or hearing preservation is a goal. When the tumor is small, 1.5 cm or less, and hearing preservation cannot be a goal, the translabyrinthine route is satisfactory and very safe for the patient. A translabyrinthine exposure for a radical intracapsular removal in an exceptionally large tumor in an elderly or ill patient is also useful

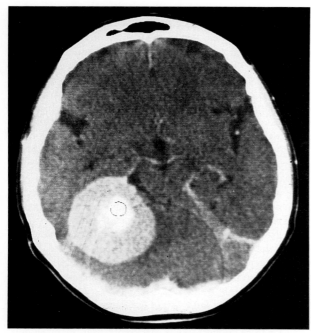

Figure 28-6 This is a typical giant vascular acoustic schwannoma. The tumor had recurred after two previous attempts at removal. Preoperative embolization followed by a radical posterior fossa approach resulted in total removal.

occasionally. We have virtually given up the middle fossa exposure. It has been advocated for small intracanalicular tumors where hearing preservation is a realistic goal.[35,38,41]

The Translabyrinthine Exposure

The translabyrinthine technique has been elaborated upon at great length by a number of authors over the past 20

years. Those interested should consult the specialized articles which detail this operative approach.[24,25]

The principal role of the translabyrinthine approach in our practice is the treatment of small tumors which have already destroyed hearing. The translabyrinthine procedure, while it takes longer than direct intracranial exposure, does provide great safety and very small morbidity. It is also useful in the elderly patient with a large tumor. Sometimes total removal is not feasible because of the medical status of the patient. An intracapsular removal may decompress the brain stem and provide long-term palliation for such elderly patients, avoiding the risk of facial nerve paralysis or other significant morbidity.[16]

The Posterior Fossa Approach

The standard neurosurgical approach to tumors of the cerebellopontine angle has also been described in great detail.[36] These approaches are familiar enough that they need little description. Most surgeons now use a lateral or supine position with the head turned and a unilateral retromastoid posterior fossa exposure. A limited craniectomy is carried out on the side of the tumor. The amount of bony removal will relate to the size of the lesion. Once the tumor is exposed, cranial nerves are dissected free and the anterior inferior cerebellar artery and its branches are removed from the capsule.[40] Most surgeons employ an intracapsular removal to reduce the bulk of the tumor and then dissect the tumor capsule free from all surrounding vessels. At some point in the removal, the porus acusticus must be drilled open for 10 to 12 mm and the tumor then dissected free from all cranial nerves medially and laterally. Surgeons vary in their preference about lateral-to-medial or medial-to-lateral dissection to preserve the VIIth nerve. Some monitor VIIth nerve function, while others do not. The goal of the posterior fossa removal is cure of the tumor, and this is now accomplished routinely. Even the largest tumors can be treated at a single stage, and intracapsular removal is

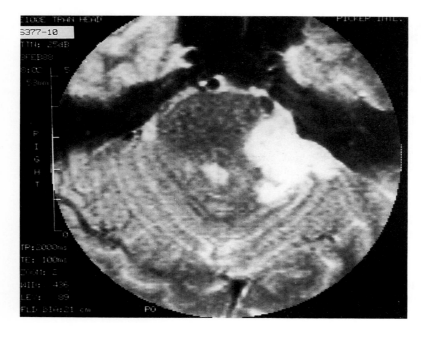

Figure 28-7 The typical features of a cerebellopontine-angle meningioma are apparent. The tumor is irregular, broadly based, and highly vascular. Brain stem compression and the insinuation of tumor into the cerebellopontine angle are typical.

rarely indicated except in the most fragile of patients or the most difficult of tumors.[18]

Current neurosurgical practice focuses upon the preservation of hearing. How often this can be accomplished is not yet certain, but optimistic reports have appeared.[35,38,41]

Preservation of VIIth nerve function is now routine.[47] A significant percentage of patients develop temporary paresis, but anatomic preservation of the nerve is accomplished most of the time, and virtually all of these patients have satisfactory recovery of function. Occasionally a VIIth nerve is divided deliberately or accidentally. There is now good evidence that intracranial suturing with or without grafting provides recovery of function in most of these patients.[4,14]

The major question with cerebellopontine angle tumors are no longer technical. Total removal is virtually always possible. The problems in management relate to decision making about what to do with certain kinds of patients.

The most frustrating of these patients are those that harbor bilateral tumors. It is the usual practice of most individuals to allow the tumors to grow, retaining useful hearing as long as possible, and then to advocate tumor removal when hearing is lost. Patients are educated in sign language during the interval period. As preservation of hearing becomes feasible, there is an increasing tendency to try to remove these tumors and preserve hearing in so doing. When this becomes feasible, a more aggressive approach to the bilateral tumor is indicated.

The very small tumor discovered almost accidentally is another management problem. These can be observed with repeat scanning on a regular basis, since MRI is available. It is our practice to operate only when they begin to grow. However, there are some risks to this approach, and an occasional tumor will grow very rapidly. Strict monitoring with regular scans is required if these patients are not operated upon.

The small tumor in the elderly patient is a particular problem. It is our general practice not to operate on these tumors and to follow the patients until the tumors become symptomatic.

The huge tumor in the elderly patient is another major problem. Some patients are simply not able to withstand the formidable operation required for the total removal of these large tumors. In this situation an intracapsular removal by the translabyrinthine route is a way to palliate the symptoms and provide a long period of functional survival for these elderly patients. Even repeat intracapsular removal is a reasonable way to maintain such patients. Another possibility is intracapsular removal followed by intracranial removal of a tumor which has been greatly reduced in bulk. Many elderly patients who could not have total tumor removal at one sitting can tolerate it well after the brain stem has returned to its normal position and hydrocephalus has come under control.

Preoperative Angiography and Embolization

Many of these skull base tumors are avascular. However, some, particularly meningiomas, angioneurofibromas, and an occasional schwannoma, may be very vascular (Fig. 28-6). The MRI and enhanced CT scan usually give a clue to vascularity. If the tumor appears to have an abundant blood supply, then preoperative angiography is useful. This should be coordinated with surgery so that the major feeding vessels of the tumor can be obliterated no more than 48 h before the operation. Occasionally one of these tumors will swell following embolization, necessitating urgent surgery. It is our usual practice to perform the angiography and embolization the day before the proposed operation to maximize the reduction in blood flow. Adequate embolization will often so devascularize these tumors that they become necrotic and the matter of removal is aided greatly.

These extracranial and combined intracranial-extracranial approaches to paracranial tumors are unusual for neurosurgeons. They require a detailed understanding of the anatomy of the skull base. The surgeon must also understand the intracranial anatomy in the same detail and be able to visualize the intracranial anatomy with the dura intact. The surgeon must be skilled in the use of high speed surgical drills, capable of handling intracranial extensions, and prepared to repair transected cranial nerves and injured cerebral vessels. While there is no reason why one surgeon cannot manage all of these factors as they relate to the orbit, petrous bone, clivus, and cranial contents, most current training programs do not provide the knowledge to do so. For this reason we have elected to approach these complex lesions through the use of a surgical team which includes neurosurgery, neuro-ophthalmology, and neuro-otology. The surgical duties are shared, with each surgeon responsible for that portion of the procedure within that specialty's domain. These lesions are the most complex and surgically demanding of all three disciplines. Improvement in their management is one of the major challenges confronting neurosurgery.

References

1. Al-Mefty O, Fox JL, Rifai A, et al. A combined infratemporal and posterior fossa approach for the removal of giant glomus tumors and chondrosarcomas. *Surg Neurol* 1987; 28:423–431.
2. Al-Mefty O, Fox JL, Smith RR. Petrosal approach for petroclival meningiomas. *Neurosurgery* 1988; 22:510–517.
3. Brackmann DE. A review of acoustic tumors: 1979–1982. *Am J Otol* 1984; 5:233–244.
4. Brackmann DE, Hitselberger WE, Robinson JV. Facial nerve repair in cerebellopontine angle surgery. *Ann Otol Rhinol Laryngol* 1978; 87:772–777.
5. Brammer RE, Graham MD, Kemink JL. Glomus tumors of the temporal bone: contemporary evaluation and therapy. *Otolaryngol Clin North Am* 1984; 17:499–512.
6. Britton BH. Glomus tympanicum and glomus jugulare tumors. *Radiol Clin North Am* 1974; 12:543–551.
7. Catz A, Reider-Groswasser I. Acoustic neuroma and posterior fossa meningioma: clinical and CT radiologic findings. *Neuroradiology* 1986; 28:47–52.
8. Cherington M, Schneck SA. Clivus meningiomas. *Neurology* 1966; 16:86–92.
9. Cophignon J, Lucena J, Clay C, et al. Limits to radical treatment of spheno-orbital meningiomas. *Acta Neurochir (Wien)* 1979; 28(suppl):375–380.
10. Deen HG Jr, Scheithauer BW, Ebersold MJ. Clinical and pathological study of meningiomas of the first two decades of life. *J Neurosurg* 1982; 56:317–322.

11. Derome PJ. Surgical management of tumours invading the skull base. *Can J Neurol Sci* 1985; 12:345–347.

12. Ferrara P, Cimino A, Tortorici M. Role of radiation therapy in glomus tumor. *Am J Otol* 1987; 8:390–395.

13. Fisch U. Infratemporal fossa approach for glomus tumors of the temporal bone. *Ann Otol Rhinol Laryngol* 1982; 91:474–479.

14. Fisch U, Dobie RA, Gmür A, et al. Intracranial facial nerve anastomosis. *Am J Otol* 1987; 8:23–29.

15. Gagnon NB, Lavigne F, Mohr G, et al. Extracranial and intracranial meningiomas. *J Otolaryngol* 1986; 15:380–384.

16. Gardner G, Robertson JH, Clark WC. 105 patients operated upon for cerebellopontine angle tumors: experience using combined approach and CO_2 laser. *Laryngoscope* 1983; 93:1049–1055.

17. Glasscock ME III, Harris PF, Newsome G. Glomus tumors: diagnosis and treatment. *Laryngoscope* 1974; 84:2006–2032.

18. Glasscock ME III, Hays JW, Jackson CG, et al. A one-stage combined approach for the management of large cerebellopontine angle tumors. *Laryngoscope* 1978; 88:1563–1576.

19. Glasscock ME III, Miller GW, Drake FD, et al. Surgery of the skull base. *Laryngoscope* 1978; 88:905–923.

20. Goin DW. Surgical management of petrous apex meningioma. *Laryngoscope* 1979; 89:204–213.

21. Grand W, Bakay L. Posterior fossa meningiomas: a report of 30 cases. *Acta Neurochir (Wien)* 1975; 32:219–233.

22. Hakuba A, Nishimura S. Total removal of clivus meningiomas and the operative results. *Neurol Med Chir (Tokyo)* 1981; 21:59–73.

23. Henderson JW, Campbell RJ. Primary intraorbital meningioma with intraocular extension. *Mayo Clin Proc* 1977; 52:504–508.

24. House WF, de la Cruz A, Hitselberger WE. Surgery of the skull base: transcochlear approach to the petrous apex and clivus. *Otolaryngology* 1978; 86:770–779.

25. House WF, Hitselberger WE. The transcochlear approach to the skull base. *Arch Otolaryngol* 1976; 102:334–342.

26. Karp LA, Zimmerman LE, Borit A, et al. Primary intraorbital meningiomas. *Arch Ophthalmol* 1974; 91:24–28.

27. Leipzig B, English J. Sphenoid wing meningioma occurring as a lateral orbital mass. *Laryngoscope* 1984; 94:1091–1093.

28. Lloyd GAS. Primary orbital meningioma: a review of 41 patients investigated radiologically. *Clin Radiol* 1982; 33:181–187.

29. Lloyd GAS, Phelps PD. The investigation of petro-mastoid tumours by high resolution CT. *Br J Radiol* 1982; 55:483–491.

30. Mafee MF, Aimi K, Valvassori GE. Computed tomography in the diagnosis of primary tumors of the petrous bone. *Laryngoscope* 1984; 94:1423–1430.

31. Mawhinney RR, Buckley JH, Worthington BS. Magnetic resonance imaging of the cerebello-pontine angle. *Br J Radiol* 1986; 59:961–969.

32. Mayberg MR, Symon L. Meningiomas of the clivus and apical petrous bone: report of 35 cases. *J Neurosurg* 1986; 65:160–167.

33. McFadzean RM, Gowan ME. Orbital tumours: a review of 34 cases. *J R Coll Surg Edinb* 1983; 28:361–364.

34. Morrison AW, King TT. Space-occupying lesions of the internal auditory meatus and cerebellopontine angle. *Adv Otorhinolaryngol* 1984; 34:121–142.

35. Nadol JB Jr, Levine R, Ojemann RG, et al. Preservation of hearing in surgical removal of acoustic neuromas of the internal auditory canal and cerebellar pontine angle. *Laryngoscope* 1987; 97:1287–1294.

36. Nedzelski JM, Tator CH. Surgical management of cerebellopontine angle tumors. *J Otolaryngol* 1980; 9:105–112.

37. Nedzelski J, Tator C. Other cerebellopontine angle (non-acoustic neuroma) tumors. *J Otolaryngol* 1982; 11:248–252.

38. Nedzelski JM, Tator CH. Hearing preservation: a realistic goal in surgical removal of cerebellopontine angle tumors. *J Otolaryngol* 1984; 13:355–360.

39. Penzholz H. Development and present state of cerebellopontine angle surgery from the neuro- and otosurgical point of view. *Arch Otorhinolaryngol* 1984; 240:167–174.

40. Perneczky A, Perneczky G, Tschabitscher M, et al. The relationship between the caudolateral pontine syndrome and the anterior inferior cerebellar artery. *Acta Neurochir (Wien)* 1981; 58:245–257.

41. Rosenberg RA, Cohen NL, Ransohoff J. Long-term hearing preservation after acoustic neuroma surgery. *Otolaryngol Head Neck Surg* 1987; 97:270–274.

42. Sekhar LN, Schramm VL Jr, Jones NF. Subtemporal-preauricular infratemporal fossa approach to large lateral and posterior cranial base neoplasms. *J Neurosurg* 1987; 67:488–499.

43. Slooff JL. Pathological anatomical findings in the cerebellopontine angle. *Adv Otorhinolaryngol* 1984; 34:89–103.

44. Stein BM. Operative approaches to midline tumors. *Acta Neurochir (Wien)* 1985; 35(suppl):42–49.

45. Stern WE. Meningiomas in the cranio-orbital junction. *J Neurosurg* 1973; 38:428–437.

46. Susac JO, Smith JL, Walsh FB. The impossible meningioma. *Arch Neurol* 1977; 34:36–38.

47. Tator CH, Nedzelski JM. Facial nerve preservation in patients with large acoustic neuromas treated by a combined middle fossa transtentorial translabyrinthine approach. *J Neurosurg* 1982; 57:1–7.

48. Thomsen J. Cerebellopontine angle tumours, other than acoustic neuromas: a report on 34 cases; a presentation of 7 bilateral acoustic neuromas. *Acta Otolaryngol (Stockh)* 1976; 82:106–111.

49. Valavanis A, Schubiger O, Hayek J, et al. CT of meningiomas on the posterior surface of the petrous bone. *Neuroradiology* 1981; 22:111–121.

50. Valvassori GE. Benign tumors of the temporal bone. *Radiol Clin North Am* 1974; 12:533–542.

51. Weisman PA. Meningioma of the sphenoid ridge: palliative surgery for facial involvement. *Panminerva Med* 1969; 11:117–122.

29

Craniofacial Osteotomies to Facilitate the Resection of Tumors of the Skull Base

Ian T. Jackson

One of the main problems confronting those who, in the past, attempted to excise skull base tumors was exposure of the involved area. Without adequate exposure, *en bloc* resection is next to impossible, and when attempted can be highly dangerous. In an attempt to improve on this situation, structures were sacrificed which could produce adverse functional effects together with facial deformity. Experience in the correction of congenital craniofacial anomalies led to the development of "exposure osteotomies," methods of preventing infection (e.g., galeal frontalis myofascial flap[3]), and techniques of reconstruction (e.g., free cranial bone grafts[4,6] and vascularized cranial bone grafts[1,7]). Armed with these new developments, skull base tumor surgery has taken on a completely new look; exposure is usually adequate, and *en bloc* resection is frequent, with minimal complications.

Exposure Osteotomies

Exposure osteotomies have been described previously in a systematic fashion,[2–5] and these continue to be a convenient series of techniques to learn initially; however, after these techniques have been mastered, improvization is the key. The type of osteotomy performed is that which is necessary and possible to expose the tumor. Basically, anterior and lateral approaches are used.

The Anterior Approach

Under this heading, only upper face osteotomies will be discussed. The mandibular swing technique is used to resect infratemporal fossa tumors extending to the base of the middle cranial fossa; it is a good approach in selected cases, but it is unlikely that a neurosurgeon would ever choose to use it. By contrast, the upper face approaches, if studied on the skull or, better still, on the cadaver, could fall within the sphere of the neurosurgeon. This is not advocated. A team approach involving the head and neck surgeon is strongly advised. The surgery is accomplished more expeditiously and safely.

Supraorbital Osteotomy

For tumors lying in the superior or cranial segment of the orbit (Fig. 29-1), the approach should be a combined intra- and extracranial one, particularly if they are malignant. There is nothing to recommend and everything to deprecate a subcranial approach through the upper lid. This approach virtually ensures inadequate resection with its inevitable consequences.

The orbit is exposed through a bicoronal flap. This should be raised using an incision from ear to ear. The older incision just within the hairline can cause an unacceptable and uncorrectable aesthetic problem and should be abandoned. To claim that this allows better exposure is illogical. The frontal craniotomy should be that which gives adequate exposure and no more. This ensures that any problem such as infection will result in the loss of the smallest possible area of bone. If the tumor lies within the periorbitum, e.g., a neurilemoma, the periorbitum is elevated from the orbital walls medially, cranially, and laterally without disturbing the medial and lateral canthal ligaments. If the periorbitum of the orbital roof is involved, the uninvolved area only is dissected. The frontal lobe is elevated.

Using an air drill with a side cutting burr, or a saw (sagittal or reciprocal), the supraorbital rim is cut through vertically, medially, and laterally. If the periorbitum is intact, the orbital and cranial contents are protected with malleable retractors and the osteotomies are extended posteriorly through the roof near the orbital apex—usually a distance close to 4 cm. The cuts are joined and the osteotomy segment is removed.

When the periosteum is involved, the bony segment anterior to this area is removed. The involved posterior segment of the orbital roof will be removed *en bloc* with the orbital contents.

With this exposure, resection can be performed safely and accurately under direct vision. At the completion of the resection, the osteotomy is wired or miniplated back into position. If necessary, any orbital roof defect is reconstructed with a split cranial bone graft. This is also stabilized with wires or miniplates. If an orbital exenteration has been performed, the osteotomy is exposed in the orbit and must be covered with vascularized tissue. This is accomplished using the temporalis muscle taken through an ostectomy in the lateral orbital wall—the "letter box" technique. A split skin graft applied to the transposed temporalis muscle will give a very adequate socket.

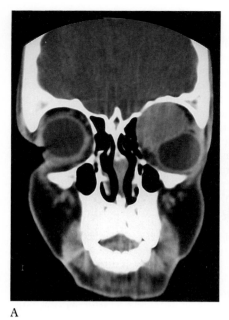

A

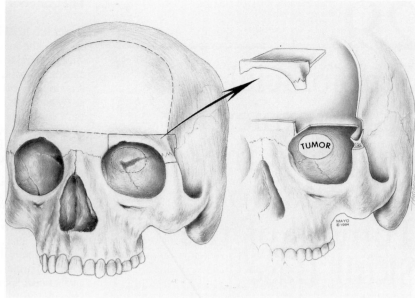

B

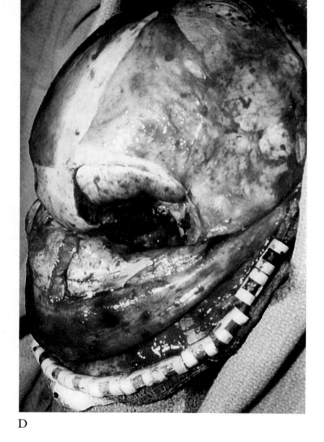

C

D

Figure 29-1

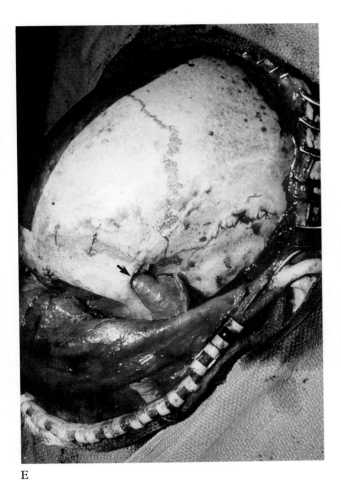

E

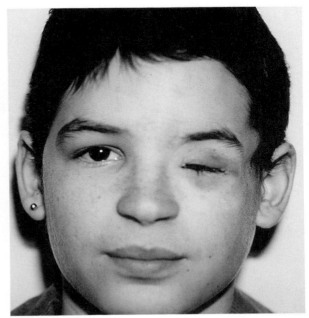

F

Figure 29-1 Supraorbital osteotomy. *A.* Coronal CT scan showing recurrent post radiotherapy rhabdomyosarcoma of right orbit. *B.* Diagram illustrating the supraorbital exposure osteotomy. *C.* The osteotomy cuts have been outlined. *D.* The osteotomy has been removed for exposure. Following this, orbital exenteration in continuity with the roof of the orbit has been performed. *E.* Orbital roof bone grafted. The osteotomy has been wired back in position, and the temporalis muscle has been taken through a defect of the lateral orbital wall to line the socket (letter box technique; *arrow*). *F.* Result at 1 year. *G.* Split skin graft covering the transposed temporalis muscle.

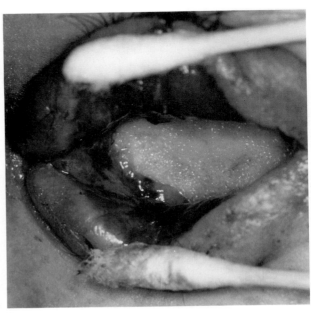

G

Glabellar Osteotomy

Midline tumors which need only a limited bony exposure can be approached by midline trephination (Fig. 29-2). Associated skull base resection will result in a communication with the nasopharynx; infection was a problem in the past, and therefore removal of as little bone as possible is strongly advocated. The frontal lobes are elevated, and the contents of both orbits are dissected subperiosteally. This may have to be limited because of tumor extension into the periorbita.

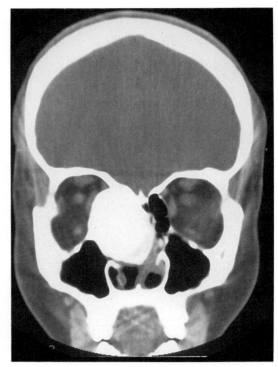

B

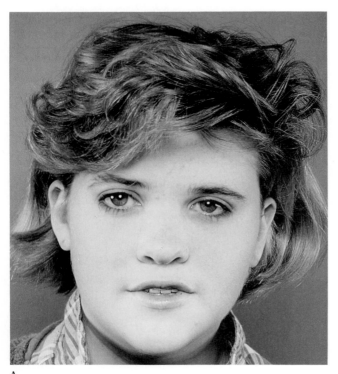

A

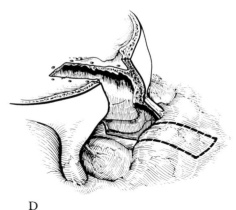

D

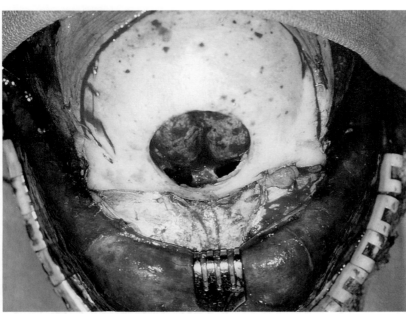

C

Figure 29-2 Glabellar exposure osteotomy. *A, B.* Patient with fibrous dysplasia involving cribriform fossa, medial orbital wall, and nasal cavity. *C.* Trephine craniotomy. *D.* Diagram showing removal of glabellar region with resection of tumor. Galeal frontalis flap being elevated. *E.* Galeal frontalis flap ready to be inserted into the floor of the anterior cranial fossa. *F.* Diagram to show galeal frontalis flap sutured in anterior cranial fossa using drill holes illustrated in *D*. *G.* Glabellar osteotomy and trephine craniotomy wired back in position. Note galeal frontalis flap placed through "letter box" under the glabellar osteotomy (*arrows*). *H.* Result after 1 year.

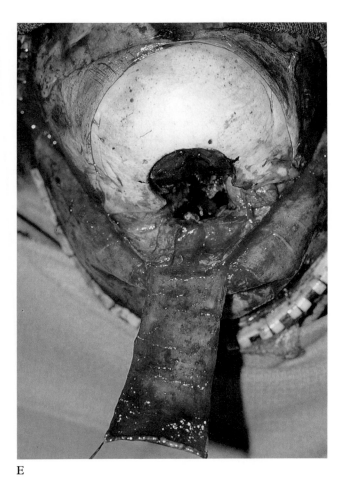

E

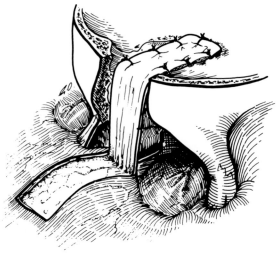

F

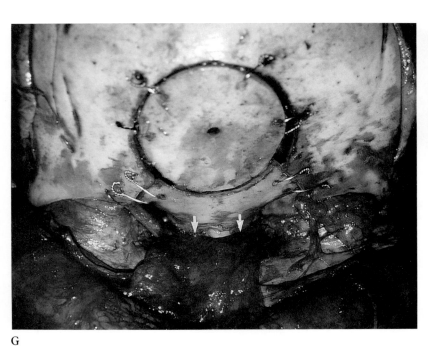

G

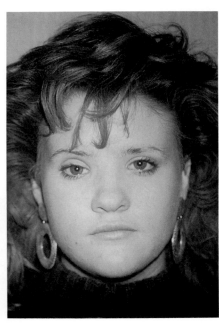

H

Figure 29-2 Continued

Osteotomies are now made vertically from the edge of the trephine defect through the superior orbital rims into the orbits. Their cuts are taken back just in front of the crista galli and are then joined transversely. Anteriorly, the nasal mucoperiosteum is dissected off the undersurface of the nasal bones and medial orbital walls. With the mucoperiosteum protected, cuts are made into the nose at the desired level and the glabellar and nasal bone block is removed.

This osteotomy gives excellent exposure, and it is possible to resect medial orbital walls, septum, ethmoid sinuses, cribriform plate, and sphenoid sinuses back to their posterior wall as a single block. At the completion of the procedure, holes are drilled through the edges of the anterior cranial base defect and a galeal frontalis myofascial flap is sutured carefully and securely to separate the anterior cra-

nial fossa from the nasopharynx. When the glabellar bone segment is reinserted, a portion is removed transversely from its lower end so that the pedicle of the flap is not constricted—the "letter box" technique. All replaced bone segments are stabilized with wires or miniplates. It is possible to carry out medial and orbital wall reconstruction with split cranial bone grafts. A second galeal frontalis myofascial flap may be necessary to cover these grafts, since otherwise they would be exposed into the nose.

Frontonasomaxillary Osteotomy

In a frontonasomaxillary osteotomy (Fig. 29-3), when midline lesions are positioned deep in the anterior cranial fossa and are extensive, a wider exposure may be necessary to ensure safety during the resection.

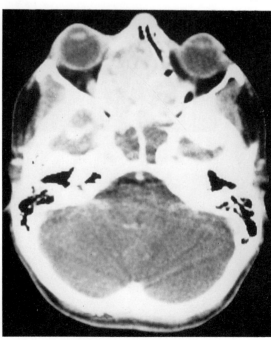

A

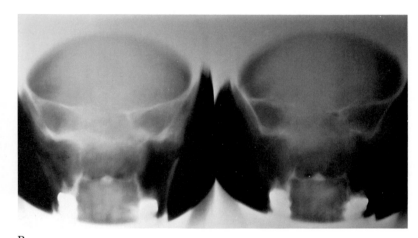

B

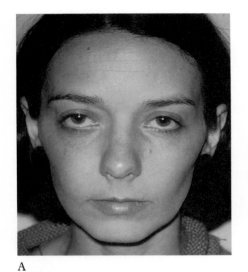

C

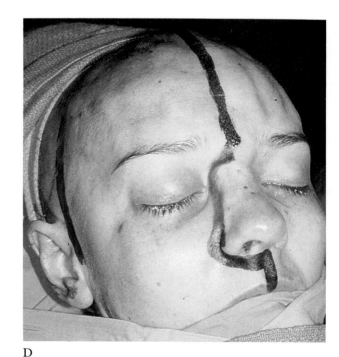

D

Figure 29-3

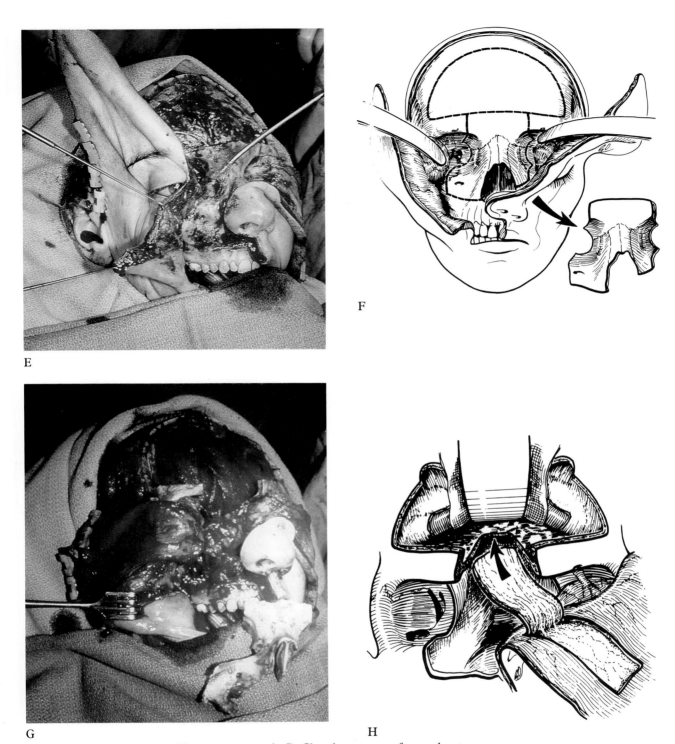

E

F

G

H

Figure 29-3 Frontonasomaxillary osteotomy. *A, B*. Chondrosarcoma of central anterior skull base. Its extent can be seen on tomography. *C*. Coronal CT scan. *D*. Planned approach. Coronal flap and face splitting incision. *E*. Exposure of nasomaxillary area through face splitting incision and anterior cranial fossa through a frontal craniotomy. *F*. Diagram of frontomaxillary exposure osteotomy. *G*. The osteotomy has been completed to give good exposure of the tumor. *H*. Following resection, a galeal frontalis flap is used to separate anterior cranial fossa from nasopharynx. *I*. Osteotomy is replaced and wired or plated in position. *J*. Patient 3 years after resection.

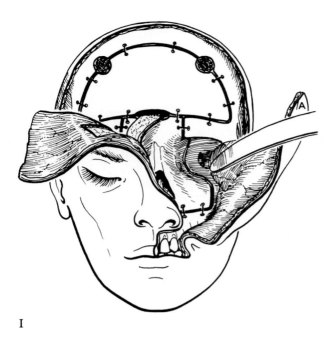

I

Figure 29-3 Continued

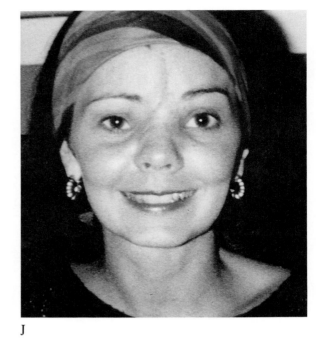

J

The approach is again by the bicoronal flap, but on this occasion, a standard bifrontal cranial bone flap is removed. The approach to the face is greatly facilitated by a "face splitting" incision. This will usually result in a satisfactory scar. The orbital contents are dissected as completely as possible superiorly, medially, and inferiorly, depending on the tumor pathology and its extension. The frontal lobes and orbital contents are protected. Vertical osteotomies are taken through the medial third of the supraorbital rims into the orbits. These are taken back as far as possible in the orbital roof and are joined by a horizontal cut. The osteotomy is then taken down the medial wall of the orbit unilaterally or bilaterally; this continues into the floor of the orbit, stopping medial to the infraorbital nerve. The cut is then brought through the inferior orbital rim vertically down the maxilla to the same level as the pyriform aperture floor. It is then taken transversely to the lateral wall of the pyriform aperture. An osteotome introduced through the anterior cranial fossa osteotomy will, with gentle tapping, mobilize this whole bony segment and allow it to be removed without difficulty.

The tumor can now be safely removed under direct vision. If an orbit is involved in such a way that exenteration is judged to be necessary, this can be accomplished very easily in continuity with the central block. At the completion of the resection, the segment of osteotomized bone is replaced, and using the "letter box" technique, the connection between the extradural space and the nasopharynx is closed as described earlier. The interior of the replaced bone is covered by a contralateral galeal frontalis myofascial flap. In this way, resection can be readily accomplished without the complications which were so prone to occur in the past as a result of these procedures.

Le Fort I Osteotomy

The Le Fort I osteotomy (Fig. 29-4) is used to approach chordomas. It affords excellent exposure to the posterior aspect of the upper nasopharynx and central skull base (clivus) area.

Through an upper buccal sulcus incision extending between the first molars, the periosteum of the maxilla is elevated. This dissection is taken up to the infraorbital nerves. The mucoperiosteum of the pyriform aperture is elevated completely from anterior to posterior along the nasal floor and lateral walls. Laterally, the dissection is taken to the retrotuberosity area. A saw cut is made from the lateral margin of the pyriform aperture, with the mucoperiosteum protected, to the tuberosity and the pterygomaxillary groove. The lateral pyriform wall is cut completely from front to back, the cartilaginous septum is elevated from the vomerine ridge, and the vomer is cut with a notched osteotome.

A curved osteotome is placed in the pterygopalatine groove and separates the bony connection with the pterygoid plates. The maxillary fragment is now downfractured to gain posterior exposure.

When the resection has been completed, the maxilla is placed back in its correct position and held there with miniplates on the lateral margins of the pyriform fossa and the zygomaticomaxillary buttress. The patient is maintained on a soft diet for 1 month.

The Lateral Approach

Tumors involving the middle cranial fossa and the lateral orbit are exposed by a lateral approach.

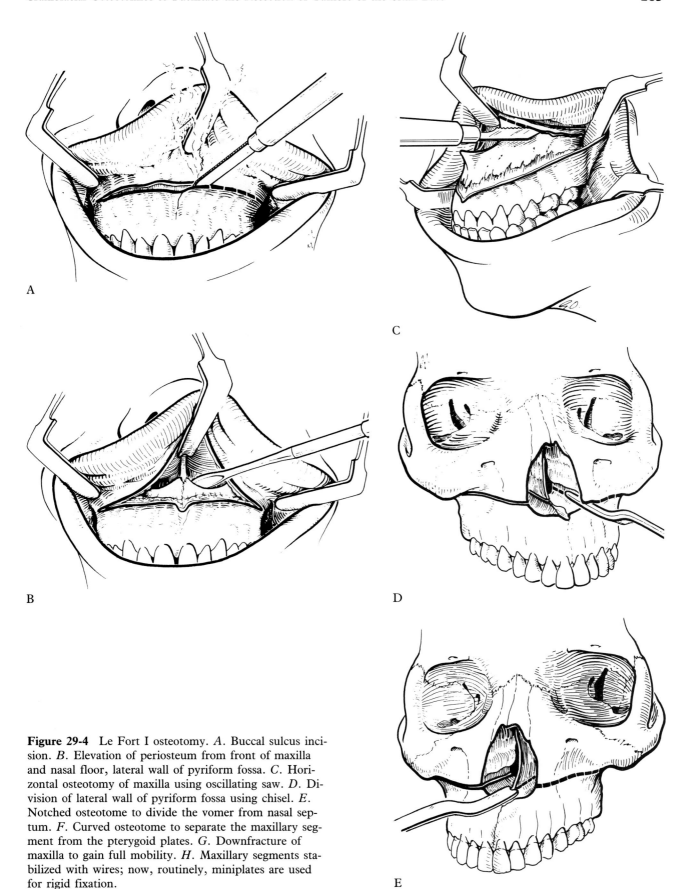

A

B

C

D

E

Figure 29-4 Le Fort I osteotomy. *A.* Buccal sulcus incision. *B.* Elevation of periosteum from front of maxilla and nasal floor, lateral wall of pyriform fossa. *C.* Horizontal osteotomy of maxilla using oscillating saw. *D.* Division of lateral wall of pyriform fossa using chisel. *E.* Notched osteotome to divide the vomer from nasal septum. *F.* Curved osteotome to separate the maxillary segment from the pterygoid plates. *G.* Downfracture of maxilla to gain full mobility. *H.* Maxillary segments stabilized with wires; now, routinely, miniplates are used for rigid fixation.

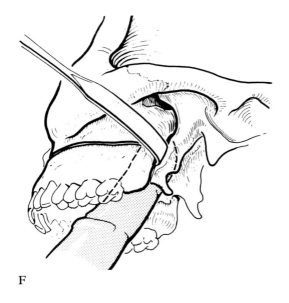

F

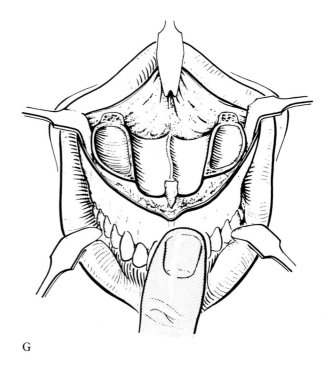

G

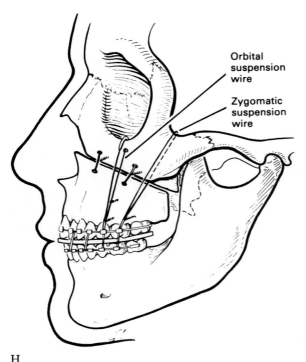

H

Figure 29-4 Continued

Orbitozygomatic Osteotomy

The two lesions most commonly approached using the orbitozygomatic osteotomy (Fig. 29-5) have been sphenoid ridge meningiomas and fibrous dysplasia of that region. A coronal flap is again used, since this is most aesthetically acceptable. On the affected side, the incision is taken down to below the zygomatic arch. In the temporal area, the flap is elevated just above the deep temporal fascia to prevent damage to the frontal branch of the facial nerve. The temporalis

muscle with the pericranium cranial to it is dissected off the skull and lateral orbital wall to expose the temporal fossa. The periosteum is elevated over the lateral orbital rim, the zygomatic arch, and the anterior surface of the maxilla. The periorbita is elevated superiorly, laterally, and inferiorly. A limited frontotemporal craniotomy is performed, and the frontal lobe is elevated. The supraorbital rim is cut through where indicated for exposure, as is the orbital roof with the periorbita protected. The most posterior part of the lateral orbital wall is cut vertically to the inferior orbital fissure. The osteotomy cuts are varied depending on how much maxilla and zygoma needs to be removed for exposure. The infraorbital rim is cut through onto the anterior aspect of the maxilla. From here a horizontal osteotomy is taken to under the zygomatic arch; the arch is cut through. The bony segment is mobilized and removed. Any involved temporal and orbital bone is resected, as is the main lesion. During this procedure, the temporal lobe is protected. Since the exposure is good, an *en bloc* removal is possible on most occasions. The temporal bony defect is reconstructed with split bone grafts, and the exposure osteotomy is replaced. Stabilization is achieved with miniplates. The temporalis muscle is returned to its original position and is held in place using sutures through drill holes in the lateral orbital rim and temporal ridge.

Orbitozygomatic Mandibular Osteotomy

The orbitozygomatic mandibular osteotomy (Fig. 29-6) is used for infratemporal fossa lesions. These may be maxillary or intraoral tumors invading the skull base, or intracra-

Orbital
suspension
wire

Zygomatic
suspension
wire

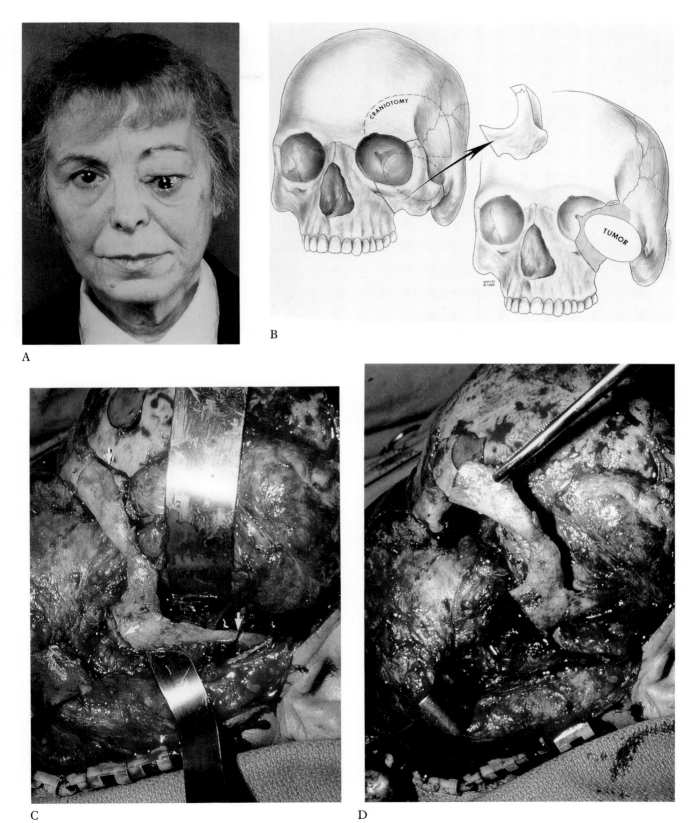

Figure 29-5 Orbitozygomatic osteotomy. *A*. Patient with left sphenoid wing meningioma invading the orbit. *B*. Diagram of orbitozygomatic exposure osteotomy. *C*. The cuts for the osteotomy can be seen *(arrows)*. *D*. Osteotomized segments being removed. *E*. The meningioma has been excised completely. *F*. Result 2 years later.

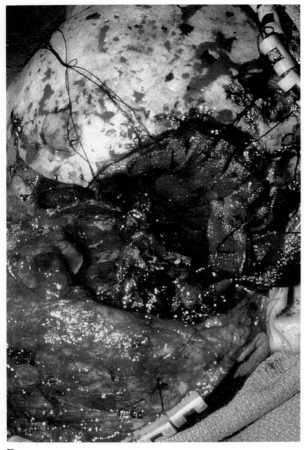

E

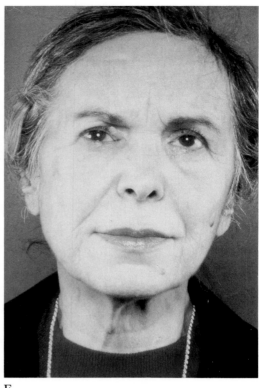

F

Figure 29-5   Continued

nial tumors escaping through a foramen into the infratemporal fossa.

The skin incision begins in the anterior temporal area and curves superiorly and posteriorly to then run down in the preauricular region into the neck where it is fashioned as a lazy S. After the skin and scalp have been elevated, as for a face-lift, the temporalis muscle is dissected up as described in the preceding section. A limited temporal craniotomy is used for access to the tumor to confirm resectability or otherwise. A total parotidectomy with preservation of all branches of the facial nerve is performed. The zygomatic arch with or without a portion of the maxilla and lateral orbital wall is removed. If the mandible is involved by the tumor, the ascending ramus is sacrificed. If, however, this is not the case, an osteotomy is made through the angle after the periosteum has been elevated. The temporal mandibular joint is disarticulated, and the ascending ramus removed or, if possible, simply hinged forward on the masseter and/or pterygoid muscles.

A neck dissection with preservation of the sternomastoid muscle is usually performed. This allows identification of the jugular and carotid vessels, which makes for safer dissection in the skull base region. This specimen is then removed with an in-continuity resection of the infratemporal fossa contents and base of skull. On occasion, it may be necessary to include a portion of the maxilla with or without the orbital contents in the resected specimen.

The sternomastoid is divided inferiorly and swung up on its superior pedicle to fill dead space in the infratemporal fossa. In selected cases, i.e., without prior radiotherapy, nonmalignant tumors, or less aggressive malignant tumors, the osteotomies can be replaced and stabilized with miniplates. The temporalis muscle is replaced as described in the previous section. The patient is kept on a soft diet for 1 month.

Figure 29-6   Orbitozygomatic mandibular osteotomy. *A, B.* Patient with left infratemporal fossa liposarcoma well seen on coronal CT scan (*B*). *C.* Planned skin incision. *D.* Total parotidectomy with preservation of facial nerve and all of its branches and modified radical neck dissection preserving sternomastoid with good exposure of internal carotid artery and external jugular vein. *E.* Diagram of the orbitozygomatic mandibular exposure osteotomy with small temporal craniotomy. *F.* Zygomatic and maxillary segment being removed. *G.* Defect following resection of tumor involving orbit and maxilla. Facial nerve intact (*arrow*). *H.* Sternomastoid muscle divided inferiorly to be swung up in its superior pedicle to fill up infratemporal dead space. *I.* Result 1 year later. Patient died 18 months postoperatively with spinal metastasis.

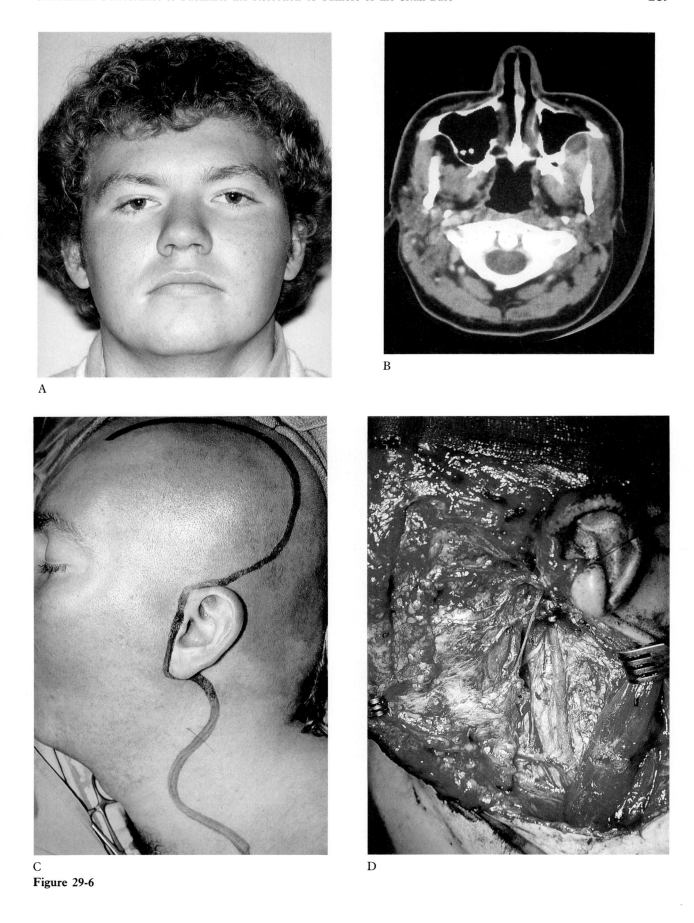

A

B

C

D

Figure 29-6

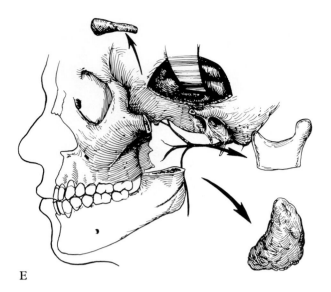

E

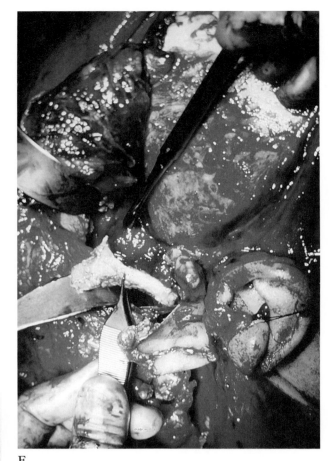

F

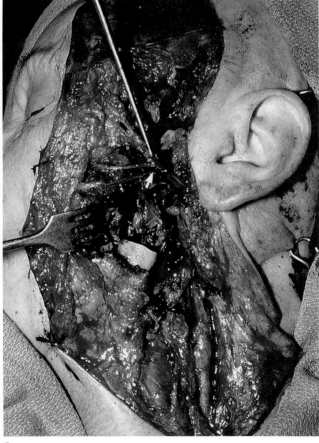

G

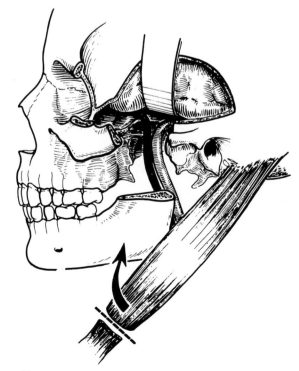

H

Figure 29-6 Continued

significant infections and no surgical deaths. What cannot be claimed at the moment is whether the improved exposure and consequently better resection will lead to an increase in survival rates. In 123 malignant tumors of widely varying pathology, the majority of which were recurrent after surgery and radiotherapy, the 5-year survival rate was 48 percent. This is encouraging, but a larger number of cases with a longer follow-up need to be studied.

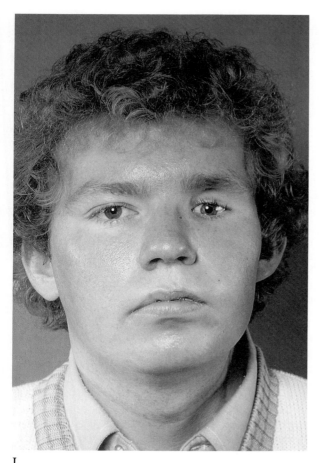

I

Figure 29-6   Continued

Conclusion

These exposure osteotomies have made skull base surgery less complex and safer. In 168 cases in which malignant tumors outweighed nonmalignant by 2 to 1, there were no

References

1. Bite U, Jackson IT, Wahner HW, et al. Vascularized skull bone grafts in craniofacial surgery. *Ann Plast Surg* 1987; 19:3–15.
2. Jackson IT. Craniofacial surgery for congenital deformities: its contribution to surgery of the skull. In: Chretien PB, Johns ME, Shedd DP, et al. (eds.), *Head and Neck Cancer*. St Louis: Mosby, 1985; 1:263–272.
3. Jackson IT, Adham MN, Marsh WR. Use of galeal frontalis myofascial flap in craniofacial surgery. *Plast Reconstr Surg* 1986; 77:905–910.
4. Jackson IT, Helden G, Marx R. Skull bone grafts in maxillofacial and craniofacial surgery. *J Oral Maxillofac Surg* 1986; 44:949–955.
5. Jackson IT, Marsh WR, Bite U, et al. Craniofacial osteotomies to facilitate skull base tumour resection. *Br J Plast Surg* 1986; 39:153–160.
6. Tessier P. Autogenous bone grafts taken from the calvarium for facial and cranial applications. *Clin Plast Surg* 1982; 9:531–538.
7. van der Meulen JCH, Hauben DJ, Vaandrager JM, et al. The use of a temporal osteoperiosteal flap for the reconstruction of malar hypoplasia in Treacher Collins syndrome. *Plast Reconstr Surg* 1984; 74:687–693.

30

An Extended Frontal Approach to Tumors Involving the Skull Base

Laligam N. Sekhar
Chandra Nath Sen

A combined transcranial and transfacial approach to orbital tumors first was described by Ray and McLean in 1943.[8] Smith et al., in 1954, reported the use of a combined approach for the treatment of cancers of the paranasal sinuses.[11] Their main problem appeared to be inadequate delineation of the tumor preoperatively. Ketcham et al., in 1966,[6] and Van Buren et al., in 1968,[12] reported their 10-year experience in the treatment of tumors of the paranasal sinuses by a combined approach. The intracranial portion of

their procedure was done through an enlarged frontal burr hole. In the 31 patients that they reported, cerebral complications were frequent, including cerebrospinal fluid (CSF) leaks and cerebral edema. In 1972, Derome et al. described the subfrontal transbasal approach to extensive tumors involving the ethmoidal and sphenoidal sinuses, along with techniques of reconstruction.[1] This was an extension of Tessier's work on craniofacial surgery for congenital deformities. Schramm et al. used a formal craniotomy as a part of a craniofacial resection; this provided better exposure for complete resection and a better opportunity for reconstruction, thus reducing the incidence of CSF leaks.[9]

The concept of removing the supraorbital rim to provide a basal approach to minimize brain retraction is an old one. In 1913, Frazier described a unilateral frontal craniotomy along with removal of the supraorbital rim and the orbital roof to approach the pituitary gland.[3] Jane et al. extended the application of this technique for approaching a variety of lesions.[5]

This chapter details the use of a basal subfrontal approach to lesions involving the anterior cranial base, the sphenoid bone, the sphenoidal sinus, and the clivus.

This approach, along with the removal of the supraorbital rims (Fig. 30-1), allows the surgeon to minimize frontal lobe retraction, improve exposure, and allow the early interruption of the blood supply to the tumor. The clival resection can be carried down to the foramen magnum but is limited superiorly by the sella, which hides the dorsum sellae, and laterally by the optic nerves and the internal carotid arteries. Immediate reconstruction is possible using a pericranial flap or a galeal–frontalis muscle–pericranial flap. More extensive reconstruction using a microvascular free flap is also feasible. For purely intracranial lesions with some extension into the sphenoidal and ethmoidal sinuses and the clivus, the basal subfrontal approach alone is adequate (Figs. 30-2 and 30-3). However, for malignant tumors

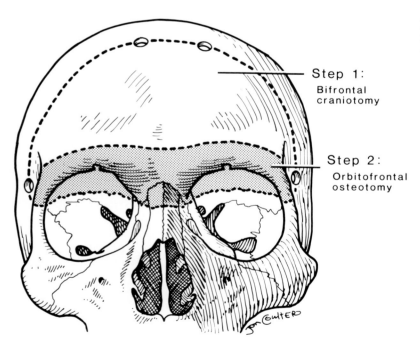

Step 1:
Bifrontal craniotomy

Step 2:
Orbitofrontal osteotomy

Figure 30-1 A bifrontal craniotomy is followed by orbitofrontal osteotomy for the extended bifrontal exposure.

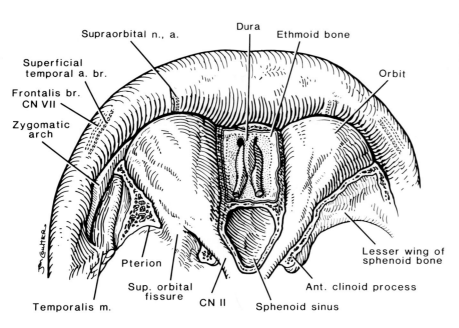

Supraorbital n., a.
Dura
Ethmoid bone
Superficial temporal a. br.
Orbit
Frontalis br. CN VII
Zygomatic arch
J. Coulter
Pterion
Sup. orbital fissure
Temporalis m.
CN II
Sphenoid sinus
Ant. clinoid process
Lesser wing of sphenoid bone

Figure 30-2 Exposure of the sphenoid sinus between the unroofed optic nerves after removing the planum spenoidale.

of the paranasal sinuses and the orbit that must be removed *en bloc*, the additional transfacial approach is necessary.

When the tumor extends into the parasellar region and into the petrous apex on one side, a combination of the basal subfrontal approach with the subtemporal and preauricular infratemporal approach[10] can be used (Figs. 30-4 and 30-5).

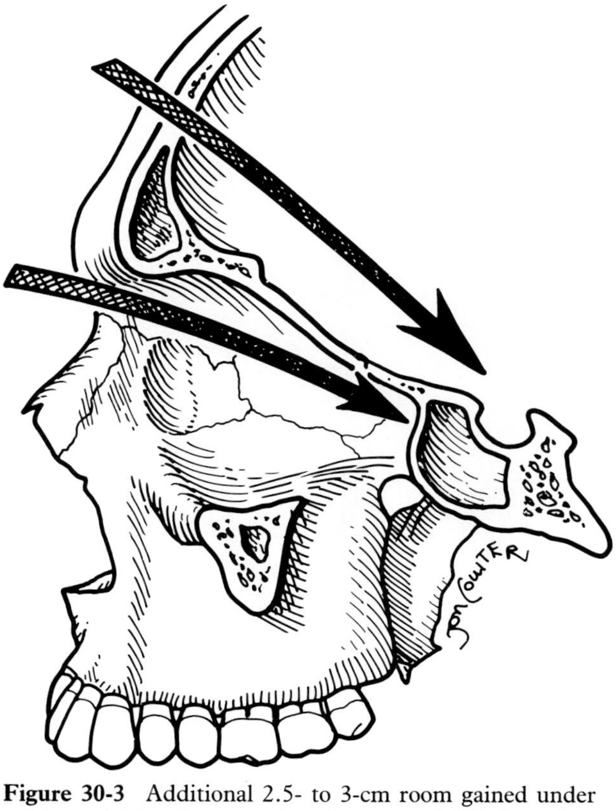

Figure 30-3 Additional 2.5- to 3-cm room gained under the frontal lobes by removing the supraorbital rims, frontal sinus, and orbital roof.

This is an excellent combination because it provides control of the petrous segment of the internal carotid artery and also adds a lateral perspective to the sphenoidal sinus, the parasellar region, and the petrous temporal bone. This exposure of extensive tumors from both the anterior and lateral directions increases the possibility of achieving a complete resection. A multidisciplinary collaboration involving an otolaryngologist and sometimes a plastic surgeon is usually necessary.

Types of Lesions

Tumors in these areas can arise from three different types of tissues. *Meningiomas* originating from the basal meninges can be of two types. The first is the en plaque type, which spreads out over a wide area of the dura. This type is associated with hyperostosis of the underlying bone, which commonly manifests microscopic invasion by tumor. Frequently, on the other side of the involved bone, tumor spreads into the air sinuses, the orbits, and the pterygoid and temporalis muscles. The second type, the en masse meningioma, is predominantly intracranial. En masse meningiomas include tumors of the olfactory groove, planum sphenoidale, and tuberculum sellae. Such tumors can extend inferiorly into the ethmoidal or sphenoidal sinuses with the destruction of the basal bony structures. Total removal of these tumors and their extensions, including the involved bone and dura, is essential to avoid recurrence. The blood supply to these tumors enters from the cranial base; thus, a very basal approach offers an excellent opportunity to interrupt the blood supply prior to the actual tumor removal.

Neoplasms that arise from the cranial bones and cartilage include chordomas, chondrosarcomas, chondromas, fibrous dysplasia of bone, ossifying fibromas, and osteogenic sarcomas. These tumors usually do not invade the dura unless they are quite advanced or have recurred after resection.

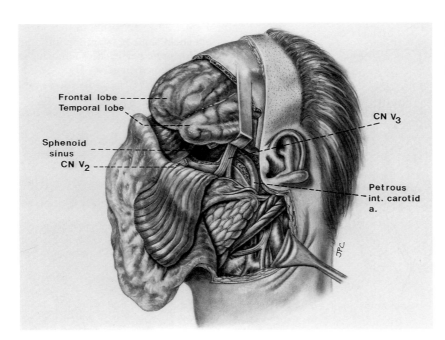

Figure 30-4 Combined basal subfrontal approach and subtemporal infratemporal approach; the petrous ICA and petrous apex region have been exposed.

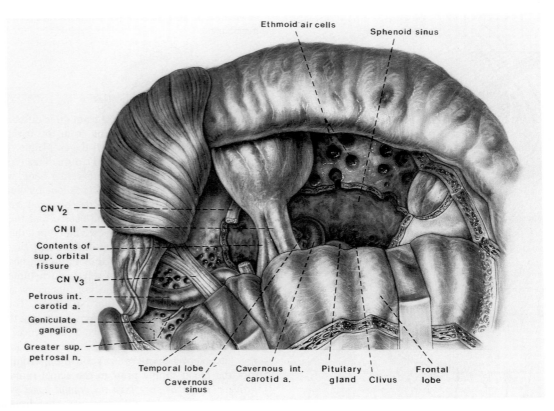

Figure 30-5 Subfrontal view in the combined anterior and lateral approach; the left orbital apex has been unroofed and the medial aspect of the left intracavernous ICA is seen through the sphenoid sinus.

However, the bony involvement can be much more extensive than apparent on the preoperative roentgenograms.

Tumors arising in the nasal cavity and the paranasal sinuses can extend superiorly to involve the cranial base and even the meninges of the brain. These include the esthesioneuroblastoma, juvenile angiofibroma, squamous cell carcinoma, adenoid cystic carcinoma, inverted papilloma, and lymphoma. The removal of these tumors requires a wide excision with normal tissue margins.

Anatomy of the Anterior Cranial Base

The anterior cranial base consists of the frontal bone (including the frontal sinus) in front, the orbital roofs laterally, the ethmoid bones in the midline, and the lesser sphenoid wings posteriorly. The foramen cecum lies immediately behind the frontal bone in the midline; the ethmoid bone forms the posterior and lateral boundaries of this foramen. The crista galli forms a bony ridge posterior to the foramen cecum. On either side of the crista lies the cribriform plate with the olfactory foramina, which transmit the anterior and posterior ethmoidal arteries and olfactory nerves, each of which carries a dural and arachnoidal sleeve. Behind the cribriform plate, the floor of the anterior cranial base is made up of the planum sphenoidale and the lesser wing of the sphenoid. The shape of the floor is important in understanding the mechanics of the approach: The cribriform plate and the planum sphenoidale are the lowest points of the floor. From there, the floor slopes upward and laterally over the orbits. Thus, removal of the orbital roofs along with the supraorbital rims and the downward retraction of the orbital contents allows a direct view with virtually no frontal lobe retraction (Fig. 30-3).

The dura covering the orbitofrontal area is quite thick except in the region of the cribriform plates. There are usually several invaginations of the dura into the bone, posterior to the cribriform area, where tears can be produced during separation. Blood supply to this part of the dura comes from the ethmoidal, the middle meningeal, and the internal carotid arteries. The anterior falcial artery, a branch of the ethmoidal, supplies the anterior falx.

The frontal, ethmoidal, and sphenoidal paranasal sinuses make up the medial part of the anterior cranial base. They are pneumatized to a varying extent and are usually very thin-walled, permitting easy passage of tumors. It must be noted that during surgery, the drainage routes of these sinuses must be preserved, or the mucosa must be denuded as thoroughly as possible, to prevent the formation of a mucocele.

The orbit is an important neighbor of the anterior cranial base, and its relationships should be well understood for operative interventions in the anterior cranial fossa. The orbital process of the frontal bone, which is pneumatized to a variable degree, forms the orbital roofs.

The lateral wall of the orbit is formed by the greater wing of the sphenoid bone and the zygomatic bone. This is the shortest wall of the orbit. Immediately beneath the greater wing is the base of the pterygoid plates. At the anterior extent of the pterygoid plates is the foramen rotundum and the

inferior orbital fissure. At the posterior extent lies the foramen ovale. These structures frequently are involved by tumors arising from the nasopharynx and the sinuses.

The medial wall of the orbit is composed of the lacrimal, ethmoid, and sphenoid bones. Important landmarks in this region are the ethmoidal foramina, usually two in number, which transmit the ethmoidal arteries. They are situated at the level of the frontoethmoidal suture and, in some cases, are on the frontal side of the suture. When approaching through the orbit, these foramina mark the floor of the medial part of the anterior cranial base. The posterior ethmoidal foramen is about 5 mm anterior to the orbital opening of the optic canal.

The optic foramen lies at the posterior limit of the anterior cranial base, from which the optic canal proceeds anteroinferolaterally at an angle of about 40 degrees to the sagittal plane. Extensions of the sphenoidal and ethmoidal sinuses can be found in the roof, floor, and medial wall of the canal.[7]

Preoperative Evaluation

The exact extent of the lesion must be defined accurately to plan the operative approach and the limits of excision to be performed. Bony definition is obtained from axial and coronal computed tomography (CT) images, using bone algorithms. Opacification of the paranasal air sinuses, which is noted frequently, may be due to obstructive changes in the sinus or actual tumor invasion. Magnetic resonance imaging (MRI) is an excellent means to differentiate this and define the soft tissue extensions of the tumor. For both benign and malignant tumors, the plane of demarcation from the brain can be visualized preoperatively, and invasion of the parenchyma of the brain can be determined. The relationship of the optic nerves to the tumor, a very important piece of information, is readily obtained from MRI. In most instances, the vascular anatomy relative to the tumor can be determined accurately with MRI. An arteriogram is obtained to determine the relationship of the major vessels to the tumor, the source of blood supply to the tumor, and the potential collateral channels (anterior and posterior communicating arteries and the ophthalmic artery) available in the event of internal carotid artery occlusion. If the tumor is very vascular, preoperative embolization can be performed to reduce intraoperative blood loss. If the internal carotid arteries are displaced or encased by the tumor, a balloon occlusion test of the artery is performed.[2] Both clinical evaluation and stable xenon CT blood flow measurement are done with the balloon inflated and deflated in the involved internal carotid artery to determine the circulatory reserve of the brain. Thus, the patient's tolerance of temporary or permanent occlusion of the artery can be predicted.

Operative Technique

Anesthesia

After induction of general anesthesia and endotracheal intubation, the tube is secured to the mandible or the lower teeth with wire. This is important to ensure that the tube will not be dislodged if the position of the head is changed intraoperatively.

When a large part of the soft palate is to be resected, a tracheostomy is performed. A balanced anesthetic technique is employed. A third-generation cephalosporin antibiotic is administered before the skin incision and is continued every 6 h during the operation. Patients who undergo resection of an intradural lesion begin receiving steroids 24 to 48 h preoperatively.

Drainage of spinal fluid allows the operation to be performed with minimal brain retraction; therefore, a spinal subarachnoid catheter is inserted after the induction of general anesthesia. However, this is avoided if a significant degree of cerebral compression is evident on the preoperative scans. Indwelling arterial and central venous catheters are used, because these operations generally are lengthy, and considerable blood loss can be anticipated.

Intermittent pneumatic compression of the lower limbs is used during the operation to reduce the incidence of deep venous thrombosis. To maintain a normothermic state, the patient lies on a foam mattress covered with a heating blanket. Osmotic dehydrating agents are avoided usually, unless a large amount of cerebral compression and edema is present. Dehydration further complicates the already difficult management of the patient's volume status during long operations if there is excessive blood loss.

Operation

Position

The patient is placed supine with the midsagittal plane of the head perpendicular to the floor. The head is elevated and slightly extended on the neck on the horseshoe headrest. Pin fixation can be used if the head does not need to be moved during the operation. The head, including the face, is shaved and prepared. The thigh is likewise prepared for the purpose of harvesting fat and/or a fascia lata graft. The eyelids then are sewn shut to avoid exposure keratitis.

Craniotomy

After the scalp is infiltrated with 1% lidocaine, a temporotemporal incision is made starting just in front of the ear, at the level of the zygoma on each side. At the temporal region, the incision is carried down to the subcutaneous fat. The superficial temporal arteries are dissected and preserved so that the scalp flap and the galeal-pericranial flap will have blood supply from the supraorbital and the superficial temporal arteries on either side. Above the temporal lines, the incision is carried down to the bone; below this, it is taken down to the temporalis fascia. The scalp flap then is elevated subperiosteally and superficial to the temporalis fascia, carrying the frontalis branch of the facial nerve and the anterior branch of the superficial temporal artery within it. The periosteum along with the periorbita are elevated over the supraorbital ridges. The supraorbital nerves and vessels are released carefully by unroofing the bony tunnel, if present. This exposes the frontal bones up to the coronal sutures, the

zygomatic arches, the supraorbital ridges out to the frontozygomatic sutures, and the frontonasal suture in the midline. If a frontal approach and a lateral approach are being combined, the exposure is carried down to the inferior orbital fissure and the maxillary-zygomatic suture on one side.[10] The temporalis muscle then is divided at the anterior part of the temporal line, leaving a small cuff of fascia to suture it back to at the end of the procedure. The temporal fascia is divided along the superior border of the anterior part of the zygomatic arch. The muscle is retracted with sutures to expose the anterior temporal fossa on both sides. Next, a standard bifrontal craniotomy is performed. While the dura is being separated from the bone flap, it is helpful to remove 20 to 50 ml of CSF from the spinal drain.

Removal of the Supraorbital Ridges

The basal frontal dura is separated to the lateral limits of the anterior cranial base. After coagulating and dividing the anterior ethmoidal artery, the periorbita is separated from the orbital roof and the lateral wall. A high speed drill is then used to enter the anterior portion of the orbital roof intracranially on both sides while the orbital soft tissue is protected with a malleable retractor. This opening is extended with Kerrison rongeurs anterior to the cribriform plate and laterally to the frontozygomatic suture. Care should be taken not to violate the periorbita during bone removal in this region. Herniation of the orbital fat not only is a hindrance to the further progress of dissection but also increases the risk of injury to the orbital contents. While the osteotomy is being extended medially, the basal extension of the frontal sinus may be entered. With a reciprocating saw, the frontozygomatic suture is divided, completing the osteotomy in the orbital roof laterally; in the midline, a horizontal cut is made in the region of the frontonasal suture to meet the osteotomy made from the inside in front of the cribriform plate. The entire supraorbital rim then is removed, to be replaced at the end of the procedure. If a combined anterior and lateral approach is being used, the zygomatic arch on one side is removed with the supraorbital rims.

Intracranial Procedure

This portion of the procedure depends on the type of tumor being resected and its location. The principles involved in dealing with each category are discussed in the examples below.

Meningioma Coagulation of the ethmoidal vessels at the medial aspect of the orbits will reduce the blood supply to the tumor. The dura is opened and the tumor is debulked, working from its base. When the optic nerves are markedly stretched over the tumor, the bony optic nerve canals are unroofed early (working intradurally rather than extradurally), and the dural sheath around each nerve is opened. This releases the pressure on the nerves markedly and allows for safer manipulation. After this, the tumor is carefully dissected away from the optic nerves and the anterior cerebral arteries. Occasionally the anterior cerebral artery complex may be encased by tumor. In these patients it is best to find the artery near the carotid artery bifurcation and follow it into the tumor. Attention is then directed to the basal dura and bony structures. If hyperstosis is seen around the optic nerves, the optic nerve canal is unroofed completely. The optic nerve sheath must be opened to make sure that there is no tumor in that area. The involved dura and bone are removed as thoroughly as possible, because this is usually the site of recurrence.

Chordoma or Other Osseous Tumor The olfactory nerves are divided at the cribriform plate. Multiple dural openings result commonly, and these holes are sutured. The entire dura of the anterior cranial base is elevated as far back as the tuberculum sellae. The optic nerves and the superior orbital fissures are unroofed, and the sphenoidal sinus is entered by drilling through the planum sphenoidale (Fig. 30-2). The tumor then is removed progressively medial to the internal carotid arteries. There is usually a good plane between the dura, the arteries, and tumor. It is possible to reach down to the foramen magnum in the midline and to the petrous apex laterally by this approach.[1] If the tumor extends lateral to the internal carotid arteries, the subtemporal-preauricular infratemporal approach can be combined with the bifrontal approach (Figs. 30-4 and 30-5). Bone must be removed aggressively beyond apparent tumor margins.

Paranasal Sinus Carcinoma As far as possible, an *en bloc* resection of the tumor is planned. The bifrontal dura is opened, and the olfactory tracts are divided. The dura superior to the cribriform plates of the ethmoid is left attached to the specimen. The basal dura is incised around this area, and elevated posteriorly over the planum sphenoidale, and laterally over the orbital roofs. The optic nerve canals are unroofed, and the sphenoid sinus is entered through the planum sphenoidale. Bone is also removed along the medial wall of the orbit at the orbital apex area. For an ethmoidectomy, the remainder of the tumor excision is completed by a transfacial approach. If the orbital contents are to be removed *en bloc*, the optic nerve and contents of the superior orbital fissure are coagulated and divided from the intracranial approach.

Transfacial Resection

This portion of the operation is performed by the otolaryngologist. It begins with a Weber-Fergusson incision, which can be extended down to the upper lip, if required. Osteotomies in the maxilla and the palate are made through this approach. If the orbital walls have shown signs of invasion by a malignant neoplasm on the initial scans, the orbital contents are removed along with the tumor specimen. The bicoronal incision allows access to the pterygoid plates when the tumor extends that far posteriorly. After a small temporal craniectomy is made, the maxillary and mandibular nerves are identified extradurally to locate the base of the pterygoid plates. The pterygoid plates are removed along with their base in the middle fossa using a reciprocating saw while protecting the temporal dura.

Reconstruction

This is a critical part of the operation, because inadequate reconstruction can result in CSF leakage, infection,

and cosmetic deformities. Some authors do not advocate definitive construction at the time of tumor removal because it can mask tumor regrowth,[4] but we have found MRI to be sensitive enough to demonstrate a recurrence when such scans are performed serially.

The dura is closed meticulously under magnification and in a watertight manner (if possible) with a fascia lata or a pericranial patch taken from the posterior scalp. Following meningioma removal, a watertight closure may not be possible, but the dural graft is carefully approximated circumferentially to the edges of the defect in the dura with 7-0 sutures under the operating microscope. When only the orbital roofs or one medial orbital wall have been removed, bony reconstruction is not usually necessary. Loss of the orbital floor or both medial walls necessitates bony reconstruction. A flap consisting of the pericranium alone; the pericranium and the galea; or the pericranium, galea, and frontalis muscle is created from the bifrontal scalp flap, based on the blood supply from the two supraorbital arteries and at least one of the superficial temporal arteries. This flap is folded backward over the orbits to lie between the frontal dura and the anterior cranial base.

On occasion the flap may be pedicled on the superficial temporal artery on one side while the other side is divided and rotated posteriorly. It provides an adequate barrier between the pharnyx, the sinuses, and the dura. Depending upon the length needed, the flap may be brought above or below the orbital rims, which are replaced. If the orbital contents also are removed, the temporalis muscle is rotated on its attachment to the coronoid process and placed to fill the orbital cavity. When combined anterior and lateral approaches have been used, the galeal-pericranial or galeal-frontalis-pericranial flap can be brought into the sphenoid sinus anterosuperiorly, then out through the lateral opening of the sphenoid sinus into the infratemporal fossa and returned to the temporal dura. The pericranial flap is held in place by a few sutures through the dura as far posteriorly as possible, at least behind the deepest dural tear. If a much larger defect is present, a vascularized tissue transfer using a rectus abdominis or a latissimus dorsi muscle (or myocutaneous) flap is performed by the plastic surgery team. We do not use a skin graft to line the lower aspect of the galeopericranial flap on the nasal side, since it is unnecessary and creates a greater problem with crusting and malodor. If the oral cavity is exposed, however, a myocutaneous flap is used with skin lining the oral cavity. The facial skeleton and the bone flap are replaced and held with sutures, with care being taken to trim the lower border of the frontal bone or the supraorbital rim osteotomy segment so that they do not strangle the anterior blood supply to the galeal flap.

Postoperative Care

Antibiotics are continued until the wound drains and the spinal fluid catheter are removed postoperatively. If there are doubts about the adequacy of the dural closure, spinal drainage is continued for a maximum of 48 h postoperatively. Whenever spinal drainage is continued into the postoperative period, drainage is restricted to 50 ml every 8 h to avoid problems associated with overdrainage. A subgaleal drain is left in to drain by gravity; no suction drains are used, to avoid an accentuation of CSF leakage. This drain also is removed within 48 h. A CT scan is done on the first postoperative day to check for intracranial air, edema, and hematomas. The pneumatic compression stockings are maintained until the patient can walk. Serum electrolytes and anticonvulsant levels must be monitored closely in the postoperative period.

Illustrative Cases

Between 1985 and 1987, we used this approach either alone or in combination with a subtemporal infratemporal approach in 35 cases (Table 30-1). The following cases demonstrate the use of this technique.

Case 1   A 72-year-old woman had a chordoma involving the sphenoidal sinus and the upper and middle clivus. She had a prior partial tumor removal by a trans-sphenoidal route and had received 6000 rad of external beam radiotherapy. Because of continued tumor growth (Fig. 30-6A and B), she underwent an extended subfrontal approach in which the tumor was removed through an entirely extradural route. The tumor was dissected off the medial aspect of both cavernous sinuses, and the clival dura was removed piecemeal. A free fat graft was packed into the sphenoid sinus, enclosed within the folded galeal-pericranial flap (Fig. 30-7A and B). This patient has not had a tumor regrowth during a 1-year follow-up but has had a delayed optic neuropathy due to the radiation.

Case 2   This patient was involved in an automobile accident, and a CT scan revealed an asymptomatic lesion which had not been present on skull roentgenograms obtained many years previously. The chordoma involved the sphenoid and petrous bones, the clivus, and the cavernous sinus (Fig. 30-8A and B). Extension of the tumor around the petrous internal carotid artery (ICA) and into the

TABLE 30-1   Neoplasms Operated Upon Using an Extended Frontal Approach (1985–1987)

Squamous cell carcinoma	10
Adenoid cystic carcinoma	3
Meningioma	4
Chordoma	2
Chondrosarcoma	2
Chondroblastoma	1
Pituitary adenoma	2
Adenocarcinoma	1
Juvenile angiofibroma	1
Osteogenic sarcoma	2
Ossifying fibroma	1
Esthesioneuroblastoma	3
Melanoma	1
	35

medial aspect of the cavernous sinus necessitated the addition of a lateral approach to the anterior one. The tumor was resected using a combination of an extended subfrontal and a subtemporal pre-auricular infratemporal approach (Figs. 30-4 and 30-5). A galeal-pericranial flap was brought under the frontal lobes into the sphenoid sinus (Fig. 30-9A and B). The temporalis muscle was rotated to fill the space in the infratemporal fossa. No recurrence has been seen during a 1½-year follow-up.

The Extended Frontal Approach

Advantages

1. It provides excellent exposure for all lesions involving the anterior cranial base as well as midline clival lesions.
2. Reconstruction of the anterior cranial base is easier to perform than through a smaller opening.
3. Frontal lobe retraction is greatly minimized.
4. Radical excision of malignant lesions can be performed adequately and under direct vision, thus improving the chance of cure.

Limitations

1. Lesions involving the internal carotid artery require an additional lateral approach.
2. When using this approach for clival lesions, the lateral limits of resection are determined by the internal carotid arteries and the optic nerves on either side.

Complications

1. **Cerebral edema**   With the use of spinal drainage, hyperventilation, and the extended bifrontal approach, the incidence of this problem has been very low. However, if it occurs, it is treated in the usual manner.
2. **Syndrome of inappropriate ADH secretion**   A more common reason for the patient's confused state may be a hyponatremic state in the face of normo- or hypervolemia. Thus the serum electrolytes must be closely monitored for several days postoperatively, and a trend must be watched for. Fluid restriction is usually sufficient to correct this hyponatremia, which presumably results from the inappropriate secretion of antidiuretic hormone (ADH).
3. **Pneumocephalus**   This has been observed in some patients in whom the spinal drain was left in place postoperatively to achieve a good dural seal and excessive CSF drainage occurred inadvertently. Air is trapped in the epidural space, and overdrainage of CSF does not allow the space to be refilled. The patient may be obtunded or even stuporous without any focal deficits. The CT images show the air displacing the frontal lobes posteriorly and effacing the ventricles. Stopping the spinal drainage

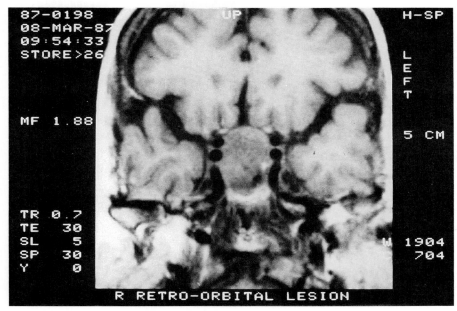

A

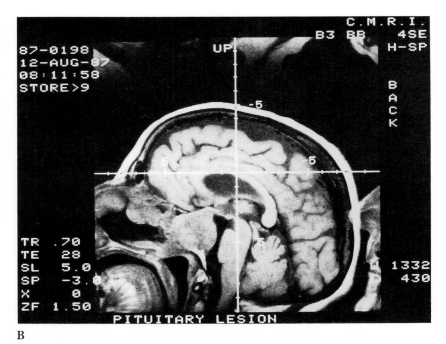

B

Figure 30-6 *A, B.* Coronal and sagittal MRI showing the chordoma medial to the cavernous ICA on either side and destroying the superior and middle clivus.

is usually sufficient to rectify this condition, but occasionally, the pressure may have to be relieved by insertion of a needle through a burr hole under strict antiseptic conditions. This has been seen in three patients earlier in our series. For these reasons, we employ postoperative CSF drainage sparingly, and if we do, we use volume regulation (50 to 75 ml every 8 h) rather than drainage regulated by raising or lowering the bag.

4. **CSF leaks** If meticulous care has been exercised in repairing the dura and reinforcing the floor of the anterior cranial fossa, CSF leaks can be reduced drastically. A small leak can be treated by spinal fluid drainage for a short time; otherwise, reexploration is required to repair the leak. None of our patients required reexploration for CSF leakage.

5. **Epidural infection** Because of the communication cre-

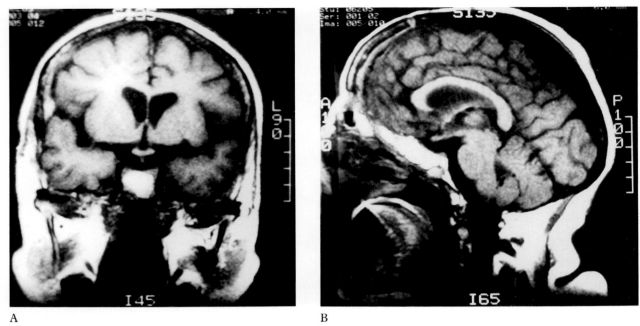

A   B

Figure 30-7 *A, B.* Postoperative MRI showing the high signal intensity from the fat graft and galeal-pericranial flap.

ated between the intracranial contents and the air sinuses and the nasal cavity, this problem remains a distinct possibility. The patient may show all the signs of an epidural infection including fever and mental status changes or may be asymptomatic except for some fullness of the frontal scalp and some periorbital edema. Careful aspira-

tion and culture of the fluid reveals the diagnosis. Open debridement and removal of the bone flap must be performed, and a prolonged course of antibiotics must be administered. This complication occurred in only one of our patients.

6. **Scalp flap necrosis**   Mobilization of a galeal-pericranial

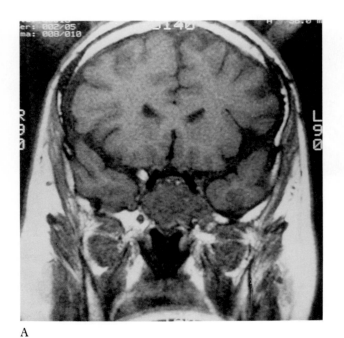
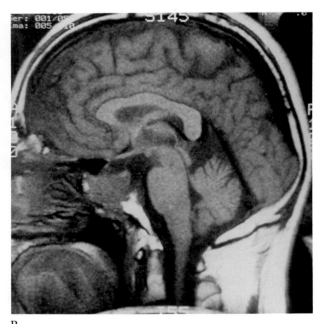

A   B

Figure 30-8 *A, B.* Clivus chordoma extending lateral to the left petrous ICA requiring a combined anterior and lateral approach.

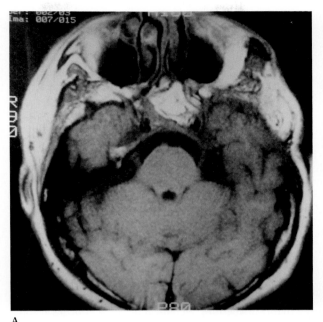

A

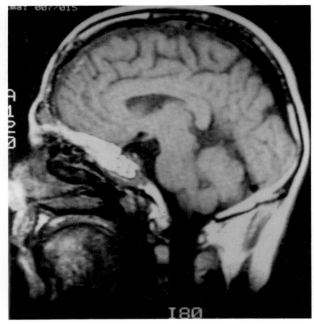

B

Figure 30-9 *A*, *B*. After tumor removal the reconstruction with the fat and galeal pericranial graft is well seen.

flap, or a galeal-pericranial-frontalis flap can devascularize the remainder of the flap. This can set the stage for a deeper infection. We have encountered this problem in one patient in whom a galeal flap was raised from the thin scalp of a patient who had a prior operation and pericranial flap reconstruction and who had received postoperative radiation therapy.

References

1. Derome P, Akermàn M, Anquez C, et al. Les tumeurs sphéno-ethmoidales: possibilités d'exérèse et de réparation chirurgícales. *Neurochirurgie* 1972; 18(Suppl 1):1–164.
2. Erba SM, Horton JA, Latchaw RE, et al. Balloon test occlusion of the internal carotid artery with stable xenon/CT cerebral blood flow imaging. *AJNR* 1988; 9:533–538.
3. Frazier CH. An approach to the hypophysis through the anterior cranial fossa. *Ann Surg* 1913; 57:145–150.
4. Jackson IT, Marsh WR, Hide TAH. Treatment of tumors involving the anterior cranial fossa. *Head Neck Surg* 1984; 6:901–913.
5. Jane JA, Park TS, Pobereskin LH, et al. The supraorbital approach: technical note. *Neurosurgery* 1982; 11:537–541.
6. Ketcham AS, Hoye RC, Van Buren JM, et al. Complications of intracranial facial resection for tumors of the paranasal sinuses. *Am J Surg* 1966; 112:591–596.
7. Lang J. Anterior cranial base anatomy. In: Sekhar LN, Schramm VL Jr (eds.), *Tumors of the Cranial Base: Diagnosis and Treatment*. Mt Kisco, New York: Futura, 1987: 247–264.
8. Ray BS, McLean JM. Combined intracranial and orbital operation for retinoblastoma. *Arch Ophthalmol* 1943; 30:437–445.
9. Schramm VL Jr, Myers EN, Maroon JC. Anterior skull base surgery for benign and malignant disease. *Laryngoscope* 1979; 89:1077–1091.
10. Sekhar LN, Janecka IP, Jones NF. Subtemporal-infratemporal and basal subfrontal approach to extensive cranial base tumours. *Acta Neurochir (Wien)* 1988; 92:83–92.
11. Smith RR, Klopp CT, Williams JM. Surgical treatment of cancer of the frontal sinus and adjacent areas. *Cancer* 1954; 7:991–994.
12. Van Buren JM, Ommaya AK, Ketcham AS. Ten years' experience with radical combined craniofacial resection of malignant tumors of the paranasal sinuses. *J Neurosurg* 1968; 28:341–350.

31

Midface Degloving Approach to Tumors Involving the Skull Base

Wayne M. Koch
John C. Price

Tumors involving the anterior and central skull base present the surgeon with a particularly difficult challenge. Access to the region is limited by the desire to preserve vital function and to achieve a cosmetically acceptable repair of the surgical defect. In order for resection to be complete while normal structures are protected, exposure must provide maximal visualization and accommodate necessary instrumentation. Lesions in this area are best addressed by a team of specialists including an otolaryngologist–head and neck surgeon approaching via the paranasal sinuses or nasopharynx and a neurosurgeon arriving at the skull base via a frontal or lateral craniotomy.

Since the introduction of the midfacial degloving procedure by Casson et al. in 1974,[3] otolaryngologists have found that it offers exposure of the nasal vault and paranasal sinuses equal to or surpassing that of other approaches while avoiding the creation of a facial scar. Midfacial degloving consists of rhinoplastic release of nasal soft tissues combined with bilateral anterior maxillary exposure. In combination with medial maxillectomy and ethmoidectomy, it provides a nearly ideal method for reaching the cribriform plate, inferomedial orbital apex, nasopharynx, and clivus from below.

The existence of a large number of alternative approaches to the anterior and central skull base attests to the complexity of surgical management of tumors in this area. Splitting the palate to gain access to the nasopharynx was described by Wilson in 1951.[15] In 1968, Doyle proposed the use of an incision along the nasofacial groove, the lateral rhinotomy, to enter the nasal cavity.[5] These reports were followed by proposals to combine various incisions to extend access.[6] The nasopharynx may also be approached laterally via a periauricular incision with splitting of the zygoma, mandible, and pterygoid plates,[12] or anteriorly via the midline, splitting the mandible, tongue, and palate.[2]

Late in the nineteenth century, George Caldwell and Henri Luc provided the foundation for the midfacial degloving procedure by describing a sublabial incision to reach the maxillary antrum.[14] Further incipient work was reported in 1927 by Portmann and Retrouvey, who performed a peroral maxillectomy.[10] After the first published account of the midfacial degloving procedure by Casson et al.,[3] Conley and Price applied the technique to the management of neoplastic disease.[4] Many others have subsequently attested to the merits of this approach.[1,9,13] Recently, Price reported a series of 29 cases of skull-base tumors managed by the degloving approach in combination with frontal or temporal craniotomy.[11]

Relevant Anatomy

The anterior wall of the maxilla and the bony nasal (pyriform) aperture are encountered immediately upon sublabial incision. The nasal skeleton has fibrous attachments at the pyriform aperture laterally and the anterior nasal spine in the midline. The cartilaginous skeleton, including the lower and upper lateral cartilages and the septal cartilage, projects rostrally from the bony aperture. It is the lower lateral cartilages which determine the shape of the nasal tip. The other cartilages provide support, projection, and supratip morphology. At the tip, the skin is firmly attached to the cartilages, but it becomes loose and mobile more superiorly. A dense fibrous band holds the upper lateral cartilages to the nasal bones. Within the nasal aperture, keratinizing, stratified squamous epithelium containing skin appendages abruptly changes to the ciliated columnar epithelium of the mucous membranes approximately 1 cm deep to the alar margin at a line known as the limen vestibule.

The midface is supported by a series of strong bony struts including the maxillary-frontal process medially, the zygomaticofrontal process laterally, and the pterygoid plates posteriorly. The fibrous bone between these struts becomes paper-thin in most areas. Inferiorly, the anterior maxillary wall contains the roots of the maxillary teeth, including any unerupted permanent teeth. The anterior maxilla is penetrated near the orbital rim by the infraorbital nerve, a sensory terminal branch of the maxillary division of the trigeminal nerve. The lacrimal duct courses deep to the maxillary-nasal suture on its way from the medial canthus to the nasal cavity. In adults, the maxillary sinus floor is at roughly the same level as the floor of the nose. The inferior turbinate joins the medial wall of the sinus. Posterosuperiorly, the maxillary sinus ostium opens into the middle meatus of the nose. The internal maxillary artery passes through the infratemporal fossa deep to the posterior wall of the maxillary sinus, branching into the sphenopalatine, posterior superior alveolar, pharyngeal, and greater palatine arteries behind the inferoposteromedial corner of the antrum. Superiorly, the infraorbital nerve crosses the roof of the sinus within a bony canal, although the bone may be dehiscent. Ciliated columnar epithelium rich in mucus-producing goblet cells lines the sinus walls. The midportion of the ethmoidal labyrinth is easily reached via the maxillary antrum. The frontoethmoidal recess and the sphenoid sinus are encountered when the ethmoidal air cells are opened anteriorly and posteriorly. The ethmoidal arteries, after crossing the roof of the orbit, enter the ethmoid sinuses and nasal roof at the level of the cribriform plate.

Surgical Technique

General anesthesia is administered using a precurved oral endotracheal tube fixed to the midline of the chin. The patient is positioned so as to allow intraoperative maneuvering of the head, permitting both flexion and extension and side to side movements. Topical 4% cocaine hydrochloride on cotton pledgets is placed intranasally to provide vasoconstriction, and the areas of planned incisions are injected with 1% lidocaine and 1:100,000 epinephrine. The patient's eyes are protected by a tarsorrhaphy stitch or corneal shields. A standard surgical scrub is performed. Draping is coordinated with the neurosurgical team but must permit access to the upper lip, nose, malar region, eyes, and eyebrows.

A complete nasal septal transfixion and intercartilaginous incisions separate the nasal tip including its lower lateral cartilage skeleton from the septum, upper lateral cartilages, and nasal dorsum (Fig. 31-1). Extension of the incision circumferentially within the nasal vestibule at the skin-mucosal junction completes the release of the nasal soft tissue at the pyriform aperture. Soft tissues of the nasal dorsum are widely elevated in the subperiosteal plane (Fig. 31-2). Elevation must extend to the maxillary-nasal suture on each side, joining across the midline, and from the nasal supratip to the glabella.

A sublabial incision from the first molar tooth across the midline to the opposite first molar is carried down to bone (Fig. 31-3). The soft tissue of the anterior maxilla is elevated in the subperiosteal plane, sparing each infraorbital nerve as it exits its foramen. Elevation is wide, from the zygomatic buttress to join the nasal elevation medially, extending as

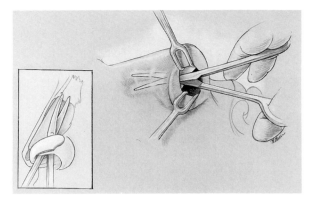

Figure 31-2 Elevation of nasal soft tissue. Elevation in a subperiosteal plane is carried out through the intercartilaginous incisions bilaterally. Care must be taken not to separate the upper lateral cartilages from the nasal bones. (From Price JC, Holliday MJ, Johns ME, et al. The versatile midface degloving approach. *Laryngoscope* 1988; 98:291–295, with permission.)

high as the infraorbital rim. Inferiorly, the soft tissues of the nasal floor and attachments at the anterior maxillary spine are separated, working through the nasal incisions in order to avoid creating a secondary entrance into the vestibule. Facial soft tissues including the lip, cheeks, intact nasal tip, columella, and nasal skin may then be retracted (Fig. 31-4).[8]

Bone is resected next, in order to visualize the tumor. The anterior wall of the maxilla is entered via a small chisel cut and the sinusotomy is widened with rongeurs from the zygomatic buttress to the medial wall of the nose and from the sinus floor to the infraorbital rim. The bone immediately around the infraorbital nerve is spared. Medially the opening is extended to the sinus roof by removing the frontal process of the maxilla. Osteotomies across the strut of bone remaining at the pyriform margin inferiorly and superiorly, followed by division of the corresponding soft tissues of the nose complete the medial maxillectomy. The maxillary an-

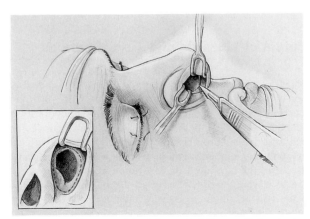

Figure 31-1 Intranasal incisions. A full transfixion incision is connected with intercartilaginous, pyriform, and nasal floor incisions bilaterally. (From Price JC, Holliday MJ, Johns ME, et al. The versatile midface degloving approach. *Laryngoscope* 1988; 98:291–295, with permission.)

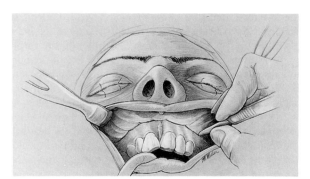

Figure 31-3 Sublabial incision. This incision extends to the first molar tooth on each side. Incision placement is such that a cuff of loose labial mucosa remains on the gingival side to facilitate closure. (From Price JC, Holliday MJ, Johns ME, et al. The versatile midface degloving approach. *Laryngoscope* 1988; 98:291–295, with permission.)

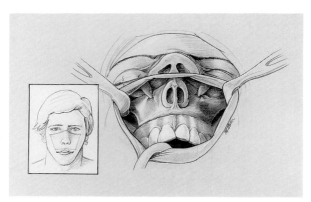

Figure 31-4 Elevation of malar soft tissue. Wide subperiosteal dissection permits the elevation of the midfacial soft tissue. Adhesions between the maxillary and nasal tunnels must be released. *Inset*: Region exposed by the midfacial degloving technique. (From Price JC, Holliday MJ, Johns ME, et al. The versatile midface degloving approach. *Laryngoscope* 1988; 98:291–295, with permission.)

trum on the contralateral side may be opened for inspection and access to the ethmoid sinuses, but resection of the maxillary-frontal process bilaterally may result in collapse of the midface. Ethmoidectomy and sphenoidectomy are then performed under direct vision. The entire nasal septum may be released inferiorly and swung to the side away from the lesion. Alternatively, the septum may be resected, although it is highly desirable to leave dorsal and caudal struts to support the nose. The cribriform plate is then well exposed, and safe resection of a tumor in the anterior skull base may be performed working in conjunction with the neurosurgery team after frontal craniotomy and elevation of the frontal lobes.

Full access to the pterygoid plates and muscles, posterior sphenoid, nasopharynx, and clivus requires removal of the posterior wall of the maxilla and the ascending process of the palatine bone. Brisk bleeding of the greater palatine and sphenopalatine arteries must be anticipated and controlled. After the resection of bulk tumor, an otologic drill with large diamond burr is useful to resect residual bone of the pterygoid plates and clivus, approaching the optic chiasm, carotid canals, pituitary, and posterior fossa dura. Use of the operating microscope during this step is essential. All bone spicules are smoothed. Hemostasis is achieved by temporary packing with gauze soaked in a vasoconstricting agent, followed by bipolar cautery. Extensive areas of dural repair performed via the craniotomy are covered from below by dermal grafts. The cavity is packed with antibiotic-soaked petrolatum gauze that is brought out through the nares.

Closure is begun by redraping the facial soft tissue and carefully repositioning the nasal tip using a transfixion stitch. The vestibular incisions are then accurately approximated using interrupted, absorbable 4-0 sutures. An interlocking, running closure of the sublabial incision is performed. After the skin is cleansed, tincture of benzoin is applied to the nose and cheeks, and the nose is taped and splinted as after a rhinoplasty.

Packing is gradually removed after 3 to 5 days using twice-daily advances of the gauze strip. Intranasal crusting occurs for several months and must be controlled with saline irrigation and repeated mechanical cleaning in the clinic.

Advantages and Limitations

Benign and malignant neoplasms which occupy the anterior or central skull base may be addressed via the midfacial degloving procedure. For most lesions, exposure is equivalent or superior to that achieved by lateral rhinotomy, transpalatal, or other approaches. The bilateral access obtained is useful for large tumors or when the disease crosses the midline. Hemostasis is facilitated by this approach in that both internal maxillary arteries may be easily exposed. The technique does not involve any external incisions, and there is little risk of palatal dysfunction.

Midfacial degloving does not provide sufficient exposure of the lateral maxilla for some cases. When the disease extends to the zygomatic buttress, lateral rhinotomy with elevation of a large, unilateral cheek flap is preferable. Tumor within the soft tissues of the medial canthus, nasolacrimal, and frontal regions is not easily managed via midfacial degloving alone. An incision immediately below the eyebrow may be combined with a midfacial degloving approach in that situation, or the lateral rhinotomy incision may be extended to the brow. The frontal sinus ostia may be enlarged via the midfacial degloving approach, but tumors invading this sinus must be managed in conjunction with the frontal craniotomy bone flap or by a separate frontal sinusotomy using a coronal or brow incision. Controlled elevation of a partial-thickness cheek flap in the setting of malar soft tissue invasion by tumor is best performed under the more direct vision obtained by lateral rhinotomy. Finally, midfacial degloving does not permit access to the petrous apex due to the location of the internal carotid canals and optic chiasm. A lateral skull base approach is required to safely reach this area.[7]

Potential Hazards and Complications

Bleeding may be profuse during the osteotomies and resection of nasal and paranasal sinus soft tissues. Once the tumor has been removed, hemorrhage is controlled temporarily by packing followed by meticulous use of bipolar electrocautery and absorbable thrombostatic collagen. Preoperative angiography and embolization of feeding vessels significantly decreases the bleeding from the tumor in many cases. Failure to elevate nasal soft tissue in the proper subperiosteal plane will result in excessive avoidable blood loss before tumor resection.

When wide sinusotomies are not performed on all sinuses exposed or approached during the procedure, postoperative edema and crusting may result in obstruction and sinusitis. Residual bony spicules are a nidus for osteitis. Crusting is an expected result of the stripping of mucous membranes and will continue until full reepithelization occurs. Even after that, irregular nasal airflow and the breakdown of normal mucociliary transport causes crusting and a sense of dryness in the nose. Ozena has not been a problem after midfacial degloving in our experience, however.

Malar (infraorbital) and maxillary dental numbness or paresthesias are common postoperative complaints. Unless the nerves in question have been sacrificed to achieve adequate tumor resection, sensation should return within 3 to 6 months.

Hyperplastic scarring and contraction beneath the nasomalar flap may result in a "sneer" deformity of the upper lip and columella. Misplacement of the nasal transfixion stitch may cause a "polly-beak" deformity or excessive show of the nasal apertures. Vestibular stenosis is the result of inaccurate closure of the intranasal sutures. These problems will evolve and may correct themselves during the initial postoperative period. Thus, attempts at surgical correction should not be made for at least 6 months. A small amount of CSF drainage may be seen immediately postoperatively in the setting of extensive dural repair and is managed conservatively with lumbar drainage and bed rest. If CSF leakage persists or occurs when the dura had not been violated, surgical exploration and repair may be required. Blindness, cerebrovascular accident, cavernous sinus thrombophlebitis, epiphora, oronasal or oroantral fistulae, and disturbances in the facial growth patterns (in pediatric cases) are theoretically possible but have not been reported after midfacial degloving.

Results

Nearly 100 midfacial degloving procedures have been performed by members of our department from 1985 to the present. Approximately one quarter of these cases involved tumor resection at the anterior or central skull base. In each case, exposure was adequate for tumor resection in conjunction with a craniotomy. Although this represents a small patient population with limited follow-up information available to date, it is our conviction that local control of tumor and long-term survival for these patients is as good as in published series using any alternative surgical approach.

The midfacial degloving technique is a versatile, effective approach to the anterior and central skull base. It is rela-

tively easy to master, requires only 2 to 3 h to accomplish and repair, and offers superior cosmetic results compared to the alternative methods available for managing tumors in this location. With appropriate patient selection, we believe that it has become the method of choice for surgical management of neoplasms of the nasal roof and midskull base.

References

1. Allen GW, Siegel GJ. The sublabial approach for extensive nasal and sinus resection. *Laryngoscope* 1981; 91:1635–1640.
2. Biller HF, Lawson W. Anterior mandibular-splitting approach to the skull base. *Ear Nose Throat J* 1986; 65:134–141.
3. Casson PR, Bonanno PC, Converse JM. The midfacial degloving procedure. *Plast Reconst Surg* 1974; 53:102–103.
4. Conley J, Price JC. Sublabial approach to the nasal and nasopharyngeal cavities. *Am J Surg* 1979; 138:615–618.
5. Doyle PJ. Approach to tumors of the nose, nasopharynx and paranasal sinuses. *Laryngoscope* 1968; 78:1756–1762.
6. Doyle PJ, Riding K, Kahn K. Management of nasopharygeal angiofibroma. *J Otolaryngol* 1977; 6:224–232.
7. Fisch U. Infratemporal fossa approach for extensive tumors of the temporal bone and base of the skull. In: Silverstein H, Norrell H (eds.), *Neurological Surgery of the Ear*. Birmingham: Aesculapius, 1977:34–53.
8. Kahn JM, Hilsinger RL Jr, Korol HW. A method for hands-free retraction when performing the midfacial degloving surgical approach. *Otolaryngol Head Neck Surg* 1989; 100:83–84.
9. Maniglia AJ. Indications and techniques of midfacial degloving: a 15-year experience. *Arch Otolaryngol Head Neck Surg* 1986; 112:750–752.
10. Portmann G, Retrouvey H. *Le Cancer du Nez, des Fosses Nasales, de Cavités Accessoires et du Naso-pharynx*. Paris: Gaston Doin, 1927.
11. Price JC. The midfacial degloving approach to the central skull base. *Ear Nose Throat J* 1986; 65:174–180.
12. Ross DE, Sukis AE. Nasopharyngeal tumors: a new surgical approach. *Am J Surg* 1966; 111:524–530.
13. Sacks ME, Conley J, Rabuzzi DD, et al. The degloving approach for total excision of inverted papilloma. *Laryngoscope* 1984; 94:1595–1598.
14. Tobin HA. Surgery of the maxilla and mandible. In: Paparella MM, Shumrick DA (eds.), *Otolaryngology*, 2d ed. Philadelphia: Saunders, 1980: 2716–2757.
15. Wilson CP. The approach to the nasopharynx. *Proc R Soc Med* 1951; 44:353–358.

32

Transoral Approach to the Clivus and Upper Cervical Spine

Arnold H. Menezes

The first pathologic description of abnormalities affecting the craniovertebral junction (CVJ) was given by Meckel in 1815.[6] After this initial description, autopsy studies were reported in reference to these abnormalities. It was only after Chamberlain's classic radiographic study of basilar invagination in 1939[2] that bony abnormalities of the CVJ were considered for antemortem recognition and treatment, rather than being regarded as pathologic and anatomic curiosities.

The early surgical treatment of CVJ compressive pathology was posterior enlargement of the foramen magnum and removal of the posterior arches of the atlas and axis vertebrae.[7,10] The postoperative mortality and morbidity associated with such treatment of irreducible ventral compressive abnormalities of the brain stem and high cervical cord were high.[4,7] In 1951, Scoville and Sherman stated that "the angulation of the medulla over an abnormally high odontoid process is the chief offender and causation of neurologic

signs and disability in platybasia. Future surgical advance lies in the development of successful removal of the odontoid, possibly through the mouth."[13] A transoral approach, through the posterior pharyngeal wall, was an operation that had been in use for drainage of retropharyngeal abscess for many years. Although this route provided access to the CVJ, it had not gained its well-deserved place in the neurosurgical armamentarium, because of initial reports of infection, limited exposure, CSF leakage, vertebral artery injury, and unacceptable patient morbidity and mortality. Fang and Ong, in 1962, published their direct anterior approach to the upper cervical spine for atlanto-axial instability and fusion, as well as for tuberculous lesions.[5] Over the past three decades, the value of the anterior cervical approach to lesions of the ventral spinal canal has been defined in several disorders including abnormalities of the clivus and the upper cervical spine with ventral compression of the cervicomedullary junction (CMJ).[5,7,12,15] Variations of the transoral operation include combinations with the transbasal procedure as described by Derome, the trans-sphenoidal operation, lateral rhinotomy, and mandibular splitting with a median glossotomy.

In 1977, a surgical physiologic approach to correct pathology secondary to abnormality of the CVJ was formulated.[10] Using these guidelines, the high morbidity and mortality previously attendent with posterior decompression of ventrally placed lesions was not seen.[9] The factors which influenced specific treatment were (1) the etiology of the lesion—whether it was bony, granulation or soft tissue, tumor or vascular; (2) whether the bony abnormality could be reduced to its normal position; (3) the direction and the mechanics of compression; and (4) the associated neural abnormalities present.

The primary treatment of CVJ lesions that can be reduced is stabilization (Table 32-1). Surgical decompression of the CMJ is required in patients with irreducible pathology. The transoral-transpharyngeal approach has been the procedure of choice for ventral decompression of the CMJ.[1,3,7–9,11,12] This approach has been utilized in 91 individuals ranging in age from 6 to 82 years, 33 of whom were children.

TABLE 32-1 Summary of Surgical Treatment at the Craniovertebral Junction in 378 Patients (1977–1988)

Stability	Compression	Operative Approach	Postoperative Stability	Posterior Fusion
Reducible 191 (60)	—	Immobilization 25(23)		166(37)
Nonreducible 187 (75)	Ventral 91(33)	Anterior	Stable 21(5)	
			Unstable 70(28)	70(28)
	Dorsal 96(42)	Posterior	Stable 30(11)	
			Unstable 66(31)	66(31)

NOTE: Numbers in parentheses refer to number of children.

TABLE 32-2 Pathology in 91 Patients Who Underwent Transoral-Transpalatine Clivus-Odontoid Resection

Primary basilar invagination	48
Rheumatoid irreducible cranial settling	17
Basilar invagination after malunion, O-C1 dislocation	4
Upward migration of nonfused odontoid fracture (C1-C2 posterior fusion)	4
Dystopic os odontoideum	7
Granulation mass	4
Calcium pyrophosphate mass	1
Osteoblastoma, C1	1
Chordoma, lower clivus	4
Chondroma, clivus-C1	1
Total (1977–1988)	91

The primary indication for the transoral-transpalatine approach to the clivus and upper cervical spine is ventral irreducible compression of the CMJ. This includes bony abnormalities, soft tissue epidural masses such as granulation tissue and tumor, and rarely an intradural ventral mass at the foramen magnum that defies other surgical approaches (Table 32-2). It is important that mere identification of a ventral abnormality at the CVJ, such as in rheumatoid cranial settling, does not form an indication for a transoral operation.[3] A ventral operative decompression is of questionable value unless the reducibility of the lesion has been attempted by cervical traction (except in tumor). Thus, of the 75 patients in our series with rheumatoid basilar invagination and cranial settling, only 17 required a ventral decompression. The remaining 58 patients of this group had reduction of the odontoid invagination with cervical traction and required only a posterior stabilization procedure.

Patients with a Chiari malformation and atlas-occipital assimilation with basilar invagination require first a ventral decompression and subsequently a dorsal decompression procedure together with rerouting of the CSF pathways to improve the CSF circulation (Fig. 32-1). Intra-arachnoid lesions should not be approached by the transoral route as the primary procedure unless other approaches prove ineffective. Numerous patients with clivus chordoma, meningioma, and schwannoma, referred to our facility for an anterior transoral resection, underwent suboccipital or posterolateral approaches combined with middle fossa and posterior operations, with complete surgical resection of the tumor.

Investigative Studies

Plain roentgenograms of the skull and cervical spine are essential for recognition of bony pathology as well as identification of oral pharyngeal abnormalities that have a bearing on the surgical technique to be utilized. Paget's disease, osteogenesis imperfecta, platybasia, basilar invagination, Klippel-Feil syndrome, os odontoideum, and osseous tumors of the skull base and upper cervical spine are easily visualized on these plain films.[8,9] In addition, instability of the CVJ and upper cervical spine is readily recognized by documenting reducibility with the flexed and extended positions.[9,14] The neuroimaging procedure of choice is magnetic resonance imaging (MRI). This is accomplished in the coronal, sagittal, parasagittal, and axial views with thin sections to best identify the neural as well as osseous abnormalities (Figs. 32-2A and B). The flexed and extended positions must be viewed in the midsagittal plane in both the T1-weighted and T2-weighted images. The drawback here is suboptimal bone detail which is best supplemented by dynamic pleuridirectional polytomography in the frontal and lateral planes, including the lateral flexed and extended positions (Fig. 32-2C). These studies define the bone abnormalities in detail, as well as demonstrate abnormal biomechanical and translation forces and the effects of cervical traction.[16] In rheumatoid involvement of the CVJ, as well as

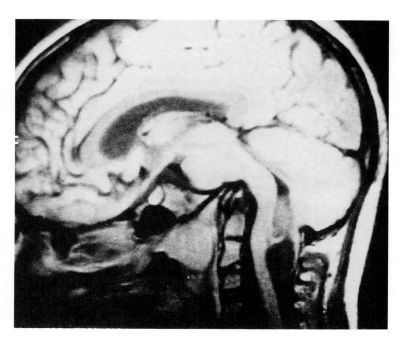

Figure 32-1 Midsagittal T1-weighted MRI of brain reveals extreme ventral indentation of the pontomedullary junction by the clivus-atlas and odontoid complex. There is basilar invagination and atlas occipitalization. The cystic cerebellar tonsils extend to the C3 level. The patient presented with lower cranial nerve palsies and spastic quadriparesis.

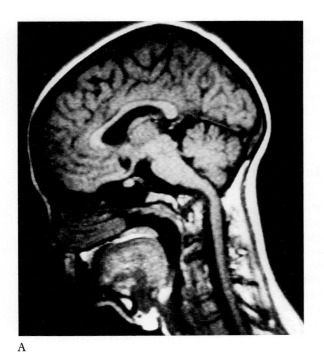

A

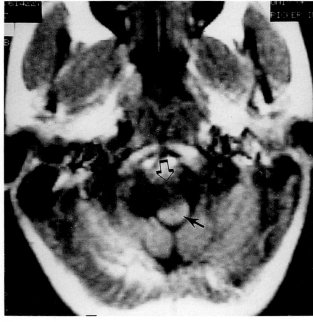

B

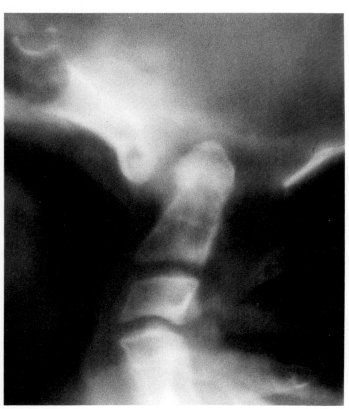

C

Figure 32-2 *A*. Midsagittal T1-weighted MRI of the head and cervical spine shows odontoid invagination into the foramen magnum, compressing the cervico-medullary neural tissue ventrally. This 26-year-old woman complained of "lightning" paresthesias in the trunk and limbs with attempted head extension. *B*. Axial T1-weighted MRI, 15 mm above the plane of the foramen magnum. There is compression of the medulla (*arrow*) by bone and granulation tissue from a ventral direction (*open arrow*). *C*. Lateral midline pleuridirectional tomography of the craniovertebral junction (CVJ). This illustrates the bony abnormalities of occipitalization of the atlas, odontoid invagination into the foramen magnum, and abnormal clivus-odontoid angulation. There is an increased interspinous distance between the dorsal foramen magnum and the axis. *D*. Lateral midline pleuridirectional tomogram of the CVJ after a transoral operation documents the bony resection of the clivus-atlas anterior arch and odontoid. *E*. Midsagittal T1-weighted MRI of the CMJ 5 days after transoral resection of the ventral CVJ. There is no neural compression. Prevertebral swelling is noted. The patient had recovered neurologic function.

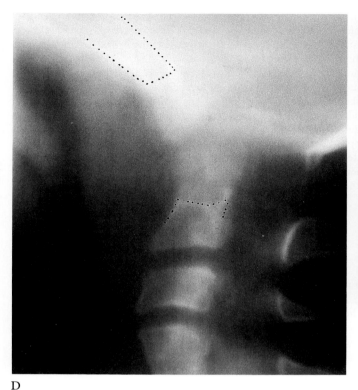

D

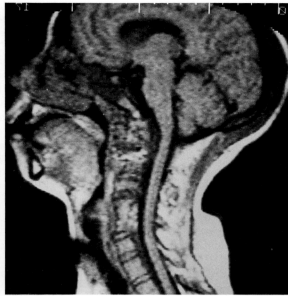

E

Figure 32-2 Continued

with os odontoideum and atlanto-axial instability with associated ventral cervicomedullary compression, it is important that an MRI-compatible halo traction device is utilized to document the effects of cervical traction and an attempt to achieve reduction. In addition, the preoperative halo traction in such situations provides familiarity to the patient regarding traction which would more than likely be required for the stabilization procedure and subsequent halo vest immobilization should this be required. Median nerve somatosensory evoked responses are obtained during this time as a baseline to provide the added safety required during the operative procedure. Occasionally CT myelography of the CVJ is essential to identify the precise location and nature of the invaginating mass such as with neurofibromas, sequestered bone from odontoid rheumatoid basilar invagination, and intradural tumors.[9,14]

Relevant Anatomy

In order to understand craniovertebral abnormalities and their treatment, it is necessary to possess a knowledge of the embryologic development of this area as well as its complex anatomy and biomechanics.[8,16]

The occipito-atlanto-axial joints are approximated by multiple ligamentous structures that are responsible for its complex movement and stability. The ventral ligaments include the anterior atlanto-occipital membrane (which is the rostral extension of the anterior longitudinal ligament) and its insertions on the anterior clivus. The principal stabilizer of the atlanto-axial joint, the transverse ligament, approximates the dens to the atlas and inserts on the mesial aspect of each atlas lateral mass. The atlas is connected to the occiput by the apical dens ligament, the cruciate ligament, the tectorial membrane, and the oblique alar ligaments. The posterior stabilizing tissues include the ligamentum flavum, ligamentum nuchae, the posterior atlanto-occipital membrane, the supraspinous ligaments, and the paracervical musculature.

The occipito-atlanto-axial articulations are lined by synovial membrane which is embryologically derived from the same unit. The lymphatic drainage of the occipito-atlanto-axial joints is into the retropharyngeal glands and then into the deep cervical chain.

Each hypoglossal nerve exits from the condylar foramen $1\frac{3}{4}$ to 2 cm from the midline, at the base of the skull. This limits the lateral extent of the exposure of the clivus with a transoral operative procedure. Likewise, the medial opening of the eustachian tubes at the upper level of the pharynx prevents exposure at the CVJ from being more than $1\frac{1}{2}$ to 2 cm to either side of the midline. It is important to realize that the posterior pharyngeal musculature is devoid over the clivus, and the posterior nasopharyngeal mucosa is extremely thin in this location. The circular sinus, also known as the marginal sinus, circumscribes the foramen magnum and thus is the first structure to be encountered behind the clivus at the foramen magnum. Opening of one of the leaves of this dural sinus requires cauterization of both its leaves or tamponade with hemostatic agents.

The angle of approach in a transoral operation is dependent on (1) the ability to open the oral cavity to its maximum, and thus the integrity of the temporomandibular joints; (2) the presence of abnormal tonsillar and adenoid tissue; and (3) severe basilar invagination with platybasia which can place the CVJ higher than the dorsum sellae. This creates a narrow channel of approach which may require resection of a portion of the hard palate to gain access into this area. The inferior limit of a transoral operation is the C2-C3 junction. Caudal exposure is obtained by either midline splitting of the tongue or a combination of mandibular splitting and median glossotomy.[1] Should an intradural operative procedure be envisioned through the transoral route, vertebral angiography is mandatory to identify the location of abnormal vascular structures and the vascularity of the tumor.

Operative Procedure

Nasopharyngeal cultures are obtained 3 days before the proposed surgery. If no pathologic flora are identified, then 2 million units of penicillin G are administered 6 h before the operation, intraoperatively, and every 4 h for the first day. The patient is positioned supine on the operating table using 5 to 7 lb of skeletal traction in an MRI-compatible halo ring. Fiber-optic awake oral endotracheal intubation is then accomplished, and the patient is repositioned and examined awake to ensure no change in neurologic status due to the positioning. General endotracheal and intravenous anesthesia then ensues. A tracheostomy is preferred to provide for better operative exposure and to ensure an adequate airway after the operation. This is an important step in the procedure. It keeps the endotracheal tube away from the oral cavity as well as provides for postoperative safety if lingual swelling occurs after the operation. It also allows for ease of ventilation and respiratory toilet, especially in patients who have impaired brain stem function.

Following tracheostomy, dental rolls soaked in 5% cocaine topical anesthetic are placed into the nasal passages to prevent drainage of nasal sinus secretions into the high nasopharynx during the operation. A pharyngeal gauze packing is also placed in the laryngopharynx to prevent fluid going into the stomach. This also allows free cleansing of the nasopharynx, oropharynx, laryngopharynx, as well as the oral cavity with 10% PVP iodine solution and with hydrogen peroxide. A normal saline rinse completes the preparation. Previously made teeth guards are then placed over the upper and lower dentition and a self-retaining Dingman mouth retractor is placed for tongue depression and lateral retraction of the cheeks. A midline incision in the soft palate is made extending from the hard palate to the base of the uvula, skirting away from the midline. Stay sutures are then placed in the soft palate and retracted over the springs of the Dingman mouth retractor. The operating microscope is now brought in for magnification and a concentrated light source.

The posterior pharyngeal mucosa is anesthetized with topical cocaine, and infiltration of the median raphe with 0.5% lidocaine solution with 1:200,000 epinephrine. A midline incision in the posterior pharyngeal median raphe is carried through the mucosa, the constrictor muscles, and the buccopharyngeal fascia. The prevertebral fascia is swept away and retracted with stay sutures. The longus colli muscles are separated from their ligamentous osseous attachment to expose the caudal half of the clivus and the atlas and axis vertebrae as far laterally as the eustachian tubes. The anterior longitudinal ligament and the occipital ligaments are cauterized and sharply dissected free of the caudal clivus, the anterior arch of the atlas, and the ventral aspect of the axis body. Stay sutures help in maintaining lateral retraction of the soft tissues. When necessary, the caudal half of the clivus is removed using a high speed air drill. The bony resection is then carried down to the anterior arch of the atlas, which is removed for a width of 3 cm in the midline to visualize the proximal odontoid process. Depending on the pathology, granulation tissue may be present behind the anterior atlas arch. This prevents visualization of the proximal odontoid process. During resection of the caudal clivus, it is necessary to separate the dura from the posterior aspect to prevent bleeding from the marginal sinus. All soft tissue anterior to the odontoid process is now removed, and the odontoid is resected in a rostral-caudal direction using a high speed drill with a diamond burr. The shell of odontoid process is finally removed with fine Kerrison rongeurs, and the additional granulation tissue is cauterized and subsequently removed far laterally toward the occipital condyles. The extent of exposure is 3 to $3\frac{1}{2}$ cm in its transverse dimension. It is only after resection of the tectorial membrane and additional granulation tissue that an adequate decompression is accomplished. This is heralded by the dura becoming pulsatile and occupying the decompression site. The caudal resection should be taken down to the midportion of the body of the axis and is limited at the central vein exit from the C2 body. Should further exposure into the ventral spinal canal be required, this is easily carried out far laterally as well as caudally.

If an intradural exposure is planned, a lumbar subarachnoid drain is installed prior to the operation.[3,9,12] CSF is now removed, relieving the turgidity of the ventral dura and allowing intradural exposure. A cruciate incision is then made in the dura caudal to the foramen magnum and then extended upward in the vertical direction. Hemostatic clips are applied to the dura at the marginal sinus and sutures are used for self-retaining dural retraction for exposure of the intradural contents. The marginal sinus may be cauterized. The intradural operative procedure must be carried out with the highest power of the operating microscope. Dural closure is performed with 0000 polygalactin suture to be as complete as possible. The ideal closure is made by placing fascia (harvested from the external oblique aponeurosis) adjacent to the dural closure. Following this, a fat pad is then used to reinforce the fascia. The longus colli muscles, the pharyngeal musculature, and the pharyngeal mucosa are then approximated with dyed 000 polygalactin sutures in individual layers. The soft palate is closed in two layers. The nasal mucosa of the soft palate is approximated with interrupted sutures, and the oral mucosa, together with the muscularis, is brought together with horizontal mattress sutures.

Intraoperative somatosensory evoked potentials and brain stem auditory evoked responses act as supplementary neurophysiologic monitors during the operation.[18] Before closure of the posterior pharyngeal wall, aerobic and anaerobic cultures are obtained from the depths of the wound.

Subsequent to the surgery, the patient is maintained in 5 to 7 lb of skeletal traction. The patient is nursed in a 15- to 20-degree head-up position, and care is taken to avoid pharyngeal suctioning. Intravenous hyperalimentation is maintained for 5 to 6 days, after which oral intake of clear liquids is permitted. This is followed by gradual increased feelings to a regular diet by the end of the third week.

If the dura was opened and a fascial graft used for repair, intravenous antibiotics for both aerobic and anaerobic coverage is continued for 10 days, as is the spinal drainage. It is possible that a lumboperitoneal shunt may be required, as experienced by others. A fenestrated tracheostomy tube allows for speech by the third postoperative day.

Evaluation of Postoperative Stability

Between the 5th and 7th days after the ventral operation, pleuridirectional lateral tomography of the CVJ is obtained to visualize the resection and determine craniovertebral stability (Fig. 32-2D). This is done both with and without traction in the flexed and extended positions. The tomography must envisage both of the facet joints to identify an offset at the lateral occipital atlantoaxial articulations during flexion and extension. Excessive displacement of the craniospinal axis without and with halo traction is indicative of instability. MRI of the CMJ is performed during this time before any other surgical intervention (Fig. 32-2E). If instability is identified, a posterior occipitocervical or atlanto-axial fusion using bone, acrylic, or bone plus acrylic is done at the identified unstable site. In those individuals with bone fusion, occipitocervical immobilization is provided by a halo brace for 6 months. In children, the transverse portion of the cruciate ligament is not interrupted, to provide for stability.

A dorsal fixation is usually necessary after the transoral clivus odontoid resection for abnormalities associated with atlas assimilation and segmentation failures of the upper cervical spine. By definition, rheumatoid cranial settling is an unstable situation and all such patients will require occipitocervical fixation. Similarly, patients with dystopic os odontoideum require fixation.

Discussion

The advantages of the transoral-transpalatine approach to the craniovertebral junction compared to other operative approaches in irreducible ventral pathology is that (1) the extended position is utilized, thus decreasing the angulation of the brain stem during surgery as opposed to a flexed position necessary for a posterior approach or a rotated angled approach for the lateral extrapharyngeal approaches[15]; (2) the surgery is performed through the avascular pharyngeal median raphe and through the clivus; and (3) the impinging bony pathology and accompanying granulation tissue that accompanies chronic instability is accessible only via the ventral route.

The disadvantages of a posterior decompression of the CVJ in the presence of existing ventral pathology is that neurologic deterioration can occur due to

1. The progressive angulation of the pons, medulla, and cervical cord over the peglike ventral invasive complex
2. Sagging of the cerebellum into the dorsally created enlargement, resulting in an increased angulation of the lower brain stem
3. Increased neural tissue impaction that occurs at the foramen magnum, thus increasing the chances of craniospinal CSF pressure dissociation, as with Chiari malformations, that leads to increasing communicating syringohydromyelia[17]

The extent of lateral surgical exposure of the anterior CVJ via the transoral-transpalatine approach is limited by the emergence of the hypoglossal nerves $1\frac{1}{2}$ to 2 cm lateral to the clivus midline, by the vertebral arteries, and by the eustachian tubes just below the base of the skull. However, this in itself allows a total of 3 to 4 cm of transverse exposure, which is sufficient for removal of pathologic lesions from the lower half of the clivus to the upper portion of the body of C3 (Figs. 32-3A and B). Due to the inherent possibility of infection through oral contamination, intra-arachnoid lesions should not be approached via the transoral route unless other approaches are ineffective. The median labiomandibular glossotomy combined with a transoral approach adds exposure to lesions caudal to the C3 vertebra.

The importance of a tracheostomy cannot be overemphasized. It obviates the need for patient reintubation in the postoperative period in those who have had respiratory insufficiency secondary to brain stem dysfunction and also provides a safeguard against obstruction from postoperative lingual swelling. In addition, it allows for increased operative exposure during the transoral procedure.

The soft palate incision provides direct access to the lower clivus and the high craniovertebral junction. The technique of suture of the soft palate and retraction into the nasal cavity, as advocated by some, is not beneficial for exposure at the CVJ.

The experience with otolaryngologic procedures indicates that it is safe to conduct major operations in the upper airway using appropriate antibiotic coverage only when pathogenic flora are identified. There appears to be an inherent host immunity of the nasopharyngeal structures to normal oral flora. Needless to say, the primary potential hazard is infection. This may be bacterial or fungal. Thus, it is important to have precise indications for the operation as well as to limit as far as possible the procedure to extradural compressive phenomena.

Injury to the vertebral arteries is avoided by precise preoperative localization of the vessels on coronal and parasagittal magnetic resonance images and by limitation of the lateral dissection during operation. Secondary involvement of the vertebral artery may occur with osteomyelitis that can occur postoperatively due to an epidural retropharyngeal abscess. Treatment of this is immediate evacuation of the

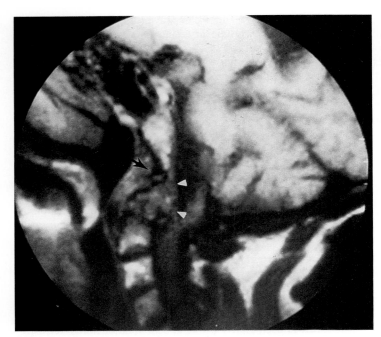

A

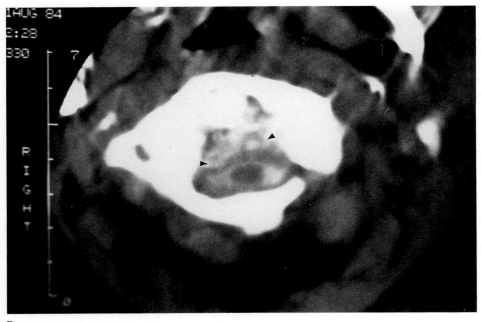

B

Figure 32-3 *A*. Midsagittal T1-weighted MRI of the CMJ. The caudal clivus and odontoid area is replaced by a chordoma (*white arrowheads*) kinking the CMJ. The prevertebral mass is located by the *arrow*. *B*. CT-metrizamide myelogram. Axial view at the level of the atlas. The neural tissue at the CMJ is dorsally displaced by the extradural chordoma (*between the black arrowheads*).

abscess and appropriate antibiotic coverage with adequate attention to the nutritional status of the patient. This can become difficult in rheumatoid patients who have been on a high dosage of steroids over a long term.

Dehiscence of the pharyngeal closure is treated by utilizing a pharyngeal flap, and at times closure by secondary intention if infected. The key to wound healing during this time is nutrition.

Most patients do develop a serous otitis media and a transient sinusitis due to the supine position, which must be alleviated as soon as possible. Failure to identify postoperative cranivertebral instability can be disastrous. It is thus imperative to avoid this by investigating for postoperative stability by the end of the first week. Should the integrity be preserved, it is advisable to recheck the postoperative stability at the end of 6 to 8 weeks. Most patients with brain stem dysfunction will require tube feedings to prevent aspiration. Recovery has been the rule.

Results

The youngest patient in our series was 5 years old, and the oldest was 82. There were 33 children below the age of 16 who underwent the ventral operation for primary basilar invagination, abnormal clivus-odontoid articulation, or dystopic os odontoideum. The transverse portion of the cruciate ligament and the periosteum of the dens was not interrupted in eight children below 12 years. These children were immobilized postoperatively in a halo brace or a sterno-occipito-mandibular immobilizing brace for 3 months. Three of these eight children later showed craniovertebral instability and required dorsal fixation. The other five have remained stable, and three of these demonstrate new bone formation replacing the odontoid process.

Intradural lesions were evident in nine individuals. In five of these patients a sequestered odontoid process was found indenting into the pons and medulla secondary to rheumatoid upward invagination of the odontoid process. In one patient with a clivus chordoma, a previous dorsal operative procedure allowed the tumor to grow into an intra-arachnoid location. Post-traumatic odontoid invagination and abnormal location of the occipital condyles and lateral masses of the atlas with disruption of the dura were recognized in three individuals.

Of the 91 patients who underwent a ventral transoral-transpalatine decompression of the CVJ, 72 required a dorsal fixation procedure. In these individuals, postoperative immobilization was maintained for an average of 6 months.

Neurologic recovery was the rule in all patients. Eight individuals who were dependent on a ventilator before the operation after either a previous primary posterior decompression or trauma, had recovery of their neurologic deficit during the immediate postoperative period. Brain stem dysfunction was a prominent presenting feature in 19 individuals with basilar invagination and a Chiari malformation; this regressed following a ventral decompressive procedure. Ten patients with a Chiari malformation and occipitalization with basilar invagination had undergone a primary operation consisting of a posterior fossa and upper cervical canal decompression. Rapid deterioration or initial improvement followed by progressive deterioration in neurologic function ensued. All of these patients improved after the ventral decompression. It is more than likely that the improvement is secondary to relief of brain stem angulation and possibly due to improved CSF circulation, relieving the craniospinal CSF pressure dissociation. Visual abnormalities of internuclear ophthalmoplegia and cranial nerve palsies also improved.

Two patients died within the first month of operation. A 79-year-old rheumatoid man with cranial settling and basilar invagination had recovered neurologic function. He died 4 weeks after operation from a myocardial infarction. A 52-year-old woman, admitted quadriplegic after a motor vehicle accident, died 3 weeks after the operation from *Escherichia coli* sepsis that was existent at the time of her admission. She had recovered a great deal of her neurologic deficit after the transoral operation. A pharyngeal wound infection occurred in an 82-year-old man, with subsequent osteomyelitis of the atlas that responded to drainage of the retropharyngeal abscess and immobilization plus appropriate antibiotic coverage.

The ventral transoral-transpharyngeal approach to the lower clivus and upper cervical spine is a rapid, safe, and efficacious means of relieving irreducible ventral compressive pathology at the craniovertebral junction.

References

1. Arbit E, Patterson RH Jr. Combined transoral and median labiomandibular glossotomy approach to the upper cervical spine. *Neurosurgery* 1981; 8:672–674.
2. Chamberlain WE. Basilar impression (platybasia): a bizarre developmental anomaly of the occipital bone and upper cervical spine with striking and misleading neurologic manifestations. *Yale J Biol Med* 1939; 11:487–496.
3. Crockard HA, Essigman WK, Stevens JM, et al. Surgical treatment of cervical cord compression in rheumatoid arthritis. *Ann Rheum Dis* 1985; 44:809–816.
4. Dastur DK, Wadia WH, DeSai AD, et al. Medullospinal compression due to atlanto-axial dislocation and sudden haematomyelia during decompression. *Brain* 1965; 88:897–924.
5. Fang HSY, Ong GB. Direct anterior approach to the upper cervical spine. *J Bone Joint Surg [Am]* 1962; 44:1588–1604.
6. Gladstone RJ, Erichsen-Powell W. Manifestation of occipital vertebrae and fusion of the atlas with the occipital bone. *J Anat Physiol* 1915; 49:190–209.
7. Greenberg AD, Scoville WB, Davey LM. Transoral decompression of atlanto-axial dislocation due to odontoid hypoplasia: report of two cases. *J Neurosurg* 1968; 28:266–269.
8. Menezes AH. Os odontoideum: pathogenesis, dynamics and management. In: Marlin AE (ed.), *Concepts in Pediatric Neurosurgery*. Basel: Karger, 1988; 8:133–145.
9. Menezes AH, VanGilder JC. Anomalies of the craniovertebral junction. In: Youmans JR (ed.), *Neurological Surgery*, 3d ed. Philadelphia: Saunders, 1990:1359–1420.
10. Menezes AH, VanGilder JC, Graf CJ, et al. Craniocervical abnormalities: comprehensive surgical approach. *J Neurosurg* 1980; 53:444–455.
11. Mullan S, Naunton R, Hekmat-panah J, et al. The use of an anterior approach to ventrally placed tumors in the foramen magnum and vertebral column. *J Neurosurg* 1966; 24:536–543.
12. Pasztor E, Vajda J, Piffko P, et al. Transoral surgery for craniocervical space-occupying processes. *J Neurosurg* 1984; 60:276–281.
13. Scoville WB, Sherman IJ. Platybasia: report of ten cases with comments on familial tendency, a special diagnostic sign, and the end results of operation. *Ann Surg* 1951; 133:496–502.
14. Smoker WRK, Keyes WD, Dunn VD, et al. MRI versus conventional radiologic examinations in the evaluation of the craniovertebral and cervicomedullary junction. *Radiographics* 1986; 6:953–994.
15. Stevenson GC, Stoney RJ, Perkins RK, et al. A transcervical transclival approach to the ventral surface of the brain stem for removal of a clivus chordoma. *J Neurosurg* 1966; 24:544–551.
16. White AA III, Panjabi MM. The clinical biomechanics of the occipitoatlantoaxial complex. *Orthop Clin North Am* 1978; 9:867–878.
17. Williams B. Simultaneous cerebral and spinal fluid pressure recordings: II. Cerebrospinal dissociation with lesions at the foramen magnum. *Acta Neurochir (Wien)* 1981; 59:123–142.
18. Yamada T, Machida M, Tippin J. Somatosensory evoked potentials. In: Owen JH, Davis H (eds.), *Evoked Potential Testing*. New York: Grune and Stratton, 1985: 109–158.

33

Median Glossotomy, Mandibulotomy, and Transpalatal Approaches to the Clivus and Upper Cervical Spine

Richard Anthony Ruiz
Roger Lowlicht
Clarence T. Sasaki

Lesions that arise in the clivus and anterior cervical spine represent a therapeutic challenge to the surgeon, particularly with regard to adequate surgical exposure. Although many techniques have been described for approaching this region at the skull base, the midline labiomandibular glossotomy when combined with a transpalatal approach affords excellent wide-field access while preserving adjacent vital structures.

This chapter reviews the details of this approach as it relates to surgical exposure of the clivus and anterior cervical spine. While this technique has only recently been developed in its present form, it is not an entirely new one. The midline labiomandibular glossotomy had its beginnings in 1839, when Roux described splitting the lower lip and mandible in the midline to approach tumors of the anterior oral cavity.[1] In 1929, Trotter further extended this technique by splitting the tongue in its median raphe for exposure of the base of the tongue, epiglottis, and posterior oropharyngeal wall.[5] Trotter referred to this as a "median (anterior) translingual pharyngotomy." The term *median labiomandibular glossotomy* was coined in 1961 by Martin et al.,[4] who reintroduced the procedure for excision of midline lesions of the base of the tongue and posterior pharyngeal wall. In 1980, Wood et al. described the "median labiomandibular glossotomy, soft palate split, and hard palate resection for se-

lected congenital and acquired lesions of this area."[6] Wood et al. should therefore be given at least partial credit for synthesizing today's approach to the midline base of the skull.

Indications, Contraindications, and Patient Selection

Indications for this procedure include, in the broadest terms, the need for access to the midline base of the skull (clivus) and the anterior cervical spine from C-1 to C-3. The procedure therefore includes access to the pons, the medulla, and the foramen magnum. Additionally, access to the posterior pharyngeal wall is excellent.

Tumors most typically located at the clivus are the chordoma and the meningioma. Chordomas are known to arise from notochordal remnants in the clivus with subsequent clival destruction. These tumors are extradural, slow-growing, and usually present in the third to fourth decades of life.

The treatment of chordoma of the clivus has been, up until now, quite discouraging. In 1960, Zoltan and Fenyes reported eight cases of surgical excision of clivus chordomas; early tumor recurrence or death occurred in six of the eight patients.[7] Only two of the eight had remissions (of 1 and $1\frac{1}{2}$ years, respectively). Poor results were presumably due to incomplete removal of the primary tumor. With improved access and visualization of the tumor, patients with clivus chordomas will no doubt experience better long-term outcomes.

Meningiomas are also known to occur in the clival region. These tumors occur in late adult life. The literature supports the notion that nonoperative therapy leads to progressive disease that is ultimately fatal. It is well accepted that the best therapy for meningioma is complete excision. Median labiomandibular glossotomy with palatal split allows excellent surgical access for the most complete resection of clival meningiomas while yielding acceptable cosmetic and functional results.

Additional indications for the median labiomandibular glossotomy include excision of clival schwannomas, anterior foramen magnum tumors, and neurofibrosarcomas. Acquired intervertebral disc disease remains quite a common indication for anterior cervical fusion, and upper cervical fusions can be accomplished with this technique.

This approach is not indicated for lesions of the anterior cervical spine primarily below the level of C-4. Access to these lesions can easily be obtained via a standard anterior (retropharyngeal) approach which does not utilize the transoral route.

Relevant Anatomic Concept

Important to the review of the median labiomandibular glossotomy is an understanding of the neural, vascular, and muscular structures of the head and neck. Embryologically, these structures develop bilaterally, resulting in midline fusion. Therefore little or no direct communication exists across the midline. Thus, extensive midline surgical incisions are possible in the tissues of the head and neck with preservation of the major neurovascular structures. This results in a virtually bloodless field with minimal functional disability.

Surgical Technique

After adequate general endotracheal anesthesia has been obtained, a preliminary tracheotomy is performed. Tracheotomy eliminates the endotracheal tube from the operative field and allows for a secure airway postoperatively in the face of postoperative swelling of the tongue and floor of the mouth. Tracheotomy is accomplished with the patient in the supine position with the neck extended. A shoulder roll is utilized to maximize neck extension. The area of the incision is infiltrated with 0.5% lidocaine with 1:200,000 epinephrine. The skin is incised, and the soft tissues anterior to the trachea are divided in the midline. When necessary, the isthmus of the thyroid gland is divided between clamps and suture-ligated. The inferior margin of the cricoid cartilage is a good landmark to approximate the superior margin of the thyroid isthmus. Once the anterior wall of the trachea is cleared, a window of cartilage is removed from the second or third tracheal ring. A low-pressure cuffed tube is inserted into the tracheotomy and is utilized to deliver anesthesia. This tracheotomy tube is left in place postoperatively, and the patient is decannulated once oropharyngeal swelling has subsided. Once the tracheotomy is completed, the head of the operating room table is then turned 90 degrees to the patient's right and the patient is reprepped and draped for completion of the operative procedure.

A lip-splitting incision is utilized which is curved to conform to the skin creases for better cosmetic results. The skin incision is outlined on the lower lip and carried down to the level of the hyoid bone in the midline. The proposed incision is infiltrated using 0.5% lidocaine with 1:200,000 epinephrine. After injection of local anesthesia, 4 to 7 min are allowed to elapse prior to incision to allow for maximal effect of the vasoconstrictor. The lower lip is firmly grasped on each side of the outlined incision to occlude the labial artery. A through-and-through incision is made down to the periosteum of the mandible and is carried inferiorly to the level of the hyoid bone. The mucosal portion of this flap should be designed so that the closure will not directly overlie the proposed osteotomy. The periosteum of the mandible is elevated to the opposite side of the mucosal flap, in a similar fashion. This will allow for a double-layered closure away from the osteotomy and maximize periosteal blood supply to the bone segments. We prefer a stepped osteotomy to optimize mechanical integrity of the repaired mandible. The superior vertical osteotomy is placed between the central incisors and carried to at least 5 mm below the root tips to preserve the teeth. The horizontal portion is at least 1 cm in width: the remaining inferior vertical osteotomy is carried through the inferior border. We prefer a microsaggital saw

for these bone cuts because the saw blade is 0.5 mm in thickness. At the alveolar crest, a fine spatula osteotome may be necessary to preserve the incisor teeth and complete the cut. In the anterior floor of the mouth, the mucogingival flap is also designed so that the closure is not directly over the osteotomy.

Division of the tongue is carried out in the following fashion. Large 0 silk sutures are placed anteriorly and lateral to the median raphe on each side for traction. These are firmly grasped and the tongue and floor of mouth are divided exactly in the midline utilizing a handheld laser or electrocautery. The floor of the mouth is divided between Wharton's ducts and carried inferiorly to the hyoid bone. If either duct is damaged, it must be repaired by marsupialization to avoid salivary stasis. The tongue is divided to the glossoepiglottic fold. The mandibular-lingual halves are now retracted laterally with self-retaining retractors.

The soft palate and the mucosa of the hard palate are split in the midline along their entire length. Laterally based mucoperiosteal flaps are elevated from the bony palate. Sutures (of 2-0 silk) are placed in the mucoperiosteal flaps for lateral retraction. The vomerian crest is identified. Using the vomer as a landmark, a midline incision is made superiorly from the posterior border of the vomer down the posterior oropharyngeal wall to a level about 1 cm above the arytenoid cartilages. Although some surgeons suggest making the incision to the arytenoid cartilages, this will add unnecessary difficulty to the closure if access below C-2 is not needed. Two laterally based posterior pharyngeal mucosal and constrictor muscle flaps are elevated. Elevation is carried as far laterally as possible without disturbing the eustachian tubes. The remaining structures to be elevated from the clivus are the prevertebral fascia, the prevertebral muscles, and the anterior longitudinal ligament. These structures are incised in the midline and elevated laterally.

Our cadaver dissections agree with those of Wood et al., who state that when elevating the soft tissues from the clivus, the lateral margins become gutter-like depressions.[6] Within these gutters, the soft tissues become more adherent. This observation is important because just lateral to each gutter the internal carotid artery will be encountered. The location of the foramen lacerum with reference to the elevation can be verified by fluoroscopy. The upper part of the foramen lacerum is traversed by the internal carotid artery.

When the clivus has been sufficiently exposed, an air-driven drill can be utilized to remove the clivus and gain access to the primary lesion. An operative microscope will provide necessary magnification and illumination.

After resection of the primary lesion, closure of the surgical defect is accomplished in reverse fashion. The prevertebral fascia and muscles are approximated utilizing 3-0 Vicryl (polyglactin; Ethicon, Inc., Somerville, NJ) interrupted sutures. Wood et al. advocate placement of a suction drain in the retropharyngeal space. The drain is brought out through the superior aspect of the closure of the posterior pharyngeal muscle flaps and out through the nose. Thus, the two laterally based posterior pharyngeal mucosal and constrictor muscle flaps are reapproximated with interrupted 3-0 Vicryl sutures, the suction drain exiting from the superior aspect of the midline posterior pharyngotomy.

Closure of the palate is accomplished next. The muco-periosteal flaps of the bony palate are sutured using 3-0 Vicryl. The soft palate is closed in a three-layer closure. This is all accomplished utilizing interrupted sutures supported by nylon retention sutures over soft rubber bolsters. A nasogastric tube is placed under direct visualization for postoperative feeding. The tube may be sutured to the nasal columella with a large silk braid and taped to the nose for further security.

The tongue is closed from base to tip. The intrinsic musculature is reapproximated followed by the dorsal and the ventral surfaces. The floor of mouth is closed last. Wood et al. advocate using a Penrose drain at the base of the tongue, brought out through the inferior portion of the skin incision.[6]

Intermaxillary occlusion is then reestablished with temporary circumdental wiring of the bicuspid teeth. A bone plate is used at the inferior border in the compression mode. If intermaxillary fixation is to be avoided, a tension band must be established. We use either a short segment of arch bar on the mandibular incisor teeth or an interosseous wire at the most superior portion of the inferior vertical osteotomy. The principles of healing for the osteotomy are identical to those of a symphysis fracture. Thus, occlusion must be reestablished, and segment immobility must be maintained. The lip is closed using 3-0 Vicryl. The external lip and submental region are closed with a two-layer closure using interrupted Vicryl subcutaneously. The skin is closed with a 5-0 running nylon suture for optimal cosmetic results. The neck is dressed with a bulky sterile dressing to cover the Penrose drain.

Advantages and Limitations of this Technique

The median labiomandibular glossotomy to the clivus and the anterior cervical spine affords excellent exposure. The strength of this approach derives from the fact that the surgeon is able to be quite close to the operative field and is not operating through a "keyhole." This allows the surgeon wide-field access to the primary lesion.

The midline approach has the advantage of offering the most direct access while preserving major neurovascular structures. Because the major neurovascular structures do not cross the midline, they are not jeopardized, thus sparing the external carotid artery and its branches. Less blood loss and better visualization intraoperatively are permitted. Cranial nerves are also spared with this technique. Because there is no need to retract nerves and certainly no need to divide them, this results in better postoperative function. This technique does not interfere with the eustachian tubes, resulting in less postoperative middle ear effusions compared to lateral approaches.[3]

The median labiomandibular glossotomy is a somewhat limited approach, in the sense that only midline lesions of the base of the skull, posterior pharyngeal wall, and base of the tongue are accessible to complete resection. Furthermore, lesions which require *en bloc* neck dissections are more easily resected by other techniques.[3]

Potential Hazards and Complications

A major risk of this and all other transoral approaches to the base of the skull is intracranial infection secondary to contamination by intraoral organisms. While this risk cannot be altogether eliminated, it can be minimized. Preoperative cultures of the nose and the oropharynx should be obtained. The microbiology laboratory should be informed to identify the "predominant organism," since a reading of "normal flora" will not be very helpful in the selection of the most appropriate antibiotic. These results can be used to guide postoperative antibiotic therapy. Additionally, after cultures are obtained, the patient is begun on a preoperative antibiotic mouth rinse and parenteral antibiotics. These measures will decrease the oral flora and ensure adequate blood levels of the parenteral antibiotics at the time of surgery. The antibiotic mouth rinse we prefer consists of clindamycin 300 mg/500 ml of normal saline. Every 6 h the patient rinses with 30 ml for 30 s, then expectorates the solution.[2]

Mandibular malunion is a possible complication of this approach. The possibility can be minimized, however. Reduction of the mandible can be facilitated by drilling the holes for the wire, or the screws, prior to making the cuts on the mandible. Additionally, care must be taken to preserve the soft tissue adjacent to the mandibulotomy to allow for ample periosteum for closure. If a satisfactory reduction cannot be obtained with figure-of-eight wiring or bone plating techniques, then the surgeon must be prepared to apply intermaxillary fixation.

Retropharyngeal abscess is another possible complication. Placement of a suction drain for 3 to 5 days is advocated to reduce this possibility.[6]

Variation of Technique

Surgical access to the clivus and anterior cervical spine can be easily accomplished utilizing a median labiomandibular glossotomy. If access to a lower level of the anterior spine without access to the clivus is required, this can be secured to the level of C-4. In this instance the palate may not need to be split. It may be sufficient to retract the soft palate with catheters placed in the nostrils and brought out through the mouth. Additionally, when incising the posterior oropharyngeal wall, the incision should be made down to the level of C-4. This will focus the exposure to a more inferior level on the spine.

Conclusions

While the median labiomandibular glossotomy to the clivus and anterior cervical spine is limited in its usefulness to a minority of cases, it is an excellent approach to midline lesions. While reported outcomes utilizing this technique are still few in number, utilization of the median labiomandibular glossotomy with a palatal split will increase progressively as our notion of resectability is developed by improved preoperative radiographic imaging, intraoperative monitoring of neurologic function, and greater interdisciplinary cooperation.

References

1. Butlin HT, Spencer WG. *Diseases of the Tongue*. London: Cassell and Co Ltd, 1900:359.
2. Kirchner JC, Edberg SC, Sasaki CT. The use of topical oral antibiotics in head and neck prophylaxis: is it justified? *Laryngoscope* 1988; 98:26–29.
3. Krespi YP, Har EG. Surgery of the clivus and anterior cervical spine. *Arch Otolaryngol Head Neck Surg* 1988; 114:73–78.
4. Martin H, Tollefsen HR, Gerold FP. Median labiomandibular glossotomy: Trotter's median (anterior) translingual pharyngotomy. *Am J Surg* 1961; 102:753–759.
5. Trotter W. Operations for malignant disease of the pharynx. *Br J Surg* 1929; 16:485–495.
6. Wood BG, Sadar ES, Levine HL, et al. Surgical problems of the base of the skull: an interdisciplinary approach. *Arch Otolaryngol Head Neck Surg* 1980; 106:1–5.
7. Zoltan L, Fenyes I. Stereotactic diagnosis and radioactive treatment in a case of sphenooccipital chordoma. *J Neurosurg* 1960; 17:888–900.

34

Anterior Retropharyngeal Approach to the Upper Cervical Spine

Manning M. Goldsmith
Paul C. McAfee
Michael E. Johns

Disease processes of the upper cervical spine may result in spinal instability. Causes of this instability range from trauma to neoplastic disease, infection, and collagen vascular disease. Treatment may involve anterior decompression of the cervical spinal cord with bone grafting.

Several approaches to the upper cervical spine and clivus have been described. Most necessitate exposure through the oral cavity or nasopharynx. Such transoral approaches may be combined with a palatal split,[1] glossotomy and mandibulotomy,[3] mandibular dislocation,[2] or a combination of these. While providing excellent exposure as far superiorly as the clivus, these approaches have been associated with prohibitive infection rates (up to 50 percent) when utilized for bone grafting of the spine.[6]

Whitesides et al. described a lateral extrapharyngeal approach in which dissection is carried out posterior to the carotid sheath.[8,9] A tracheostomy is performed routinely. We have found that the anterior approach following mobilization of the marginal mandibular and hypoglossal nerves gives superior anterior exposure compared with the lateral approach. Anterior strut-grafting is more readily accomplished with this more direct approach to the spine. Furthermore, with flexible laryngoscopic techniques, inspection of the airway may be performed postoperatively prior to extubation. In this way, tracheostomy should be avoided in most patients, and the infection rate should theoretically be decreased.

The anterior retropharyngeal approach to the upper cervical spine that will be described provides sufficient exposure for extirpation and stabilization of lesions involving the axis and atlas.[4,5] It is a cranial extension through the same fascial planes that are utilized in the anterior cervical approach described by Riley[6] and by Southwick and Robinson.[7] The surgical approach is entirely extramucosal, and it can be used for decompression of the spinal canal as well as for stabilization with a strut graft.

Surgical Technique

Preoperative evaluation includes computed tomography (CT), magnetic resonance imaging (MRI), and angiography. The last is performed both for diagnostic reasons and for accurate localization of the vertebral arteries.

The patient is placed on an operative wedge turning frame with careful neurologic monitoring. Spinal cord monitoring via cortically recorded somatosensory evoked potentials is established and is used throughout the procedure. Gardner-Wells skull tongs with 4.5 kg (10 lb) of traction are used, as a head-halter extends too far inferiorly around the mandible. With the patient awake, the neck is extended as far as possible, but only to a point which does not cause the Lhermitte phenomenon or other neurologic symptoms or changes in monitored potentials of the spinal cord. This position of maximum allowable neck extension should not be exceeded for the remainder of the operative procedure. Awake nasotracheal intubation is accomplished under local anesthesia using a fiberoptic bronchoscope. No oral airways or esophageal stethoscopes are permitted.

A curvilinear incision is made from just inferior to the mastoid process, anterior to the sternocleidomastoid muscle, extending to the inferior border of the thyroid cartilage (Fig. 34-1). The incision is made through the platysma muscle, and the cervical flaps are elevated in a subplatysmal plane.

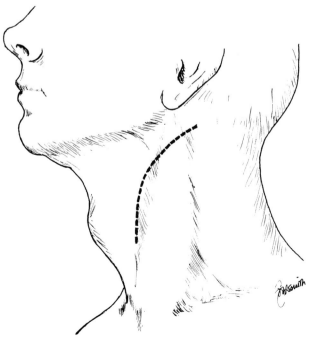

Figure 34-1 The incision for the anterior retropharyngeal approach.

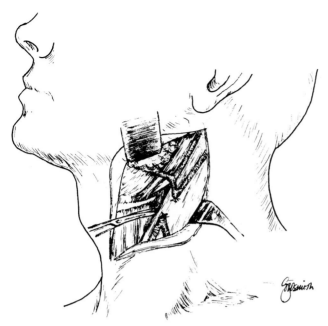

Figure 34-2 Identification of the superior laryngeal nerve at the beginning of the retropharyngeal dissection.

Care is taken to identify and preserve the marginal mandibular branch of the facial nerve as it crosses the anterior facial vein near the antegonial notch of the mandible. The anterior border of the sternocleidomastoid muscle is mobilized, and the carotid sheath is inspected. A neck dissection may be performed if indicated.

The dissection is then carried toward the thyrohyoid membrane between the carotid sheath contents laterally and the larynx and pharynx anteromedially (Fig. 34-2). External carotid artery branches including the ascending pharyngeal, superior thyroid, and lingual as well as branches of the internal jugular vein may be sacrificed to facilitate lateralization of the carotid sheath for added exposure. The superior laryngeal nerve is identified as it enters the thyrohyoid membrane just superior to the superior cornu of the thyroid cartilage. This nerve is carefully mobilized from its origin near the nodose ganglion to its entrance into the larynx and is gently retracted superiorly. The laryngopharyngeal complex is dissected from the carotid sheath laterally and the alar and prevertebral fascia overlying the cervical spine posteriorly (Fig 34-3). Retraction of the laryngopharyngeal complex anteriorly, superiorly, and medially may be facilitated by separation of the digastric tendon from the hyoid bone. Care must be taken not to damage the hypoglossal nerve during this maneuver. The prevertebral fascia as well as the longus colli muscles (which course longitudinally over the cervical spine to insert upon the anterior tubercle of the atlas) are divided in the midline, exposing the atlas and axis.

The neurosurgical/orthopedic surgical team performs the necessary decompression and stabilization procedure. The exact nature of this part of the procedure is dependent upon the extent of the lesion. The anterior atlanto-occipital membrane is not violated, but the anterior longitudinal ligament is sacrificed. A thorough C-2–C-3 discectomy is performed

and a C-2 corpectomy, if required, is accomplished with a high speed burr. Hemostasis is achieved with the bipolar cautery as well as Gelfoam (The Upjohn Company, Kalamazoo, MI) soaked with thrombin.

In the presence of an intact arch of C-1, the cord decompression is followed by an iliac or fibular graft from C-1 to C-3 or C-4. The graft is fashioned in the shape of a clothespin. The two prongs of the clothespin strut graft are placed to straddle the anterior arch of C-1. The inferior edge of the graft is tapped into the superior aspect of the C-3 or C-4 body.

Closure is begun by the reapproximation of the digastric tendon using standard tendon repair technique. Suction drains are then placed in the retropharyngeal space and in the subcutaneous space. They are brought out through separate stab incisions beneath the cervical flap. The platysma and the skin are then sutured in the standard fashion.

Posterior stabilization may be performed under the same anesthetic in a one-stage combined anterior-posterior procedure. The achievement of stability is dependent upon a good posterior cervical or posterior occipitocervical fusion. The anterior strut graft should be thought of as conferring compressive stability only.

Tracheostomy increases the risk of wound infection and therefore is avoided if possible. The decision to perform a tracheostomy is a clinical judgment based upon the amount of retraction trauma to the laryngopharyngeal complex and intraoperative fiber-optic inspection of the airway. A tracheostomy is performed to secure the airway if there is any concern at all, for it is much easier to perform this intraoperatively prior to the placement of the halo traction apparatus. If no tracheostomy is performed, a nasal cannula is placed prior to extubation, which is done at least 48 h postopera-

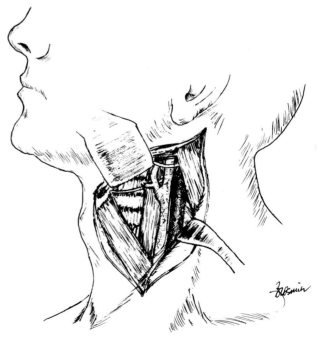

Figure 34-3 Superomedial retraction of the laryngopharyngeal complex and exposure of the cervical spine.

tively. Flexible nasopharyngoscopy is performed to ensure the adequacy of the upper airway prior to extubation.

Indications, Results, Complications

The anterior extraoral approach to the cervical spine represents an important collaborative effort between otolaryngologist–head and neck surgeons, neurosurgeons, and orthopedic surgeons. We have used the anterior retropharyngeal approach in 17 patients with lesions of the upper cervical spine.[4,5] Indications have primarily consisted of neoplastic disease (most commonly plasmacytoma and metastatic breast carcinoma), post-traumatic deformity, and involvement of the spine by rheumatoid arthritis, with atlantoaxial subluxation. Combining the series of Whitesides et al.[8,9] with the present series, multiple myeloma and metastatic breast carcinoma are the leading neoplasms involving these vertebrae.

In contrast to the reported results of transmucosal approaches to the atlas and axis,[1,2] no postoperative infections have occurred in our series. No patient had a respiratory arrest or required an emergency tracheostomy. Six patients had a prophylactic tracheostomy as part of the index operative procedure. Four patients had the nasotracheal tube removed immediately postoperatively. One patient was extubated at 24 h, two patients at 48 h, and four patients at 72 h postoperatively, without complication.

Three patients had nerve deficits postoperatively. One had a permanent unilateral injury to the hypoglossal nerve but was asymptomatic. The other two had hypoglossal neurapraxia, with one having, in addition, neurapraxia of a mandibular branch of the facial nerve. All three of the neurapraxias resolved within 3 months postoperatively.

The hypopharynx was inadvertently entered only once and there were no sequelae. This occurred in a patient who, before referral, had undergone a failed transoral approach that had resulted in more fibrosis and adhesions than are normally encountered.

There were no iatrogenic neurologic deficits of the spinal cord or nonunions of the arthrodeses. The maximum loss of blood for any of our 17 patients, including one who had an aneurysmal bone cyst and one who had a telangiectatic osteogenic sarcoma, was only 1200 ml.

We believe that the transoral route to the atlas and axis should be reserved mainly for biopsies and drainage of infections.[4,5,7] As the transmucosal approach necessitates contaminating the spine with oropharyngeal bacterial flora, bone-grafting through this approach has been reported to carry the unacceptably high risk of infection of as much as 50 percent.[1] The lateral retropharyngeal approach that was popularized and used extensively by Whitesides and Kelly also has the advantage of being extraoral. However, this approach involves a lateral dissection posterior to the carotid sheath. If an anterior decompression of the spine is performed, the approach remains close to the ipsilateral vertebral artery; and if this vessel is lacerated, bleeding is difficult to control. The contralateral vertebral artery is not approachable via the lateral approach.

An anterior approach was described by Riley.[6] A tracheostomy was performed. He found that anterior dislocation of the mandible was required to facilitate exposure. We have not found this to be necessary in the reported cases.

Conclusions

The anterior retropharyngeal approach is an anterior extraoral approach for achieving exposure to the atlas and axis. This approach may be safely performed without tracheostomy, and it provides superior exposure when compared to the lateral techniques. Because of the lower incidence of postoperative infection, the anterior retropharyngeal approach appears to be a safer procedure for grafting than the transoral approaches.

References

1. Alonso WA, Black P, Connor GH, et al. Transoral transpalatal approach for resection of clival chordoma. *Laryngoscope* 1971; 81:1626–1631.
2. Fang HSY, Ong GB. Direct anterior approach to the upper cervical spine. *J Bone Joint Surg [Am]* 1962; 44-A:1588–1604.
3. Hall JE, Denis F, Murray J. Exposure of the upper cervical spine for spinal decompression by a mandible and tongue-splitting approach: case report. *J Bone Joint Surg [Am]* 1977; 59-A:121–123.
4. McAfee PC, Bohlman HH, Riley LH Jr, et al. The anterior retropharyngeal approach to the upper part of the cervical spine. *J Bone Joint Surg [Am]* 1987; 69-A:1371–1383.
5. Nachlas NE, McAfee PC, Johns ME. Anterior extraoral approach to the atlas and axis. *Laryngoscope* 1987; 97:814–819.
6. Riley LH Jr. Surgical approaches to the anterior structures of the cervical spine. *Clin Orthop* 1973; 91:16–20.
7. Southwick WO, Robinson RA. Recent advances in surgery of the cervical spine. *Surg Clin North Am* 1961; 41:1661–1683.
8. Whitesides TE, Kelly RP. Lateral approach to the upper cervical spine for anterior fusion. *South Med J* 1966; 59:879–883.
9. Whitesides TE, McDonald AP. Lateral retropharyngeal approach to the upper cervical spine. *Orthop Clin North Am* 1978; 9:1115–1127.

35

The Middle Cranial Fossa Approach to Lesions of the Temporal Bone and Cerebellopontine Angle

William F. House
William E. Hitselberger
John T. McElveen, Jr.
Clough Shelton

The middle cranial fossa approach is an effective technique to reach lesions of the petrous apex and structures within the internal auditory canal (IAC). Although a middle fossa approach was used initially by Hartley[9] in 1891 and subsequently by Horsley[10] and Cushing[3] to treat tic douloureux, it was Parry[16] in 1904 who first used the approach to access structures within the internal auditory canal. Unfortunately, in sectioning the vestibular and cochlear nerves to relieve his patient of ear-related vertigo, Parry inadvertently transected the facial nerve.

The middle fossa approach was subsequently used for a variety of procedures, including (1) fenestration of the superior semicircular canal in patients with otosclerosis (Holmgren, 1917),[17] (2) ablation of the superior semicircular canal in patients with Meniere's disease (Putnam, 1930),[18] (3) drainage of the petrous apex in patients with apical petrositis (Kopetzky and Almour, 1930),[13] (4) sectioning of the greater superficial petrosal nerve in patients with unilateral headaches (Gardner et al., 1947),[6] and (5) grafting of the facial nerve in patients with facial paralysis following temporal bone fractures (Clerc and Batisse, 1954).[1] However, it was not until 1961 that new instrumentation, especially the operative microscope, expanded the indications for this surgery, and the approach became widely accepted.[11]

Indications

Currently, the middle cranial fossa approach is used for facial nerve repair, vestibular neurectomy, repair of dural defects, removal of intracanalicular tumors, and surgical treatment of other temporal bone lesions, including cholesterol granulomas, cholesteatomas, and petrous apex meningiomas. The middle cranial fossa approach allows the surgeon to reach areas deep within the temporal bone without destroying hearing. By staying superior to the labyrinth and medial to the middle ear structures, the surgeon can access the internal auditory canal and the geniculate ganglion.

The middle fossa approach is probably the best technique to ensure a complete section of the vestibular nerves. The retrolabyrinthine approach is more commonly used for this, but does not ensure total vestibular nerve section.[14] Those patients failing retrolabyrinthine vestibular neurectomy must have complete section of the vestibular nerve through the middle fossa approach if vestibular function is to be ablated.

In patients with spontaneous or iatrogenically induced cerebrospinal fluid otorrhea and temporal lobe herniation, the middle fossa approach allows the surgeon to extradurally resect the necrotic portion of the temporal lobe, patch the dural defect, and reinforce the floor of the middle cranial fossa.

The use of the middle fossa approach in acoustic tumor surgery is generally limited to patients with intracanalicular tumors and good residual hearing. With this approach, the lateral end of the internal auditory canal can be inspected and the facial nerve identified before entering the tumor mass. The middle fossa approach is particularly useful in resecting hemangiomas, lipomas, and neurinomas of the geniculate ganglion and exteriorizing supralabyrinthine cholesteatomas or cholesterol granulomas that are inaccessible by other hearing conservation approaches.

Anatomic Overview

The important structures of the petrous portion of the temporal bone, from the perspective afforded by the middle fossa approach, include the foramen spinosum, which transmits the middle meningeal artery and marks the anterior limit of the dural elevation; the arcuate eminence, which roughly corresponds to the location of the superior semicircular canal; the facial nerve hiatus, which transmits the greater superficial petrosal nerve from the area of the geniculate ganglion; and the petrous ridge, which is grooved by the superior petrosal sinus and forms the medial extent of the dural exposure.

Figure 35-1 illustrates the orientation of the cochlea, internal auditory canal, facial nerve, semicircular canals, and middle ear structures. Of particular importance is the close proximity of the superior semicircular canal to the basal turn

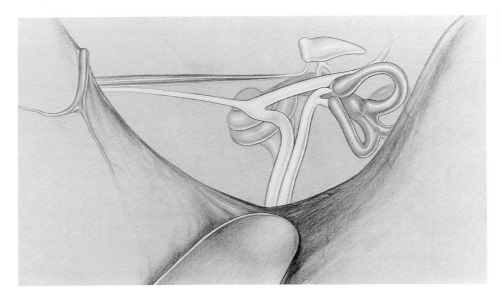

Figure 35-1 Relationship of structures within the temporal bone as viewed from the middle fossa.

of the cochlea.[15] Residual hearing is potentially sacrificed if either structure is penetrated inadvertently.

Surgical Technique

Positioning

The operation is performed under general anesthesia with the patient in a supine position and the head turned so that the involved ear is up. The surgeon is seated at the head of the table and the scrub nurse is positioned to the left of the surgeon. The microscope is brought in from the right side, and the anesthesiologist is at the foot of the table (Fig. 35-2).

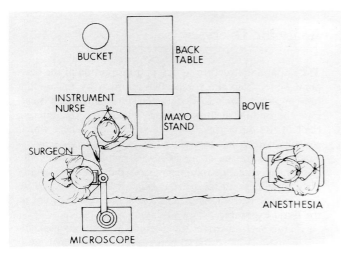

Figure 35-2 Operating room arrangement. The surgeon is seated at the head of the table.

Instrumentation and Equipment

In addition to the microscope and microsurgical instruments, a middle fossa retractor, a microdrill system, a bipolar cautery, and a suction-irrigation set-up are essential. Facial nerve and evoked auditory monitoring equipment is very useful, particularly in the removal of acoustic tumors.

Incision

Prior to the incision, the patient is usually administered mannitol to aid the retraction of the temporal lobe. The incision is made starting at the tragal notch and extending from the root of the zygoma superiorly 7 cm (Fig. 35-3). Using a monopolar cautery, a vertical incision is made through the temporalis muscle to the squama of the temporal bone.

Creation of Bone Flap and Elevation of Dura

Using a combination of cutting and diamond burrs, a 4-cm by 3-cm bone flap is created, the base of which is at the root of the zygoma. The bone flap is made two-thirds anterior and one-third posterior to the external auditory canal (Fig. 35-4). It is important not to penetrate the dura while drilling or removing the bone flap.

Once the bone flap is removed, the dura is elevated off the floor of the middle cranial fossa. The dural elevation proceeds in a posterior to anterior direction, minimizing the likelihood of inadvertent injury to an exposed facial nerve. In our experience, the facial nerve has no bony covering in the region of the geniculate ganglion in about 5 percent of cases, and it has been reported to be exposed in as many as 15 percent of cases.[19] The dural elevation should extend anteriorly to the foramen spinosum and medially to the superior petrosal sinus. Using the House-Urban retractor (Fig. 35-5), the middle fossa dura and temporal lobe are gently retracted.

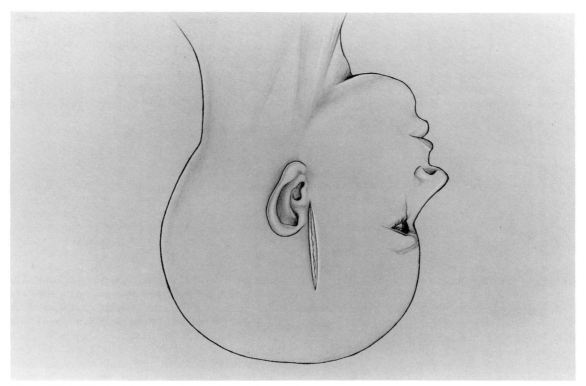

Figure 35-3 The incision is made starting at the tragal notch and extending from the root of the zygoma superiorly 7 cm.

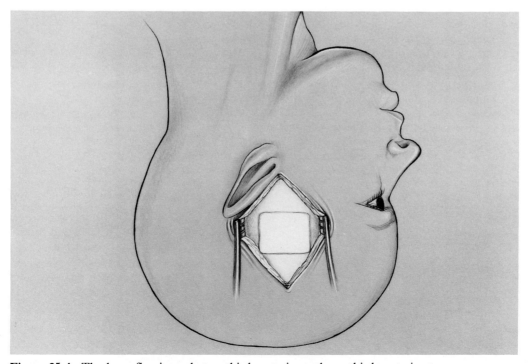

Figure 35-4 The bone flap is made two-thirds anterior and one-third posterior to the external auditory canal.

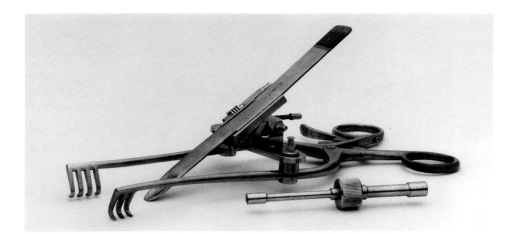

Figure 35-5 The House-Urban retractor. Three adjustments allow for desired placement of the blade.

Exposure of the Internal Auditory Canal

The IAC can be exposed by following the greater superficial petrosal nerve to the geniculate ganglion. The bone is then drilled off of the arcuate eminence until only a thin layer remains over the superior semicircular canal ("blueline") (Fig. 35-6). This marks the posterior boundary of the dissection of the IAC. The facial nerve is followed from the geniculate ganglion to the lateral end of the IAC.[12]

Two other methods for exposing the IAC have been described, but we do not commonly use them. In one, the bone is drilled off the arcuate eminence until only a thin layer remains over the superior semicircular canal. An imaginary line 60 degrees to the anterior limit of the superior semicircular canal is extended medially; this roughly corresponds to the location of the underlying IAC.[4] The other method involves locating the IAC medially, without skeletonizing the superior semicircular canal or the facial nerve. An approximate location of the IAC is made by bisecting the angle formed by the axis of the arcuate eminence and that of the greater superficial petrosal nerve. The canal is identified medially and bone removal continues laterally until the end of the internal auditory canal is identified.[5] We think that this method can be somewhat hazardous because the exact location of the facial nerve and labyrinth are not known.

It is best to leave an eggshell thickness of bone over the IAC until the drilling is completed. Extensive skeletonization of the IAC is essential when using the middle fossa approach to remove acoustic tumors. Medially, it is possible to expose 270 degrees of the IAC; however, laterally, the basal turn of the cochlea and the superior semicircular canal and vestibule limit the exposure. It is essential to identify "Bill's bar," a vertical crest of bone situated in the lateral end of the IAC and arising from the transverse crest. This key landmark separates the anteriorly situated facial nerve from the more posteriorly situated superior vestibular nerve (Fig. 35-6).

Once the facial nerve is positively identified, the remaining eggshell layer of bone overlying the IAC dura is re-

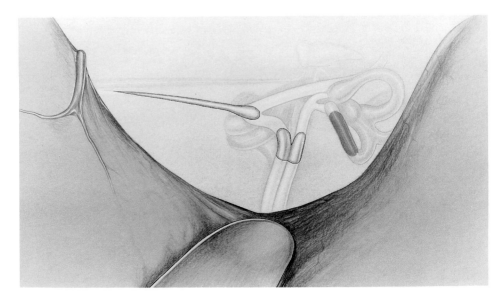

Figure 35-6 The greater superficial petrosal nerve (*left*) and superior semicircular canal (*right*) are landmarks to the lateral end of the internal auditory canal. A vertical crest of bone (Bill's bar) separates the facial and superior vestibular nerves.

moved. The dura is incised along the posterior aspect of the IAC in order to avoid injury to the facial nerve.

Acoustic Tumor Removal

An acoustic tumor is removed using a combination of delicate hooks. Beginning laterally, the superior vestibular nerve and the tumor are separated from the labyrinthine portion of the facial nerve. The tumor is then removed from the inferior compartment of the IAC. Tumor removal from this region is particularly difficult due to limited exposure of the lateralmost aspect of the inferior compartment and the need to maintain the integrity of the cochlear nerve and the vascular supply to the cochlea. The tumor, in conjunction with the vestibular nerves, is reflected medially and removed from the operative field. In this last phase of tumor removal, it is important not to injure the anterior inferior cerebellar artery, which may lie in the plane between the facial nerve and the tumor.

Closure

The remaining defect is closed with a free graft of temporalis muscle. The House-Urban retractor is removed and the temporal lobe is allowed to reexpand. The bone flap is replaced. The temporalis muscle and fascia are reapproximated and the skin is closed in a standard fashion. A modified mastoid dressing is placed, to be removed on the fourth postoperative day.

Modifications for Other Middle Fossa Procedures

The standard middle cranial fossa technique used for acoustic tumor removal can be modified for other indications. In cases of dural defects and temporal lobe herniation, no dissection of the IAC is required; the dura and temporal lobe are merely elevated. Necrotic herniated brain is cauterized and resected, and the defect in the middle fossa floor is reinforced with two layers of temporalis fascia and one layer of bone or cartilage.[7]

Cholesterol granulomas of the petrous apex, inaccessible by an infralabyrinthine approach, can be drained into the mastoid cavity, the middle ear cavity, or the eustacian tube. Using the middle fossa approach, the temporal lobe is elevated, the tegmen overlying the middle ear or mastoid is removed, and the cholesterol granuloma is exteriorized into the air spaces of the temporal bone. A similar approach can be used to exteriorize supralabyrinthine cholesteatomas.

Vestibular neurectomy via the middle fossa approach does not require the extensive exposure needed in acoustic tumor removal. However, the superior and inferior vestibular nerves and the facial nerve must be positively identified. The dissection must extend medially enough to include the resection of the singular nerve and Scarpa's ganglion.

Accessing facial nerve lesions in the area of the geniculate ganglion may require additional bone removal laterally (Fig. 35-7). This lateral exposure facilitates the following: (1) resection of perigeniculate tumors in cases of hemangiomas and neurinomas, (2) facial nerve decompression following temporal bone fractures and in selected cases of facial palsy following herpes zoster oticus, and (3) reapproximation of the facial nerve in cases of transection.

Results and Complications

Acoustic tumors removed by a middle fossa approach should be less than 10 mm in size and associated with a speech reception threshold of 30 dB or better with at least 70 percent speech discrimination. However, these criteria must be individualized to the needs of the patient.

In a series of 106 middle fossa acoustic tumor removals, postoperative facial function was normal or nearly normal (House-Brackmann grades I–II) in 89 percent of patients at

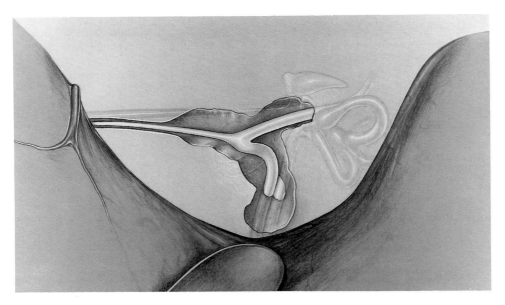

Figure 35-7 The intracranial, labyrinthine, and tympanic segments of the facial nerve can be exposed through the middle fossa.

1 year.[20] Measurable postoperative hearing remained in 59 percent of cases, with serviceable hearing (speech reception threshold ≤50 dB and speech discrimination score ≥50 percent) in 43 percent of the cases.[21] In 35 percent of cases, hearing was preserved near the preoperative level.

In Harker and McCabe's report of 10 patients undergoing acoustic tumor removal via the middle fossa approach, hearing was preserved in six.[8] Five patients had some degree of facial weakness postoperatively, and two of these had incomplete recovery after 1 year. Complications included one case of cerebrospinal fluid rhinorrhea with subsequent meningitis and one fatality. The death occurred in the postoperative period as a result of retrograde thrombosis of the anterior inferior cerebellar artery.

The middle fossa approach has been more frequently used in the treatment of ear-related vestibular disorders and facial nerve injuries. Garcia-Ibanez and Garcia-Ibanez used this approach for vestibular neurectomy in 373 patients with ear-related vertigo.[5] Of the 332 patients with Meniere's disease, 330 (99.4 percent) were completely relieved of their vertigo. Eighty-five percent (35/41) of the patients with other conditions had a resolution of vertigo. Hearing was the same or better in 105 of the 127 patients who had postoperative audiometric follow-up. However, five of the 127 experienced a complete sensorineural loss in the operated ear. In addition to the hearing loss, complications of the entire group (373 patients) included three subdural hematomas, two cerebrospinal fluid leaks, one case of meningitis, and 26 cases of facial palsy. Of the 26 patients with facial palsy, 25 had a complete recovery of function and one had a 60 percent recovery. There were no deaths in this series.

In Fisch's series of 92 patients undergoing middle fossa surgery,[4] those undergoing vestibular neurectomy obtained results similar to the cases reported by Garcia-Ibanez and Garcia-Ibanez.[5] Ninety-two percent of Fisch's patients with Meniere's disease were completely relieved of vertigo, 7 percent experienced transitory facial weakness, and only one patient experienced a complete loss of hearing in the operated ear.

Fisch's series of 92 patients included 14 cases of facial nerve disorders.[4] The nerve was successfully explored in all cases. Complications from his entire series included four cerebrospinal fluid leaks and one case of Jacksonian seizures; there were no cases of meningitis and no deaths.

The middle fossa approach, alone or in combination with a transmastoid approach, was successfully used by Coker et al. to treat intratemporal facial nerve injuries.[2] Of the 15 patients with facial paralysis following a longitudinal temporal bone fracture, 12 required a middle fossa procedure. The only reported complication was in one patient who experienced a moderate sensorineural hearing loss at frequencies above 500 Hz.

The most frequent complication in the reported series is a transitory facial paralysis. This usually develops 2 to 4 days postoperatively, but it may develop immediately postoperatively and resolve quickly. Whether this paralysis is a result of neural edema or devascularization is not clear. Fortunately, the majority of patients experience a complete recovery.

The most dangerous potential complications include posterior fossa bleeding, thrombosis of the anterior inferior cerebellar artery, and formation of an epidural hematoma. An epidural hematoma in the middle fossa is readily evacuated, but posterior fossa bleeding may be difficult to access in an emergent situation. This is a major consideration when contemplating this approach for acoustic tumors extending outside the internal auditory canal. Although temporal lobe abnormalities following retraction might be expected, this seldom has been reported.

Discussion

The middle cranial fossa approach allows the surgeon to reach structures within the petrous apex without compromising auditory, vestibular, or facial nerve function. This approach, when combined with the transmastoid approach, is the only one that enables the surgeon to evaluate the entire intratemporal course of the facial nerve without destroying hearing.

When this approach is used for vestibular neurectomy, the superior and inferior vestibular nerves can be sectioned before they join the cochlear portion of the vestibulocochlear nerve. This minimizes, although does not entirely eliminate, the possibility of an incomplete vestibular neurectomy.

For acoustic tumor removal with the possibility of hearing preservation, the main advantage of the middle fossa approach over the retrosigmoid approach is the complete exposure of the contents of the IAC. This makes blind dissection of the lateral IAC unnecessary, ensuring total tumor removal and facilitating positive facial nerve identification in its bony canal.

The middle cranial fossa approach is not without its disadvantages. Bleeding from the venules surrounding the foramen spinosum, and epidural bleeding, can impair visualization. The concentration of structures, particularly in the lateral aspect of the IAC (i.e., the vestibule, semicircular canal, cochlea, and facial nerve), requires meticulous care. Patients over 65 tend to have thin dura that is easily torn and difficult to elevate.

The facial nerve may be subjected to greater manipulation during tumor removal via the middle fossa approach than through the translabyrinthine approach. Particularly with schwannomas originating from the inferior vestibular nerve, one must dissect past the facial nerve to remove tumor. This may subject the facial nerve to more trauma than that caused during tumor removal from the translabyrinthine approach where the facial nerve is furthest from the surgeon. Thus, facial nerve results for the middle fossa approach are not quite as good as those for the translabyrinthine approach after the removal of tumors of similar size.

Another risk associated with the middle cranial fossa approach is the limited accessibility to the posterior fossa in the event of posterior fossa bleeding. This is an unlikely complication and has not occurred in our experience, although the potential exists. If such bleeding should occur, it would be necessary to drill out the labyrinth for greater access to the posterior fossa. This can be done very rapidly and allows adequate access.

With recent advances in imaging, particularly the use of gadolinium-enhanced magnetic resonance imaging, there has been a considerable increase in the detection of small acoustic tumors, with the potential for preservation of hearing. Thus, we foresee a growing need for use of the middle fossa technique because it has the advantage of allowing total exposure of the contents of the internal auditory canal.

Mastery of the middle fossa surgical approach is important for all surgeons dealing with temporal bone and cerebellopontine angle lesions. It makes possible effective management of many lesions not treatable through any other surgical approach.

References

1. Clerc P, Batisse R. Abord des organes intrapétreux par voie endo-crânienne (greffe du nerf facial). *Ann Oto-laryngol* 1954; 71:20–38.
2. Coker NJ, Kendall KA, Jenkins HA, et al. Traumatic intratemporal facial nerve injury: management rationale for preservation of function. *Otolaryngol Head Neck Surg* 1987; 97:262–269.
3. Cushing H. A method of total extirpation of the gasserian ganglion for trigeminal neuralgia: by a route through the temporal fossa and beneath the middle meningeal artery. *JAMA* 1900; 34:1035–1041.
4. Fisch U. Transtemporal surgery of the internal auditory canal: report of 92 cases, technique, indications, and results. *Adv Otorhinolaryngol* 1970; 17:203–240.
5. Garcia-Ibanez E, Garcia-Ibanez JL. Middle fossa vestibular neurectomy: a report of 373 cases. *Otolaryngol Head Neck Surg* 1980; 88:486–490.
6. Gardner WJ, Stowell A, Dutlinger R. Resection of the greater superficial petrosal nerve in the treatment of unilateral headache. *J Neurosurg* 1947; 4:105–114.
7. Graham MD. Surgical management of dural and temporal lobe herniation into the radical mastoid cavity. *Laryngoscope* 1982; 92:329–331.
8. Harker LA, McCabe BF. Iowa results of acoustic neuroma operations. *Laryngoscope* 1978; 88:1904–1911.
9. Hartley F. Intracranial neurectomy of the second and third divisions of the fifth nerve: a new method. *NY Med J* 1892; 55:317–319.
10. Horsley V. An address on the surgical treatment of trigeminal neuralgia. *Practitioner* 1900; 65:251–263.
11. House WF. Surgical exposure of the internal auditory canal and its contents through the middle cranial fossa. *Laryngoscope* 1961; 71:1363–1385.
12. House WF, Gardner G, Hughes RL. Middle cranial fossa approach to acoustic tumor surgery. *Arch Otolaryngol* 1968; 88:631–641.
13. Kopetzky SJ, Almour R. The suppuration of the petrous pyramid: pathology, symptomatology and surgical treatment. *Ann Otol Rhinol Laryngol* 1930; 39:996–1016.
14. McElveen JT Jr, House JW, Hitselberger WE, et al. Retrolabyrinthine vestibular nerve section: a viable alternative to the middle fossa approach. *Otolaryngol Head Neck Surg* 1984; 92:136–140.
15. Parisier SC. The middle cranial fossa approach to the internal auditory canal: an anatomical study stressing critical distances between surgical landmarks. *Laryngoscope* 1977; 87(suppl 4): 1–20.
16. Parry RH. A case of tinnitus and vertigo treated by division of the auditory nerve. *J Laryngol* 1904; 19:402–406.
17. Portmann G, Portmann M, Claverie G. *The Surgery of Deafness.* Sultana WA, McKenzie W (trans.-eds.). Valetta, Malta: Progress Press, 1964:47.
18. Putnam TJ. Treatment of recurrent vertigo (Ménière's syndrome) by subtemporal destruction of the labyrinth. *Arch Otolaryngol* 1938; 27:161–168.
19. Rhoton AL Jr, Pulec JL, Hall GM, et al. Absence of bone over the geniculate ganglion. *J Neurosurg* 1968; 28:48–53.
20. Shelton C, Brackmann DE, House WF, et al. Middle fossa acoustic tumor surgery: results in 106 cases. *Laryngoscope* 1989; 99:405–409.
21. Shelton C, Brackmann DE, House WF, et al. Acoustic tumor surgery: prognostic factors in hearing conservation. *Arch Otolaryngol* (in press).

36

Postauricular Infratemporal Fossa Approach to Tumors Involving the Skull Base

Derald E. Brackmann

Treatment of lesions of the skull base presents a formidable challenge. They occupy areas that are relatively inaccessible and dangerous to approach because of important surrounding neural and vascular structures. Until recently many of these lesions were considered inoperable. Development of computed cranial tomography and magnetic resonance imaging allows accurate delineation of the extent of these tumors. The development of microsurgical techniques has allowed removal of tumors heretofore considered inoperable.

One of the most significant advances in our ability to treat skull base lesions is the posterior lateral infratemporal fossa approach developed by Fisch et al.[3,4] This approach allows access to the entire infratemporal course of the internal carotid artery and to cranial nerves V through XII. It offers a possibility of complete removal of even large posterior-medially situated tumors with acceptable morbidity and preservation of a good quality of life. In this chapter, I will describe the types of infratemporal fossa approaches, discuss the indications for surgery and patient selection, and then report on the difficulties with this approach and the results in a series of patients.

Relevant Anatomy

Lesions of the skull base are in close proximity to the internal carotid artery, the major venous sinuses, and cranial nerves III through XII. The facial nerve blocks direct access to the area (Fig. 36-1). The tumors frequently extend into the posterior or middle fossa. The primary advantage of the infratemporal fossa approach is to allow direct lateral access to the internal carotid artery throughout its course from the carotid foramen to the cavernous sinus. In order to accomplish this access, the facial nerve is permanently arteriorly transposed, and this requires removal of the external auditory canal, tympanic membrane, and malleus and incus, with a resultant permanent conductive hearing impairment

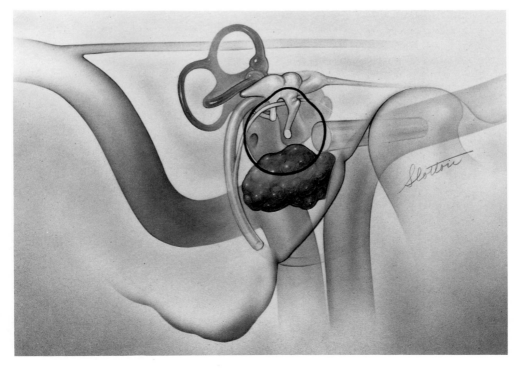

Figure 36-1 Diagram of glomus jugulare tumor contacting the internal carotid artery. The overlying tympanic ring and facial nerve prevent adequate exposure of the tumor and carotid artery.

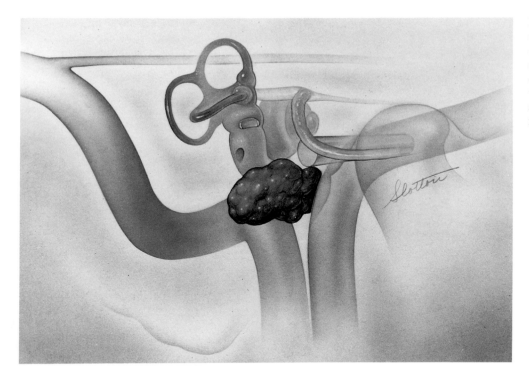

(Fig. 36-2). This is an acceptable morbidity for treatment of these difficult problems.

Surgical Techniques

Type A Approach

The type A approach is primarily used for glomus tumors of the temporal bone. The following is a description of the surgical procedure for that lesion. Hair is removed from approximately 6 cm about the ear, and an incision is made approximately 2 cm posterior to the postauricular sulcus. The incision is stopped at the mastoid tip at this point in the dissection. A simple mastoidectomy is completed, and the facial recess is opened. The incudostapedial joint is disarticulated to protect inner ear function. The external auditory canal is transected at the level of the bony cartilaginous junction. The skin of the meatus is everted and closed with 5-0 nylon sutures. The periosteum of the postauricular area is sutured behind the opening in the meatus to further reinforce the closure. The skin of the external auditory canal is removed along with the tympanic membrane, malleus, and incus. The bony external auditory canal is then removed. Following this, the facial nerve is freed of bone from the geniculate ganglion through the stylomastoid foramen.

Fisch originally described exposure of the facial nerve through the stylomastoid foramen into the parotid with permanent anterior transposition of the facial nerve.[3] In my experience, this always produced a temporary facial paralysis and sometimes a minor permanent residual facial weakness. I have modified this approach as follows.[1]

The postauricular incision is now extended into the neck along the anterior border of the sternocleidomastoid muscle. Rather than exposing the facial nerve into the parotid as Fisch described, I elevate the entire tail of the parotid along with the periosteum of the stylomastoid foramen and the nerve. The facial nerve is then carefully freed from the fallopian canal with sharp dissection. There are multiple fibrous connections which are sharply incised in the descending portion of the nerve. In the tympanic portion of the nerve, there are no adhesions, and this section elevates readily. The entire tail of the parotid with the contained facial nerve is then elevated lateral to the mandibular ramus. A large silk suture is placed through the periosteum of the stylomastoid foramen and attached to the soft tissue in the area of the root of the zygoma. This elevates the facial nerve and prevents its being stretched when the retractors are placed.

For the past 18 months, I have been using continuous monitoring of facial nerve activity during this dissection. EMG electrodes are placed into the facial muscles and the activity of the muscle is continuously monitored. Even minor manipulation of the facial nerve produces activity in the facial muscles. This technique has significantly improved postoperative facial nerve function.[5]

After the facial nerve and parotid gland are elevated, I place a large Perkins retractor beneath the angle of the mandible and retract the entire mandible forward. I have not had to resect the mandibular condyle even in large tumors extending far into the infratemporal fossa.

Transposition of the facial nerve allows exposure of the skull base in the area of the jugular foramen and carotid artery (Fig. 36-3). The common carotid artery is identified and the external carotid ligated. The internal carotid artery is then followed through the skull base to its infratemporal course. The ninth, tenth, and eleventh cranial nerves are identified in the neck and followed into the jugular foramen.

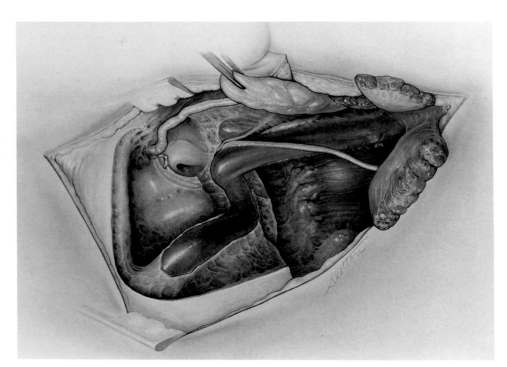

Figure 36-3 Infratemporal fossa exposure. See text for details.

The twelfth cranial nerve is also identified and followed to its foramen.

The sigmoid sinus is doubly ligated with silk sutures. The jugular vein is elevated and the tumor freed inferiorly. The tumor is then freed from the carotid artery anteriorly. Bleeding corticotympanic vessels are controlled with bipolar cautery. If the tumor is adherent to the internal carotid artery it is best to leave a portion of it on the artery at this point and remove the bulk of the tumor. Removal of the last bit of the tumor from the artery is then saved for the conclusion of the procedure. The tumor is freed superiorly and posteriorly and then medially, and total removal of the tumor is thus accomplished.

If there is intracranial extension of the tumor, a decision must be made at this point whether to attempt a total removal of the tumor. We base this decision upon the amount of blood loss to this point. If the blood loss has been limited to less than 3000 ml, we proceed with the removal of the intracranial extension of the tumor. All glomus jugulare tumors now receive preoperative embolization with polyvinyl alcohol sponge (lvalon; Pacific Medical Industry, San Diego, CA). Since utilizing this technique, blood loss is greatly reduced and we are almost always able to accomplish a total removal of tumors even with large intracranial extensions. If there has been greater than 3000 ml of blood loss, one may encounter problems with bleeding despite the replenishment of the clotting factors with fresh frozen plasma and platelet packs. In such a case we prefer a two-stage procedure with removal of the intracranial portion of the tumor approximately 6 months after the primary surgery.

The removal of the intracranial portion of the tumor is often easier than the removal of that within the temporal bone. By the time one is ready for the removal of the intracranial extension, the blood supply has often been controlled. The blood supply to the intracranial portion of the tumor is usually discrete and can be controlled with bipolar cautery as with other cerebellopontine-angle tumors. If tumor has been left along the internal carotid artery, this is now removed. Closure is accomplished by obliterating the mastoid defect with strips of abdominal fat. If the CSF space has been entered, continuous lumbar drainage is used for approximately 5 days until the wound is sealed.

Type B Approach

The most common skull base tumor requiring this approach is the clival chordoma. The description which follows describes that procedure. The incision is as for the type A approach except that it extends more forward superiorly. The external auditory canal is transected and closed and the flap anteriorly is undermined widely. The facial nerve is identified in the retromandibular fossa, and the superior branches are dissected peripherally to allow freeing and inferior displacement of the frontal ramus.

Holes that will later be used to rewire the zygoma are drilled in the arch, which is then divided between them. Posteriorly, the zygomatic arch is sectioned at the area of the temporomandibular joint. The zygomatic arch with the attached masseter muscle and freed temporalis muscle are displaced inferiorly and folded over the inferiorly displaced frontal ramus of the facial nerve to protect it. The external auditory canal and tympanic bone are then removed as described for the type A approach. The bone of the glenoid fossa is removed and the temporomandibular joint is disarticulated and retracted inferiorly with an infratemporal fossa retractor. The internal carotid artery is then exposed throughout its course to the foramen lacerum. This requires detachment of the medial cartilaginous portion of the eustachian tube.

When it is necessary to reach the anterior part of the clivus, the middle meningeal artery and the third division of the trigeminal nerve are coagulated and divided. To reach the anterior clivus, the tensor veli palatini muscle, cartilaginous eustachian tube, and pterygoid processes are displaced inferiorly.

After tumor exposure, the soft portions of the tumor are removed with suction and curettes. Diamond burrs are used until firm bone or dura is encountered. Care must be taken not to injure the contralateral internal carotid artery.

Closure is accomplished by packing with abdominal fat after the zygomatic arch has been wired in place anteriorly.

Type C Approach

The most frequent indication for the type C approach is nasopharyngeal carcinoma (failing radiotherapy) and advanced juvenile nasopharyngeal angiofibroma.

The dissection as described for the type B approach is first accomplished. After the displacement of the mandibular condyle inferiorly, the middle meningeal artery and the mandibular division of the trigeminal nerve are divided. Both pterygoid plates are removed, and the internal carotid artery is exposed from the middle ear to the foramen lacerum. The lateral wall of the nasopharynx covered by the palatal and pterygoid muscles can then be removed *en bloc* with the infiltrating tumor. Juvenile nasopharyngeal angiofibromas are dissected bluntly along their capsule. Extensions into the sphenopalatine fossa, sphenoid sinus, or nasal cavity are reached after complete removal of the pterygoid processes and division of the maxillary division of the trigeminal nerve at the foramen rotundum.

Closure is accomplished by obliteration of the anterior operative cavity with a pedicle of the temporalis muscle. Posteriorly, the mastoid cavity is obliterated with abdominal fat and the zygomatic arch is wired into its original position.

Indications

A variety of skull base lesions may be treated by the infratemporal fossa approach. Tables 36-1, 36-2, and 36-3 list the most common tumors treated by the different approaches.

Contraindications

An absolute contraindication to the infratemporal fossa approach is a malignant tumor extending across the skull base. However, Fisch et al. have stated that even in extensive carcinomas, surgery may be worthwhile for relief of trigeminal pain and general palliation.[4]

Involvement of one internal carotid artery is not a contraindication to surgery. Balloon occlusion studies are performed with continuous EEG monitoring. If this indicates that sacrifice of the internal carotid artery would not be tol-

TABLE 36-1 Type A Infratemporal Fossa Approach

Glomus tumor
Temporal bone carcinoma
Primary cholesteatoma
Jugular foramen neuroma
Meningioma
Sarcoma

TABLE 36-2 Type B Infratemporal Fossa Approach

Chordoma
Chondrosarcoma
Squamous cell carcinoma
Dermoid and primary cholesteatoma
Meningioma

TABLE 36-3 Type C Infratemporal Fossa Approach

Nasopharyngeal carcinoma
Juvenile nasopharyngeal angiofibroma
Adenoid cystic carcinoma
Meningioma
Sarcoma
Ameloblastoma

erated, plans must be made either for extracranial-intracranial bypass grafting or saphenous vein grafting of the resected internal carotid artery.

Relative contraindications to surgery include poor general health. These procedures are extensive, and the patient's general health must be carefully assessed before recommending the procedure.

In general, I do not recommend surgery for glomus tumors of the temporal bone in elderly patients. In my experience, radiation therapy is a better modality for treating the elderly person with a glomus tumor.[2]

Advantages and Limitations of the Infratemporal Fossa Approach

The advantage of the infratemporal fossa approach is the wide exposure of lesions of the skull base. Total exposure and protection of the carotid artery is a major advantage. With this technique the facial nerve is mobilized and preserved. Exposure of cranial nerves V through XII is possible and allows protection and preservation of these nerves when they are not involved by the tumor.

One disadvantage of the approach is the permanent conductive hearing impairment which results from blind sac closure of the external auditory canal and removal of the conductive hearing mechanism. Sensorineural hearing function is preserved in the majority of patients unless tumor invades the labyrinthine capsule. In such cases, complete tumor removal requires sacrifice of sensorineural hearing function.

A temporary facial paralysis may result from mobilization of the facial nerve in the type A approach. In the types B and C approaches, weakness of the musculature innervated by the frontal branch is common. As discussed previously, intraoperative monitoring of facial nerve function and not exposing the nerve at the stylomastoid foramen have greatly decreased the incidence of facial paralysis. Hypesthesia in the distribution of the second and third divisions of the fifth cranial nerve accompany the types B and C infratemporal fossa approaches.

Hoarseness of the voice and aspiration to a variable degree occur with sacrifice of the ninth and tenth cranial nerves. I do not do a preoperative tracheotomy or gastrostomy even when I know that these nerves will be sacrificed. Most patients will tolerate these deficits in the immediate postoperative period. Early Teflon injection of the vocal cord is performed. Cricopharyngeal myotomy is also beneficial to enhance swallowing and decrease aspiration. Shoulder discomfort is common with sacrifice of the eleventh cranial nerve. Exercises are beneficial for this problem.[6]

When tumors extend intracranially, a CSF leak is a potential problem. When the CSF space has been entered, a lumbar subarachnoid drain is routinely placed and remains until the wound is well sealed, which is usually about 5 days. Meningitis is an infrequent complication. Intra- and perioperative antibiotics are not routinely used.

Tumors with large intracranial extensions may involve the posterior fossa circulation, making total tumor removal impossible. Surgery in these cases may still be beneficial by decreasing the blood supply to the tumor with removal of its main bulk.

Results

As of December 1987, I have performed 60 infratemporal fossa approaches for various tumors of the skull base. The results with these cases are summarized in Table 36-4. The most common tumor that I have treated is the glomus jugulare tumor, although a variety of other lesions have also been operated upon. Total removal of the tumor was accomplished in most cases. Incomplete removal was performed on several early cases with large intracranial extensions. Second-stage procedures were planned, but follow-up has shown no growth of the tumor so they are currently being observed. Removal of the intracranial portion of the tumor will be accomplished if growth is demonstrated. Extensive involvement of the cavernous sinus has been a second indication for partial removal in three cases. These patients are also being carefully monitored, and if aggressive tumor growth is demonstrated, further surgery will be recommended.

Only one patient in the series has died from the disease. This patient had a very large meningioma of the skull base which had previously been operated upon. It extended to the cavernous sinus. We thought that a total removal had been accomplished, but recurrent disease developed. She had further surgery elsewhere but had rapid regrowth of tumor following that and died of intracranial extension of the disease. Two patients have died of other disease without evidence of residual tumor in the temporal bone or infratemporal fossa.

A number of patients have been given postoperative x-ray therapy. In general, I do not recommend this for glomus tumors unless residual tumor is left and this demonstrates growth. In that case, a relatively small dose of therapy is recommended to decrease the blood supply to the tumor.[2] Postoperative x-ray therapy of chordoma and chondrosarcoma is somewhat controversial but has been employed in three of the four patients in this series. The patient with the recurrent papillary adenoma with intracranial extension also received postoperative x-ray therapy.

The quality of life in these patients has been excellent. All have returned to full activity without the need for tracheotomy or gastrostomy, even though these measures were employed immediately postoperatively in a number of patients.

TABLE 36-4 Summary of Results ($N = 60$)

Tumor Type	Primary Surgery	Surgery for Recurrence	Total Removal	Partial Removal	Alive without Disease	Alive with Disease	Died of Disease	Died of Other Disease	Postoperative Irradiation
Meningioma, $N = 7$	5	2	6	1	6		1		1
Jugular fossa neuroma, $N = 4$	4		4		4				
Glomus jugulare tumor, $N = 39$	32	7	32	7	31	7		1	6
Glomus vagale tumor, $N = 3$	2	1	2	1	2	1			1
Chordoma, $N = 2$	2		2		1			1	2
Chondrosarcoma, $N = 2$	1	1	1	1	1	1			1
Cholesteatoma, $N = 2$	1	1	2		2				
Papillary adenoma, $N = 1$		1	1		1				1

Conclusion

The postauricular infratemporal fossa approach is a significant advance in our ability to treat extensive skull base lesions. Total removal of even large tumors is usually possible, with preservation of good quality of life.

References

1. Brackmann DE. The facial nerve in the infratemporal approach. *Otolaryngol Head Neck Surg* 1987; 97:15–17.

2. Brackmann DE, House WF, Terry R, et al. Glomus jugulare tumors: effect of irradiation. *Trans Am Acad Ophthalmol Otolaryngol* 1972; 76:1423–1431.

3. Fisch U. Infratemporal fossa approach for glomus tumors of the temporal bone. *Ann Otol Rhinol Laryngol* 1982; 91:474–479.

4. Fisch U, Fagan P, Valavanis A. The infratemporal fossa approach for the lateral skull base. *Otolaryngol Clin North Am* 1984; 17(3):513–552.

5. Leonetti JP, Brackmann DE, Prass RC. Improved preservation of facial nerve function in the infratemporal approach to the skull base. *Otolaryngol Head Neck Surg* 1989; 101:74–78.

6. Saunders WH, Johnson EW. Rehabilitation of the shoulder after radical neck dissection. *Ann Otol Rhinol Laryngol* 1975; 84:812–816.

37

Surgical Treatment of Tumors Involving the Cavernous Sinus

Laligam N. Sekhar
Chandra Nath Sen

Winslow was the first to coin the name *cavernous sinus* because he thought it resembled the corpus cavernosum of the penis.[13] Since that time, whether the cavernous sinus is a large venous space with trabeculations or is a plexus of veins has been controversial. After a review of the various published studies, and on the basis of our anatomic studies and surgical observations, we favor the concept of a venous plexus but with some large spaces in some areas of the plexus.[6,8,17,20] It is now well accepted that the oculomotor, trochlear, ophthalmic, and maxillary nerves course in the

lateral wall of the cavernous sinus and that the contents of the cavernous sinus include the internal carotid artery (ICA), the abducens nerve, and the sympathetic nerve. The complex relationship of the ICA and the various cranial nerves in the cavernous sinus region are shown in Fig. 37-1. Although Holmes (1860), Bartholomew (1872), and Foix (1920) described mass lesions and clinical syndromes of the cavernous sinus, Jefferson provided the best clinical descriptions of the various cavernous sinus syndromes (1937, 1938).[13] Krogius in 1896 was the first to remove a mass lesion of the cavernous sinus.[13] Many other surgeons had knowingly or unknowingly operated on lesions involving this area, but Parkinson was the first to systematically approach vascular and neoplastic lesions involving this area.[12,13] However, enthusiasm for such operations waned, especially with advances in treatment of carotid cavernous fistulae with balloon catheters. Dolenc, Hakuba, Sekhar, and Isamat, working independently, have revived the interest of other neurosurgeons in this area recently.[2–5,7,9–11,14,16,18,19] Neurosurgeons who wish to perform surgery in the region of the cavernous sinus should be well versed in microneurosurgery, especially in the management of cranial vessels and nerves. Before starting operations in this area, they must spend as much time as possible observing other surgeons with experience and even more time working with cadavers to learn the anatomy and surgical techniques.

Clinical Presentation and Preoperative Evaluation

Tumors involving the cavernous sinus may present with symptoms referable to cranial nerves coursing through or adjacent to this space. Such symptoms include pain in the V_1 or V_2 distribution, diplopia secondary to sixth or third nerve palsy, and visual loss. When high-resolution imaging

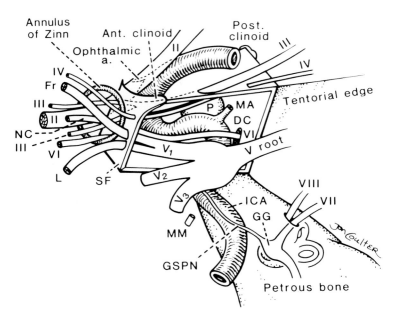

Figure 37-1 Schematic representation of the anatomy of the cavernous sinus and related structures. II, III, IV, V, V_1, V_2, V_3, VI, VII, VIII = cranial nerves; ICA = internal carotid artery; DC = Dorello's canal; GG = geniculate ganglion; GSPN = greater superficial petrosal nerve; MM = middle meningeal artery; MA = meningohypophyseal artery; P = pituitary gland; SF = superior orbital fissure; NC = nasociliary branch; L = lacrimal branch; Fr = frontal branch.

TABLE 37-1 Balloon Occlusion Test of ICA

	Neurologic Deficit	No Neurologic Deficit → Xenon CT-CBF Study		
		Incomplete Study	Reduction of CBF 15–35 ml/100 g/min	No Reduction of CBF >35 ml/100 g/min
Distribution	8% of tested	8% of tested	10% of tested	73% of tested
Hemodynamic stroke risk				
Brief temporary ICA occlusion (<2 h)	Mild-moderate		None	None
Prolonged temporary ICA occlusion (>2 h)	High		Mild	Mild
Permanent ICA occlusion	High		Moderate-high	None
Decision regarding tumor treatment	Reconsider nonoperative therapies			
Management options if artery occluded	STA-MCA bypass STA-MCA bypass + direct vein graft ECA-MCA long vein graft		STA-MCA bypass ICA-ICA short vein graft	ICA-ICA short vein graft (benign tumors) No reconstruction (malignant tumors)

ECA = External carotid artery; ICA = Internal carotid artery; MCA = Middle cerebral artery; STA = Superficial temporal artery.

studies are not used, the diagnosis of a small tumor of the cavernous sinus may be missed for years, and the patient may carry the diagnosis of atypical face pain or myasthenia gravis. Tumors extending into the cavernous sinus from other areas may not produce symptoms referable to the area, being discovered because of other symptoms such as increased intracranial pressure, seizures, proptosis, or other neurologic deficits.

During the preoperative evaluation of cavernous sinus tumors, a careful general physical and neurologic examination is conducted. Based on the findings, additional investigations such as visual field and acuity measurements, audiometry, and endocrinologic studies are performed as indicated. Radiologic studies include computed tomography (CT) in axial and coronal planes and using soft tissue and bone algorithms, and magnetic resonance imaging (MRI) with and without gadolinium enhancement. The relative value of CT and MRI is being evaluated, but at the moment, both appear to provide complementary information. Cerebral arteriography is performed to study the status of the intracavernous ICA, the blood supply of the tumor, and the potential collateral circulation in the event of ICA occlusion, i.e., the anterior and posterior communicating arteries, the ophthalmic artery, and, rarely, the trigeminal artery.

Balloon Occlusion Test

The balloon occlusion test of the ICA gives an excellent preoperative assessment of the collateral circulation in the event of temporary or permanent ICA occlusion. This test is performed at the end of arteriography. A Swan-Ganz catheter is introduced into the ipsilateral ICA, and after systemic heparinization, the balloon is inflated to occlude the artery for 15 min. The patient's neurologic status is carefully moni-

tored during this period, and if any deficits develop, the balloon is immediately deflated and the patient is considered to have failed the clinical part of the test. If no deficits develop, the patient undergoes a xenon CT-CBF study with the balloon inflated and then with it deflated. The majority of the patients exhibit very minimal or no change of cerebral blood flow (CBF) with test balloon occlusion. A smaller percentage of patients exhibit a reduction of CBF during test ICA occlusion. Based on the results of balloon occlusion tests in 154 patients, and the surgical management of these patients' arteries, an algorithm of hemodynamic risk for stroke and management options has been developed (Table 37-1). The risk of doing this test in these 154 patients included a transient ischemic attack in one patient and asymptomatic ICA dissection in two other patients.

Occasionally, both ICAs may be tested in sequence or a vertebral artery may be tested. The test is contraindicated in the event of significant occlusive vascular disease. An unruptured or a remotely ruptured ICA aneurysm is not a contraindication.

Anesthesia

After administration of sodium thiopental and short-acting muscle relaxants, the patient is endotracheally intubated and ventilated. If monitoring of cranial nerve function during the operation is important, an inhalational anesthetic such as isoflurane is used. However, if the intracranial pressure is elevated, monitoring of cranial nerve function is not used, and a thiopental infusion, narcotics, and muscle relaxants are used for anesthesia. For extradural operations, a lumbar subarachnoid drain is used to relax the brain. For intradural operations, cisternal drainage of cerebrospinal fluid is employed. If the intracranial pressure is significantly elevated, osmotic diuretics and/or the excision of the tip of the temporal lobe may be employed to avoid retraction-induced cerebral injury. During the operation, colloid replacement is preferred over crystalloid administration, to minimize postoperative brain edema. If the blood replacement exceeds 4 units of packed red cells, fresh frozen plasma and platelets should be administered as needed.

Neurophysiologic Monitoring

The goal of intraoperative neurophysiologic monitoring is to reduce or eliminate postoperative morbidity. Electroencephalographic monitoring should be considered if temporary ICA occlusion is anticipated and especially if there was significant reduction of CBF during the balloon occlusion test. Monitoring of the brain stem evoked responses (BSER) from the contralateral ear (since the majority of the supranuclear pathway crosses over in the pons) has been found to be a sensitive indicator of the pressure on the brain stem caused by temporal lobe retraction.

Monitoring of the function of cranial nerves III, VI, and VII is quite useful to locate these nerves when the anatomy is altered, and to reduce injury to them during the removal of the tumor.[16,18] Fine needle electrodes are placed transcutaneously into the orbicularis oculi and mentalis muscles for facial nerve monitoring, and inside the orbit adjacent to the appropriate extraocular muscles for third and sixth cranial nerve monitoring (Fig. 37-2). During the operation, the suspected nerve is stimulated by a monopolar stimulator at 0.3 to 2 V, and the evoked electromyographic activity is monitored for nerve identification. During the dissection of the neoplasm from a nerve, spontaneous electromyographic activity from the muscles in question may indicate irritation or injury to the nerve, sometimes allowing the surgeon to alter the operative technique. Monitoring of facial nerve function is useful during the exposure of the petrous portion of the ICA or during the removal of a tumor involving the petrous temporal bone.

Operative Technique

Exposure of the Tumor

The current techniques used in the exposure of the tumor emphasize maximal visualization of all the essential structures, minimal brain retraction, and the possibility of appropriate reconstruction after tumor removal. Control of the ICA proximal to the cavernous sinus is essential, and may involve the exposure of the cervical or the petrous ICA. Depending upon the nature of the tumor, we currently use one of three methods:

1. For predominantly intracavernous and intracranial tumors such as meningiomas, the cervical ICA is exposed, and a frontotemporal craniotomy is combined with the temporary removal of the superior and lateral rims and walls of the orbit and the zygomatic arch. However, the condyle of the temporomandibular joint is not disturbed. Structures in the floor of the middle cranial fossa which are exposed extradurally include the greater superficial petrosal nerve (which is divided), the middle meningeal artery, and the cranial nerves V_2 and V_3. The horizontal segment of the petrous ICA may be exposed if needed (Fig. 37-3).

2. For tumors which extend into the cavernous sinus from the petroclival bone or cartilage, a subtemporal-preauricular infratemporal extradural approach is combined with a frontotemporal intradural approach. The condyle of the mandible is either dislocated or excised, and the entire petrous ICA is exposed and mobilized as needed (Fig. 37-4). One can then enter the cavernous sinus by the *inferior extradural approach* by following the petrous ICA upward, or by the *anterolateral extradural approach* between V_2 and V_3 or V_1 and V_2, between the leaves of the dura (Fig. 37-5). Only the lower half of the cavernous sinus is exposed by these approaches; they are ideal for tumors such as chondrosarcomas and juvenile angiofibromas which have a small component of tumor within the cavernous sinus. It is difficult to be sure that total

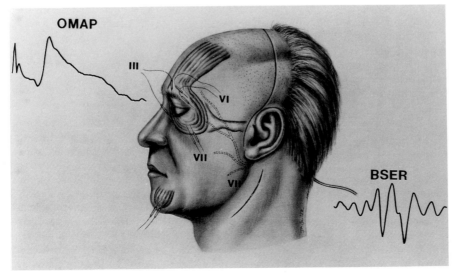

Figure 37-2 The incisions used during operations on the majority of neoplasms of the cavernous sinus and the monitoring techniques commonly employed are shown in this figure.

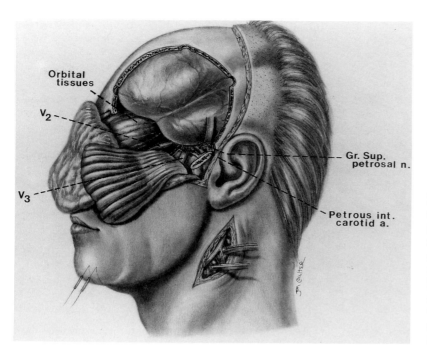

Figure 37-3 The frontotemporal craniotomy and orbitozygomatic osteotomy approach shown are used to expose predominantly intracranial cavernous sinus neoplasms (e.g., meningioma). The cervical internal carotid artery (ICA) and the horizontal segment of the petrous ICA are exposed. The superior and lateral rim and walls of the orbit and the zygomatic arch are removed temporarily. (From Sekhar et al.,[19] with permission.)

tumor removal has been achieved unless intradural exposure of the cavernous sinus is performed or by postoperative imaging studies.

3. For tumors which extend into the cavernous sinus from the sphenoid sinus, a basal subfrontal approach is performed. A bifrontal craniotomy is combined with the temporary removal of the orbital rim and superior walls. The optic nerves are decompressed from their bony canals and the sphenoid sinus is entered. The cavernous sinus is then exposed after removal of the lateral wall of the body of the sphenoid bone. This is the *medial extradural approach* to the cavernous sinus, exposing the medial and inferior aspects of the intracavernous ICA (Fig. 37-6). This approach destroys the olfactory sense. Only small medial intracavernous extensions of tumors can be removed by this route. This approach is ideally combined with the inferior and anterolateral extradural approaches.

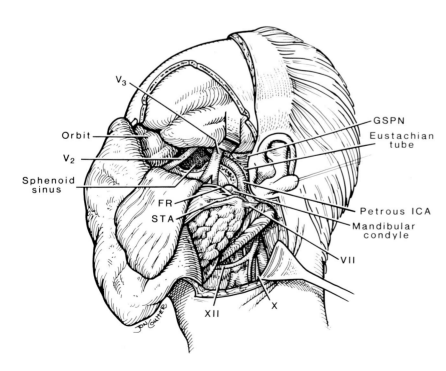

Figure 37-4 For tumors arising in the cranial bones or cartilage (e.g., chondrosarcoma) but extending into the cavernous sinus, the entire petrous ICA is exposed and displaced from its bony canal. The dislocation or excision of the mandibular condyle is necessary for this. V_1, V_2, V_3, VII, X, XII = cranial nerves, Fr = frontalis branch of facial nerve, STA = superficial temporal artery, GSPN = greater superficial petrosal nerve. (From Sekhar et al.,[19] with permission.)

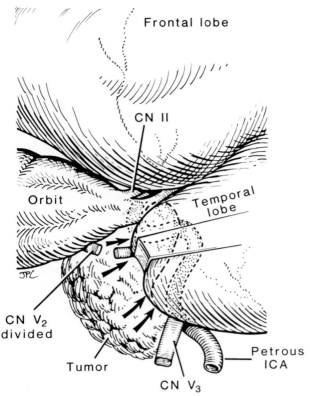

Figure 37-5 The inferior and anterolateral extradural approaches to the cavernous sinus are illustrated. (Modified from Sekhar et al.,[19] with permission.)

Intradural Approaches

After the dura is opened, the optic nerve and carotid cisterns are opened if the tumor is small. However, if the tumor is large and may encase the supraclinoid ICA or middle cerebral artery (MCA), the sylvian fissure is opened from a lateral to a medial direction and the MCA and its branches are traced medially (Fig. 37-7). Bridging veins draining the temporal lobe tip will have to be coagulated and divided. After inspection of the extent of the tumor and its nature, removal of the intradural portion is performed first. Removal of the cavernous sinus tumor is performed next, working under the frontal lobe, under the anterior temporal lobe, or through the sylvian fissure. If considerable temporal lobe retraction is necessary, it is better to remove the anterior 3 cm of the temporal tip, to minimize postoperative problems. The cavernous sinus is entered by a superior or lateral approach for tumor removal.

Superior Approach

After excising the dura over the optic nerve canal and the anterior clinoid process, the optic nerve canal is unroofed and the anterior clinoid process and the optic strut are removed. The dural sheath of the optic nerve is opened. The anterior bend and the anterior vertical segment of the intra-

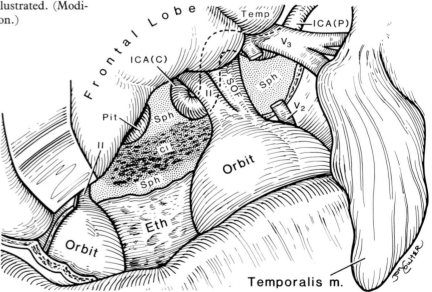

Figure 37-6 For tumors of the sphenoidal or ethmoidal areas that extend into the cavernous sinus, a bifrontal craniotomy is combined with the temporary removal of the superior rims and walls of both orbits. Proximal control of the ICA is essential, preferably in the petrous segment. Thus, this approach ideally is combined with that illustrated in Fig. 37-4. The lateral wall of the body of the sphenoid bone is removed, exposing the cavernous ICA and sinus. The close relationship of the intracavernous ICA to the optic nerve anteriorly is apparent. II, V_2, V_3, = cranial nerves, SOF = superior orbital fissure structures, Temp = temporal lobe, ICA (P) = petrous internal carotid artery, ICA (C) = cavernous internal carotid artery, Pit = pituitary gland, Cl = clivus seen through the sphenoid sinus, Sph = sphenoid sinus. (From Sekhar et al.,[19] with permission.)

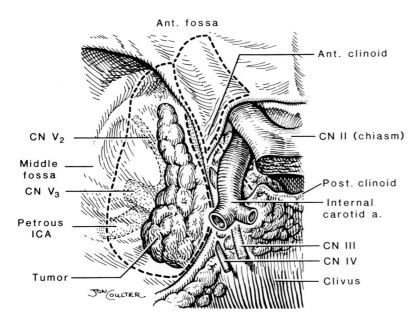

Ant. fossa

Ant. clinoid

CN V₂

CN II (chiasm)

Middle fossa

Post. clinoid

CN V₃

Internal carotid a.

Petrous ICA

CN III

CN IV

Tumor

Clivus

Figure 37-7 Figures 37-7 through 37-10 illustrate the steps in the removal of a meningioma of the cavernous sinus, tentorial notch, and upper clivus. Figure 37-7 shows the initial appearance of the meningioma. The dotted lines illustrate the dural incisions used. CN = cranial nerves, ICA = internal carotid artery. (From Sekhar et al.,[19] with permission.)

cavernous ICA will be exposed. The ICA is attached at the point of its exit from the cavernous sinus by a dense fibrous ring which will need to be divided to mobilize the artery (Fig. 37-8). The superior wall of the cavernous sinus (which is devoid of cranial nerves) is then opened back to the posterior clinoid process. Venous bleeding from the anterior and posterior ends of the cavernous sinus can be controlled by packing with Surgicel (oxidized regenerated cellulose; Johnson & Johnson, New Brunswick, NJ). The ICA is followed back into the cavernous sinus. The superior and medial aspects of the cavernous sinus, the superior and medial walls of the horizontal portion of the intracavernous ICA and its anterior bend, and the lateral aspect of the pituitary gland are well exposed by this approach.

Lateral Approach

This approach differs according to whether the tumor is a meningioma, or a chordoma, chondrosarcoma, or neurilemoma. For meningiomas, the entire lateral wall of the cavernous sinus is peeled away (Fig. 37-8), exposing cranial nerves III, IV, and V, imbedded in the lateral wall. The cavernous sinus is then entered between the ophthalmic and trochlear nerves (Parkinson's triangle) or between V₁ and V₂ to remove tumor. The dissection of the ICA and the identification of the abducens nerve are the more difficult parts of tumor removal. Electrical stimulation and anatomic landmarks such as the posterior clinoid process and the petroclinoid ligament are useful for identifying the abducens

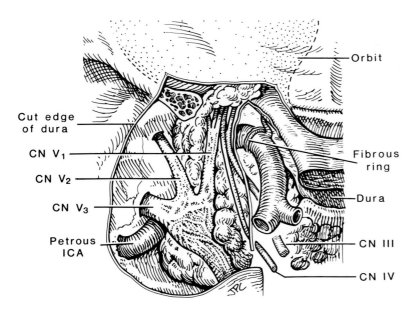

Orbit

Cut edge of dura

CN V₁

CN V₂

Fibrous ring

CN V₃

Dura

Petrous ICA

CN III

CN IV

Figure 37-8 The optic nerve has been unroofed, and the anterior clinoid process has been removed to expose the anterior bend and anterior vertical segment of the intracavernous ICA. The fibrous ring at the exit of the intracavernous ICA is shown. The tentorium has been divided, and the neoplasm-invaded lateral wall of the cavernous sinus has been removed. (From Sekhar et al.,[19] with permission.)

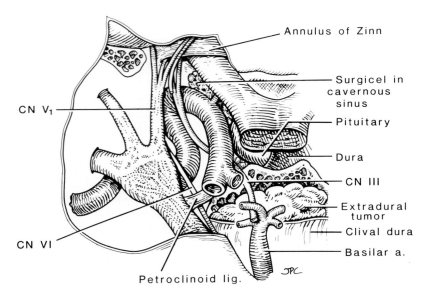

Figure 37-9 Appearance after resection of tumor from within the cavernous sinus. The fourth cranial nerve has been divided. The neoplastic dura covering a portion of the pituitary gland has been removed. The neoplastic bone of the upper clivus also has been removed. Tumor is now seen extradurally in the clival area, as was commonly observed in our patients. (From Sekhar et al.,[19] with permission.)

nerve (Fig. 37-9). When the ICA is completely encased (360-degree circumference) by a meningioma, it is futile to attempt dissection of the tumor. Instead, the intracavernous ICA is occluded and excised with tumor, with or without vein graft reconstruction. Such reconstruction usually is performed with a 5- to 6-cm long saphenous vein graft extracted from the thigh, anastomosed end-to-side or end-to-end to the supraclinoid ICA, and end-to-end to the petrous ICA. The anastomosis is performed with 7-0 prolene or 8-0 nylon interrupted sutures and takes about 90 to 120 min to complete. A good pulse in the graft indicates a good technical anastomosis that is not likely to cause any postoperative problems (Fig. 37-10).

For tumors such as chordomas, chondrosarcomas, or neurilemomas, the dura of the lateral wall is often incised in a cruciate fashion over the most prominent areas. The oph-

thalmic, maxillary, and sometimes the trochlear nerves need to be dissected, but the oculomotor nerve need not be dissected. Tumor removal can be adequately performed through this opening into the cavernous sinus (Figs. 37-11 and 37-12).

Transcavernous Approach to the Clivus and Sella

After the removal of a large tumor component within the cavernous sinus, or after the excision of the intracavernous ICA, a transcavernous approach to the sphenoid, upper clivus, and the sella is possible (Fig. 37-12). Intracavernous meningiomas often involve the dura of the sella, the dura of the clivus (extradural and subdural tumor extension), the dura of the tentorial notch–petrous area, the bone of the

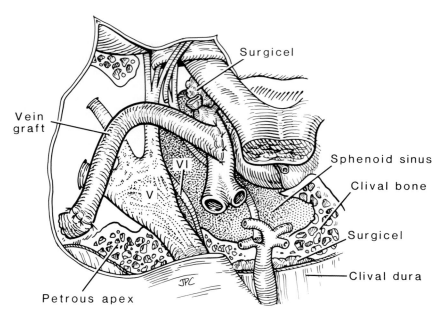

Figure 37-10 This step is used only in some tumor operations. The intracavernous ICA has been excised. A vein graft has been used for reconstruction. The tumor-invaded bone of the sphenoid, petrous apex, and upper clivus has been removed. Extradural and subdural meningioma has been removed from the clival area. The sphenoid sinus will be packed with fat after removal of any tumor within. A fascia lata graft will be sutured over it. (From Sekhar et al.,[19] with permission.)

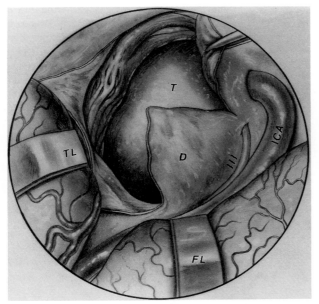

Figure 37-11 Steps in the removal of a cartilaginous tumor (chondrosarcoma or chordoma) or a neurilemoma of the cavernous sinus. The sylvian fissure has been split, the dura has been incised in a cruciate fashion and peeled away to expose the tumor and the trigeminal nerve. The oculomotor nerve is not dissected extensively. TL = temporal lobe, FL = frontal lobe, T = tumor, III = oculomotor nerve. (Modified from Sekhar and Møller,[18] with permission.)

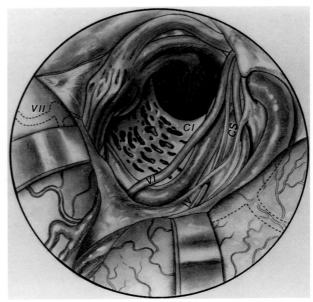

Figure 37-12 Appearance after the removal of an extensive chordoma involving the petroclival-cavernous sinus area. The intracavernous ICA and the displaced sixth cranial nerve are now visible. VII = the approximate location of the seventh cranial nerve, which is not exposed during this operation, IV, VI = cranial nerves, Cl = clivus, CS = what remains of the cavernous sinus after tumor resection. (Modified from Sekhar and Møller,[18] with permission.)

clivus and the sphenoid, and the sphenoid sinus itself. Removal of all this tumor is possible through the cavernous sinus when the intracavernous ICA has been excised, without or with vein graft reconstruction. The same can be achieved with large chordomas and chondrosarcomas even when the intracavernous ICA has not been excised. The tentorium must be divided, and the upper basilar artery and the brain stem must be visualized and protected during such tumor resection.

Management of the Cranial Nerves

The most important cranial nerves passing through the cavernous sinus in their order of importance are the oculomotor, ophthalmic, and abducens. Patients will readily compensate for the loss of trochlear nerve function, and minor degrees of third and sixth cranial nerve dysfunction can be corrected with strabismus surgery. Permanent loss of corneal sensation produces a long-term risk for neurotrophic keratitis and corneal ulceration. Dissection of cranial nerves (especially the third and the sixth) from the tumor can be aided by neurophysiologic monitoring. Occasionally a tumor-invaded nerve will have to be excised. If feasible, reconstruction should be attempted by direct suture or with an interposition nerve graft. We performed reconstruction of the oculomotor nerve in one patient with partial recovery, the ophthalmic nerve in one patient with partial recovery,

and the abducens nerve in one patient with no recovery to date.[19]

Management of the ICA

If the intracavernous ICA is partially encased (180 degrees or less of circumference) by a meningioma, or even totally encased by a cartilaginous or nerve sheath tumor, it can be dissected free of tumor. Total encasement by a meningioma, or even partial encasement by a highly malignant tumor will require excision with or without vein graft reconstruction, based on the patient's life expectancy and the results of the balloon occlusion test. We have occluded the intracavernous ICA in seven patients and performed vein graft reconstruction in three patients with tumors (and other patients with vascular lesions). None had a permanent cerebral deficit postoperatively.

Management of Venous Bleeding

Venous bleeding can always be controlled by packing with Surgicel. Slight head elevation may also be helpful. When the patient's arterial oxygen tension is much higher than normal levels, confusion may occur between venous and arterial bleeding. On this occasion, lowering the Pa_{O_2} to normal levels is helpful.

We have not encountered any problems caused by venous occlusion of the cavernous sinus. However, when the dominant venous drainage of the temporal lobe is anteriorly directed, postoperative swelling and hematomas can develop. This can be prevented by careful review of preoperative arteriograms and the judicious use of temporal tip excision during the operation.

Reconstruction of the Cranial Base

Appropriate cranial base reconstruction will prevent postoperative complications of cerebrospinal fluid leakage and infection. A dural closure is always performed using autologous pericranium or fascia lata. Although a watertight closure is not always possible, circumferential suturing of the dural graft is helpful for healing. When the eustachian tube orifice is exposed at the end of tumor resection, it is occluded with fat and a flap of temporalis muscle. If the sphenoid sinus is exposed to the cranial cavity, its mucosa is removed, it is packed with fat, and a free fascial graft is used to reconstruct the clival dura. However, when the sphenoid sinus has been previously communicated with the nasal cavity by ethmoidectomy, a vascularized flap reconstruction is necessary. If the intracranial contents and/or the ICA may

be exposed to the upper aerodigestive tract at the end of resection of malignant neoplasms, a vascularized flap reconstruction is needed to avoid ascending infection. Such flaps may be regional or distant. Regional flaps include the pericranial flap, galeofrontalis flap, temporalis muscle flap, and scalp rotation flaps. Distant flaps include the pectoralis myocutaneous flap, the trapezius flap, rectus abdominis microvascular free flap, or the latissimus dorsi microvascular free flap. For the more extensive surgical procedures, collaboration with specialists from otolaryngology and plastic surgery is essential.[19]

Surgical Results

During the period 1983–1988, 52 intracavernous neoplasms and 5 vascular lesions of the cavernous sinus (aneurysms and carotid-cavernous fistulae) were operated upon. The pathology of the operated neoplasms, the completeness of their removal, previous and postoperative adjuvant therapy, and follow-up data are summarized in Table 37-2. In addition to the patients with tumor who have been operated upon, 13 patients have also been followed without surgery. The reasons for a nonoperative management have included the min-

TABLE 37-2 Surgical Management of Intracavernous Neoplasms, 1983–1988 (*n* = 52)

| | | Excision | | | Radiation Therapy | | | | | | Follow-up |
	No.	Total	Subtotal	Residue	Preoperative	Postoperative	AS̃D	AW̄D	DOD	DOC	Average (Months)
Benign tumors											
Meningioma	20	16	4	Cavernous sinus 1 / Clivus 2 / Orbital apex 1	EB 5	EB 1 / GK 2	15	4	—	1	22
Neurilemoma	5	5	—		—	—	5	—	—	—	18
Juvenile angiofibroma	2	1	1	Pterygopalatine fossa 1	—	—	1	1	—	—	23
Chondroblastoma	1	1	—	—	—	—	1	—	—	—	18
Hemangioma	1	1	—	—	—	—	1	—	—	—	10
	29	24	5				23	5	0	1	
Malignant tumors											
Meningioma	1	—	1	Cavernous sinus, orbital apex	—	EB	—	1	—	—	9
Pituitary adenoma, invasive	2	2	—	—	—	EB 2	1	—	—	1	12
Chordoma	6	3	3	Cavernous sinus 2 / Clivus 2	EB 2 / PB 1	PB 2	3	3	—	—	23
Chondrosarcoma	5	2	3	Clivus 2 / Cavernous sinus 1	—	EB 2	2	3	—	—	51
Adenoid cystic carcinoma	3	3	—	—	EB 2	EB 2	3	—	—	—	31
Squamous cell carcinoma	2	1	1	Cervical nodes	—	EB 2	1	1	—	—	35
Plasmycytoma	1	—	1	Cavernous sinus	—	EB 1	—	1	—	—	11
Hypernephroma (metastatic)	1	1	—	—	—	EB 1	1	—	—	—	21
Basal cell carcinoma	1	1	—	—	—	EB 1	1	—	—	—	2
Osteogenic sarcoma	1	1	—	—	EB 1	Chemo	1	—	—	—	1
	23	14	9				13	9	0	1	

AS̃D = Alive without disease; AW̄D = Alive with disease; Chemo = Chemotherapy; DOC = Died of other causes; DOD = Died of disease; EB = External beam radiotherapy; GK = Gamma knife; PB = Proton beam radiotherapy.

imality of symptoms and the absence of radiographically documented growth in the case of benign tumors, the unfeasibility of total tumor resection in the case of highly malignant tumors (e.g., bilateral cavernous sinus invasion with sarcoma or carcinoma), or the refusal of a patient to undergo surgery that was recommended.

Meningiomas were technically the most difficult tumors to excise. The operative difficulties depended upon whether the tumor encased the ICA partially or totally, the consistency of the tumor (fibrous or soft), the extension of the tumor to various other areas of the cranial base (orbit, sphenoid bone and sinus, infratemporal fossa, temporal bone, clival bone, and petroclival dura), and whether the patient had undergone prior operative procedures. *Neurilemomas* of the trigeminal nerve often involve the cavernous sinus, although the trigeminal nerve runs in the lateral wall. They were technically easier to remove. *Chordomas and chondrosarcomas* were also technically easier tumors to remove from the cavernous sinus region. However, because of their cartilaginous consistency, it is easy to leave behind residual tumor. For highly malignant tumors such as *squamous cell carcinoma*, we have increasingly adopted a strategy of removing all the contents of the cavernous sinus including the cranial nerves and the ICA along with the tumor. An intracavernous operation is performed only if the tumor can be totally removed from other areas of the cranial base.

Extraocular Muscle Function

Many patients sustain a partial or total paralysis of cranial nerves III, IV, V, and VI after the removal of an intracavernous neoplasm. However, if the cranial nerve was well preserved during the operation, postoperative recovery occurs within 3 to 12 months. The extent of recovery is dependent on the preoperative level of function.[19] In 42 earlier patients in whom the extraocular muscle function has been evaluated postoperatively, the pre- and postoperative functional levels are compared in Table 37-3. Table 37-4 lists permanent injuries to cranial nerves during intracavernous operations. Some of these were intentional, because the patient had longstanding paralysis of the third cranial nerve or had a highly malignant tumor.

TABLE 37-3 Extraocular Muscle (EOM) Function in Patients with Surgical Removal of Cavernous Sinus Neoplasms ($n = 42$)

	Excellent	Good	Fair	Poor
Preoperative	21	6	9	7
Postoperative				
Excellent	16	2	2	—
Good	3	4	2	2
Fair	1	—	5	—
Poor	—	—	—	5
Cannot assess	1	—	—	—
Too soon	—	—	—	—
	21	6	9	7

Excellent = No EOM weakness.
Good = Mild EOM weakness (correctable).
Fair = Moderate EOM weakness (correctable).
Poor = Severe EOM weakness or complete paralysis.

TABLE 37-4 Neurologic Worsening and Improvement in Patients with Cavernous Sinus Tumors

	Permanent Postoperative Worsening		Postoperative Improvement
	Total	Unintentional	
Mental status	—	—	2
Motor function	—	—	3
Sensory function	—	—	3
Cerebellar function	—	—	1
Cranial nerves			
I	3	0	0
II	1	1	1
III	1	1	7
IV	7	0	2
V_1	4	0	2
V_2	7	0	3
V_3	6	1	—
VI	6	3	6

All patients with extraocular muscle palsies should be seen preoperatively and postoperatively by a neuro-ophthalmologist. At the end of a year, some patients may benefit from oculoplastic surgery to correct minor impairments of extraocular muscle function.

Other Postoperative Complications

One patient sustained an ascending wound infection with gram-negative organisms and a carotid pseudoaneurysm (with sentinel hemorrhage). This occurred because the wound was inadequately excluded from the oropharynx by a rectus abdominis free flap. It was successfully treated by balloon occlusion of the ICA, removal of the bone flap, debridement, and antibiotic therapy. A subdural hematoma occurred from a middle meningeal artery branch which had been inadequately coagulated. Both CSF leaks through the sphenoid sinus occurred prior to the practice of packing an open sinus with fat. They both required reoperation. The rest healed with spinal fluid drainage. Transient diabetes insipidus occurred in patients in whom the pituitary gland was dissected free of partially encasing tumor. It lasted 1 to 5 days. All these patients were tested for endocrinologic deficits postoperatively. None developed new hormonal problems. (See Table 37-5.)

TABLE 37-5 Cavernous Sinus Neoplasms—Other Surgical Complications

Wound infection and carotid pseudoaneurysm	1
Subdural hematoma	1
Temporal lobe edema	2
Seizures, postoperative	2
Diabetes insipidus, transient	4
Cerebrospinal fluid leakage	
Sphenoid sinus	2 (reoperated)
Wound	2
Ear canal (eustachian tube)	2
Deep vein thrombosis	2

Management Controversies

The current controversies regarding tumors involving the cavernous sinus center around whether or not anything should be done, when to operate, and the role of radiation therapy versus surgery.[1,15,19,21] Much of the fear with regard to operations in the cavernous sinus relates to venous bleeding, which technically is the easiest to deal with. The major potential problems during intracavernous operations relate to the intracavernous ICA and the cranial nerves that traverse the cavernous sinus. We and others have now demonstrated that cavernous sinus operations can be performed with a low mortality and cerebral morbidity. The use of the balloon occlusion test of the ICA and a systematic plan for the exposure and management of the intracavernous ICA has greatly reduced the morbidity related to it. In our experience, cranial nerve morbidity does not seem to be as significant a problem as popularly believed. However, the eventual outcome is closely related to the preoperative status. Based on current experience, an algorithm for management of cavernous sinus neoplasms has been developed (Table 37-6).

From our material it appears that minimally symptomatic benign tumors within the cavernous sinus can remain dormant for many years. Therefore operations are performed only for tumors that are enlarging, with or without progressive symptomatology. When a large intracranial benign tumor has a small intracavernous component, we prefer to remove the cavernous sinus portion of the tumor if the patient is physiologically healthy and tolerates the balloon occlusion test of the ICA. Malignant cartilaginous neoplasms are technically the easiest to remove, and one can be

more aggressive with their resection even if there is bilateral cavernous sinus involvement. Highly malignant cavernous sinus lesions are operated on only if there is a prospect of total overall surgical resection.

There are two alternative forms of therapy. The first is stereotactically directed radiation therapy using either the gamma knife or the linear accelerator. This modality of treatment is possible only for lesions less than 2.5 cm in diameter. The long-term effects on cavernous sinus neoplasms in terms of tumor control and cranial nerve and vascular morbidity are as yet not known. If radiotherapy is elected, such stereotactic methods are preferred for the treatment of benign lesions, since the adverse effects on surrounding brain structures can be expected to be minimal.

The second form of therapy is external beam radiotherapy. This relies on the differential sensitivity of the tumor cells to radiation effects in comparison with the brain cells. The use of such radiation for benign tumors is controversial. There are many reports of the variable response of meningiomas and neurilemomas to radiation, although the larger series have not documented control of tumor growth by imaging studies.[1,15,21] Unfortunately, once the adverse effects of radiation set in there is not much that can be done to reverse them. In our institution, we have been impressed with the adverse effects of radiation therapy of cranial base neoplasms. We, therefore, reserve external beam radiation therapy for malignant neoplasms.

The operative techniques for the management of intracavernous neoplasms, the intracavernous ICA, and the related cranial nerves are continuously evolving at the present time. The small number of patients with such tumors and the complex surgical techniques required to treat them preclude randomized controlled studies. However, careful pro-

TABLE 37-6 Management Algorithm for Cavernous Sinus Neoplasms (Operation Only on Tumors That Are Enlarging ± Progressive Symptoms)

	Benign Tumors*	Malignant Cartilaginous Tumors†	Highly Malignant Tumors‡
Small, restricted to CS (<3 cm)	Surgical removal (alternative: gamma knife)	Surgical removal	Surgical removal if lesion can be totally removed
Large with small portion within cavernous sinus (>3 cm)	Remove large part first; consider removal of intracavernous component in physiologically healthy patient (alternative: gamma knife for small residue)	Attempt total removal; adjuvant radiotherapy for residue	Surgical removal of cavernous sinus if total resection can be accomplished
Bilateral cavernous sinus tumor	Remove tumor from one CS first; if results are good, opposite CS lesion may be operated on or treated with gamma knife (alternative: external beam radiation therapy)	Surgical removal in stages; adjuvant radiotherapy for any residue	No operation
Failed balloon occlusion test of ICA clinically	Consider radiotherapy; if operation is elected, consider prior STA-MCA bypass and intraoperative vein graft replacement of ICA	Surgical removal with preparation for STA-MCA bypass and vein graft to ICA	Operation not preferred; consider alternatives

* For example, meningioma and neurilemoma.
† For example, chordoma and chondrosarcoma.
‡ For example, squamous cell carcinoma and basal cell carcinoma.

spective studies of the outcome of such operations are necessary in institutions which treat significant numbers of such patients.

References

1. Barbaro NM, Gutin PH, Wilson CB, et al. Radiation therapy in the treatment of partially resected meningiomas. *Neurosurgery* 1987; 20:525–528.
2. Dolenc V. Direct microsurgical repair of intracavernous vascular lesions. *J Neurosurg* 1983; 58:824–831.
3. Dolenc VV, Kregar T, Ferluga M, et al. Treatment of tumors invading the cavernous sinus. In: Dolenc VV (ed.), *The Cavernous Sinus: A Multidisciplinary Approach to Vascular and Tumorous Lesions.* New York: Springer-Verlag, 1987: 377–391.
4. Hakuba A, Nishimura S, Shirakata S, et al. Surgical approaches to the cavernous sinus: report of 19 cases. *Neurol Med Chir (Tokyo)* 1982; 22:295–308.
5. Hakuba A, Suzuki T, Jin TB, et al. Surgical approaches to the cavernous sinus: report of 52 cases. In: *Proceedings of the International Symposium on Cavernous Sinus.* Ljubljana, Yugoslavia, 1986: 302–327.
6. Harris FS, Rhoton AL Jr. Anatomy of the cavernous sinus: a microsurgical study. *J Neurosurg* 1976; 45:169–180.
7. Isamat F, Ferrer E, Twose J. Direct intracavernous obliteration of high-flow carotid-cavernous fistulas. *J Neurosurg* 1986; 65:770–775.
8. Lang J. *Clinical Anatomy of the Head: Neurocranium, Orbit, Craniocervical Regions,* Translated by Wilson RR, Winstanley DP. New York: Springer-Verlag, 1983.
9. Laws ER Jr, Onofrio BM, Pearson BW, et al. Successful management of bilateral carotid-cavernous fistulae with a transsphenoidal approach. *Neurosurgery* 1979; 4:162–167.
10. Lesoin F, Pellerin P, Clarisse J, et al. Direct microsurgical approach to intracavernous tumors. In: *Proceedings of the International Symposium on Cavernous Sinus.* Ljubljana, Yugoslavia, 1986: 290–300.
11. MacKay A, Hosobuchi Y. Treatment of intracavernous extensions of pituitary adenomas. *Surg Neurol* 1978; 10:377–383.
12. Parkinson D. A surgical approach to the cavernous portion of the carotid artery: anatomical studies and case report. *J Neurosurg* 1965; 23:473–484.
13. Parkinson D, West M. Lesions of the cavernous plexus region. In: Youmans JR (ed.), *Neurological Surgery,* 2d ed. Philadelphia: Saunders, 1982: 3004–3023.
14. Perneczky A, Knosp E, Matula C. Cavernous sinus surgery: approach through the lateral wall. *Acta Neurochir (Wien)* 1988; 92:76–82.
15. Petty AM, Kun LE, Meyer GA. Radiation therapy for incompletely resected meningiomas. *J Neurosurg* 1985; 62:502–507.
16. Sekhar LN. Operative management of tumors involving the cavernous sinus. In: Sekhar LN, Schramm VL Jr (eds.), *Tumors of the Cranial Base: Diagnosis and Treatment.* Mount Kisko, New York: Futura, 1987: 393–419.
17. Sekhar LN, Burgess J, Akin O. Anatomical study of the cavernous sinus emphasizing operative approaches and related vascular and neural reconstruction. *Neurosurgery* 1987; 21:806–816.
18. Sekhar LN, Møller AR. Operative management of tumors involving the cavernous sinus. *J Neurosurg* 1986; 64:879–889.
19. Sekhar LN, Sen CN, Jho HD, et al. Surgical treatment of intracavernous neoplasms: a four-year experience. *Neurosurgery* 1989; 24:18–30.
20. Taptas JN. The so-called cavernous sinus: a review of the controversy and its implications for neurosurgeons. *Neurosurgery* 1982; 11:712–717.
21. Wallner KE, Sheline GE, Pitts LH, et al. Efficacy of irradiation for incompletely excised acoustic neurilemomas. *J Neurosurg* 1987; 67:858–863.

38

Trigeminal Neurinomas

Kalmon D. Post
Paul C. McCormick

Incidence and Classification

Neurinomas arising from the intracranial portion of the trigeminal nerve are rare. They account for 0.07 to 0.36 percent of intracranial tumors and 0.8 to 8 percent of intracranial neurinomas.[1,4,9,11,13,16,17] These tumors are occasionally encountered in conjunction with multiple intracranial neurinomas as a manifestation of neurofibromatosis. In most of these cases, however, the trigeminal neurinoma does not represent the clinically significant pathology and is usually described as an incidental radiographic, operative, or postmortem finding.

Neurinomas can arise from the root, ganglion, or rarely, a proximal division of the trigeminal nerve. Since the intracranial course of the trigeminal nerve is closely applied to the skull base of both posterior and middle fossae, Jefferson classified trigeminal neurinomas into three types: (1) tumors mainly in the middle fossa, (2) predominantly posterior fossa tumors, and (3) tumors with significant components in both posterior and middle fossae.[8] This classification scheme has functional significance from a clinical, radiographic, and surgical perspective. A review of reported cases indicates that slightly more than 50 percent of trigeminal neurinomas arise within the middle fossa, with variable degrees of tumor extension into the posterior fossa. Approximately one-third are totally or predominantly confined to the posterior fossa, and less than 20 percent are dumbbell-shaped with significant tumor components in both middle and posterior fossae.

The data presented in this chapter reflect the experience at our institution with a series of 14 patients with trigeminal neurinoma managed operatively since 1970. To better define the clinical, radiographic, and pathologic aspects of these rare tumors, an additional 106 reported cases were analyzed.[11]

Surgical Anatomy and Pathology

The trigeminal root, consisting of a larger sensory root and a smaller medially situated motor root, arises from the lateral aspect of the rostral pons and courses in a lateral, anterior, and slightly superior direction through the anterior part of the cerebellopontine angle in the pontocerebellar cistern. The superior cerebellar artery usually passes above and the anterior inferior cerebellar artery below the root, but this relationship is not constant owing to the frequent anatomic variations and loops of these vessels. The petrosal vein lies lateral and posterior to the trigeminal root. The root passes under the trochlear nerve and free edge of the tentorium and enters the middle fossa through a dural cleft, the porus trigeminus, located just inferior to the lateral tentorial attachment and superior petrosal sinus. The root is then essentially extradural in location and terminates in the trigeminal ganglion.

The crescent-shaped trigeminal ganglion occupies a shallow bony recess on the anterior surface of the petrous apex known as Meckel's cave. Because the sensory root rotates anteriorly as it enters the trigeminal ganglion, the motor root becomes related to its inferior surface and passes under the ganglion before being incorporated into the mandibular nerve. Just anterior to Meckel's cave the connective tissue–filled foramen lacerum separates the distal part of the ganglion from the horizontal petrous segment of the internal carotid artery and the eustachian tube. The greater superficial petrosal nerve courses anteriorly beneath the trigeminal ganglion and is frequently injured during removal of neurinomas involving the ganglion. The dural covering of the trigeminal ganglion is continuous anteriorly with the posterolateral wall of the cavernous sinus.

The pathologic relationship of these tumors to the trigeminal root and ganglion is variable. The trigeminal ganglion is usually not visualized with tumors arising in Meckel's cave, although compressed remnants of ganglionic tissue may occasionally be identified after tumor removal. Although trigeminal nerve fibers may be seen on the surface of the tumor, in most cases, at least portions of the root appear to course through the tumor mass.

Microscopically, these tumors show the typical neurinoma appearance of bipolar elongated cells with fusiform darkly staining nuclei arranged in compact interlacing fascicles with a tendency toward palisade formation. A looser arrangement of cells, separated by a collagenous or hyalinized matrix, the Antoni B pattern, is less common. Thickened hyalinized blood vessels, occasionally thrombosed, and hemosiderin-laden macrophages (foam cells) are frequently present. Histologically malignant neurinomas and melanotic neurinomas are rare but have been described.[6,11]

Clinical Features

The peak incidence occurred during the fourth decade of life, and the mean age at the time of diagnosis was 37 years (range, 13 to 67 years). The tumors were only slightly more common in women. The duration of symptoms preceding diagnosis ranged from 6 days to 16 years, with a mean of 39 months.

The initial symptom was recorded in 114 of the 120 cases. Subjective complaints of trigeminal nerve dysfunction were the initial symptoms in 59 percent (67 of 114) of the cases. These complaints included numbness (34 cases), pain (26 cases), and paresthesias (7 cases). Frequently, the complaint was initially localized to a portion of the sensory field in the distribution of one trigeminal division. In most cases, however, the entire trigeminal distribution was involved by the time of diagnosis. The remaining initial symptoms are listed in Table 38-1.

Eventual involvement of the trigeminal nerve was the general rule, so that, by the time of diagnosis, 87 percent (104 of 120) had either subjective or objective evidence of trigeminal nerve dysfunction. Varying degrees of hypesthesia, hypalgesia, and a diminished or absent corneal reflex were the most common findings. Complete anesthesia was distinctly rare, and although one division of the trigeminal nerve was commonly more severely affected, there was usually diminished sensation in the entire trigeminal nerve distribution.

Weakness in the muscles of mastication was recorded in 50 (42 percent) patients. The paresis was generally mild, and atrophy of the masseter and temporalis muscles was noted only occasionally.

Facial pain was a prominent complaint on admission history in 45 (36 percent) patients. It was more common with tumors involving the trigeminal ganglion (52 percent) than with tumors arising from the trigeminal root (28 percent). The quality and intensity of the pain was variable, ranging from a dull ache to a severe burning pain. In most cases, the pain was constant and usually progressed in severity. Episodes of severe lancinating exacerbations of facial pain, suggestive of trigeminal neuralgia, were noted by one-third of these patients. True trigeminal neuralgia, characterized by trigger zones, prolonged pain-free periods, and the absence of objective trigeminal nerve deficits, however, was an initial symptom in only six patients. Three of these patients had tumors arising from the trigeminal root, and three patients had trigeminal ganglion tumors.

Neurologic deficits, other than trigeminal nerve abnormalities, were present in over 75 percent of patients by the time of diagnosis (Table 38-2). The majority of these deficits were in the form of cranial nerve palsies and were related to the location the tumor. The abducens nerve was most com-

TABLE 38-2 Abnormal Findings on Admission Examination in 120 Patients with Trigeminal Neurinoma*

Neurologic Abnormality	No. of Cases	Percent
Trigeminal nerve		
Decreased sensation	89	74
Diminished or absent corneal reflex	86	72
Pain	45	36
Motor weakness	50	42
Other cranial nerve deficits		
II	12	10
III	18	15
IV	8	7
VI	42	35
VII	27	23
VIII	37	31
IX, X	9	8
XI	2	1
XII	4	3
Cerebellar signs	28	23
Long tract signs	19	16
Exophthalmos	20	17
Papilledema	12	11

*Only 26 patients (22%) had abnormal findings limited to the trigeminal nerve.

monly affected by ganglion tumors, probably as a result of the proximity of the intracavernous portion of the nerve to the medial aspect of the trigeminal ganglion. Posterior fossa tumors frequently caused deficits in the seventh and eighth cranial nerves. Large posterior fossa tumors were usually also associated with cerebellar and pyramidal tract signs.

A few patients with tumors located solely within the middle fossa were noted to have conductive hearing loss or facial weakness. The hearing loss was probably the result of compression of the eustachian tube as it passes under the cartilaginous floor of Meckel's cave. The facial paresis seen with middle fossa tumors is most likely due to traction on the greater superficial petrosal nerve.

Radiologic Investigation

Plain films of the skull, frequently with thin section tomography, were performed in 99 patients. Anteroposterior, base, and Stenver's views were the most useful projections in defining the bony changes associated with trigeminal neurinomas.

Erosion of the anteromedial portion of the petrous pyramid was the most common bony abnormality and was present in 60 cases. The defect was usually described as a sharply delineated amputation of the petrous apex with smooth, rarely sclerotic, margins (Fig. 38-1).[5,7,10,14] This finding was generally seen with Meckel's cave or dumbbell-shaped tumors.

Epidermoids, meningiomas, acoustic neurinomas, and primary bone tumors of the skull base, such as chordomas and osteochondromas, also have been reported to produce erosion of the petrous apex.[4,12,18] In most cases, however, associated bony abnormalities serve to distinguish these

TABLE 38-1 Initial Symptom in 114 Patients with Trigeminal Neurinoma

Symptom	No. of Cases	Percent
Trigeminal nerve dysfunction	67	59
Numbness	34	30
Pain	26	23
Paresthesias	7	6
Headache	18	16
Diplopia	10	9
Hearing loss/tinnitus	7	6
Visual loss	5	4.5
Ear pain	4	3.5
Other*	5	4.5
Total	116†	

*Other symptoms = Subarachnoid hemorrhage, vertigo, seizure, exophthalmos, gait difficulty (1 patient each).
†Three patients presented with more than one initial complaint; one patient was asymptomatic.

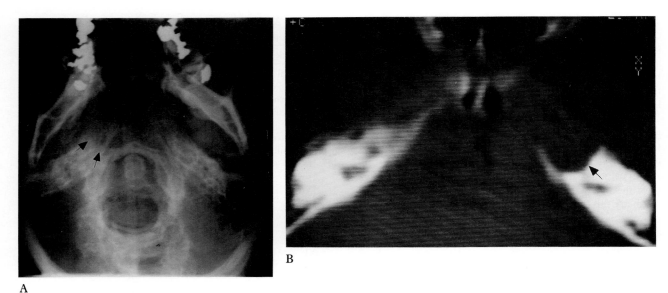

A

B

Figure 38-1 *A*. Skull roentgenogram; base view demonstrates amputation of the right petrous apex (*arrows*). *B*. Axial CT correlate on a different patient demonstrates similar erosion of the left petrous apex (*arrow*).

tumors from trigeminal neurinomas. Meningiomas frequently produce bone erosion with irregular margins or hyperostosis and may have visible intratumoral calcification. Acoustic neurinomas usually cause enlargement of the internal auditory meatus, a finding not seen with trigeminal neurinomas. Primary bone tumors of the skull base generally show more extensive destructive bony changes and are frequently calcified. Epidermoids, however, arising either in Meckel's cave or in the cerebellopontine angle, may produce bony changes identical to those seen with trigeminal neurinomas. Sclerosis at the margins of the bone defect, frequently seen with epidermoids, may help to distinguish between these tumors. Finally, aneurysms arising from the petrous, precavernous, or cavernous portions of the internal carotid artery may produce isolated erosion of the petrous apex.[12]

Additional bony abnormalities generally reflect a slowly expanding mass in the middle fossa. These findings include erosion of the floor of the middle fossa, enlargement of the basal foramina, and occasional erosion of the pterygoid plates. Medial and anterior tumor growth is associated with erosion of the lateral aspect of the sella turcica, dorsum sellae, anterior clinoid process, superior orbital fissure, and the inferolateral aspect of the optic canal.

The extradural location of these tumors in the middle fossa, growing under pressure exerted by the dura, may be responsible for the frequency and extent of bone erosion associated with these slow-growing benign tumors.

Bony changes are infrequently seen with trigeminal neurinomas in the posterior fossa. Although amputation of the petrous apex is occasionally seen, flattening of the posterior surface of the petrous apex is more common. This erosion may extend laterally to involve the anteromedial lip of the internal auditory meatus. Other bony abnormalities seen

with posterior fossa neurinomas include erosion of the lateral aspect of the clivus and diffuse changes produced by increased intracranial pressure.

Cerebral angiography was performed in 49 patients. The results were reported as normal in seven patients. All of these patients had small tumors arising either in Meckel's cave or from the trigeminal root. The remaining 42 patients exhibited abnormalities in the form of blood vessel displacement related to the location of the tumor.

Medial displacement of the initial extradural portion of the carotid siphon, the so-called ganglial or precavernous segment, was the most commonly reported abnormality associated with tumors originating in Meckel's cave (Fig. 38-2A). In most cases, there was associated anterior and inferior displacement of this portion of the siphon (Fig. 38-2B), but superior and posterior displacement, indicating tumor growth anterior to the ascending portion of the carotid siphon, was noted in some patients. Although displacement of the precavernous extradural segment of the carotid siphon may rarely be seen with large intra-axial masses arising in the temporal lobe, this finding is fairly specific for extracerebral, particularly extradural, masses arising from the skull base.[3,8]

Early posterior fossa extension through the porus trigeminus of a tumor arising in Meckel's cave was heralded by medial displacement of the proximal segments of the posterior cerebral and superior cerebellar arteries (Fig. 38-2C). Both of these vessels may also be elevated. Large posterior fossa trigeminal neurinomas, in addition, produce depression of the anterior inferior cerebellar artery and elevation or nonfilling of the petrosal vein. The basilar artery may be stretched and displaced contralaterally. Posterior displacement of the basilar artery may occasionally be seen and results from tumor growth ventral to the brain stem.

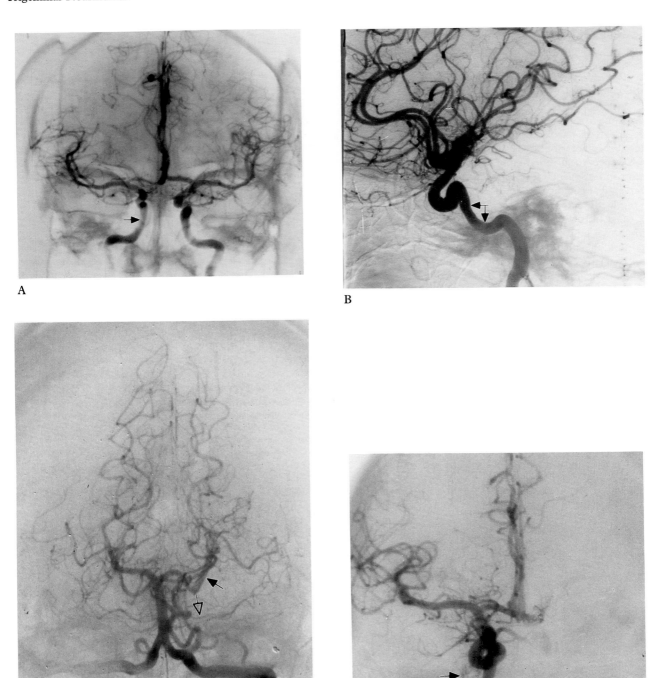

A

B

C

D

Figure 38-2 *A*. Subtraction films from bilateral internal carotid artery angiogram (superimposed) shows relative medial displacement of the precavernous segment of the right internal carotid artery (*arrow*). *B*. Lateral projection of internal carotid angiogram shows anterior and inferior displacement of the precavernous (ganglial) segment of the internal carotid artery (*arrows*). *C*. Subtraction angiogram of left vertebral artery injection shows medial displacement of the proximal segments of the superior cerebellar and posterior cerebral arteries (*arrow*). The left anterior inferior cerebellar artery is displaced inferiorly (*open arrow*). *D*. Subtraction film (anteroposterior projection) from internal carotid artery angiogram shows slight but definite neovascularity associated with a Meckel's cave neurinoma (*arrow*).

About 20 percent of trigeminal neurinomas demonstrate abnormal tumor vascularity consisting of enlarged feeding vessels or a tumor stain. The abnormal vessels are derived from the precavernous and cavernous segments of the carotid siphon (Fig. 38-2D).

Most of the cases in this review were published before the development of computed tomography (CT). Ten of the 14 patients in our series underwent preoperative CT scanning. Six tumors appeared as isodense or slightly hypodense with respect to surrounding brain and enchanced uniformly with contrast agents. The four other cases showed areas of decreased attenuation after contrast administration believed to represent either necrosis or cystic degeneration (Fig. 38-3). Axial and coronal sections of the skull base were particularly useful in identifying the extent of bone destruction in both middle and posterior fossae (Fig. 38-3B).

Although coronal CT sections provide important information in defining the relationship of the tumor to the cavernous sinus, tentorial notch, and extracranial tissues, magnetic resonance imaging (MRI) has thus far proved superior in these respects (Fig. 38-4).

Differential Diagnosis

The differential diagnosis from a radiologic standpoint has been discussed. From a clinical perspective there is no distinct clinical syndrome produced by trigeminal neurinomas. Careful examination of the motor and sensory components of the trigeminal nerve will ultimately reveal deficits in the majority of patients harboring trigeminal neurinomas, but in about 10 percent of patients, no evidence of trigeminal nerve dysfunction will be found. Additional deficits are related to the location of the tumor. Neurinomas arising in Meckel's cave frequently produce various forms of a parasellar or paratrigeminal (Raeder's) syndrome.[15] Trigeminal neurinomas confined to the posterior fossa generally will produce some form of a cerebellopontine angle syndrome with facial paresis, hearing loss, and occasional long tract and cerebellar signs. Early involvement of the trigeminal nerve tends to distinguish these tumors from acoustic neurinomas, as will the early appearance of hearing loss generally seen with acoustic neurinomas. This distinction, however, may not always be possible since up to 10 percent of patients with acoustic neurinomas initially present with symptoms related to trigeminal nerve dysfunction. Conversely, hearing loss as an initial complaint was seen in 6 percent of patients with trigeminal neurinomas.

Although facial pain may occur early in the clinical course of the patient, its atypical nature is frequently misin-

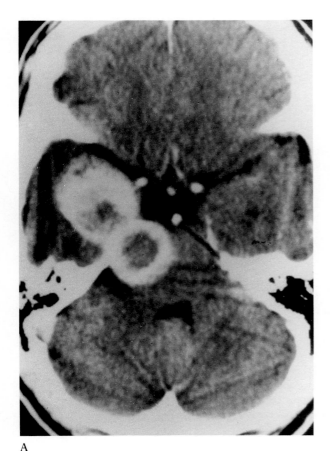

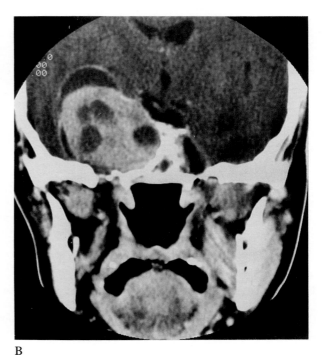

A   B

Figure 38-3 *A.* Contrast-enhanced CT scan of a dumbbell-shaped tumor shows areas of decreased attenuation representing either necrosis or cystic degeneration. *B.* Contrast-enhanced coronal CT scan shows a large inhomogeneous mass in the right middle fossa with marked erosion of the dorsum sellae and upper clivus. Note the marked atrophy of the masseter and pterygoid muscles on the right side.

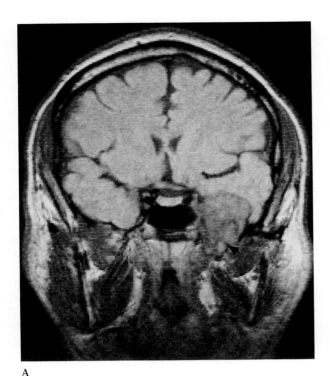

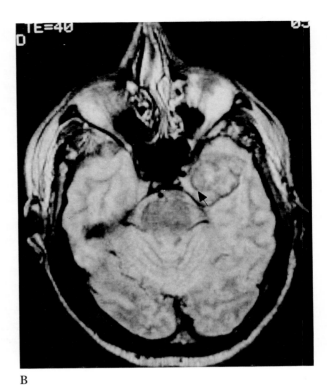

A   B

Figure 38-4 *A*. T1-weighted coronal MR image demonstrates an extra-axial mass eroding through the floor of the middle fossa into the pterygoid fossa (*arrow*). The tumor is inhomogeneous in signal intensity and somewhat hypointense with respect to the surrounding brain. *B*. T1-weighted axial MR image demonstrates the relationship of the tumor to the cavernous sinus. Note the integrity of the dura which clearly demarcates the tumor from the cavernous sinus (*arrow*).

terpreted as being caused by local processes such as tooth, temporomandibular joint, or paranasal sinus pathology. The acceptance that associated sensory deficits may be seen with trigeminal neuralgia further delays diagnosis, despite the fact that these patients respond poorly or not at all to medical treatment with carbamazepine or phenytoin.[2] Isolated paroxysms of facial pain are common, but the absence of trigger zones and the prolonged duration of these paroxysms, frequently lasting 30 min or longer, further differentiate the facial pain caused by tumors from true trigeminal neuralgia. It seems likely that minimal pressure on the trigeminal root or ganglion is capable of producing trigeminal neuralgia. With increasing pressure on either structure, the brief paroxysms of pain may give way to constant facial pain and the appearance of trigeminal nerve sensory deficits.

Surgical Techniques

The surgical approach to these tumors is dependent on their anatomic location. Accurate preoperative delineation of the tumor mass is essential in choosing the most appropriate surgical route. Much of this information can be obtained

during the radiologic evaluation. Thin-section axial CT through the skull base, posterior fossa, and parasellar region, with and without bone windows, is the most useful study because it defines the relationship of the tumor to the skull base, quantifies the degree of bone erosion, and allows an accurate estimation of the size of the tumor in both middle and posterior fossae. Coronal sections, either with CT or MRI, more precisely define the relationship of the tumor to the cavernous sinus and will identify extracranial tumor extension into the pterygoid fossa or paranasal sinuses, which occurs in about 10 percent of patients with trigeminal neurinomas (Fig. 38-4*A*).

Cerebral angiography is routinely performed in the preoperative evaluation of patients with parasellar tumors, both to rule out a petrous, precavernous, or cavernous carotid artery aneurysm, and to define the relationship of the tumor to these segments of the carotid artery. This second point is of particular importance, since there is frequently no intervening bone between the trigeminal ganglion and these segments of the carotid artery.

A subtemporal intradural approach is the preferred route in most cases, because it offers excellent exposure of the middle fossa floor and allows access into the posterior fossa. Alternatively, a predominantly extradural approach may be used, but this necessitates extensive bony removal of the skull base. Lumbar CSF drainage and mannitol are used to assist in temporal lobe retraction.

Access into the posterior fossa is obtained by incising the tentorium and ligating the superior petrosal sinus. The amount of tumor that can be removed from the posterior fossa through the subtemporal exposure depends largely on the degree of brain relaxation and the amount of erosion of the petrous apex. In most cases, significant tumor decompression can be obtained in the posterior fossa when the tumor is located primarily anteriorly in the cerebellopontine angle. Tumor extension ventral to the upper brain stem also may be removed through this exposure. Attempts to remove more caudally placed tumors below the seventh and eighth cranial nerves, especially if the tumor is closely applied to the lateral skull base (Fig. 38-5A) or ventral to the lower brain stem, will usually require an unacceptable amount of temporal lobe retraction. These portions of the tumor are more safely removed through a suboccipital route, performed either as part of a combined transtentorial approach or at a second operation.

Although a reasonable degree of access into the posterior fossa can be obtained via a subtemporal approach, only very limited access to the middle fossa can be obtained through a

suboccipital approach. Thus, the suboccipital approach is appropriate only for those tumors either entirely limited to the posterior fossa or with minimal supratentorial extension (Fig. 38-5B). The sitting or prone position is preferred. Approaching these tumors with the patient's head in a true lateral position creates certain technical difficulties because it rotates the anterior part of the cerebellopontine angle away from the surgeon and forces the surgeon to work against the long axis of the petrous pyramid, which further limits access into the middle fossa.

The combined transtentorial approach is reserved for those patients having posterior fossa tumors, the size or configuration of which prevents removal through a subtemporal approach, in which there is also tumor extension into the middle fossa (Fig. 38-5A). The position of the patient is supine with elevation of the ipsilateral shoulder and the head turned to the opposite side. The lateral sinus is not ligated when this approach is employed for tumor removal. Including the lateral sinus in the tentorial incision is a manuever which essentially allows greater retraction of the brain stem, a situation usually already created by the tumor. However, if there is significant tumor extension ventral to the brain stem then ligation of the lateral sinus may be necessary.

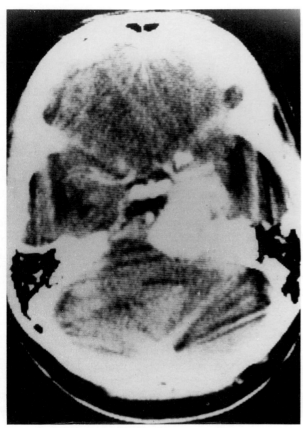

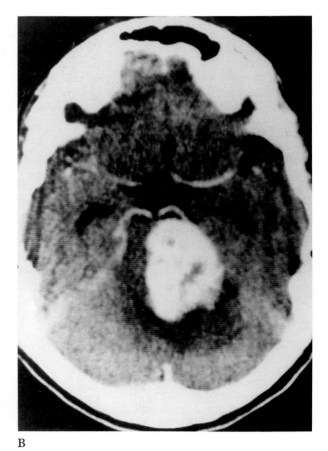

A   B

Figure 38-5 *A.* Axial CT scan demonstrating a dumbbell-shaped tumor. Although the posterior fossa tumor component is not large, its wide-based apposition to the posterior aspect of the petrous pyramid makes it unlikely that this tumor can be removed safely through a subtemporal approach. *B.* Axial CT scan shows a large trigeminal root neurinoma totally confined to the posterior fossa.

The surgical techniques for tumor removal are similar to those employed for acoustic neurinomas. Adequate illumination and magnification with the operative microscope and adherence to microsurgical principles are essential prerequisites for successful removal of these tumors. An initial subcapsular decompression minimizes tumor manipulation and protects the third, fourth, sixth, seventh, and eighth cranial nerves, which are frequently adherent to the tumor capsule. This part of the operation should be performed through a limited opening in the tumor capsule to prevent blood leakage into the subarachnoid space, which obscures the arachnoid planes surrounding the tumor capsule. The carbon dioxide laser and ultrasonic aspirator are useful in debulking the central portions of the tumor. Removal of the tumor capsule should be preceded by gentle dissection of the affected cranial nerves from the surface of the tumor. The altered anatomy of these cranial nerves depends on the size of the tumor. The trochlear nerve usually will be identified on the superior pole of the tumor, whereas the oculomotor nerve is frequently applied to the medial tumor surface. Large posterior fossa tumors will displace the seventh and eighth cranial nerves inferiorly or posteriorly. The abducens nerve may occasionally be exposed if medial extension of the extradural portion of the tumor elevates the dura from the petrous tip.

The obvious goal at operation is complete extirpation. This may not be possible, because the inferomedial portion of the tumor is frequently particularly adherent to the posterolateral wall of the cavernous sinus. Overly aggressive attempts to remove this part of the tumor pose a significant risk of injury to the cavernous sinus, carotid artery, and abducens nerve. A similar situation may exist in the posterior fossa, where part of the tumor capsule may be densely adherent to the brain stem. Rather than risking injury to these structures, the surgeon is probably better advised to accept a near-total removal in these cases. Long-term "tumor-free" intervals generally can be expected even when these portions of the tumor have been left behind.

Postoperative Course

In the immediate postoperative period, the appearance of additional cranial nerve deficits was common but usually transient, resolving in 3 weeks to 4 months. Abnormalities of trigeminal nerve function, either of new onset or worsening of existing defects, were frequently seen and tended to be permanent. Improvement of preoperative deficits was also common. Diplopia resolved in 67 percent of patients, hearing returned to a functional level in 75 percent, and facial weakness improved in 67 percent of patients. Cerebel-

lar and pyramidal tract signs resolved in all patients. Facial pain continued to be a problem in only one patient.

Some degree of trigeminal sensory loss remains in most patients. Weakness in the muscles of mastication is evident in one-third of patients. All of these patients had at least partial resection of the trigeminal root, ganglion, or peripheral divisions at operation. Tarsorrhaphy for corneal ulceration secondary to neurotropic keratitis may be necessary.

CSF shunting may be required for hydrocephalus. CSF leakage and meningitis may be complications.

Reference

1. Arseni C, Dumitrescu L, Constantinescu A. Neurinomas of the trigeminal nerve. *Surg Neurol* 1975; 4:497–503.
2. Bullitt E, Tew JM, Boyd J. Intracranial tumors in patients with facial pain. *J Neurosurg* 1986; 64:865–871.
3. Chase NE, Taveras JM. Carotid angiography in the diagnosis of extradural parasellar tumors. *Acta Radiol (Diagn)* 1963; 1:214–224.
4. De Benedittis G, Bernasconi V, Ettorre G. Tumours of the fifth cranial nerve. *Acta Neurochir (Wien)* 1977; 38:37–64.
5. Gaal A: Zur Röntgendiagnose des Neurinoma trigemini. *Röntgenpraxis* 1935; 7:546–550.
6. Hedeman LS, Lewinsky BS, Lochridge GK, et al. Primary malignant schwannoma of the gasserian ganglion: report of two cases. *J Neurosurg* 1978; 48:279–283.
7. Holman CB, Olive I, Svien HJ. Roentgenologic features of neurofibromas involving the gasserian ganglion. *AJR* 1961; 86:148–153.
8. Jefferson G. The trigeminal neurinomas with some remarks on malignant invasion of the gasserian ganglion. *Clin Neurosurg* 1955; 1:11–54.
9. Krohm G, Marguth F. Zur Sympomatik der Trigeminus-neurinome. *Zentralbl Neurochir* 1964; 25:21–29.
10. Lindgren E: Das Röntgenbild bei Tumoren des Ganglion Gasseri. *Acta Chir Scand* 1941; 85:181–194.
11. McCormick PC, Bello JA, Post KD. Trigeminal schwannoma: surgical series of 14 patients and a review of the literature. *J Neurosurg* 1988; 69:850–860.
12. Mello LR, Tänzer A. Some aspects of trigeminal neurinomas. *Neuroradiology* 1972; 4:215–221.
13. Olive I, Svien HJ. Neurofibromas of the fifth cranial nerve. *J Neurosurg* 1957; 14:484–505.
14. Palacios E, MacGee EE. The radiographic diagnosis of trigeminal neurinomas. *J Neurosurg* 1972; 36:153–156.
15. Raeder JG. "Paratrigeminal" paralysis of the oculo-pupillary sympathetic. *Brain* 1924; 47:149–158.
16. Schisano G, Olivecrona H. Neurinomas of the gasserian ganglion and trigeminal root. *J Neurosurg* 1960; 17:306–322.
17. Tönnis W. Diagnostik der intrakraniellen Geschwülste. In: Olivecrona H, Tönnis W (eds.), *Handbuch der Neurochirurgie*, Vol. 4, Pt. 3. Berlin: Springer-Verlag, 1962: 68–72.
18. Westberg G. Angiographic changes in neurinoma of the trigeminal nerve. *Acta Radiol (Diagn)* 1963; 1:513–520.

39

Microsurgical Anatomy of the Lateral Ventricles

Albert L. Rhoton, Jr.

The lateral ventricles are the site of deeply situated lesions that are commonly dealt with using microoperative techniques. The lateral ventricles also provide deep cavities through which the third ventricle and basal cisterns may be approached. The neural and vascular relationships that provide the bases for optimizing the results obtained with intraventricular operations are reviewed.

Neural Relationships

Each lateral ventricle is a C-shaped cavity situated deep within the cerebrum. The walls of each ventricle are formed predominantly by the thalamus, septum pellucidum, corpus callosum, caudate nucleus, and fornix (Figs. 39-1 through 39-3).[6,11,14]

The thalamus is located in the center of each lateral ventricle. The body of the lateral ventricle is above the thalamus, the atrium and occipital horn are posterior to the thalamus, and the temporal horn is inferolateral to the thalamus.

The caudate nucleus is an arched, C-shaped, cellular mass that wraps around the thalamus and constitutes an important part of the wall of each lateral ventricle. Its head bulges into the lateral wall of the frontal horn and body of the lateral ventricle. Its body forms part of the lateral wall of the atrium, and its tail extends from the atrium into the roof of the temporal horn.

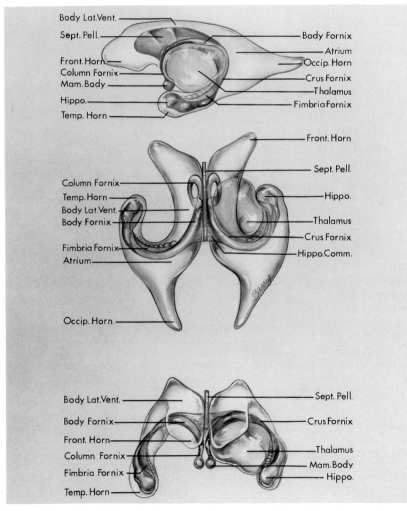

Body Lat.Vent.
Sept. Pell.
Body Fornix
Atrium
Occip. Horn
Front. Horn
Column Fornix
Crus Fornix
Mam. Body
Thalamus
Hippo.
Fimbria Fornix
Temp. Horn

Front. Horn
Sept. Pell.
Column Fornix
Temp. Horn
Hippo.
Body Lat.Vent.
Body Fornix
Thalamus
Crus Fornix
Fimbria Fornix
Hippo. Comm.
Atrium

Occip. Horn

Body Lat.Vent.
Sept. Pell.
Body Fornix
Crus Fornix
Front. Horn
Column Fornix
Thalamus
Fimbria Fornix
Mam. Body
Hippo.
Temp. Horn

A

Figure 39-1 Neural relationships of the lateral ventricles. *A.* Relationship of the septum pellucidum, thalamus, hippocampal formation, and fornix to the lateral ventricles. *Top:* Lateral view; *middle:* Superior view; *bottom:* Anterior view. Each lateral ventricle wraps around the thalamus. The frontal horn (Front. Horn) is anterior to the thalamus; the body (Body Lat. Vent.) is above the thalamus; the atrium and occipital horn (Occip. Horn) are behind the thalamus; and the temporal horn (Temp. Horn) is below and lateral to the thalamus. The septum pellucidum (Sept. Pell.) is in the medial wall of the frontal horn and body. The hippocampal formation (Hippo.) is in the floor of the temporal horn. The fornix, which arises in the hippocampal formation and wraps around the thalamus, is in the medial part of the temporal horn, atrium, and body. The fimbria of the fornix arises on the surface of the hippocampal formation in the temporal horn. The crus of the fornix is posterior to the thalamus in the wall of the atrium. The body of the fornix passes above the thalamus in the lower part of the medial wall of the body. The columns of the fornix are formed at the level of the foramen of Monro and pass inferiorly to the mamillary bodies (Mam. Body). The crura of the fornix are connected across the midline in the roof of the third ventricle by the hippocampal commissure (Hippo.

354

The fornix is another C-shaped structure that wraps around the thalamus in the wall of the ventricle. In the body of the lateral ventricle, the body of the fornix is in the lower part of the medial wall; in the atrium, the crus of the fornix is in the medial part of the anterior wall; and, in the temporal horn, the fimbria of the fornix is in the medial part of the floor. The body of the fornix crosses the thalamus approximately halfway between the medial and lateral edge of the superior surface of the thalamus. The part of the thalamus lateral to the body of the fornix forms the floor of the body of the lateral ventricle, and the part medial to the fornix forms part of the roof of the velum interpositum and third ventricle. The crus of the fornix crosses the pulvinar approximately midway between the medial and lateral edge of the pulvinar. The part of the pulvinar lateral to the crus of the fornix forms part of the anterior wall of the atrium, and the part medial to the fornix forms part of the anterior wall of the quadrigeminal cistern. The fimbria of the fornix passes below the inferolateral part of the thalamus just lateral to the medial and lateral geniculate bodies. The part of the thalamus medial to the fimbria forms the roof of the ambient cistern. The body of the fornix separates into two columns that arch along the superior and anterior margins of the foramen of Monro.

The corpus callosum, which forms the largest part of the ventricular walls, contributes to the wall of each of the five parts of the lateral ventricle. The rostrum of the corpus callosum is situated below and forms the floor of the frontal horn. The bundle of fibers in the genu, called the forceps minor, forms the anterior wall of the frontal horn. The genu and the body of the corpus callosum form the roof of both the frontal horn and the body of the lateral ventricle. The splenium contains a large fiber bundle, the forceps major, which forms a prominence, called the bulb, in the upper part of the medial wall of the atrium. Another fiber tract, the tapetum, which arises in the posterior part of the body and splenium of the corpus callosum, sweeps laterally and inferiorly to form the roof and lateral wall of the atrium and the temporal horns. The tapetum separates the fibers of the optic radiations from the temporal horn.

The septum pellucidum, which is composed of paired laminae, separates the frontal horns and bodies of the lateral ventricles in the midline. There may be a cavity, the cavum septum pellucidum, in the midline between the laminae of the septum pellucidum.

The close relationship of the internal capsule to the lateral wall of the frontal horn and body of the lateral ventricle is often forgotten in planning operative approaches to the

Figure 39-1 Continued

Comm.). *B.* Relationship of the corpus callosum (Corp. Call.), caudate nucleus (Caudate Nucl.), and hippocampal formation to the lateral ventricles. *Top:* View through the medial surface of the hemisphere; *middle:* View through the inferior surface of the hemisphere; *bottom:* View through the anterior surface of the hemisphere. The head and body of the caudate nucleus form the lateral wall of the frontal horn and body of the lateral ventricle. The tail of the caudate nucleus extends into the anterior part of the lateral wall of the atrium and into the medial part of the roof of the temporal horn to the level of the amygdaloid nucleus (Amygd. Nucl.). The corpus callosum is made up of the rostrum, which is in the floor of the frontal horn; the genu, which forms the anterior wall and roof of the frontal horn; the body, which forms the roof of the body of the lateral ventricle; and the splenium, which carries the fibers that form a prominence in the medial wall of the atrium called the bulb of the corpus callosum. The splenium also gives rise to a fiber bundle, called the tapetum, which sweeps downward to form the roof and lateral wall of the atrium and temporal horn. A prominence in the medial wall of the atrium, called the calcar avis, overlies the calcarine sulcus (Calc. Sulc.). (From Timurkaynak et al.[11])

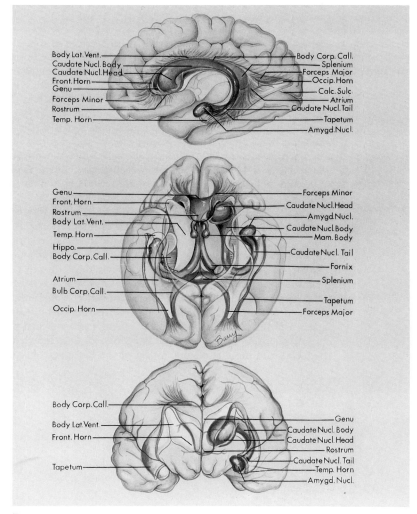

B

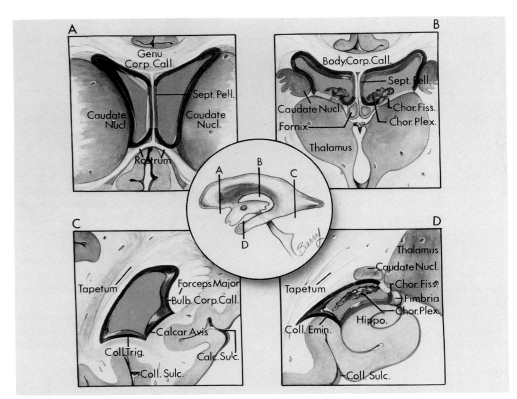

Figure 39-2 Structures in the walls of the lateral ventricles. The central diagram shows the level of the cross sections through the frontal horn (*A*), body (*B*), atrium (*C*), and temporal horn (*D*). *A*. Frontal horn. The genu of the corpus callosum (Corp. Call.) is in the roof, the caudate nucleus (Caudate Nucl.) is in the lateral wall, the rostrum of the corpus callosum is in the floor, and the septum pellucidum (Sept. Pell.) is in the medial wall. *B*. Body of the lateral ventricle. The body of the corpus callosum is in the roof, the caudate nucleus is in the lateral wall, the thalamus is in the floor, and the septum pellucidum and fornix are in the medial wall. The choroidal fissure (Chor. Fiss.), the site of the attachment of the choroid plexus (Chor. Plex.) in the lateral ventricle, is situated between the fornix and the thalamus. *C*. Atrium. The lateral wall and roof are formed by the tapetum of the corpus callosum, and the floor is formed by the collateral trigone (Coll. Trig.), which overlies the collateral sulcus (Coll. Sulc.). The inferior part of the medial wall is formed by the calcar avis, the prominence that overlies the deep end of the calcarine sulcus (Calc. Sulc.), and the superior part of the medial wall is formed by the bulb of the corpus callosum, the prominence that overlies the forceps major. *D*. Temporal horn. The medial part of the floor of the temporal horn is formed by the prominence overlying the hippocampal formation (Hippo.), and the lateral part of the floor is formed by the prominence called the collateral eminence (Coll. Emin.), which overlies the deep end of the collateral sulcus. The roof is formed by the caudate nucleus and the tapetum of the corpus callosum. The lateral wall is formed by the tapetum of the corpus callosum. The medial wall is little more than the cleft between the fimbria of the fornix and the inferolateral aspect of the thalamus. (From Timurkaynak et al.[11])

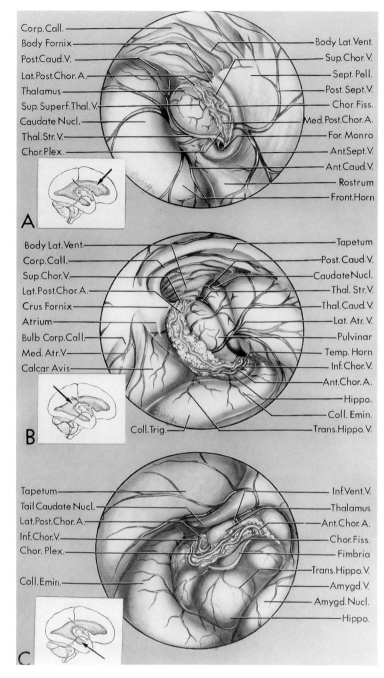

Figure 39-3 Views into the lateral ventricles. *Top:* Anterior view, along the *arrow* in the inset, into the frontal horn (Front. Horn) and body of the lateral ventricle (Body Lat. Vent.). The frontal horn is located anterior to the foramen of Monro (For. Monro) and has the septum pellucidum (Sept. Pell.) in the medial wall, the genu and the body of the corpus callosum (Corp. Call.) in the roof, the caudate nucleus (Caudate Nucl.) in the lateral wall, the genu of the corpus callosum in the anterior wall, and the rostrum of the corpus callosum in the floor. The body of the lateral ventricle has the thalamus in its floor, the caudate nucleus in the lateral wall, the body of the fornix and septum pellucidum in the medial wall, and the corpus callosum in the

roof. The choroid plexus (Chor. Plex.) is attached along the choroidal fissure (Chor. Fiss.), the cleft between the fornix and thalamus. The superior choroidal vein (Sup. Chor. V.) and branches of the lateral (Lat. Post. Chor. A.) and medial posterior choroidal arteries (Med. Post. Chor. A.) course on the surface of the choroidal plexus. The anterior (Ant. Sept. V.) and posterior septal veins (Post. Sept. V.) cross the roof and the medial wall of the frontal horn and body. The anterior (Ant. Caud. V.) and posterior caudate veins (Post. Caud. V.) cross the lateral wall of the frontal horn and body and join the thalamostriate vein (Thal. Str. V.). A superior superficial thalamic vein (Sup. Superf. Thal. V.) courses on the thalamus. *Middle:* Posterior view, along the arrow in the inset, into the atrium. The atrium has the tapetum of the corpus callosum in the roof, the bulb of the corpus callosum and the calcar avis in its medial wall, the collateral trigone (Coll. Trig.) in the floor, the caudate nucleus and tapetum in the lateral wall, and the crus of the fornix, pulvinar, and choroid plexus in the anterior wall. The temporal horn (Temp. Horn) has the hippocampal formation (Hippo.) and collateral eminence (Coll. Emin.) in the floor and the thalamus, tail of the caudate nucleus, and tapetum in the roof and the lateral wall. Branches of the anterior (Ant. Chor. A.) and lateral posterior choroidal arteries course on the surface of the choroid plexus. The thalamocaudate vein (Thal. Caud. V.) drains the part of the lateral wall of the body behind the area drained by the thalamostriate vein. The inferior choroidal vein (Inf. Chor. V.) courses on the choroid plexus in the temporal horn. The lateral (Lat. Atr. V.) and medial atrial veins (Med. Atr. V.) cross the medial and lateral walls of the atrium and temporal horn. Transverse hippocampal veins (Trans. Hippo. V.) cross the floor of the atrium and temporal horn. *Bottom:* Anterior view along the arrow in the inset, into the temporal horn. The floor of the temporal horn is formed by the collateral eminence and the hippocampal formation. The roof and lateral wall, from medial to lateral, are formed by the thalamus, the tail of the caudate nucleus, and the tapetum of the corpus callosum. The medial wall is little more than the cleft between the thalamus and the fimbria, called the choroidal fissure, along which the choroid plexus is attached. The amygdaloid nucleus (Amygd. Nucl.) bulges into the anteromedial part of the temporal horn. The fimbria of the fornix arises on the surface of the hippocampal formation. Branches of the anterior and lateral posterior choroidal arteries course on the surface of the choroid plexus. The inferior ventricular vein (Inf. Vent. V.) drains the roof of the temporal horn and receives the amygdalar vein (Amygd. V.). The inferior choroidal vein joins the inferior ventricular vein. The transverse hippocampal veins drain the floor of the temporal horn. (From Timurkaynak et al.[11])

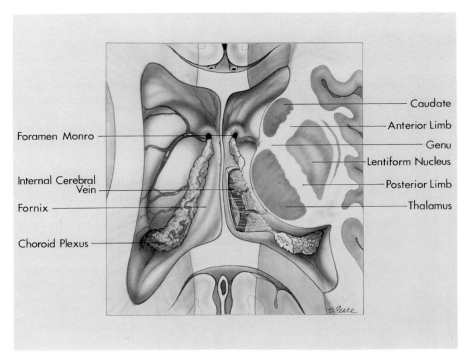

Foramen Monro

Internal Cerebral
Vein

Fornix

Choroid Plexus

Caudate

Anterior Limb

Genu

Lentiform Nucleus

Posterior Limb

Thalamus

Figure 39-4 Relationship of the internal capsule to the right lateral ventricle. The anterior limb of the internal capsule is separated from the lateral ventricle by the caudate nucleus, and the posterior limb is separated from the ventricle by the thalamus. The genu comes directly to the ventricular surface in the area lateral to the foramen of Monro in the interval between the caudate nucleus and thalamus. The right half of the body of the fornix has been removed to expose the internal cerebral veins in the roof of the third ventricle.

ventricles. The anterior limb of the internal capsule, which is located between the caudate and lentiform nuclei, is separated from the frontal horn by the head of the caudate nucleus, and the posterior limb, which is situated between the thalamus and the lentiform nucleus, is separated from the body of the lateral ventricle by the thalamus and body of the caudate nucleus. However, the genu of the internal capsule comes directly to the ventricular surface and touches the wall of the lateral ventricle immediately lateral to the foramen of Monro in the interval between the caudate nucleus and the thalamus (Fig. 39-4).

Ventricular Walls

Frontal Horn

The frontal horn, the part of the lateral ventricle located anterior to the foramen of Monro, has a medial wall formed by the septum pellucidum, an anterior wall formed by the genu of the corpus callosum, a lateral wall composed of the head of the caudate nucleus, and a narrow floor formed by the rostrum of the corpus callosum (Figs. 39-2 and 39-3). The columns of the fornix, as they pass anterior and superior to the foramen of Monro, are in the posteroinferior part of the medial wall.

Body

The body of the lateral ventricle extends from the posterior edge of the foramen of Monro to the point where the septum

pellucidum disappears and the corpus callosum and fornix meet (Figs. 39-2 and 39-3). The roof is formed by the body of the corpus callosum, the medial wall by the septum pellucidum above and the body of the fornix below, the lateral wall by the body of the caudate nucleus, and the floor by the thalamus. The caudate nucleus and thalamus are separated by the striothalamic sulcus, the groove in which the stria terminalis and the thalamostriate vein course.

Atrium and Occipital Horn

The atrium and occipital horn together form a roughly triangular cavity, with the apex posteriorly in the occipital lobe and the base anteriorly on the pulvinar (Figs. 39-2 and 39-3). The roof of the atrium is formed by the body, splenium, and tapetum of the corpus callosum. The medial wall is formed by two horizontal prominences that are located one above the other. The upper prominence, called the bulb of the corpus callosum, overlies and is formed by the large bundle of fibers called the forceps major, and the lower prominence, called the calcar avis, overlies the deepest part of the calcarine sulcus. The lateral wall has an anterior part, formed by the caudate nucleus, and a posterior part, formed by the fibers of the tapetum. The anterior wall has a medial part, composed of the crus of the fornix, and a lateral part, formed by the pulvinar of the thalamus. The floor is formed by the collateral trigone, a triangular area that bulges upward over the posterior end of the collateral sulcus.

The occipital horn extends posteriorly into the occipital lobe from the atrium. It varies in size from being absent to extending far posteriorly in the occipital lobe, and it may vary in size from side to side. Its medial wall is formed by the bulb of the corpus callosum and the calcar avis, the roof and lateral wall are formed by the tapetum, and the floor is formed by the collateral trigone.

Temporal Horn

The temporal horn extends forward from the atrium below the pulvinar into the medial part of the temporal lobe and ends blindly in an anterior wall that is situated immediately behind the amygdaloid nucleus (Figs. 39-2 and 39-3). The floor of the temporal horn is formed medially by the hippocampus, the smooth prominence overlying the hippocampal formation, and laterally by the collateral eminence, the prominence overlying the collateral sulcus which separates the parahippocampal and occipitotemporal gyri on the inferior surface of the temporal lobe. The roof is formed medially by the inferior surface of the thalamus and the tail of the caudate nucleus, and laterally by the tapetum of the corpus callosum. The medial wall is little more than a narrow cleft, the choroidal fissure, situated between the inferolateral part of the thalamus and the fimbria of the fornix.

Choroid Plexus and Choroidal Fissure

The choroid plexus in the lateral ventricle has a C-shaped configuration that parallels the fornix (Figs. 39-1 to 39-3).[4,11] It is attached along the choroidal fissure, the narrow C-shaped cleft that is situated between the fornix and the thalamus. The choroid plexus from each lateral ventricle extends through the foramen of Monro and is continuous with the two parallel strands of choroid plexus in the roof of the third ventricle. In the atrium, the choroid plexus forms a prominent triangular tuft called the glomus. The edges of the thalamus and fornix bordering the choroidal fissure have small ridges, called the teniae, that anchor the choroid plexus to the fornix and thalamus. The tenia on the thalamic side is called the tenia choroidea. The tenia on the fornical side of the fissure is called the tenia fornicis except in the temporal horn, where it is referred to as the tenia fimbriae.

The choroidal fissure extends in a C-shaped arc from the foramen of Monro through the body, atrium, and temporal horn to its inferior termination, called the inferior choroidal point, which is located just behind the uncus and amygdaloid nucleus and just lateral to the lateral geniculate body.[6] The choroidal fissure is divided into body and atrial and temporal parts. The body portion of the choroidal fissure is situated in the body of the lateral ventricle between the body of the fornix and the thalamus. The velum interpositum through which the internal cerebral veins course is located on the medial side of the body portion of the fissure in the roof of the third ventricle. Opening through the choroidal fissure from the body of the ventricle will expose the velum interpositum and the roof of the third ventricle. The atrial part is located in the atrium of the lateral ventricle between the crus of the fornix and the pulvinar. Opening through the fissure from the atrium exposes the quadrigeminal cistern, the pineal region, and the posterior portion of the ambient cistern. The temporal part is situated in the temporal horn between the fimbria of the fornix and the inferolateral surface of the thalamus. Opening through the choroidal fissure from the temporal horn exposes the structures in the ambient and posterior part of the crural cisterns. The fissure is the thinnest site in the wall of the lateral ventricle bordering the basal cisterns and the roof of the third ventricle.

Velum Interpositum

The velum interpositum is located in the roof of the third ventricle below the body of the fornix and between the superomedial surfaces of the thalami (Fig. 39-5).[8] The upper and lower walls of the velum interpositum are formed by the two membranous layers of tela choroidea in the roof of the third ventricle. The upper wall is formed by the layer that is attached to the lower surface of the fornix and the hippocampal commissure. The anterior part of the lower wall is attached to the small ridges on the free edge of the striae medullaris thalami. The posterior part of the lower wall is attached to the superior surface of the pineal body. The internal cerebral veins arise in the anterior part of the velum interpositum just behind the foramen of Monro, and they exit the velum interpositum above the pineal body to enter the quadrigeminal cistern, where they join the great vein.

Tentorial and Cisternal Relationships

The lateral ventricles are situated above the tentorial incisura, the triangular space situated between the free edges of the tentorium and the dorsum sellae (Fig. 39-6). The midbrain is situated in the center of the incisura. The area between the midbrain and the free edges is divided into (1) an anterior incisural space located in front of the brain stem, (2) paired middle incisural spaces situated lateral to the midbrain, and (3) a posterior incisural space located behind the midbrain. The frontal horns are located above the anterior incisural space; the bodies of the lateral ventricles are located directly above the central part of the incisura, where they sit on and are separated from the central part of the incisura by the thalamus; the atria are located above the posterior incisural space; and the temporal horns are situated superolateral to the middle incisural space. The three incisural spaces contain some of the basal cisterns and are so intimately related to the lateral ventricles that some operative approaches to the basal cisterns situated within the incisura are directed through the lateral ventricles.

The anterior incisural space, which is situated anterior to the midbrain, extends obliquely upward around the optic chiasm to the area below the frontal horn. It contains the interpeduncular and chiasmatic cisterns and the cisterna lamina terminalis. The middle incisural space is located between the temporal lobe and the midbrain. It contains the crural cistern, which is located between the cerebral peduncle and the uncus, and the ambient cistern, which is situated between the midbrain and the parahippocampal and dentate gyri. The ambient cistern opens laterally through the cho-

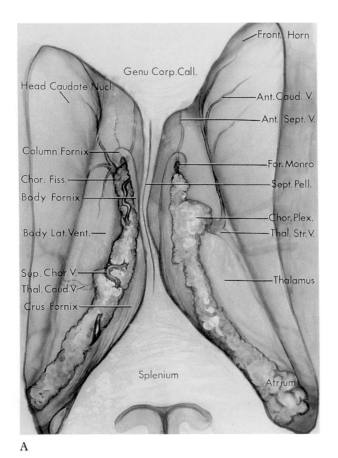

A

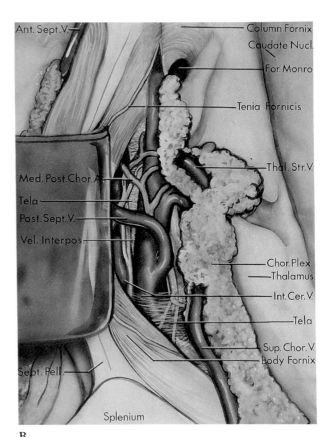

B

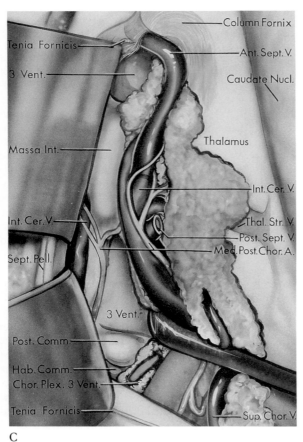

C

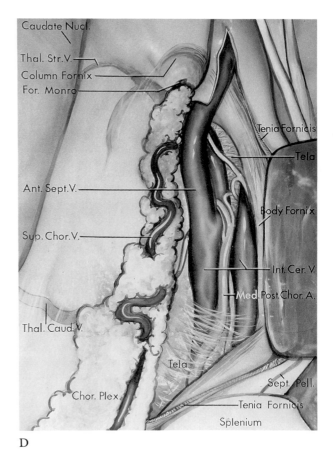

D

Figure 39-5

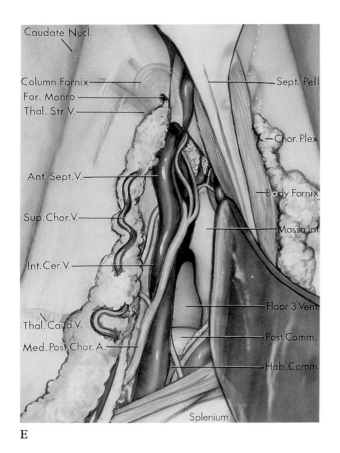

E

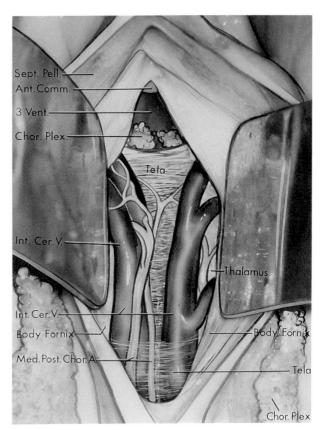

F

Figure 39-5 Comparison of left and right transchoroidal and transfornical routes to the third ventricle. *A.* The superior part of the cerebral hemispheres have been removed to expose the frontal horns (Front. Horn), bodies (Body Lat. Vent.), and atria of the lateral ventricles. The choroid plexus (Chor. Plex.) is attached along the choroidal fissures (Chor. Fiss.). The structures forming the walls of the lateral ventricle include the corpus callosum (Corp. Call.), fornix, thalamus, septum pellucidum (Sept. Pell.), and caudate nucleus (Caudate Nucl.). The anterior septal (Ant. Sept. V.), anterior caudate (Ant. Caud. V.), and superior choroidal veins (Sup. Chor. V.) join the thalamostriate veins (Thal. Str. V.) near the foramen of Monro (For. Monro). A thalamocaudate vein (Thal. Caud. V.) crosses the walls of the left lateral ventricle. *B.* Right transchoroidal approach to the third ventricle. The right choroidal fissure has been opened by incising along the tenia fornicis. The fornix has been retracted to the left in order to expose the paired internal cerebral veins (Int. Cer. V.), which course through the velum interpositum (Vel. Interpos.). The anterior septal, thalamostriate, superior choroidal, and posterior septal veins (Post. Sept. V.) empty into the right internal cerebral vein. The medial posterior chorodial arteries (Med. Post. Chor. A.) course in the velum interpositum with the internal cerebral veins. A layer of tela choroidea is located above and below the internal cerebral veins. *C.* The lower layer of tela choroidea has been opened to expose the third ventricle (3 Vent.), massa intermedia (Massa Int.), habenular (Hab. Comm.) and posterior commissures (Post. Comm.) and choroid plexus in the third ventricle (Chor. Plex 3 Vent.). *D.* Left transchoroidal approach to the third ventricle in the same speciman. The left choroidal fissure has been opened by incising along the tenia fornices, and the fornix has been retracted toward the left side. *E.* The internal cerebral veins have been separated, and the lower layer of the tela choroidea has been opened to expose the third ventricle. *F.* Transfornical approach to the third ventricle in the same specimen. The velum interpositum has been opened by incising the body of the fornix in the midline along the direction of its fibers. The upper layer of tela choroidea has been opened to expose the internal cerebral veins and the medial posterior chorodial arteries in the velum interpositum. The anterior commissure (Ant. Comm.) is exposed in the anterior part of the third ventricle. *G.* The lower layer of tela choroidea has been opened to expose the interior of the third ventricle. (From Nagata et al.[6])

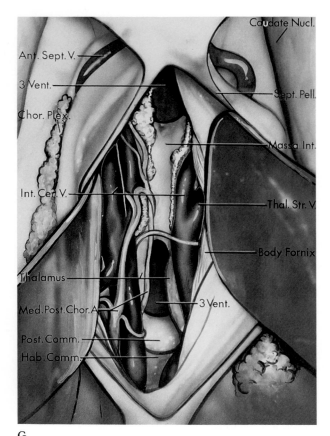

G

Figure 39-5   Continued

roidal fissure into the temporal horn. The posterior incisural space lies below the atria of the lateral ventricles and contains the quadrigeminal cistern. The atrium is separated from the quadrigeminal cistern by the crus of the fornix and the cortical gyri located below the splenium.

Figure 39-6   Superior view showing the relationship of the lateral ventricles to the tentorial incisura. The tentorial incisura surrounds the midbrain and is divided into the anterior (Ant.), middle (Mid.), and posterior (Post.) incisural spaces. The anterior incisural space lies between the dorsum sellae and the cerebral peduncles and extends forward above the diaphragma sellae and around the optic chiasm to the subcallosal area. The paired middle incisural spaces are situated between the lateral surface of the brain stem and the tentorial incisura and approximate the area of the crural and ambient cisterns. The posterior incisural space lies posterior to the midbrain and corresponds to the quadrigeminal cistern and pineal region. The frontal horns (Front. Horn) are situated above the anterior incisural space. The bodies of the lateral ventricles (Body Lat. Vent.) are situated above the thalami and the central part of the incisura. The atria and occipital horn (Occip. Horn) are situated above the posterior incisural space in the area lateral to the pineal body. The temporal horn (Temp. Horn) sits above the medial edge of the tentorium and opens through the choroidal fissure into the middle incisural space. (From Timurkaynak et al.[11])

Arterial Relationships

Each part of the lateral ventricle has surgically important arterial relationships: all of the arterial components of the circle of Willis are located below the frontal horns and bodies of the lateral ventricles; the internal carotid arteries bifurcate into the anterior and middle cerebral arteries in the area below the frontal horns and give rise to the anterior choroidal arteries, which send branches through the choroidal fissures to the choroid plexus; the posterior part of the circle of Willis and the apex of the basilar artery are situated below the thalami and bodies of the lateral ventricles; the anterior cerebral arteries pass around the floor and anterior wall of the frontal horns to reach the roof of the frontal horns and bodies; and the posterior cerebral arteries pass medial to the temporal horns and atria in the ambient and quadrigeminal cisterns and give rise to the posterior choroidal arteries, which supply the choroid plexus in the temporal horns, atria, and bodies (Fig. 39-7).[4,6]

The arteries most intimately related to the lateral ventricles and choroidal fissures are the choroidal arteries which supply the choroid plexus in the lateral and third ventricles. They arise from the internal carotid and posterior cerebral arteries in the basal cisterns and reach the choroid plexus by passing through the choroidal fissures. The most common pattern is for the anterior choroidal artery to supply a portion of the choroid plexus in the temporal horn and atrium; the lateral posterior choroidal arteries to supply a portion of the choroid plexus in the atrium, body, and posterior part of the temporal horn; and the medial posterior choroidal arteries to supply the choroid plexus in the roof of the third ventricle and part of that in the body of the lateral ventricle.

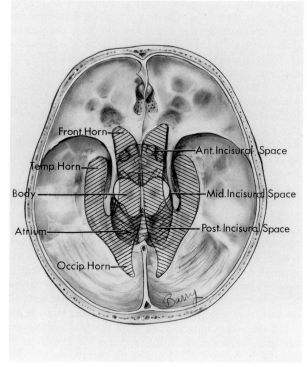

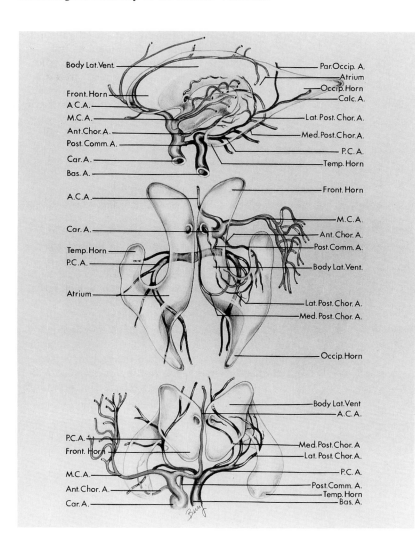

Figure 39-7 Arterial relationships of the lateral ventricles. Lateral (*top*), superior (*middle*), and anterior (*lower*) views. The carotid artery (Car. A.) bifurcates into the anterior (A.C.A.) and middle cerebral branches (M.C.A.) in the area below the posterior part of the frontal horn (Front. Horn). The origins of the middle cerebral arteries are situated below the frontal horns. The anterior cerebral arteries pass anteromedial below the frontal horns and give rise to the pericallosal and callosomarginal branches which curve around the anterior wall and roof of the frontal horn. The anterior choroidal arteries (Ant. Chor. A.) enter the choroid plexus in the anterior part of the temporal horns (Temp. Horn.). The posterior communicating arteries (Post. Comm. A.) are situated below the thalami and bodies of the lateral ventricles (Body Lat. Vent). The basilar artery (Bas. A.) bifurcates below the bodies of the lateral ventricles into the posterior cerebral arteries (P.C.A.), which course below the thalami and near the medial aspect of the temporal horns and atria. The medial posterior choroidal arteries (Med. Post. Chor. A.) arise from the proximal part of the posterior cerebral arteries and encircle the brain stem below the thalami and pass forward in the roof of the third ventricle, where they give branches to the choroid plexus in the roof of the third ventricle and the body of the lateral ventricle. The lateral posterior choroidal branches (Lat. Post. Chor. A.) of the posterior cerebral arteries pass laterally through the choroidal fissures to enter the temporal horns and atria. The middle cerebral arteries course on the insulae in the area above the temporal horns and lateral to the bodies of the lateral ventricles. The posterior cerebral arteries bifurcate into the calcarine (Calc. A.) and parieto-occipital (Par. Occip. A.) in the area medial to the atria and occipital horns (Occip. Horn). (From Timurkaynak et al.[11])

The anterior choroidal artery arises from the internal carotid artery, courses between the cerebral peduncle and uncus and below the optic tract, passes through the choroidal fissure near the inferior choroidal point, and courses along the medial border of the choroid plexus in the temporal horn.

The lateral posterior choroidal arteries are the one to six branches that arise in the ambient and quadrigeminal cisterns from the posterior cerebral artery. They pass laterally around the pulvinar and through the choroidal fissure to reach the choroid plexus in the temporal horn, atrium, and body.

The medial posterior choroidal arteries arise as one to three branches from the proximal part of the posterior cerebral artery in the interpeduncular and crural cisterns, encircle the midbrain medial to the main trunk of the posterior cerebral artery, turn forward at the side of the pineal gland to enter the roof of the third ventricle, and course in the velum interpositum adjacent to the internal cerebral veins. They supply the choroid plexus in the roof of the third ventricle and sometimes pass through the foramen of Monro or choroidal fissures to supply the choroid plexus in the lateral ventricles.

Venous Relationships

The deep venous system of the brain collects into channels that course in a subependymal location through the walls of the lateral ventricles and pass through the margins of the choroidal fissure to reach the internal cerebral, basal, and great veins (Fig. 39-8).[7] In general, the veins draining the frontal horn and body of the lateral ventricle drain into the internal cerebral vein as it courses through the velum inter-

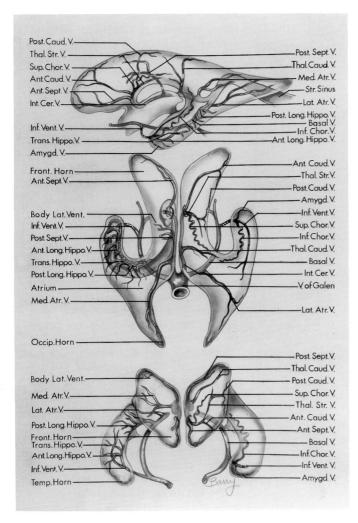

Post. Caud. V.
Thal. Str. V.
Sup. Chor. V.
Ant. Caud. V.
Ant. Sept. V.
Int. Cer. V.
Inf. Vent. V.
Trans. Hippo. V.
Amygd. V.
Front. Horn
Ant. Sept. V.
Body Lat. Vent.
Inf. Vent. V.
Post. Sept. V.
Ant. Long. Hippo. V.
Trans. Hippo. V.
Post. Long. Hippo. V.
Atrium
Med. Atr. V.
Occip. Horn
Body Lat. Vent.
Med. Atr. V.
Lat. Atr. V.
Post. Long. Hippo. V.
Front. Horn
Trans. Hippo. V.
Ant. Long. Hippo. V.
Inf. Vent. V.
Temp. Horn

Post. Sept. V.
Thal. Caud. V.
Med. Atr. V.
Str. Sinus
Lat. Atr. V.
Post. Long. Hippo. V.
Basal V.
Inf. Chor. V.
Ant. Long. Hippo. V.
Ant. Caud. V.
Thal. Str. V.
Post. Caud. V.
Amygd. V.
Inf. Vent. V.
Sup. Chor. V.
Inf. Chor. V.
Thal. Caud. V.
Basal V.
Int. Cer. V.
V of Galen
Lat. Atr. V.
Post. Sept. V.
Thal. Caud. V.
Post. Caud. V.
Sup. Chor. V.
Thal. Str. V.
Ant. Caud. V.
Ant. Sept. V.
Basal V.
Inf. Chor. V.
Inf. Vent. V.
Amygd. V.

Figure 39-8 Venous relationships of the lateral ventricles. Lateral *(top)*, superior *(middle)*, and anterior *(lower)* views. The ventricular veins are divided into medial and lateral groups. The ventricular veins drain into the internal cerebral (Int. Cer. V.), basal (Basal V.), and great veins (V. Galen). The lateral group consists of the anterior caudate vein (Ant. Caud. V.) in the frontal horn (Front. Horn); the thalamostriate (Thal. Str. V.), posterior caudate (Post. Caud. V.), and thalamocaudate veins (Thal. Caud. V.) in the body (Body Lat. Vent.); the lateral atrial veins (Lat. Atr. V.) in the atrium and occipital horn (Occip. Horn); and the inferior ventricular (Inf. Vent. V.) and amygdalar veins (Amygd. V.) in the temporal horn (Temp. Horn). The medial group is formed by the anterior septal vein (Ant. Sept. V.) in the frontal horn, the posterior septal veins (Post. Sept. V.) in the body, the medial atrial veins (Med. Atr. V.) in the atrium, and the transverse hippocampal veins (Trans. Hippo. V.) in the temporal horn. The transverse hippocampal veins drain into the anterior (Ant. Long. Hippo. V.) and posterior longitudinal hippocampal veins (Post. Long. Hippo. V.). The superior choroidal veins (Sup. Chor. V.) drain into the thalamostriate and internal cerebral veins, and the inferior choroidal vein (Inf. Chor. V.) drains into the inferior ventricular vein. The great vein drains into the straight sinus (Str. Sinus). (From Timurkaynak et al.[11])

positum; those draining the temporal horn drain into the segment of the basal vein coursing through the ambient cistern; and the veins from the atrium drain into the segments of the basal, internal cerebral, and great veins coursing through the quadrigeminal cistern.

The ventricular veins are divided into medial and lateral groups based on whether they course through the thalamic or fornical side of the choroidal fissure: the lateral group passes through the thalamic or inner side of the fissure, and the medial group passes through the outer or fornical circumference of the fissure. The veins constituting the medial and lateral groups frequently join near the choroidal fissure to form a common stem before terminating.

The medial group of veins in the frontal horn and body is formed by the anterior and posterior septal veins, and the lateral group consists of the thalamostriate, thalamocaudate, and anterior and posterior caudate veins. The veins of the lateral group are larger than those of the medial group. The veins in the lateral group penetrate the tenia choroidea to reach the velum interpositum.

The anterior septal veins course in the frontal horn on the septum pellucidum and the posterior septal veins course on the septum pellucidum in the body. They terminate by joining the internal cerebral vein. The anterior caudate veins course on the lateral wall of the frontal horn and terminate in

the thalamostriate vein. The posterior caudate veins cross the lateral wall of the body and terminate in the thalamostriate or thalamocaudate veins.

The thalamostriate vein passes forward in the sulcus between the caudate nucleus and thalamus toward the foramen of Monro, where it turns sharply posterior through the posterior margin of the foramen of Monro and enters the velum interpositum to join the internal cerebral vein. The angle formed by the junction of the thalamostriate and internal cerebral veins, called the venous angle, as seen on the lateral view of the cerebral angiogram, approximates the site of the foramen of Monro. In some cases, this venous angle will not approximate the site of the foramen of Monro because the thalamostriate vein passes through the choroidal fissure well behind the foramen of Monro. If the thalamostriate vein is small or absent, the thalamocaudate vein will drain the same area. The thalamocaudate vein courses medially across the caudate nucleus and thalamus behind the posterior extent of the thalamostriate vein and ends in the internal cerebral vein.

The medial group of veins in the atrium and occipital horn consists of the medial atrial veins, and the lateral group is composed of the lateral atrial veins. The medial atrial veins course forward on the medial wall of the atrium and pass through the margin of the choroidal fissure to terminate within the velum interpositum or quadrigeminal cistern by joining the internal cerebral, basal, or great vein. The lateral atrial veins course forward on the lateral wall of the atrium, turn medially on the pulvinar, and pass through the choroidal fissure to reach the quadrigeminal cistern, where they join the internal cerebral, basal, or great vein.

The lateral group in the temporal horn is formed by the inferior ventricular and amygdalar veins, and the medial group is formed by the transverse hippocampal veins. The inferior ventricular vein crosses the roof of the temporal horn and exits the temporal horn just behind the inferior choroidal point to join the basal vein. The amygdalar vein courses across the ventricular surface of the amygdaloid nucleus and terminates in the inferior ventricular or basal vein. The transverse hippocampal veins are a group of very fine veins that course medially across the hippocampal formation and collateral eminence and join tributaries of the basal vein.

The superior and inferior choroidal veins are the largest veins on the choroid plexus. The superior choroidal vein runs forward on the choroid plexus in the body of the lateral ventricle and terminates near the foramen of Monro in the internal cerebral vein or its tributaries. The inferior choroidal vein courses anteriorly in the temporal horn along the inferior end of the choroid plexus and terminates by passing through the choroidal fissure near the inferior choroidal point to terminate in the basal vein or its tributaries. The superior and inferior choroidal veins frequently anastomose on the choroid plexus in the atrium.

The venous relationships in the quadrigeminal cistern medial to the atria are the most complex in the cranium because the internal cerebral, basal, and great veins and many of their tributaries converge on this area. The union of the paired internal cerebral veins to form the great vein may be located above or posterior to the pineal body and inferior or posterior to the splenium. The basal vein is formed on the anterior perforated substance below the frontal horn, proceeds posteriorly between the midbrain and temporal lobe to drain the walls of the crural and ambient cisterns, and terminates within the quadrigeminal cistern by joining the internal cerebral or great vein. The great vein passes below the splenium to enter the straight sinus at the tentorial apex.

Operative Considerations

The selection of the best operative approach to a lesion in the lateral ventricles will be determined by the site of the lesion, the size of the lateral ventricles, and the relationship of the lesion to the third ventricle and basal cisterns (Fig. 39-9). This section reviews some general principles applicable to all of the operative approaches to the lateral ventricles.

Neural Incisions

It is impossible to reach the lateral ventricles without opening some neural structures. The surgical approaches to the lateral ventricle may require cortical incisions in the frontal, parietal, or temporal lobes and the anterior or posterior part of the corpus callosum, division or displacement of the fornix, and opening of the choroidal fissure and septum pellu-

cidum. The brain may be retracted to expose an external wall of the ventricle such as the corpus callosum, but then the wall must be incised to reach the ventricle. After reaching the lateral ventricles, another neural incision through a site such as the fornix or opening of the choroidal fissure is needed to expose those lesions which extend into the third ventricle or the basal cisterns.

In opening the choroidal fissure, it is better to open through the tenia fornicis and tenia fimbriae than through the tenia choroidea, because fewer arteries and veins pass through the teniae fimbriae and fornicis than through the tenia choroidea.[6] Opening through the choroidal fissure in the body of the ventricle will expose the velum interpositum and the roof of the third ventricle, opening through it in the atrium will expose the quadrigeminal cistern and the pineal region, and opening through it in the temporal horn will expose the crural and ambient cisterns.

The incision and retraction of neural structures in order to reach the lateral ventricles produce variable results: in some cases there has been no deficit, and in others the deficit has been transient or permanent or has resulted in the loss of life.[3,12,15] Structures sacrificed with variable results include the anterior and posterior parts of the corpus callosum and various parts of the fornix. Callosal incisions have resulted in disorders of the interhemispheric transfer of information, visuospatial transfer, the learning of bimanual motor tasks, and memory, and also in deficits including alexia, apraxia, and astereognosis. The cerebral retraction needed for the anterior and posterior transcallosal approaches and the cortical incisions for the transcortical approaches have caused convulsions, hemiplegia, mutism, impairment of consciousness, and visual field loss. Manipulation of lesions extending into the walls of the third ventricle may cause hypothalamic dysfunction as manifested by disturbances of temperature control, respiration, consciousness, and hypophyseal secretion; visual loss due to damage of the optic chiasm and tracts; and memory loss due to injury to the body and columns of the fornix. Dissection medial to the atrium in the area of the quadrigeminal plate may cause disorders of eye movement, edematous closure of the aqueduct of Sylvius, blindness from edema in the colliculi or geniculate bodies, and extraocular palsies due to edema of the nuclei of the nerves or the central pathways in the brain stem.

Opening the choroidal fissure carries the risk of damaging the fornix. However, unilateral damage to the fornix produces no deficit, and damage to the forniceal fibers from both hemispheres does not usually produce a permanent memory loss.[1,8–10] This is evidence that lesions in the crus and hippocampal commissure have a more deleterious effect on memory than lesions in the body or columns.[5] Opening the temporal part of the choroidal fissure risks damaging the fimbria and hippocampal formation. However, unilateral damage of the hippocampal formation produces no deficit.[13,15]

Arterial Considerations

Intraventricular tumors and arteriovenous malformations are commonly supplied by the choroidal arteries. The fact that the choroidal arteries converge on and pass through the choroidal fissure assists in identifying this fissure. Opening

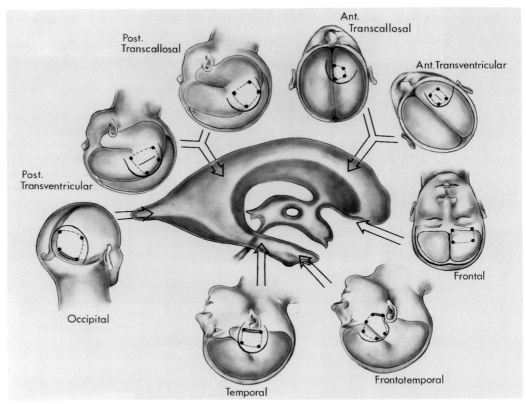

Figure 39-9 Surgical approaches to the lateral ventricles. The site of the skin incision (*solid line*) and the bone flap (*interrupted line*) are shown for each approach. The anterior part of the lateral ventricle may be reached by the anterior transcallosal, anterior transcortical, and frontal approaches. The posterior routes to the lateral ventricle are the posterior transcallosal, posterior transcortical, and occipital approaches. The inferior part of the lateral ventricle is reached using the frontotemporal and temporal approaches. (From Timurkaynak et al.[11])

through the fissure in the body of the ventricle will expose the medial posterior choroidal arteries in the velum interpositum and the roof of the third ventricle, opening through the fissure in the atrium will expose the medial and lateral posterior choroidal arteries in the quadrigeminal cistern and the pineal region, and opening through it in the temporal horn will expose the anterior and medial and lateral posterior choroidal arteries in the ambient cistern.

Other arteries which may also be exposed in removing tumors of the lateral ventricle are the anterior cerebral and anterior communicating arteries in the region of the frontal horns and bodies; the posterior part of the circle of Willis, the apex of the basilar artery, and the proximal part of the posterior cerebral arteries in the area medial to the temporal horns; the distal part of the posterior cerebral arteries in the area medial to the atria; and branches of both the anterior and the posterior cerebral arteries into the roof of the bodies and atria. Extreme effort should be made to avoid sacrificing any of these arteries. Occlusion of the perforating branches of these arteries at the anterior part of the circle of Willis is likely to result in disturbances of memory and personality, and occlusion of those at the posterior part of the circle of

Willis is more likely to result in disorders of the level of consciousness.

Venous Considerations

The ventricular veins provide valuable landmarks in directing one to the foramen of Monro and choroidal fissure during operations on the ventricles. This is especially true if hydrocephalus, as commonly occurs with ventricular tumors, is present, because the borders between the neural structures in the ventricular walls become less distinct as the ventricles dilate.

The number of veins sacrificed in approaching a ventricular lesion should be kept to a minimum because of the undesirable consequences of their loss. Obliteration of the deep veins, including the great, basal, and internal cerebral veins and their tributaries, and the bridging veins from the cerebrum to the dural sinuses is inescapable in reaching and removing some tumors in or near the ventricles. Before sacrificing these veins, one should try placing them under moderate or even severe stretch (accepting the fact that they may be torn) if it will allow satisfactory exposure and yield some possibility of the veins being saved. Before sacrificing the basal, internal cerebral, and great veins, try working around them or displacing them out of the operative route, or try dividing only a few of their small branches, which may allow the displacment of the main trunk out of the operative field.

Sacrifice of branches of the superficial and deep venous systems has produced inconstant deficits.[2,8] Dandy noted that one internal cerebral vein may be sacrificed without effect, and on a few occasions both veins and even the great vein of Galen had been ligated with recovery without any apparent disturbance of function.[3] On the other hand, it seems that injury to this venous network may cause diencephalic edema, mental symptoms, coma, hyperpyrexia, tachycardia, tachypnea, miosis, rigidity of limbs, and exaggeration of deep tendon reflexes. Occlusion of the thalamostriate and other veins at the foramen of Monro may cause drowsiness, hemiplegia, mutism, and hemorrhagic infarction of the basal ganglia. Obliteration of veins coursing between the cerebrum and the superior sagittal sinus anterior or posterior to the rolandic vein, as may be required in the transcallosal approaches, although usually not causing a deficit, may be accompanied by hemiplegia. Sacrificing the internal occipital vein or the bridging veins from the occipital pole to the superior sagittal or transverse sinuses may cause hemianopsia.

Selection of Approach

The routes to the lateral ventricles are divided into anterior, posterior, and inferior approaches (Fig. 39-9). The anterior approaches are directed to the frontal horn and body of the lateral ventricle. The posterior approaches are directed to the atrium, and the inferior approaches are directed to the temporal horn.

Lesions within the anterior portion of the lateral ventricle are most commonly reached by the anterior transcallosal and anterior transcortical approaches. This anterior transcallosal approach is suitable for lesions in the frontal horn and body of the lateral ventricle and for reaching the anterosuperior part of the third ventricle through the lateral ventricle. The transcallosal approach is easier to perform than the transcortical approach if the ventricles are of a normal size or are minimally enlarged. This anterior transcortical approach is suitable for reaching tumors in the anterior part of the lateral ventricle and the anterosuperior part of the third ventricle, especially if the tumor is situated predominantly in the lateral ventricle on the side of the approach. It is more difficult to expose the lateral ventricle on the opposite side through the transcortical than through the transcallosal approach. The transcortical approach is facilitated if the lateral ventricles are enlarged. Routes through the lateral ventricles to the third ventricle, other than by incising the ipsilateral column of the fornix, are by the transfornical approach in which the body of the fornix is split longitudinally, in the midline, or by the transchoroidal approach in which the choroidal fissure is opened, thus allowing the fornix to be pushed to the opposite side in order to expose the structures in the roof of the third ventricle.[1,6,12] The transchoroidal and transforni-

cal approaches have the advantage of giving access to the central portion of the third ventricle behind the foramen of Monro by displacing, rather than transecting, the fibers in the fornix. The transfornical and transchoroidal routes provide a satisfactory view into the third ventricle when the ventricle is exposed through the corpus callosum. On the other hand, the transchoroidal opening provides a better view into the third ventricle than the transfornical approach when the ventricle is exposed through the middle frontal gyrus. An anterior frontal approach may infrequently be considered for a lesion that involves the region of the rostrum and lower half of the genu of the corpus callosum or that extends from the rostrum into the third ventricle behind the lamina terminalis.

The posterior transcortical approach is the preferred route for exposing lesions situated entirely within the atrium, or arising in the glomus of the choroid plexus. Selected lesions may be exposed by the posterior transcallosal or the occipital approach. The transcallosal approach would be considered for a lesion that arises in the splenium and extends into the ventricle from the roof or the upper part of the medial wall of the atrium. The occipital approach directed along the falcotentorial junction would be used if the lesion arises in the medial wall of the atrium or extends from the atrium to the cisternal surface of the medial wall.

The temporal horn may be approached by the posterior frontotemporal, temporal, or subtemporal approach. The posterior frontotemporal approach would be used for a lesion involving the anterior portion of the temporal horn, which could be exposed through a small cortical incision in the anterior part of the temporal lobe or through a temporal lobectomy. The temporal and subtemporal routes to the temporal horn would be used for a lesion in the middle or posterior one-third of the temporal horn or for selected lesions in the cisterns medial to the temporal horn. The subtemporal route using a cortical incision in the occipitotemporal gyrus on the inferior surface of the temporal lobe is preferred. The opening into the temporal horn will expose the choroidal fissure. Opening through the choroidal fissure in the temporal horn will provide a transventricular view of the posterior cerebral artery and basal vein in the ambient cistern.

References

1. Apuzzo MLJ, Giannotta SL. Transcallosal interforniceal approach. In: Appuzzo MLF (ed.), *Surgery of the Third Ventricle.* Baltimore: Williams & Wilkins, 1987:354–379.
2. Bailey P. Peculiarities of the intracranial venous system and their clinical significance. *Arch Neurol Psychiatry* 1934; 32:1105.
3. Dandy WE. Operative experience in cases of pineal tumor. *Arch Surg* 1936; 33:19–46.
4. Fujii K, Lenkey C, Rhoton AL Jr. Microsurgical anatomy of the choroidal arteries: lateral and third ventricles. *J Neurosurg* 1980; 52:165–188.
5. Garretson HD. Memory in man: a neurosurgeon's perspective. In: Apuzzo MLF (ed.), *Surgery of the Third Ventricle.* Baltimore: Williams & Wilkins, 1987:209–212.
6. Nagata S, Rhoton AL Jr, Barry M. Microsurgical anatomy of the choroidal fissure. *Surg Neurol* 1988; 1:3–59.

7. Ono M, Rhoton AL Jr, Peace D, et al. Microsurgical anatomy of the deep venous system of the brain. *Neurosurgery* 1984; 15:621–655.

8. Rhoton AL Jr. Microsurgical anatomy of the third ventricular region. In: Apuzzo MLF (ed.), *Surgery of the Third Ventricle.* Baltimore: Williams & Wilkins, 1987:92–166.

9. Rhoton AL Jr, Yamamoto I, Peace DA. Microsurgery of the third ventricle: Part 2. Operative approaches. *Neurosurgery* 1981; 8:357–373.

10. Stein BM. Transcallosal approach to third ventricle tumors. In: Schmidek HH, Sweet WH (eds.), *Operative Neurosurgical Techniques: Indications, Methods, and Results.* New York: Grune & Stratton, 1982:575–584.

11. Timurkaynak E, Rhoton AL Jr, Barry M. Microsurgical anatomy and operative approaches to the lateral ventricles. *Neurosurgery* 1986; 19:685–723.

12. Viale GL, Turtas S. The subchoroid approach to the third ventricle. *Surg Neurol* 1980; 14:71–76.

13. Woolsey RM, Nelson JS. Asymptomatic destruction of the fornix in man. *Arch Neurol* 1975; 32:566–568.

14. Yamamoto I, Rhoton AL Jr, Peace DA. Microsurgery of the third ventricle: Part 1. Microsurgical anatomy. *Neurosurgery* 1981; 8:334–356.

15. Zaidel D, Sperry RW. Memory impairment after commissurotomy in man. *Brain* 1974; 97:263–272.

40

Microsurgical Anatomy of the Region of the Tentorial Incisura

Albert L. Rhoton, Jr.
Michio Ono

The neurovascular relationships in the region of the tentorial incisura are among the most complex in the cranium. The incisural area contains the bifurcation of the carotid and basilar arteries, the circle of Willis, and the convergence of the deep intracranial venous system to form the vein of Galen. It is intimately related to the depths of the cerebrum and cerebellum, six cranial nerves, and the upper brain stem. The incisura is exposed during many operations for aneurysms, deep tumors, arteriovenous malformations, trigeminal neuralgia, and epilepsy.

Anatomy of the Tentorium

The tentorium covers the cerebellum, supports the cerebrum, and forms a tight collar around the brain stem (Fig. 40-1). The incisura provides the only communication between the supratentorial and infratentorial spaces. The tentorium slopes downward from its apex, located just behind the pineal gland. All of the tentorial margins, except the free edges bordering the incisura, are rigidly attached to the skull.

The anterior end of each free edge is attached to the petrous apex and the anterior and posterior clinoid processes (Fig. 40-1). The attachment to the petrous apex and the clinoid processes forms three dural folds—the anterior and posterior petroclinoid and the interclinoid folds. Between these folds is located the oculomotor trigone, a depressed area through which the oculomotor and trochlear nerves enter the cavernous sinus (Fig. 40-1). The posterior petroclinoid fold extends from the petrous apex to the posterior clinoid process, the anterior petroclinoid fold extends from the petrous apex to the anterior clinoid process, and the interclinoid fold covers the ligament extending from the anterior to the posterior clinoid process. The oculomotor nerve

penetrates the dura in the central part of this triangle, and the trochlear nerve enters the dura at the posterolateral edge of this triangle.

Tentorial Incisura

The incisura is roughly triangular and has its anterior edge or base on the dorsum sellae and its apex dorsal to the midbrain, behind the pineal gland (Figs. 40-1 to 40-4). The incisura, when viewed from above after removal of the cerebral hemispheres, is filled by the midbrain and cerebellum. The free edges skirt the cerebral peduncles, either touching or being separated from them by a variable distance. The amount of cerebellar cortex visible between the midbrain and the free edge varies from none when the free edge hugs the tectum, to a large amount when the incisura extends far posteriorly. The incisura, when viewed from below after removal of the cerebellum, is filled by the midbrain, the uncus, and the parahippocampal gyrus. The amount of parahippocampal gyrus visible from below varies from none when the free edge hugs the tectum, to a large amount when the incisura is very wide.

The area between the brain stem and the free edges is divided into an anterior incisural space located in front of the brain stem, paired middle incisural spaces situated lateral to the brain stem, and a posterior incisural space located behind the brain stem (Figs. 40-1 to 40-5).

Anterior Incisural Space

Neural Relationships

The anterior incisural space is located anterior to the midbrain and pons. It extends inferiorly between the brain stem and clivus and upward around the optic chiasm to the subcallosal area. It opens laterally into the sylvian fissure, and posteriorly, between the uncus and the brain stem, into the middle incisural space (Figs. 40-1, 40-2, and 40-5). The posterior wall of the part located below the optic chiasm is formed by the pons and cerebral peduncles, and the posterolateral wall is formed by the bulbous prominence on the anterior part of the uncus, which hangs over the free edge above the oculomotor trigone. The part above the optic chiasm extends in front of the lamina terminalis and is limited superiorly by the rostrum of the corpus callosum. The anterior limb of the internal capsule is located above the anterior incisural space.

Cisternal Relationships

The anterior incisural space contains the interpeduncular cistern, which is located between the cerebral peduncles; the part of the sylvian cistern situated below the anterior perforated substance; the chiasmatic cistern, which is located below the optic chiasm; and the cisterna laminae terminalis, which lies anterior to the lamina terminalis. The interpe-

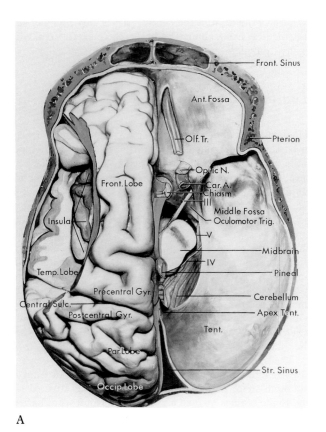

A

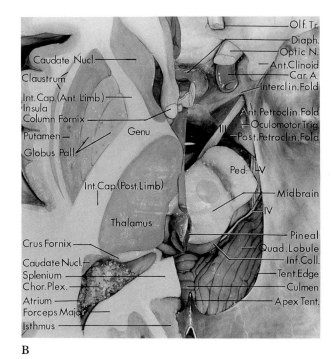

B

C

Figure 40-1 Tentorium and incisura: *A.* Superior view. The right cerebral hemisphere has been removed to expose the tentorium (Tent.). The midbrain is in the center of the incisura. The anterior incisural space is located anterior to the midbrain. The middle incisural space is located lateral to the midbrain. The posterior incisural space is located between the apex of the tentorium (Apex Tent.) and the midbrain. Structures in the exposure include the frontal (Front. Lobe), parietal (Par. Lobe), occipital (Occip. Lobe), and temporal lobes (Temp. Lobe); olfactory tract (Olf. Tr.); optic (Optic N.), oculomotor (III), trochlear (IV), and trigeminal nerves (V); central sulcus (Central Sulc.); precentral (Precentral Gyr.) and postcentral gyri (Postcentral Gyr.); carotid artery (Car. A.); straight sinus (Str. Sinus); anterior cranial fossa (Ant. Fossa); frontal sinus (Front. Sinus); and oculomotor trigone (Trig.). *B.* The superior part of the left cerebral hemisphere has been removed to expose the lateral ventricle and thalamus. The frontal horn (Front. Horn) is above the anterior incisural space. The atrium is above the posterior incisural space. The oculomotor nerve enters the roof of the cavernous sinus through the oculomotor trigone, which is situated between three dural folds: the interclinoid fold (Interclin. Fold), which extends from the posterior (Post. Clinoid), to the anterior clinoid process (Ant. Clinoid), forms the medial margin; the anterior petroclinoid fold (Ant. Petroclin. Fold), which extends

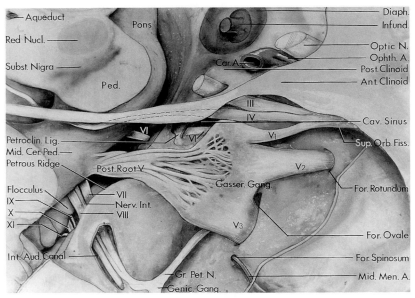

D

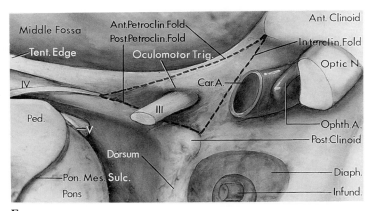

E

Figure 40-1 Continued

from the petrous apex to the anterior clinoid process, forms the lateral margin; and the posterior petroclinoid fold (Post. Petroclin. Fold), which extends from the petrous apex to the posterior clinoid process, forms the posterior margin. The anterior limb (Ant. Limb) of the internal capsule (Int. Cap.) is located above the anterior incisural space, and the posterior limb (Post. Limb) is located above the middle incisural space. Other structures in the exposure include the caudate nucleus (Caudate Nucl.), choroid plexus (Chor. Plex.), globus pallidus (Globus Pall.), diaphragma sellae (Diaph.), cerebral peduncle (Ped.), quadrangular lobule (Quad. Lobule), inferior colliculus (Inf. Coll.), and tentorial edge (Tent. Edge). *C.* Enlarged view of the incisura. The cerebellomesencephalic fissure (Cer. Mes. Fiss.) extends inferiorly between the midbrain and the cerebellum. Structures exposed include the central lobule (Cent. Lobule), vein of Galen (V. of Galen), substantia nigra (Subst. Nigra), red nuclei (Red Nucl.), and infundibulum (Infund.). *D.* Right superolateral view. The dura forming the lateral

wall of the cavernous sinus (Cav. Sinus) has been removed. The trochlear nerve enters the dura in the anteromedial edge of the tentorium (*dotted lines*). The abducent nerve (VI) enters the cavernous sinus by passing below the petroclinoid ligament (Petroclin. Lig.). Other structures exposed include the posterior clinoid process (Post. Clinoid); trigeminal root (Post. Root V.); middle cerebellar peduncle (Mid. Cer. Ped.); gasserian ganglion (Gasser. Gang.); foramen ovale (For. Ovale), rotundum (For. Rotundum), and spinosum (For. Spinosum); superior orbital fissure (Sup. Orb. Fiss.); facial (VII), vestibulocochlear (VIII), greater petrosal (Gr. Pet. N.), glossopharyngeal (IX), vagus (X), and accessory nerves (XI); nervus intermedius (Nerv. Int.); internal auditory canal (Int. Aud. Canal); ophthalmic (Ophth. A.) and middle meningeal arteries (Mid. Men. A.); and the geniculate ganglion (Genic. Gang.). *E.* Superior view. Enlarged view of the oculomotor trigone on the left side. The trochlear nerve passes forward at the level of the pontomesencephalic sulcus (Pon. Mes. Sulc.). (From Ono et al.[7])

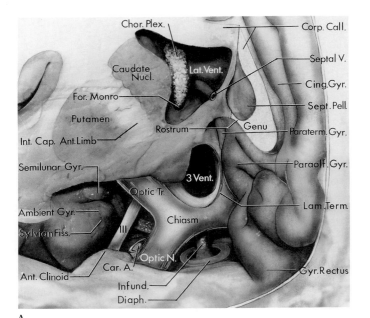

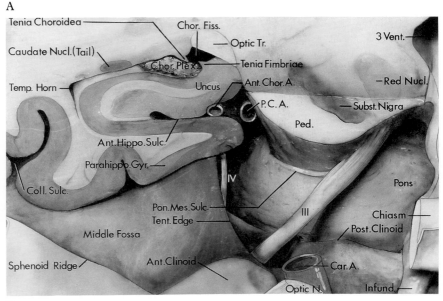

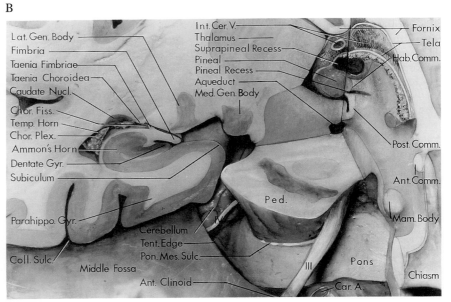

Figure 40-2 Tentorial incisura: Stepwise dissection, anterior-superior view. *A.* The anterior part of the frontal lobe has been removed to expose the anterior incisural space. The anterior incisural space extends upward around the optic chiasm, lamina terminalis (Lam. Term.), and the anterior part of the third ventricle (3 Vent.). Other structures in the exposure include the septum pellucidum (Sept. Pell.); corpus callosum (Corp. Call.); caudate nucleus (Caudate Nucl.); lateral ventricle (Lat. Vent.); choroid plexus (Chor. Plex.); foramen of Monro (For. Monro); optic tract (Optic tr.); optic (Optic N.) and oculomotor nerves (III); infundibulum (Infund.); diaphragma sellae (Diaph.); carotid artery (Car. A.); septal vein (Sept. V.); cingulate (Cing. Gyr.), paraterminal (Parater. Gyr.), paraolfactory (Paraolf. Gyr.), semilunar (Semilunar Gyr.), and ambient gyri (Ambient Gyr.); gyrus rectus (Gyr. Rectus); sylvian fissure (Sylvian Fiss.); internal capsule (Int. Cap. Ant. Limb); and anterior clinoid (Ant. Clin.). *B.* The transverse section has been extended behind the foramen of Monro to include part of the cerebral peduncle (Ped.). The posterior part of the right optic nerve and the right half of the optic chiasm have been removed to expose the posterior part of the anterior incisural space. The middle incisural space is located between the uncus and the midbrain. Other structures in the exposure include the substantia nigra (Subst. Nigra); red nucleus (Red Nucl.); parahippocampal gyrus (Parahippo. Gyr.); tentorial edge (Tent. Edge); temporal horn (Temp. Horn); collateral (Coll. Sulc.) and anterior hippocampal sulci (Ant. Hippo. Sulc.); choroidal fissure (Chor. Fiss.); anterior choroidal (Ant. Chor. A.) and posterior cerebral arteries (P.C.A.); pontomesencephalic sulcus (Pon. Mes. Sulc.); posterior clinoid (Post. Clinoid); and trochlear nerve (IV). *C.* The coronal section is located immediately behind the posterior (Post. Comm.) and habenular commissures (Hab.

Figure 40-2 Continued Comm.). The internal cerebral veins (Int. Cer. V.) course in the velum interpositum (Velum Interpos.). The mesial temporal structures form the lateral wall of the middle incisural space. Other structures in the exposure include the anterior commissure (Ant. Comm.); medial (Med. Gen. Body), lateral geniculate (Lat. Gen. Body), and mammillary bodies (Mam. Body); and the dentate gyrus (Dent. Gyr.). *D.* The level of the section has been extended behind the pineal body to expose the posterior incisural space and the vein of Galen (V. of Galen). The parahippocampal gyrus overlies the free edge. Other structures in the exposure include the massa intermedia (Massa. Int.), and hippocampal (Hippo. Sulc.) and fimbriodentate sulci (Fimb. Dent. Sulc). *E.* The right cerebral hemisphere has been removed. The posterior incisural space is located between the apex of the tentorium (Apex Tent.) and the midbrain. Structures in the exposure include the inferior colliculus (Inf. Coll.); cerebellomesencephalic fissure (Cer. Mes. Fiss.); anterior (Ant. Paraolf. Sulc.) and posterior paraolfactory sulci (Post. Paraolf. Sulc.); cingulate (Cing. Sulc.), lateral mesencephalic (Lat. Mes. Sulc.), and callosal sulci (Call. Sulc.); infundibular recess (Infund. Recess); striae medullaris thalami (Str. Med. Thal.); and interpeduncular fossa (Interped. Fossa). (From Ono et al.[7])

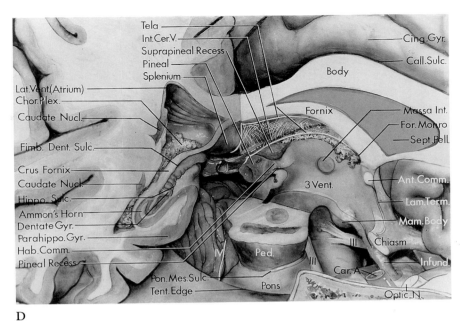

duncular and chiasmatic cisterns are separated by Liliequist's membrane, an arachnoidal sheet extending from the dorsum sellae to the anterior edge of the mammillary bodies.

Ventricular Relationships

The anterior part of the third ventricle projects into the anterior incisural space. The frontal horns of the lateral ventricles are located above the anterior incisural space (Figs. 40-1 and 40-2).

Cranial Nerves

The optic nerves and chiasm cross the anterior incisural space (Fig. 40-2). The optic nerves emerge from the optic canals medial to the attachment of the free edge to the anterior clinoid processes. The optic chiasm is usually located above the diaphragma sellae but may be prefixed and lie over the tuberculum sellae or postfixed and lie over the dorsum sellae. From the chiasm, the optic tract continues around the cerebral peduncle to enter the middle incisural space (Fig. 40-3). The oculomotor nerve crosses the anterior

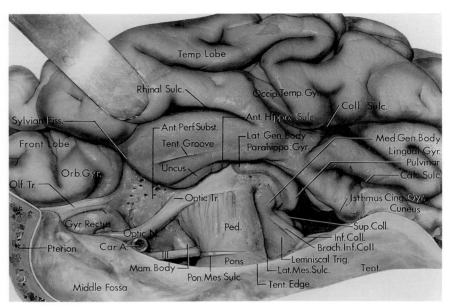

A

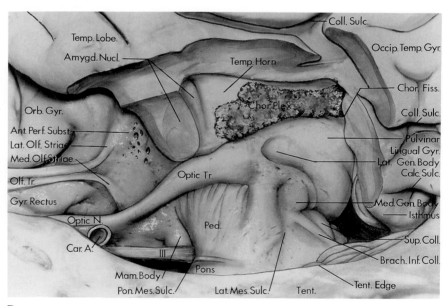

B

Figure 40-3 Tentorial incisura: Neural relationships.
A. Lateral view. The frontal (Front. Lobe) and temporal
lobes (Temp. Lobe) have been retracted away from the
tentorium (Tent.). The free edge (Tent. Edge) has
grooved (Tent. Groove) the lower surface of the uncus.
Structures in the exposure include the rhinal (Rhinal
Sulc.), anterior hippocampal (Ant. Hippo. Sulc.), calcarine (Calc. Sulc), collateral (Coll. Sulc.), pontomesencephalic (Pon. Mes. Sulc.), and lateral mesencephalic
sulci (Lat. Mes. Sulc.); anterior perforated substance
(Ant. Perf. Subst.); sylvian fissure (Sylvian Fiss.);
parahippocampal (Parahippo. Gyr.), occipitotemporal
(Occip. Temp. Gyr.), orbital (Orb. Gyr.), and lingual
gyri (Lingual Gyr.); carotid artery (Car. A.); optic
(Optic N.) and oculomotor nerves (III); olfactory (Olf. Tr.)

and optic tracts (Optic Tr.); cerebral peduncle (Ped.);
medial (Med. Gen. Body) and lateral geniculate (Lat. Gen.
Body) and mammillary bodies (Mam. Body.); brachium
of the inferior colliculus (Brach. Inf. Coll.); inferior (Inf.
Coll.) and superior colliculi (Sup. Coll.); gyrus rectus
(Gyr. Rect.); isthmus of the cingulate gyrus (Isthmus
Cing. Gyr.); and lemniscal trigone (Lemniscal Trig.).
B. The anteromedial part of the temporal lobe has been
removed to expose the temporal horn (Temp. Horn). The
removal crosses the amygdaloid nucleus (Amygd. Nucl.),
which lies deep to the uncus. Other structures include
the choroid plexus (Chor. Plex.), choroidal fissure (Chor.
Fiss.), and the medial (Med. Olf. Striae) and lateral olfactory striae (Lat. Olf. Striae). *C.* Inferior view. Neural
structures above the incisura. The uncus extends medial

incisural space between the posterior cerebral and the superior cerebellar arteries and passes inferomedial to the uncus to enter the oculomotor trigone.

Arterial Relationships

The arterial relationships of the anterior incisural space are among the most complex in the head, since it contains all the components of the circle of Willis (Figs. 40-5 and 40-6). The internal carotid artery enters the anterior incisural space by passing along the medial surface of the anterior clinoid process. The posterior communicating artery courses supero-

medial to the oculomotor nerve in the anterior incisural space. The anterior choroidal artery originates in the anterior incisural space and courses below the optic tract before passing between the uncus and the cerebral peduncle to enter the middle incisural space. The anterior cerebral artery arises in the anterior incisural space and courses above the optic chiasm and in front of the lamina terminalis. The middle cerebral artery courses laterally below the anterior perforated substance and bifurcates in the lateral part of the anterior incisural space.

The basilar artery ascends and gives rise to the posterior cerebral and superior cerebellar arteries in the posterior part of the anterior incisural space. The position of the basilar tip

C

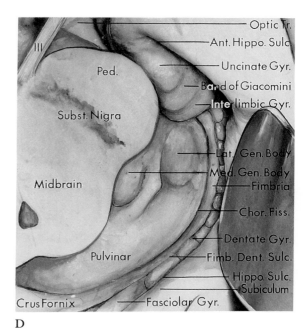

D

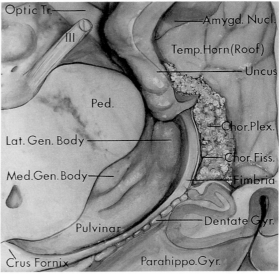

E

Figure 40-3 Continued
to, and is grooved by, the tentorial edge. Structures in the exposure include the posterior perforated substance (Post. Perf. Subst.), infundibulum (Infund.), red nucleus (Red Nucl.), and substantia nigra (Subst. Nigra.).
D. Roof of the middle incisural space. The subiculum of the parahippocampal gyrus has been retracted to expose the dentate gyrus (Dentate Gyr.) and the fimbria of the fornix. The choroidal fissure opens into the temporal horn. Other structures include the fimbriodentate (Fimb. Dent. Sulc.) and hippocampal sulci (Hippo. Sulc.) and the fasciolar (Fasciolar Gyr.), uncinate (Uncinate Gyr.), and interlimbic gyri (Interlimbic Gyr.). E. The medial part of the temporal lobe except for the fimbria has been removed to expose the temporal horn. (From Ono et al.[7])

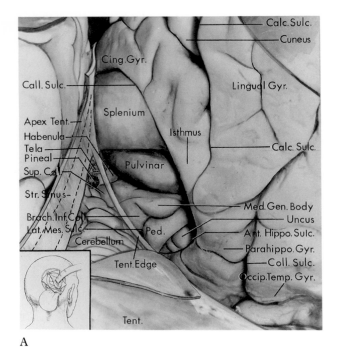

A

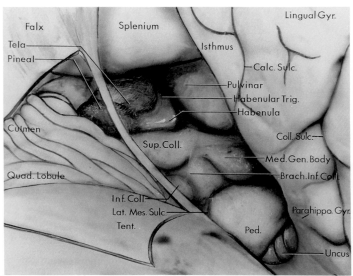

B

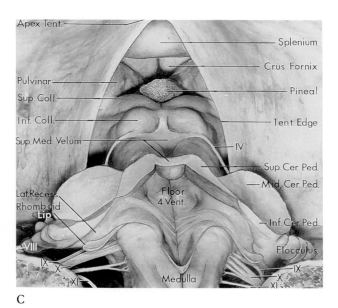

C

Figure 40-4 Neural relationships: Posterior views.
A. Posterior incisural space. (Inset, *lower left*, shows orientation.) The right occipital lobe has been retracted and the tentorium (Tent.) opened adjacent to the tentorial edge (Tent. Edge) and straight sinus (Str. Sinus). Structures in the exposure include the tentorial apex (Apex. Tent.); cerebral penduncle (Ped.); lingual (Lingual Gyr.), parahippocampal (Parahippo. Gyr.), cingulate (Cing. Gyr.), and occipitotemporal gyri (Occip. Temp. Gyr.); calcarine (Calc. Sulc.), anterior hippocampal (Ant. Hippo. Sulc.), collosal (Call. Sulc.), collateral (Coll. Sulc.), and lateral mesencephalic sulci (Lat. Mes. Sulc.); brachium of the inferior colliculus (Brach. Inf. Coll.); inferior (Inf. Coll.) and superior colliculi (Sup. Coll.); and the medial geniculate body (Med. Gen. Body).
B. Enlarged view. The pineal body protrudes inferiorly between the superior colliculi. Structures in the exposure include the habenular trigone (Habenular Trig.) and quadrangular lobule (Quad. Lobule). *C.* Posterior view below the tentorium. The cerebellum was removed by dividing the superior (Sup. Cer. Ped.), middle (Mid. Cer. Ped.), and inferior cerebellar peduncles (Inf. Cer. Ped.) just dorsal to the floor of the fourth ventricle (4 Vent.). The trochlear nerves (IV) arise below the inferior colliculi. Other structures include the superior medullary velum (Sup. Med. Velum); lateral recess (Lat. Recess); and the vestibulocochlear (VIII), glossopharyngeal (IX), vagus (X), and accessory nerves (XI). (From Ono et al.[7])

and bifurcation varies from as far caudal as 1.3 mm below the pontomesencephalic sulcus to as far rostral as the mammillary bodies.[11] The posterior cerebral artery courses around the cerebral peduncle above the oculomotor nerve and enters the middle incisural space by coursing between the uncus and cerebral peduncle. The superior cerebellar artery usually originates rostral to the level of the free edge in the anterior incisural space, then courses below the oculo-

motor nerve and dips below the tentorium to reach the cerebellum.

Venous Relationships

The main venous trunk related to the anterior incisural space is the basal vein (Fig. 40-5 and 40-7). It courses

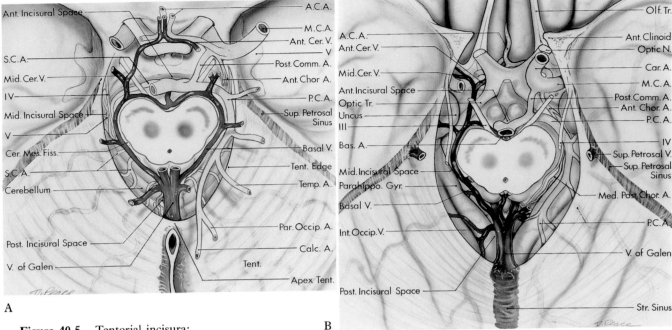

A

B

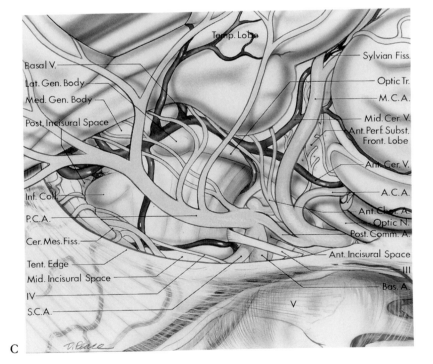

C

Figure 40-5. Tentorial incisura: Neural, arterial, and venous relationships. The tentorium is translucent to show the relations both above and below the tentorium. *A.* View from above with the cerebrum removed. *B.* View from below with the cerebellum removed. *C.* Lateral view with the temporal and frontal lobes elevated. *D.* Anterolateral view. The anterior two-thirds of the right cerebral hemisphere have been removed. *E.* Lateral view. Tentorial arteries. *A–E.* The tentorium (Tent.) slopes downward from its apex (Apex Tent.). The free edges (Tent. Edge) are attached to the petrous apex and the anterior (Ant. Clinoid) and posterior clinoid processes. The anterior (Ant.) incisural space is located anterior to the midbrain and extends upward around the optic chiasm. The middle (Mid.) incisural space is located between the lateral surface of the brain stem and the free edge. The posterior (Post.) incisural space is located between the tentorial apex and the midbrain. The oculomotor (III) and optic nerves (Optic N.) cross the anterior incisural space. The middle incisural space extends into the supratentorial area between the temporal lobe (Temp. Lobe) and the midbrain and into the infratentorial area between the cerebellum and midbrain. The lateral wall of the supratentorial part of the middle incisural space is formed by the parahippocampal (Parahippo. Gyr.) and dentate gyri (Dentate Gyr.). The medial (Med. Gen. Body) and lateral geniculate bodies (Lat. Gen. Body) and the optic tract (Optic Tr.) are in the roof of the middle incisural space. The trigeminal nerve (V) arises in the infratentorial part of the middle incisural space. The trochlear nerve (IV) arises below the inferior colliculus (Inf. Coll.) and passes forward in the cerebellomesencephalic fissure (Cer. Mes. Fiss.) and enters the free edge just be-

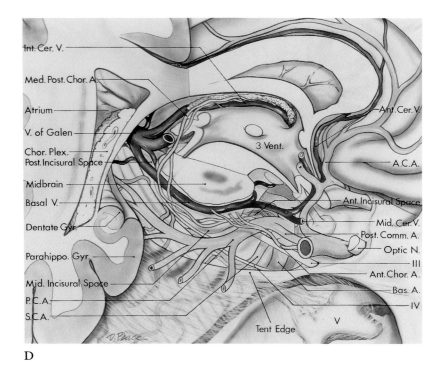

D

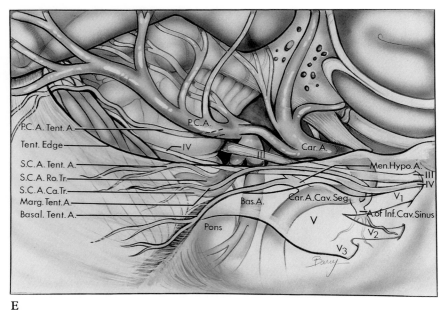

E

Figure 40-5. Continued hind the posterior clinoid process. In the anterior incisural space, the carotid arteries (Car. A.) give rise to the posterior communicating (Post. Comm. A.), anterior choroidal (Ant. Chor. A.), the middle (M.C.A.) and anterior cerebral arteries (A.C.A.), and the basilar artery (Bas. A.) gives rise to the superior cerebellar (S.C.A.) and posterior cerebral arteries (P.C.A.). The posterior cerebral artery encircles the midbrain and gives off lateral (Lat. Post. Chor. A.) and medial posterior choroidal (Med. Post. Chor. A.), temporal (Temp. A.), parieto-occipital (Par. Occip. A.), and calcarine arteries (Calc. A.). The superior cerebellar artery arises and splits into rostral (Ro. Tr.) and caudal trunks (Ca. Tr.) near where it passes below the tentorium. The meningohypophyseal branch (Men. Hypo. A.) of the carotid artery gives rise to the basal tentorial artery (Bas. Tent. A.), and the artery of the inferior cavernous sinus (A. of Inf. Cav. Sinus) gives rise to the marginal tentorial artery (Marg. Tent. A.). Tentorial branches also arise from the superior cerebellar (S.C.A. Tent. A.) and posterior cerebral arteries (P.C.A. Tent. A.). The middle (Mid. Cer. V.) and anterior cerebral veins (Ant. Cer. V.) join to form the basal vein (Basal V.) in the anterior incisural space. The basal vein passes through the middle incisural space. The basal and internal cerebral veins (Int. Cer. V.) join the vein of Galen (V. of Galen) in the posterior incisural space. The superior petrosal sinus (Sup. Pet. Sinus) receives the superior petrosal veins (Sup. Petrosal V.). The choroid plexus (Chor. Plex.) is exposed in the atrium and third ventricle (3 Vent.).

through the anterior and middle incisural spaces to empty into the great vein of Galen in the posterior incisural space. It originates in the anterior incisural space below the anterior perforated substance from the union of the anterior and middle cerebral veins. It courses below the optic tract and between the uncus and cerebral peduncle to enter the middle incisural space.

Middle Incisural Space

Neural Relationships

The middle incisural space is located lateral to the brain stem (Figs. 40-1 to 40-4). This narrow space extends upward

Figure 40-6 Arterial relationships. *A.* Right lateral view. The temporal lobe (Temp. Lobe) has been retracted to expose the upper surface of the tentorium (Tent.) and the tentorial edge (Tent. Edge). The arteries related to the tentorial incisura include the carotid (Car. A.); posterior communicating (Post. Comm. A.); anterior (A.C.A.), middle (M.C.A.), and posterior cerebral (P.C.A.); anterior choroidal (Ant. Cho. A.); basilar (Bas. A.); superior cerebellar (S.C.A.); long (Long Circ. A.) and short circumflex (Short Circ. A.); anterior (Ant. Temp. A.), middle (Mid. Temp. A.), and posterior temporal (Post. Temp. A.); medial posterior choroidal (Med. Post. Chor. A.); and calcarine arteries (Calc. A.). Structures in the exposure include the collateral (Coll. Sulc.), rhinal (Rhinal Sulc.), lateral mesencephalic (Lat. Mes. Sulc.), and pontomesencephalic sulci (Pon. Mes. Sulc.); parahippocampal (Parahippo. Gyr.) and occipitotemporal gyri (Occip. Temp. Gyr.); anterior perforated substance (Ant. Perf. Subst.); sylvian fissure (Sylvian Fiss.); frontal lobe (Front. Lobe); optic (Optic N.) and oculomotor nerves (III); optic (Optic Tr.) and olfactory tracts (Olf. Tr.); rostral (Ro. Tr. S.C.A.) and caudal trunks (Ca. Tr. S.C.A.) of the superior cerebellar artery; superior (Sup. Coll.) and inferior colliculi (Inf. Coll.); and cerebral peduncle (Ped.). *B.* Enlarged view. The temporal lobe has been removed. The carotid and basilar bifurcations are in the anterior incisural space. Structures exposed include the anterior (Ant. Clinoid) and posterior clinoid processes (Post. Clinoid), recurrent (Rec. A.) and lenticulostriate arteries (Lent. Str. A.), mamillary body (Mam. Body), and choroid plexus (Chor. Plex.). *C.* Inferior view. The tentorium, except for the free edge, has been removed. The inferior part of the right temporal lobe has been removed to expose the temporal horn (Temp. Horn). Structures exposed include the straight sinus (Str. Sinus), infundibulum (Infund.), lateral posterior choroidal (Lat. Post. Chor. A.) and thalmogeniculate arteries (Thal. Gen. A.), and the medial (Med. Gen. Body) and lateral geniculate bodies (Lat. Gen. Body). (From Ono et al.[7])

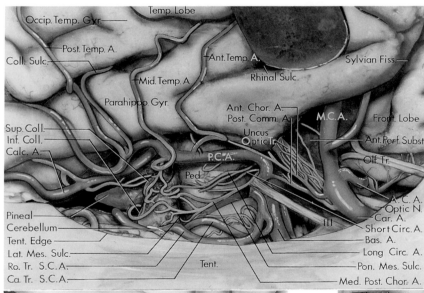

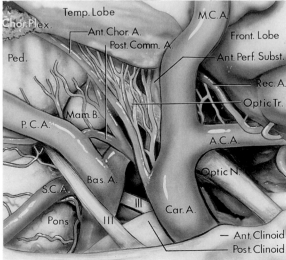

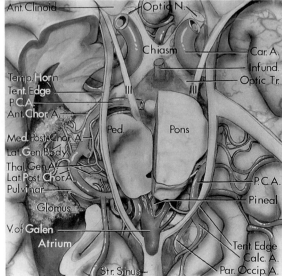

Figure 40-7 Venous relations. *A.* Anterior incisural space. The frontal lobes (Front. Lobe) have been retracted to expose the anterior part of the tentorium (Tent.). The anterior incisural space extends around the optic chiasm and along the lamina terminalis (Lam. Term.). The deep middle (Deep Mid. Cer. V.) and anterior cerebral veins (Ant. Cer. V.) join to form the basal vein (Basal V.). Other structures in the exposure are the olfactory (Olf. V.), paraterminal (Paraterm. V.), anterior pericallosal (Ant. Pericall. V.), anterior communicating (Ant. Comm. V.), and peduncular veins (Ped. V.); cerebral peduncle (Ped.); tentorial edge (Tent. Edge); ophthalmic (Ophth. A.) and carotid arteries (Car. A.); optic nerves (Optic N.); anterior clinoid (Ant. Clinoid); olfactory (Olf. Tr.) and optic tracts (Optic Tr.); infundibulum (Infund.); and orbital gyri (Orb. Gyr.). *B.* Lateral view. The left temporal lobe (Temp. Lobe) has been elevated. The basal vein arises in the anterior incisural space below the anterior perforated substance (Ant. Perf. Subst.), passes around the cerebral peduncle, through the middle incisural space, and converges on the vein of Galen in the posterior incisural space. Structures in the exposure include the inferior striate (Inf. Str. V.), lateral mesencephalic (Lat. Mes. V.), inferior ventricular (Inf. Vent. V.), anterior hippocampal (Ant. Hippo. V.), anterior longitudinal hippocampal (Ant. Long.

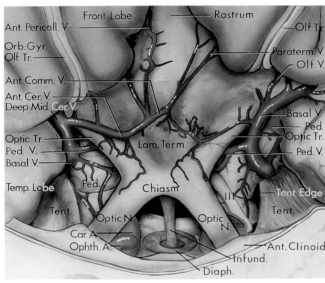

A

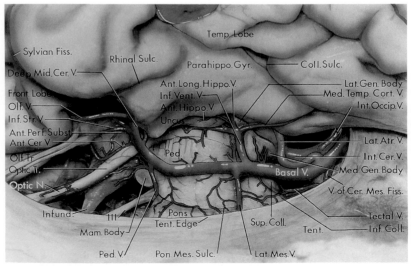

B

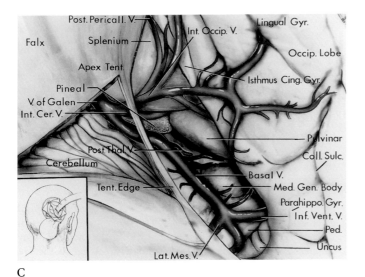

C

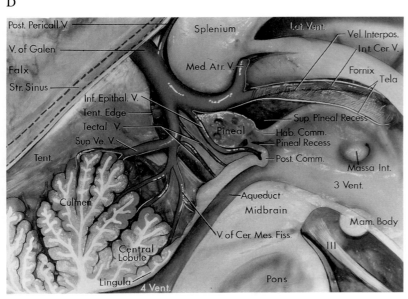

D

E

Figure 40-7 Continued
Hippo. V.), medial temporal cortical (Med. Temp. Cort. V.), lateral atrial (Lat. Atr. V.), tectal (Tectal V.), internal occipital (Int. Occip. V.), and internal cerebral veins (Int. Cer. V.); vein of the cerebellomesencephalic fissure (V. of Cer. Mes. Fiss.); sylvian fissure (Sylvian Fiss.); lateral (Lat. Gen. Body) and medial geniculate (Med. Gen. Body) and mammillary bodies (Mam. Body); parahippocampal gyrus (Parahippo. Gyr.); collateral (Coll. Sulc.), rhinal (Rhinal Sulc.), and pontomesencephalic sulci (Pon. Mes. Sulc.); and the inferior (Inf. Coll.) and superior colliculi (Sup. Coll.). C. Posterior view, with the occipital lobe (Occip. Lobe) retracted and the tentorium opened to expose the basal vein in the posterior incisural space. Inset indicates the orientation. Structures in the exposure include the posterior thalamic (Post. Thal. V.) and posterior pericallosal veins (Post. Pericall. V.), vein of Galen (V. Galen), the isthmus of the cingulate gyrus (Isthmus Cing. Gyr.), and lingual gyrus (Lingual Gyr.). D. Inferior view. The cerebellum has been removed by dividing the superior (Sup. Cer. Ped.) and middle cerebellar peduncles (Mid. Cer. Ped.) behind the fourth ventricle (4 Vent.). Other structures include the superior medullary velum (Sup. Med. Velum), trochlear nerves (IV), tentorial sinus (Tent. Sinus), inferior epithalamic (Inf. Epithal. V.) and posterior mesencephalic veins (Post. Mes. V.), and the paired veins of the superior cerebellar peduncle (V. of Sup. Cer. Ped.). E. Midsagittal section through the posterior incisural space. The internal cerebral veins course in the velum interpositum (Velum Interpos.), which is located between the layers of tela choroidea (Tela) in the roof of the third ventricle (3 Vent.). Other structures include the superior vermian (Sup. Ve. V.) and medial atrial veins (Med. Atr. V.), lateral ventricle (Lat. Vent.), posterior (Post. Comm.) and habenular commissures (Hab. Comm.), suprapineal recess (Sup. Pineal Recess), massa intermedia (Massa Int.), and mamillary bodies (Mam. Body). (From Ono et al.[7])

between the temporal lobe and the midbrain and downward between the cerebellum and the upper brain stem. The medial wall is formed by the lateral surface of the midbrain and upper pons. The junction of the pons and midbrain is situated at the level of the free edge. The roof has a narrow anterior part formed by the optic tract, which is flattened between the cerebral peduncle and the uncus, and a wider posterior part formed by the inferior surface of the pulvinar (Fig. 40-3). The medial and lateral geniculate body protrudes from the interior surface of the pulvinar into the roof of the middle incisural space.

The lateral wall of the supratentorial part of the middle incisural space is formed by the medial surface of the temporal lobe. The uncus and parahippocampal gyrus form a curved border around the middle incisural space. The uncus bulges medially at the anterior end of the parahippocampal gyrus. The amygdaloid nucleus is situated just lateral to the medial surface of the uncus (Fig. 40-3).

The uncus commonly prolapses into the incisura anteriorly and has a groove along its undersurface marking the free edge. This groove usually disappears at the lateral margin of the peduncle because the free edge often hugs the peduncle at this site, but it may reappear posterior to the peduncle on the lower surface of the parahippocampal gyrus as the space between the brain stem and the free edge increases. These grooves are commonly present on the uncus and anterior part of the parahippocampal gyrus without being seen on the posterior part of the parahippocampal gyrus. They are only rarely present posteriorly, and not anteriorly.

Posterior to the uncus, the surface of the temporal lobe facing the middle incisural space is formed by three longitudinal strips of neural tissue, one located above the other, which are interlocked with the hippocampal formation (Figs. 40-2 and 40-3). The most inferior strip is formed by the subiculum, the rounded medial edge of the parahippocampal gyrus; the middle strip is formed by the dentate gyrus; and the superior strip is formed by the fimbria of the fornix.

The choroidal fissure, the cleft along which the choroid plexus in the lateral ventricle is attached, is situated at the junction of the roof and lateral wall of the middle incisural space between the fimbria and the pulvinar.[14] The inferior choroidal point, the inferior end of the choroidal fissure, is located beside the lateral geniculate body. The middle incisural space extends below the tentorium to communicate with the cleft, called the cerebellomesencephalic fissure, located between the cerebellum and midbrain.

Cisternal Relationships

The supratentorial part of the middle incisural space contains the crural and ambient cisterns (Figs. 40-2 and 40-3). The crural cistern is located between the cerebral peduncle and the uncus. The crural cistern opens posteriorly into the ambient cistern, which is demarcated medially by the midbrain; above by the pulvinar; and laterally by the subiculum, dentate gyrus, and fimbria. The ambient cistern is continuous posteriorly with the quadrigeminal cistern.

Ventricular Relationships

The temporal horn extends into the temporal lobe lateral to the middle incisural space (Figs. 40-2 and 40-3). Opening through the choroidal fissure from the temporal horn exposes the ambient cistern. The paired bodies of the lateral ventricles are located directly above the central part of the incisura. They sit on, and are separated from, the central part of the incisura by the thalamus.

Cranial Nerves

The trochlear and trigeminal nerves are related to the middle incisural space (Figs. 40-1, 40-2, and 40-4). The trochlear nerve has the longest course within the incisura of any nerve. It is the nerve most intimately related to the free edge. The trochlear nerve arises in the posterior incisural space and passes forward through the middle incisural space between the posterior cerebral and superior cerebellar arteries. Its initial course around the midbrain is medial to the free edge. It reaches the lower margin of the free edge at the posterior edge of the cerebral peduncle. It pierces the free edge in the posterior part of the oculomotor trigone.

The trigeminal nerve courses in the infratentorial part of the middle incisural compartment and passes above the petrous apex to enter Meckel's cave. The medial edge of the posterior trigeminal root is seen just medial to the tentorial edge if one looks from straight superior through the incisura with the cerebrum removed, but it is hidden below the free edge in the lateral view provided by the subtemporal operative exposure.

Arterial Relationships

The major arteries in the middle incisural space, the anterior choroidal, posterior cerebral, and superior cerebellar arteries, arise in the anterior incisural space and reach the middle incisural space by coursing around the brain stem parallel to the free edge (Figs. 40-5 and 40-6). The anterior choroidal artery enters the superior part of the middle incisural space below the optic tract and passes through the choroidal fissure near the inferior choroidal point to supply the choroid plexus in the temporal horn.

The posterior cerebral artery enters the middle incisural space by passing between the cerebral peduncle and uncus and passes straight posteriorly between the midbrain and subiculum. It gives off several cortical branches which cross the free edge to reach the temporal and occipital lobes and the medial and lateral posterior choroidal and thalamogeniculate arteries, which course medial to the free edge. The lateral posterior choroidal arteries course through the choroidal fissure and around the pulvinar to reach the choroid plexus in the temporal horn and atrium. The thalamogeniculate branches arise below the pulvinar and pass upward through the geniculate bodies to reach the thalamus and internal capsule. The medial posterior choroidal artery arises from the proximal part of the posterior cerebral artery in the anterior incisural space, and courses medial to the posterior cerebral artery through the middle incisural space to reach the posterior incisural space.

The superior cerebellar artery passes below the level of the free edge and bifurcates into rostral and caudal trunks as it passes around the lateral margin of the cerebral peduncle to enter the middle incisural space. It passes above the trigeminal nerve and enters the cerebellomesencephalic fissure in the anterior part of the middle incisural space before dividing into hemispheric and vermian arteries. The artery may dip caudally to touch the superior surface of the trigeminal nerve.[2]

Venous Relationships

The venous relationships in the middle incisural space are relatively simple (Figs. 40-5 and 40-7). The basal vein courses along the upper part of the cerebral peduncle and below the pulvinar to reach the posterior incisural space. It may infrequently terminate in a tentorial sinus in the free edge at this level. The veins draining the medial and lateral wall of this space terminate above in the basal vein and below in the veins that drain into the superior petrosal sinus.

Posterior Incisural Space

Neural Relationships

The posterior incisural space lies posterior to the midbrain and extends backward to the level of the tentorial apex. It corresponds to the pineal region (Figs. 40-1 to 40-4). Its anterior wall is formed by the quadrigeminal plate, pineal body, and habenular complex. The roof is formed by the lower surface of the splenium. Each lateral wall is formed by the part of the medial surface of the hemisphere located below the splenium and the part of the pulvinar located beside the pineal body. The floor is formed by the anterior superior part of the cerebellum. It extends inferiorly into the cerebellomesencephalic fissure, the cleft between the cerebellum and the midbrain.

Cisternal Relationships

The quadrigeminal cistern is situated in and has the same walls described above for the posterior incisural space (Figs. 40-1 to 40-4). The quadrigeminal cistern may communicate with the velum interpositum, a space which extends forward into the roof of the third ventricle between the splenium and the pineal body (Fig. 40-2). The internal cerebral veins enter the velum interpositum just behind the foramen of Monro and exit it above the pineal body to enter the posterior incisural space.

Ventricular Relationships

The posterior portion of the third ventricle and the cerebral aqueduct are anterior, and the atria and occipital horns are lateral to the posterior incisural space (Figs. 40-1 and 40-2). The suprapineal recess extends posteriorly between the pineal body and the inferior wall of the velum interpositum toward the posterior incisural space. The atrium is separated from the posterior incisural space by the crus of the fornix and the cortical gyri located in the lateral wall of the posterior incisural space. Opening the choroidal fissure, which in the atrium is situated between the crus of the fornix and the pulvinar, exposes the quadrigeminal cistern.

Arterial Relationships

The trunks and branches of the posterior cerebral and superior cerebellar arteries enter the posterior incisural space anteriorly (Figs. 40-5 and 40-6). The posterior cerebral artery courses through the lateral part of the posterior incisural space and bifurcates into the calcarine and parietooccipital arteries near where it crosses above the free edge. The medial posterior choroidal arteries enter the posterior incisural space from anteriorly, turn forward beside the pineal body, enter the velum interpositum and supply the choroid plexus in the roof of the third ventricle and the body of the lateral ventricle. The superior cerebellar artery is coursing within the cerebellomesencephalic fissure when it reaches the posterior incisural space. Before leaving the fissure, it gives rise to its cortical branches to the vermis and hemisphere. These branches, upon exiting the cerebellomesencephalic fissure, are anterior to the free edge, but they pass below the free edge to reach the surface of the vermis and hemisphere.

Venous Relationships

The venous relationships in the posterior incisural space are the most complex in the cranium because the internal cerebral and basal veins and many of their tributaries converge on the vein of Galen within this area (Figs. 40-5 and 40-7). The internal cerebral veins exit the velum interpositum, and the basal veins exit the ambient cistern, to reach the posterior incisural space, where they join the vein of Galen. The vein of Galen passes below the splenium and joins the straight sinus at the tentorial apex. The largest vein from the infratentorial part of the posterior incisural space, the vein of the cerebellomesencephalic fissure, originates from the union of the paired veins on the superior cerebellar peduncles and courses forward through the cerebellomesencephalic fissure to terminate with the superior vermian vein in the great vein.

Tentorial Arteries

The tentorial arteries arise from three sources (Fig. 40-5).[8,9,12,15] The first source, the cavernous segment of the carotid artery, provides two arteries: the basal tentorial artery (the artery of Bernasconi-Cassinari) from the meningohypophyseal trunk and the marginal tentorial artery from the artery of the inferior cavernous sinus. The basal tentorial artery arises from the meningohypophyseal trunk and courses along the medial part of the tentorial attachment to the petrous ridge. The marginal tentorial artery arises from the artery of the inferior cavernous sinus, passes laterally over the abducens nerve, then superoposteriorly to enter the tentorial edge. If this artery is absent, a branch from the meningohypophyseal artery may replace it. The second source is the superior cerebellar artery. This tentorial branch originates near where the artery passes under the tentorium. Approximately one in four superior cerebellar arteries give rise to a tentorial branch.[7] The third source is the proximal part of the posterior cerebral artery. This branch courses around the brain stem to enter the tentorium near the apex.

Tentorial Herniation

Tentorial herniation is the most common and most important form of brain herniation.[3–8,13] In descending herniation caused by supratentorial lesions, the uncus and the parahippocampal gyri herniate downward through the incisura, and in ascending herniation resulting from infratentorial masses, the superior part of the cerebellum herniates upward through the incisura. These herniations cause direct effects due to neural compression and indirect effects due to vascular compromise. Symptoms may result from displacement, compression, and stretching of the brain stem and cranial nerves; hemorrhage and infarction due to compression and tearing of arteries and veins; increasing edema and intracranial pressure due to venous obstruction; hydrocephalus due to obstruction of the aqueduct and subarachnoid space at the incisura; and strangulation of the prolapsed tissue.

The type of herniation depends on the position and rate of expansion of the lesion and the size and shape of the incisura. The signs appear early when structures are deformed rapidly, while advanced distortion may occur before the appearance of signs if the herniation develops slowly. A wide space between the free edge and brain stem facilitates cerebral herniation, since more tissue can herniate into the space.[8] A low position of the anterior portion of the free edge also facilitates descending herniation.[8]

Descending herniations are divided into anterior, posterior, and complete types. In the anterior type, the uncus herniates into the interpeduncular and crural cisterns. This shift carries the brain stem to the opposite side, thus increasing the space between the free edge and the brain stem and facilitating further shift of tissue through the aperture. Eventually, the parahippocampal gyrus, from the splenium to the uncus, may be forced through the opening, and the incisura becomes plugged with herniated temporal lobe, deformed hypothalamus, and compressed midbrain. The amygdaloid nucleus is involved with the uncus in the herniated mass. Distortion and compression of the midbrain reticular activating pathways cause a decreased level of consciousness. Compression of the ipsilateral cerebral peduncle causes contralateral pyramidal signs, and, if the lateral displacement of the brain stem is severe, the contralateral cerebral peduncle may be forced against the free edge, thus pro-

ducing a groove on the peduncle called a Kernohan's notch, with ipsilateral pyramidal signs.[13] In the terminal stage, deformation of the midbrain causes decerebrate rigidity. Distortion and compression of the posterior hypothalamus may cause cardiovascular, respiratory, and thermoregulatory disturbances. The pituitary stalk may be stretched and compressed against the dorsum sellae, causing diabetes insipidus. The oculomotor nerve courses between the medial border of the uncus and the posterior petroclinoidal fold, and may be kinked or compressed here or between the posterior cerebral and superior cerebellar artery, or it may be stretched as the hernia displaces the midbrain posteriorly. Initially, the pupilloconstrictor fibers, which are concentrated on the superior surface of the nerve, are compressed. Later, somatic fibers to the extraocular muscles are disturbed. In the early stages, irritation of the pupilloconstrictor fibers may cause pupillary constriction, but this usually gives way to a paralytic effect with pupillary dilation as the hernia enlarges. The optic tract is displaced medially and downward, but the resulting visual loss is often masked by deepening coma. Compression of the uncus, amygdaloid nucleus, parahippocampal gyrus, and hippocampal formation against the free edge may cause memory, behavior, and personality changes. Residual scarring of the hippocampal formation may cause seizures. The trochlear nerve usually escapes involvement in such herniations, but caudal displacement of the brain stem may result in a palsy of the abducens nerve by stretching it in the subarachnoid space or strangling it in its course around the anterior inferior cerebellar artery.

Stretching or compression of the anterior choroidal and posterior cerebral arteries between the temporal lobe and the peduncle, or obstruction of the posterior cerebral artery as it crosses the free edge, may cause a visual field loss due to ischemia of the optic tract, optic radiation, or lateral geniculate body; contralateral hemiplegia due to involvement of the cerebral peduncle and midbrain; changes in personality and behavior due to damage to the amygdaloid nucleus or hippocampal formation; unconsciousness and decerebrate rigidity due to midbrain ischemia; and contralateral sensory loss due to ischemia of the ventral thalamic nuclei. Brain stem hemorrhage frequently accompanies tentorial herniation.

In the posterior type of tentorial herniation, the posterior portion of the parahippocampal and lingual gyri and the isthmus of the cingulate gyrus may shift through the incisura into the quadrigeminal cistern and compress and displace the dorsal half of the midbrain. Tectal compression may cause vertical gaze disturbances. Compression and obstruction of the aqueduct causes hydrocephalus and raises the intracranial pressure. In posterior herniation, the posterior cerebral artery or its calcarine branch is pressed against the free edge and may be obstructed, causing infarction of the occipital cortex and hemianopsia. The basal vein may be compressed between the midbrain and herniated temporal lobe, and the vein of Galen may be obstructed as it curves around the splenium, thus aggravating the venous congestion, edema, and intracranial tension. The complete type of herniation yields a combination of symptoms and signs seen with anterior and posterior herniations. Hemorrhage into the brain stem due to tearing of arteries and veins without cerebral herniation may occur if the incisura hugs the brain stem so tightly that it prevents cerebral herniation while allowing axial displacement of the brain stem.

In ascending herniation due to a posterior fossa mass lesion, the superior part of the cerebellar vermis and hemispheres herniates upward through the incisura into the quadrigeminal cistern. Cerebellar infarction may result from compression of the branches of the superior cerebellar artery where they pass under the free edge. The hernia may compress the great vein against the splenium which is fixed above by the falx, thus increasing the venous congestion, edema, and intracranial pressure.

Operative Considerations

The selection of the best operative approach for a lesion of the incisura depends on the space involved (Fig. 40-8).[7,10,14]

Anterior Incisural Space

Nearly 95 percent of saccular arterial aneurysms arise within the anterior incisural space. The aneurysms arising from the part of the circle of Willis located anterior to Liliequist's membrane, are approached through a frontotemporal (pterional) craniotomy. Aneurysms located behind Liliequist's membrane may be exposed through either a frontotemporal or subtemporal craniotomy if they are located above the dorsum, but those located below the dorsum usually require a subtemporal craniotomy.

Incision and retraction of the tentorium are commonly required to gain access to lesions around the incisura. The incision in the tentorium to expose the interpeduncular and prepontine cisterns is usually located just posterior to the point where the trochlear nerve enters the free edge. The free edge may be retracted by means of sutures placed near it, but special care is required to avoid stretching and damaging the trochlear nerve. The tentorial arteries and venous sinuses may be encountered in sectioning the tentorium. Sectioning of the tentorium has been used to alleviate pressure on the brain stem caused by giant aneurysms and incisural tumors that cannot be removed.[1]

Tumors in the anterior incisural space may be approached by the bifrontal, subfrontal, frontal-interhemispheric, frontotemporal, subtemporal, and trans-sphenoidal routes. Tumors located anterior to Liliequist's membrane between the optic chiasm and the diaphragma are commonly operated on by the trans-sphenoidal or subfrontal approach. The trans-sphenoidal approach is preferred if the tumor extends upward out of an enlarged sella turcica and is located above a pneumatized sphenoid sinus. The subfrontal intracranial approach is reserved for those tumors in the chiasmatic cistern that are located entirely above the diaphragma or extend upward out of a normal or small sella, or are located above a nonpneumatized (conchal) type of sphenoid sinus. The subfrontal approach permits exposure of the

tumor within the anterior incisural space by four routes: (1) the subchiasmatic approach between the optic nerves and below the optic chiasm, (2) the opticocarotid route directed between the optic nerve and carotid artery, (3) the lamina terminalis approach directed above the optic chiasm through a thinned lamina terminalis, and (4) the transfrontal–trans-sphenoidal approach obtained by entering the sphenoid sinus and sella through the transfrontal craniotomy. The subchiasmatic approach is used if the subchiasmatic opening is enlarged by the tumor. The opticocarotid route is selected if the tumor widens the space between the carotid artery and the optic nerve and the tumor cannot be reached by the subchiasmatic approach. The lamina terminalis approach is selected if the tumor has pushed the chiasm into a prefixed position and stretches the lamina terminalis so that the tumor is visible through it. The transfrontal–trans-sphenoidal approach is selected if the tumor grows upward out of the sella, the sphenoid sinus is pneumatized, and the tumor does not stretch the lamina terminalis or widen the optico-carotid space, and a prefixed chiasm blocks the subchiasmatic exposure. A bifrontal craniotomy may be used if the tumor extends forward in both anterior cranial fossae. A frontal interhemispheric approach directed along the anterior part of the falx is used for lesions just below the rostrum.

The frontotemporal approach is used for a tumor arising from the sphenoid ridge or anterior clinoid process, or if it arises above the diaphragma and extends along the sphenoid ridge or into the middle cranial fossa, or if the lesion is accessible through the spaces between the optic nerve and carotid artery or between the carotid artery and the oculomotor nerve. The frontotemporal approach may be combined with a temporal lobectomy to expose lesions extending into the middle incisural space.

Middle Incisural Space

Approaches to the middle incisural space include the frontotemporal, subtemporal, temporal-transventricular, and lateral suboccipital routes. The subtemporal approach with elevation of the temporal lobe is commonly used to expose lesions in the cisterns around the incisura. Hemorrhage, venous infarction, and edema following retraction of the temporal lobe during this approach are minimized by avoiding occlusion of the bridging veins, especially the vein of Labbé. The tentorium is frequently divided to increase the exposure or to decompress the brain stem when mass lesions are impacted in the incisura. Resection of part of the parahippocampal gyrus facilitates exposure of the upper part of the middle incisural space.

A transventricular approach using a cortical incision in the nondominant inferior or middle temporal gyrus may be used if the lesion involves the temporal horn, choroidal fissure, hippocampal formation, or upper part of the middle incisural space. A cortical incision directed through a sulcus on the inferior surface of the temporal lobe has been used to minimize visual and speech deficits in exposing the temporal horn of the dominant hemisphere. After entering the temporal horn, the choroidal fissure is opened to expose the mid-

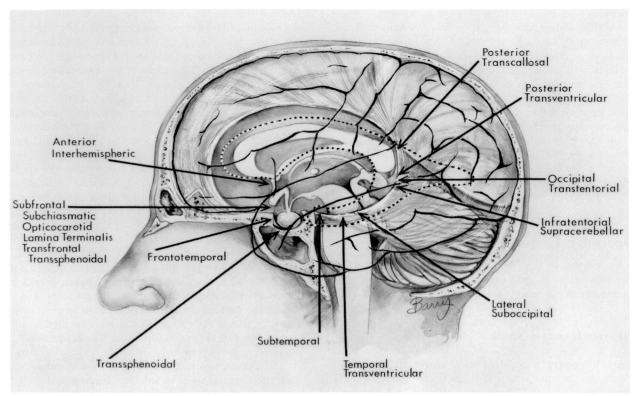

A

Figure 40-8 Lateral (*A*) and superior (*B*) views to show the operative approaches to the anterior, middle, and posterior incisural spaces. In the lateral view, the major cerebral fissures and sulci are shown on the surface, and the lateral (*dotted lines*) and third ventricles are shown in the deep areas. In the superior view, the cerebral hemisphere has been removed on the right side, and on the left side, the internal capsule (Int. Cap.), frontal horn (Front. Horn), thalamus, and caudate nucleus (Caudate Nucl.) are shown above the incisura. The approaches to the anterior incisural space are the anterior interhemispheric, trans-sphenoidal, subfrontal, and frontotemporal. The subfrontal route is divided into four different approaches: the lamina terminalis approach through the lamina terminalis, the opticocarotid approach through the opticocarotid triangle, the subchiasmatic approach below the optic chiasm between the optic nerves, and the transfrontal–trans-sphenoidal approach through the planum sphenoidale and the sphenoid sinus. The approaches to the middle incisural space are the subtemporal, temporal transventricular, and the lateral suboccipital. The operative approaches to the posterior incisural space are the posterior transcallosal, posterior transventricular, occipital transtentorial, and the infratentorial supracerebellar. (From Ono et al.[7])

dle incisural space.[12] The subtemporal craniectomy may be combined with a suboccipital craniectomy with sectioning of the tentorium and transverse sinus to remove lesions in the prepontine or cerebellopontine cisterns. The trochlear nerve is the cranial nerve most frequently injured in the middle incisural space. It can be injured in dividing the free edge and is so thin and friable that it may rupture from gentle retraction on the leaves formed by dividing the tentorium.

The posterior trigeminal root is frequently exposed through a lateral suboccipital craniectomy in the infratentorial part of the middle incisural space for rhizotomy or microvascular decompression operations. The exposure is di-

rected along the angle formed by the insertion of the tentorium to the petrous ridge. The posterior root proximal to Meckel's cave may also be exposed through a subtemporal craniectomy combined with incision of the tentorium.

Posterior Incisural Space

Lesions in the posterior incisural space or pineal region may be approached from above the tentorium using an occipital transtentorial approach directed along the medial surface of

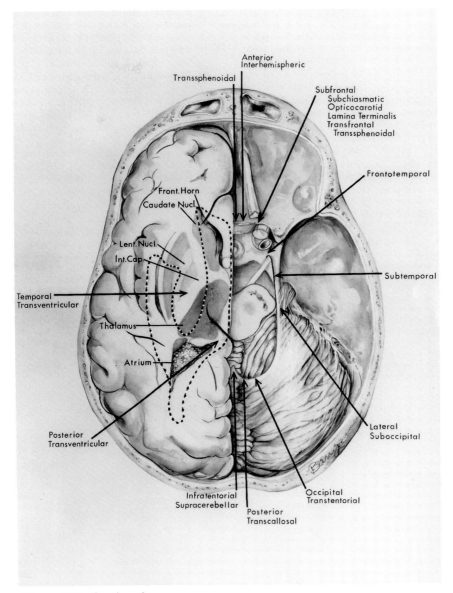

Figure 40-8   Continued

the occipital lobe; a posterior transventricular approach directed through the superior parietal lobule, atrium, and choroidal fissure; or a posterior interhemispheric transcallosal approach directed through the corpus callosum. They may also be approached from below the tentorium through an infratentorial supracerebellar approach directed between the tentorium and cerebellum. The infratentorial supracerebellar and occipital transtentorial approaches, which are most commonly selected for pineal tumors, may be combined with incision of the tentorium lateral to the straight sinus. Venous sinuses are more commonly encountered in the posterior than in the anterior parts of the tentorium. Part of the tentorium may be removed in resecting tumors that arise from or invade it.

The infratentorial supracerebellar approach is best suited to tumors that depress the quadrigeminal plate and elevate the great vein and are situated in the midline in the lower half of the posterior incisural space.[10,14] The occipital transtentorial approach is preferred for lesions centered at or above the tentorial edge and for those located above the vein of Galen. The posterior transcallosal approach, in which the splenium is divided, would be used only if the lesion appears to arise in the splenium above the vein of Galen and extends into the posterior incisural space. The posterior transventricular approach directed through the superior parietal lobule provides adequate exposure of the atrium and would be the preferred approach to a tumor that extends into the posterior incisural space from the atrium.

References

1. Fox JL. Tentorial section for decompression of the brain stem and a large basilar aneurysm: case report. *J Neurosurg* 1968; 28:74–77.
2. Hardy DG, Peace DA, Rhoton AL Jr. Microsurgical anatomy of the superior cerebellar artery. *Neurosurgery* 1980; 6:10–28.
3. Howell DA. Upper brain-stem compression and foraminal impaction with intracranial space-occupying lesions and brain swelling. *Brain* 1959; 82:525–550.
4. Klintworth GK. The comparative anatomy and phylogeny of the tentorium cerebelli. *Anat Rec* 1968; 160:635–641.
5. Klintworth GK. Paratentorial grooving of human brains with particular reference to transtentorial herniation and the pathogenesis of secondary brain-stem hemorrhages. *Am J Pathol* 1968; 53:391–408.
6. Mastri AR. Brain herniations: section I. Pathology. In: Newton TH, Potts DG (eds.), *Radiology of the Skull and Brain: Angiography.* Vol. 2, book 4. St. Louis: Mosby, 1974:2659–2670.
7. Ono M, Ono M, Rhoton AL Jr, et al. Microsurgical anatomy of the region of the tentorial incisura. *J Neurosurg* 1984; 60:365–399.
8. Plaut HF. Size of the tentorial incisura related to cerebral herniation. *Acta Radiol (Diagn)* 1963; 1:916–928.
9. Rhoton AL Jr, Hardy DG, Chambers SM. Microsurgical anatomy and dissection of the sphenoid bone, cavernous sinus and sellar region. *Surg Neurol* 1979; 12:63–104.
10. Rhoton AL Jr, Yamamoto I, Peace DA. Microsurgery of the third ventricle: part 2. Operative approaches. *Neurosurgery* 1981; 8:357–373.
11. Saeki N, Rhoton AL Jr. Microsurgical anatomy of the upper basilar artery and the posterior circle of Willis. *J Neurosurg* 1977; 46:563–578.
12. Schnürer LB, Stattin S. Vascular supply of intracranial dura from internal carotid artery with special reference to its angiographic significance. *Acta Radiol (Diagn)* 1963; 1:441–450.
13. Sunderland S. The tentorial notch and complications produced by herniations of the brain through that aperture. *Br J Surg* 1958; 45:422–438.
14. Timurkaynak E, Rhoton AL Jr, Barry M. Microsurgical anatomy and operative approaches to the lateral ventricles. *Neurosurgery* 1986; 19:685–723.
15. Weinstein M, Stein R, Pollock J, et al. Meningeal branch of the posterior cerebral artery. *Neuroradiology* 1974; 7:129–131.

41

Surgical Approaches to Pineal Tumors

Bennett M. Stein
Jeffrey N. Bruce
Michael R. Fetell

History

Walter Dandy was the first to make a concerted effort at operating on pineal region tumors with an attempt to extricate them.[2] He also did animal studies attempting to elucidate the function of the pineal gland. For the most part, Dandy's approach was supratentorial and parafalcine. The exact position of the head during this operative intervention is difficult to tell from his writings. It appears that some of his cases were done in a semisitting position and others were done with the hemisphere on the side of the approach up-

permost, retracting it against gravity. In any event, upon reaching the region of the pineal, this operative approach required sectioning the corpus callosum and dissecting the deep venous system, during which there was often venous damage and central cerebral edema. Without an operating microscope, steroids, and sophisticated anesthesia, the mortality rate was prohibitively high from these interventions. Other, just as illustrious, neurosurgeons at that time did not think that operative intervention for pineal tumors was feasible because of the technical difficulties encountered and the probability that many of these tumors were malignant and invasive and therefore could not be totally removed.

It is amazing that before Dandy's numerous efforts to surgically treat pineal tumors, Krause in 1926 operated on three patients with lesions in the area of the pineal gland which were probably astrocytomas (perhaps one was a teratoma).[4] He had no operative mortality, and the operations were done through the posterior fossa over the cerebellum. Considering the limited instrumentation, lack of microscope or good lighting, and borderline anesthesia, these must have been operative triumphs.

Since that time a number of different approaches have been advocated (Fig. 41-1) such as those around the occipital lobe and over the tentorium as advocated by Poppen.[9] The approach through a dilated lateral ventricle proposed by Van Wagenen was difficult and not adopted by neurosurgeons.[16]

Because of the continued difficulty in obtaining successful surgical results, a more conservative approach was advocated for the treatment of pineal area tumors.[1] This conservative approach consisted of a shunt for hydrocephalus and radiotherapy for presumed malignancy. Unfortunately, this resulted in numerous articles containing anecdotal information and a golden opportunity was lost to study in detail the natural history of the infinite types of pineal region tumors.

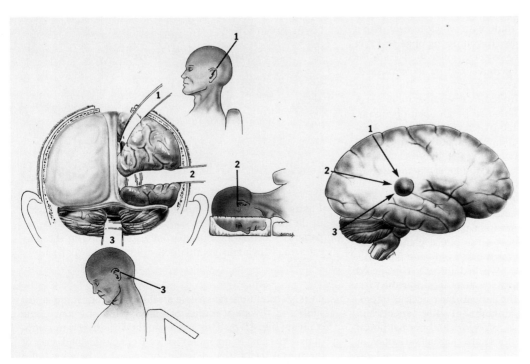

Figure 41-1 Illustration of the three basic routes to pineal region tumors: (1) the parafalx approach of Dandy; (2) the paraoccipital lobe, supratentorial approach of Poppen; (3) the infratentorial supracerebellar approach of Krause.

In the 1970s, interest in a direct surgical approach developed concomitant with the increasing use of the operative microscope.[5,7,10,12] The Japanese were active in this field, as were a number of American neurosurgeons. Debate raged as to the best surgical route to the pineal region.[10] The important issue, however, was not the route but the fact that the renewed interest in operating upon these tumors, identifying their nature, and removing the tumor wherever possible was brought about by this interest.[3,6,11,14] More recently, stereotactic biopsy has been advocated as a procedure preliminary to radiation, chemotherapy, or surgical removal, depending upon the nature of the tumor.[8]

It is generally agreed that the tumor types form a wide histologic variance, with some of the tumors being mixed in nature, containing benign elements as well as malignant elements. The diagnosis from small specimens is often difficult even for an experienced pathologist. It is also recognized that the combination of preoperative diagnostic tests cannot lead to accurate histologic typing before operative intervention.

Patient Selection

In over 100 cases of pineal region tumor which have been operated on, the age spectrum is broad, ranging from one patient 2 years of age to a number of patients in their 60s. The majority of the latter cases were meningiomas of the pineal region without dural attachment. We have seen as many patients over the age of 16 as we have under the age of 16.

The indications for operation are simple.[14] In all symptomatic patients or in patients who are asymptomatic but with aqueductal compromise and hydrocephalus, we advise operation. This is based on the assumption that the histologic diagnosis cannot be made without operation and that open operation provides the best route with which to deal with a tumor (removing it, if feasible). In comparing open or direct operation with stereotactic biopsy, we prefer the former for the following reasons: (1) If removal can be accomplished, then it is best done at the primary operation. (2) Bleeding, if it occurs, can be better controlled by open operation. (3) A sufficient specimen can be obtained by an open operation, where this may not be feasible by stereotactic biopsy. Frozen tissues are studied by both methods, but the larger specimen obtained by open surgery makes the identification easier for the neuropathologist. (4) With modern neurosurgical techniques, an open operation is reasonably safe.

With the increasing use of computed tomography (CT) scanning and especially magnetic resonance imaging (MRI), we are now encountering a group of patients, not insignificant in number, where lesions of the pineal gland are encountered which are for the most part cystic and contain a small amount of solid tissue. We had initially considered these to be low-grade cystic astrocytomas. The aqueduct has not been compromised, and the patients have been asymptomatic. We have operated on a number of these patients and found combinations of normal astrocytes and normal pineal cells. It is difficult to tell if these are normal variations of cystic change in the pineal gland or low-grade mixed tu-

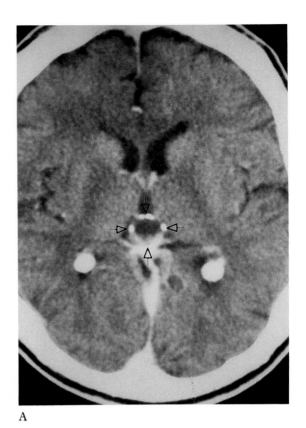

A

B

Figure 41-2 *A*. Axial enhanced CT scan showing a cyst in the pineal gland (*arrows*). *B*. Sagittal MRI view (same patient) showing a cystic, partially solid lesion in the pineal area, which was an enlarged cystic normal gland (*arrows*).

mors. A recent operative case established in our mind a possibility of a wide variation of pineal gland size and cystic content (Fig. 41-2). This was a patient with irrelevant symptoms who came to operation with a 1-cm cystic-solid mass of the pineal region that definitively proved to be a cyst of a normal gland. We are now looking at additional cases with a more conservative viewpoint. These are being followed by periodic MRI. This apparent variation on a normal gland has not been recognized through routine CT scanning.

As will be discussed later, the mortality has been most frequent with the highly cellular and extremely vascular malignant pineal cell tumors. These tend to hemorrhage spontaneously, and bleeding is difficult to control during the operative procedure, leading to postoperative hemorrhages. However, the technique of stereotactic biopsy in these cases would presumably also be associated with hemorrhage. If we could identify these tumors before operation, then we could avoid these complications. However, with our current diagnostic armamentarium, this has been impossible.

Diagnosis

The standard diagnostic workup includes a CT scan with and without contrast, an MRI scan, rarely arteriography, and measurement of biologic markers (beta human chorionic gonadotrophin, alpha fetoprotein, and carcinoembryonic antigen) from serum and CSF, if obtainable. The MRI has proven to be the most accurate diagnostic examination (Fig. 41-3) and provides information not only on the tumor type, but also on the anatomic relationships of the tumor. Angiography is only performed if the MRI suggests a vascular lesion such as a vein of Galen aneurysm or arteriovenous malformation (AVM) (Fig. 41-4A and B). Despite this broad diagnostic armamentarium, it is still difficult to determine the exact histologic nature of the tumor before operative exposure. However, some of the teratomas, especially those containing multiple germ layers, are suspected from the appearance of the scans (Fig. 41-5).

The diagnostic battery does provide relevant information about the following:

1. Size of tumor; lateral and superior extent.

2. Vascularity of the lesion and nature of its contents (whether homogeneous or heterogeneous).
3. Irregularities of margination and the probability of invasion.
4. Most importantly, the anatomic relationships of the tumor and surrounding structures. These include involvement of the third ventricle and position within the third ventricle, extension into or above the corpus callosum, superior or lateral extension to the region of the ventricular trigone, involvement or compression of the quadrigeminal region and aqueduct, and relationship to the anterior cerebellar vermis and medullary velum.

Anatomy

The vast majority of tumors arise and are attached to the undersurface of the velum interpositum, which includes choroid plexus, deep venous system, and choroidal arteries (Fig. 41-6). This attachment may be minimal or comprehensive, with the tumor invading these important midline structures. Rarely do the tumors extend above the velum interpositum for any significant distance. Therefore, the blood supply to the tumor comes from the arteries contained in the velum interpositum, mainly, the posterior medial and lateral choroidal arteries with an anastomosis to the pericallosal arteries and quadrigeminal arteries.

Some tumors extend to the foramen of Monro, but most are centered at the pineal gland and extend to the midportion of the third ventricle and posteriorly to compress the anterior portion of the cerebellum. In rare instances, the internal cerebral veins are ventral to the tumor, and this can be recognized through the MRI (Fig. 41-7). For the most part, the vein of Galen, internal cerebral veins, veins of Rosenthal, and precentral cerebellar vein surround or cap the periphery of these tumors. The quadrigeminal plate may give rise to an exophytic astrocytoma or be infiltrated by the more malignant tumors of the pineal region, encompassing

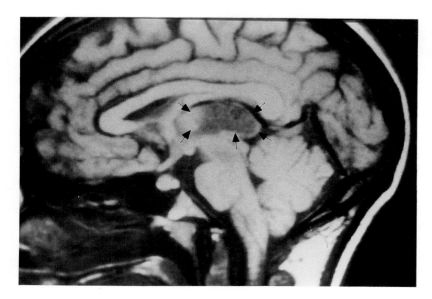

Figure 41-3 Sagittal MRI view showing a large pineal tumor (*arrows*). The anatomic relationships of the tumor are well identified, including the third ventricle, aqueduct, and quadrigeminal region.

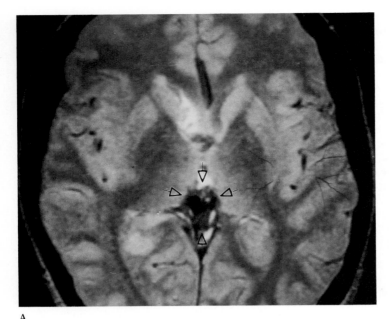

A

Figure 41-4 *A.* Axial MRI view showing typical signal voids of a vascular lesion (AVM) of the pineal region (*arrows*). *B.* Vertebral arteriogram, lateral view, showing the AVM (*arrow*) of the pineal region ventral to the vein of Galen and internal cerebral vein. This lesion was successfully removed via an infratentorial supracerebellar approach to the pineal region.

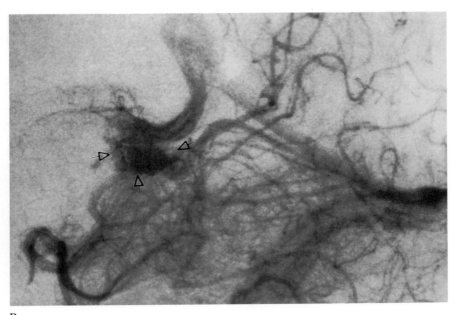

B

the aqueduct in the course of tumor growth. Tumors of this region are not highly vascular with the exception of the malignant pineocytoma, hemangioblastoma, and hemangiopericytoma or angioblastic meningioma.

The most important aspects of the anatomy as gleaned by the diagnostic scan screen are the relationship of the tumor to the third ventricle and quadrigeminal cistern, and the lateral and superior extent of the tumor. It is these features that determine the route of the operation and the degree of difficulty that may be assumed in the surgery.[17]

Surgery

The route which we prefer in most of the cases, with certain exceptions that will be discussed later, is that proposed by Krause through the posterior fossa over the cerebellum, the subtentorial supracerebellar approach to the pineal region.[13] The position of the patient is critical to the smooth performance of this operation. The patient's body in conforming to a C configuration is basically in a sitting-slouch position with the head flexed and held forward by a pin-vise type of head holder. The aim is to position the patient's tentorium as close to the horizontal as possible.

The operative microscope is essential to this operation because of the depth of the exposure and the need for magnification and excellent illumination. The angled eye pieces are reversed, and the objective used ranges between 275 mm and 300 mm, with the former being the most utilitarian. Armrests for the surgeon must be provided as the surgeon is seated during the operative procedure.

A midline incision is utilized, and a modest craniectomy not extending to the foramen magnum but extending at least to the upper edge of the transverse sinuses and torcular is performed. This is done in order to provide slight upward retraction upon the midline of the tentorium. If the patient has hydrocephalus, this must be relieved either by mannitol administration, a previous shunt insertion, or a ventricular drainage procedure. If the cerebellum is under pressure and the dura tense, the operation cannot be performed. The dura is opened in three-flap fashion with the central flap being the most important; it is reflected upward (Fig. 41-8). Assuming that decompression has been obtained upon opening the dura in the aforementioned fashion, the upper surface of the entire cerebellar hemispheres and vermis should be visible. In order to relax the cerebellum, it is necessary to cauterize and divide all of the bridging veins across the upper surface of the cerebellum. We have not encountered edema or permanent cerebellar damage from interrupting numerous bridging veins. Having accomplished this, the cerebellum will drop due to the action of gravity (Fig. 41-9). Telfa is placed over the superior surface of the cerebellum to protect it, and one retractor, self-retaining, is used over the vermis. It is necessary at this point to use the operative microscope, which is initially angled upward. An irrigating system using an 18–gauge spinal needle on the retractor arm is directed toward the pineal region and connected to a syringe with irrigating solution.

With the operative microscope in place, the rostral portion of the vermis is visualized (Fig. 41-10). The arachnoid of the quadrigeminal cistern is often thickened in the presence of tumor and must be opened widely. Caution is observed not to cut into the precentral cerebellar vein, which is usually in the midline, maybe rostral or caudal or maybe displaced to one or the other side, depending upon the configuration of the tumor. This vein is easily identified as the thickened arachnoid is opened. The arachnoid is opened close to the cerebellar edge, extending laterally and pursuing the free edge of the tentorial incisura. This will expose small arteries of the choroidal group supplying the posterior surface of the tumor and laterally the large veins of Rosenthal. Now the trajectory must be modified as the arachnoid is opened so as not to open the vein of Galen. The microscope is placed horizontally or angled slightly downward. Further opening of the arachnoid, use of the cautery, and division of the precentral cerebellar vein will expose the large posterior surface of the tumor; by opening the arachnoid further and cauterizing choroidal arteries to the tumor, this exposure is quite generous. The retractor is moved forward in order to retract the anterior vermis downward and posterior. If the tumor is large, the quadrigeminal plate will be obscured at

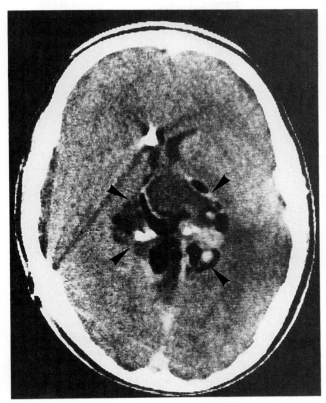

Figure 41-5 CT scan without contrast, axial view, showing the typical variegated pattern of a large benign teratoma of the pineal region (*arrows*).

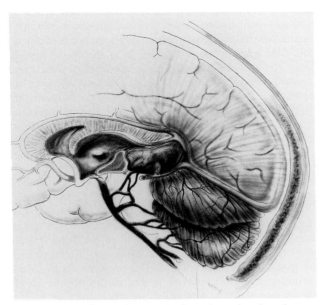

Figure 41-6 Illustration, sagittal section, showing the relationship of a typical pineal region tumor to the deep venous system, third ventricle, corpus callosum, and anterior cerebellum.

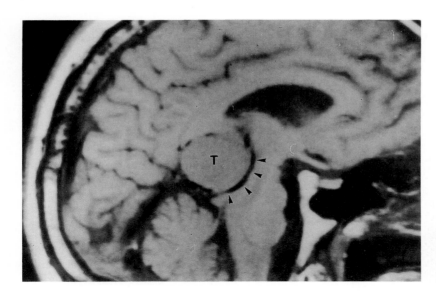

Figure 41-7 Sagittal MRI view, showing a large tumor (T) which was a meningioma situated dorsal to the internal cerebral veins (*arrows*).

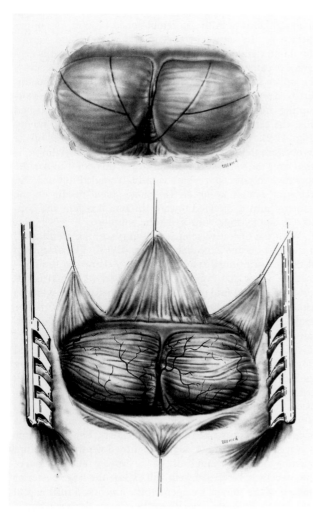

Figure 41-8 Illustration showing the pattern of the three-flap dural opening to maximize exposure of the superior cerebellum.

this point. The vascularity of the tumor is observed and biopsy taken for frozen tissue analysis. If the tumor is cystic, it may be evacuated to further decompress the area. Now the surgeon studies the encapsulation of the tumor. If a further superior view is required, then a retractor is placed under the tentorium and elevated slightly with a self-retaining system.

Work on the tumor may now commence. We have selected the usual group of instruments. However, they have been modified to longer than normal. These include cautery forceps, dissectors, suction tips, the long curved tip of the ultrasonic aspirator, and tumor forceps; trans-sphenoidal instruments are useful. Depending upon the nature of the tumor, it may be internally decompressed through the use of tumor forceps, suction, cautery, or the ultrasonic aspirator. Gradually with the decompression, if the tumor is encapsulated, the margins may be folded in to the decompressed area. The superior borders are often adherent, sometimes invading the velum interpositum. Care must be taken to cauterize and divide these connections so as not to injure the deep venous system. Inferiorly, the quadrigeminal plate tends to remain obscure and is difficult to expose or dissect from the tumor. This is because gravity is now working against the surgeon, and he or she must lift the tumor either with suction or tumor forceps and develop this plane if feasible. Finally, as much as possible, if not all, of the tumor is removed, exposing the interior of the dilated third ventricle (Fig. 41-11). The tumor may be attached to the wall of the third ventricle, representing the medial nuclei of the thalamus and the pulvinar. Occasionally there is a dense attachment to the quadrigeminal plate. However, in benign and encapsulated tumors, this is rarely a problem. At the completion of surgery, hemostasis is secured through the use of the various hemostatic agents as well as cautery.

The dura is closed and attempts made to seal the dura so that CSF will not accumulate extradurally and form a pseudomeningocele, a frequent complication to posterior fossa surgery. The muscles and fascia are closed in appropriate

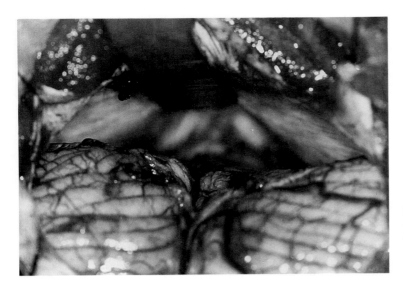

Figure 41-9 Operative photograph showing the space attained in the sitting position when all of the veins over the dorsal surface of the cerebellum are interrupted. The cerebellar hemispheres and vermis fall by gravity.

layers over a drain which is left in place for approximately 12 h. If the patient has undergone ventricular drainage, this is continued. However, in most cases, the patient has been shunted previously. In some cases the removal of a modest-sized encapsulated tumor will open the CSF pathways. The patient is extubated and goes to the intensive care unit in a semisitting position.

The advantages of the infratentorial supracerebellar approach are the following:

1. The approach is to the center of the tumor, which begins in the midline and grows eccentrically.
2. The approach is ventral to the velum interpositum and the deep venous system to which the tumor is often adherent. This avoids, for the most part, the drainage to this critical vascular region.

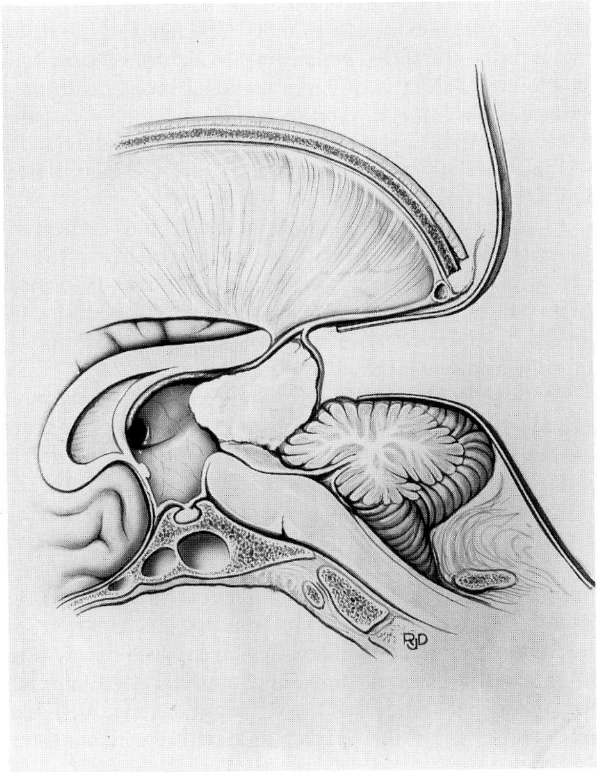

Figure 41-10 Illustration, sagittal view, showing a pineal region tumor being approached by an infratentorial supracerebellar route. Only two retractors are necessary, one on the cerebellum and one against the undersurface of the tentorium.

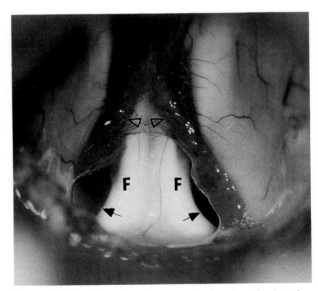

Figure 41-11 Operative photograph showing the interior of the third ventricle after total removal of a benign pineal tumor. The foramina of Monro (*closed arrows*), choroid plexus (*open arrows*), and the fornices (F) are indicated.

3. The exposure in the sitting position is comparable to that of other routes.

4. No normal tissue is violated en route to tumor.

5. If the tumor is not completely removed, a catheter can be left from the opening in the third ventricle over the cerebellum to the cisterna magna as a modified Torkildsen's procedure. If the incisura is not blocked by tumor, this may be sufficient to control hydrocephalus.

We utilize alternative approaches under the following circumstances (Figs. 41-1 and 41-12):

1. Tumors which extend superiorly, involving or destroying the posterior aspect of the corpus callosum and deflecting the deep venous system in a dorsolateral direction

2. Tumors which extend laterally to the region of the trigone

3. In rare cases where the tumor displaces the deep venous system in a ventral direction

As noted, the limitations of the posterior fossa approach are primarily related to the size of the tumor and its extension to superolateral areas that are hard to reach from the infratentorial exposure. In these instances, we prefer a modification of the classic Dandy approach. The patient is operated on in the sitting-slouch position with an approach from the nondominant posterior parietal region. The hemisphere is separated from the superior sagittal sinus and from the falx. The trajectory is toward the apex of the tentorium and posterior portion of the corpus callosum. With large tumors in which this route is used, the corpus callosum is generally thin and is resected over an area of about 2 cm from its posterior aspect. This allows visibility to the dorsal surface of the tumor. If the tumor extends into the posterior fossa,

the tentorium is incised directly from the leading edge posteriorly to the limit of the tumor. On some occasions, to reach the side opposite to the exposure, a suture placed through the tentorium adjacent to the straight sinus is used to rotate the straight sinus and tentorium so that the opposite portion of the tumor may be visualized. When this approach is used for large tumors, the deep venous system is generally displaced laterally to the region of the trigone. However, it may be necessary to divide one of the internal cerebral veins. At its best, this exposure provides a comprehensive view of the entire roof of the third ventricle, laterally to both trigones as well as to the posterior fossa in the region of the anterior medullary velum. We have utilized this exposure in about 5 percent of the tumors in the pineal region.

We have not used the occipital pole approach as advocated by Clark and others.[5,10] This approach appears to afford adequate visualization of the pineal region. However, we are concerned about the number of instances of homonymous hemianopsia from retraction of the occipital lobe and the fact that the exposure is eccentric to the bulk of the tumor and often requires sectioning of the tentorium.

Complications of Surgery

The majority of complications encountered, whatever route is utilized, are related primarily to the nature of the tumor and its potential for intra- or postoperative hemorrhage. We have found hemorrhage to be most common with the malignant pineal cell tumors, which are also associated with "pineal apoplexy," that is, preinterventional spontaneous hemorrhage. These tumors tend to be soft and highly vascular. Hemostasis is difficult to obtain both at operation and in the postoperative period. Operative mortality has been related basically to this issue.

In terms of complications from the various routes, the posterior fossa operation that we use, invariably in the sitting position, can be associated with all the complications of surgery in the sitting position, including air embolism, hypotension, and cortical collapse when hydrocephalus of significant degree is relieved by tumor removal.

We have had two unusual and unexpected complications related to the cervical spinal cord and indirectly to the flexed position of the head on the neck in the sitting position. The first occurred in a young male patient who had been in a minor automobile accident 6 weeks prior to pineal surgery. A postinjury CT scan taken for the evaluation of persistent headache had disclosed a pineal tumor, and he was referred for operation. There were no complaints of neck pain. Postoperatively, the patient had a permanent quadriplegia. Initial studies including plain and flexion/extension x-ray films of the spine and a myelogram failed to reveal any abnormalities. It was only when a CT scan was performed that fractures were noted in the pedicles and laminae which presumably compressed the spinal cord in a flexed posture resulting in spinal cord ischemia. These fractures with displacement reoriented upon straightening of the spine. The second complication occurred in an individual with an AVM of the pineal gland in which the same position was utilized. The patient awoke with a quadriparesis presumably due to spinal

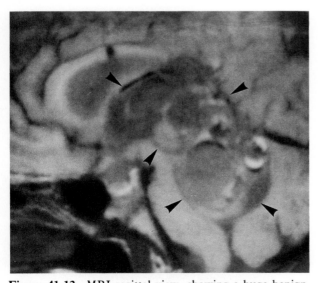

Figure 41-12 MRI sagittal view, showing a huge benign teratoma (*arrowheads*) of the pineal region extending superiorly, inferiorly, and laterally. This tumor must be approached by a supratentorial route to maximize exposure. Utilizing this route, this large tumor was totally removed and the patient cured.

cord stretching related to the intraoperative posture. Postoperative MRI was negative. Fortunately, this patient recovered completely within a week of the surgery. It would be difficult to avoid this complication, which occurs very rarely during numerous posterior fossa operations done in the sitting position with similar postures.

The problem of cortical collapse when high-grade hydrocephalus exists is a well-recognized one whenever patients are operated on in the sitting position. The only way we can conceive of reducing this complication is by preoperative shunting to allow the ventricular system to accommodate during a 1- to 2-week period before the major operation. When the phenomenon does occur, it may be of different degrees and, although striking on the postoperative CT scan, will gradually improve without major neurologic complication for the patient. It is rare that subdural shunting is required to relieve chronic hygromas resulting from this complication.

The complications of the paraparietal interhemispheric approach are related to the retraction of the parietal lobe with transient sensory or stereognostic deficits on the opposite side. These have not been serious or permanent. There have been no visual field defects. Manipulation in the environs of the third ventricle, diencephalon, and midbrain has led to impairment of consciousness and to extraocular movement derangements, but most of these complications have faded, and the patients have had no permanent deficits.

Whatever operative approach is used, when the dissection is carried out to remove the tumor from the quadrigeminal region, there may be various pupillary abnormalities, difficulty focusing or accommodating, and interocular palsies and limitation of upward gaze. These deficits improve gradually but may last for many months or for up to a year before the patient functions in a normal fashion. The fourth cranial nerve is generally caudal to the tumor and is rarely identified. However, of all the cranial nerves in the region, it is the closest, and injury may result in a specific extraocular palsy.

Ataxia has been minimal. Continued obstruction to the ventricular system is handled easily by a postoperative shunt.

Postoperative Management of Pineal Tumors

Following an operative procedure on a pineal region tumor and the identification of the tumor type, other studies are necessary to gauge possible tumor seeding (Fig. 41-13). This is most commonly seen in the malignant variety of tumors including pineocytoma, ependymoma, germinoma, and malignant germ cell tumors (embryonal carcinoma, choriocarcinoma, yolk sac tumor). When these tumors are identified, our protocol calls for a postoperative thoracic lumbosacral myelogram and a cytologic examination of the spinal fluid. If the biologic markers are abnormally elevated (this occurs rarely), then the elevation of these markers is utilized to gauge the effectiveness of therapy.

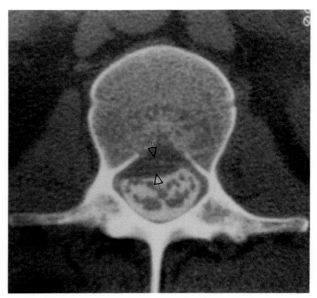

Figure 41-13 Lumbar CT scan after a myelogram, axial view, showing a metastatic deposit (*arrows*) from a malignant pineocytoma.

Most tumors except for the embryonal group are subjected to radiation therapy.[15] Standard therapy calls for 5500 rad to the tumor area and third ventricle and 3500 rad to the ventricular system, which includes most of the cerebral hemispheres. Radiation of the spinal region is reserved for those cases in which cytology or myelography is positive for tumor seeding. Chemotherapy is reserved for those tumors of the primitive germ cell group. Since some tumors may be a mixture such as benign teratoma with a small inclusion of malignancy, detailed and comprehensive evaluation of the specimen is necessary to determine the appropriate mode of therapy. One of our cases was interpreted as a germinoma. Radiation to the entire neuraxis was given. The patient returned with massive seeding and recurrence. The tumor was now an embryonal carcinoma. The radiation had eliminated the germinoma, while a small nidus of embryonal carcinoma (tumor more appropriately treated by chemotherapy) was permitted to run rampant.

Results

In 110 cases, there have been 3 deaths. Morbidity has been minor and usually temporary.

The most common tumors are astrocytoma (all grades) and germinoma. There is a 10 percent incidence of meningiomas without dural attachment and a 30 percent incidence of benign resectable tumors.

On the basis of this experience, we advocate surgery on all pineal region tumors with removal of benign encapsulated tumors and debulking of malignant tumors. Large specimens are necessary for accurate histologic typing. Ad-

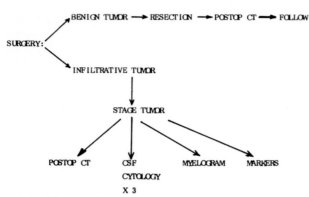

Figure 41-14 The progressive evaluation of pineal region tumors.

ditional therapy is determined from analysis of postoperative tumor staging (Fig. 41-14).

References

1. Abay EO II, Laws ER Jr, Grado GL, et al. Pineal tumors in children and adolescents: treatment by CSF shunting and radiotherapy. *J Neurosurg* 1981; 55:889–895.
2. Dandy WE. Operative experience in cases of pineal tumor. *Arch Surg* 1936; 33:19–46.
3. Fetell MR, Stein BM. Therapy of pineal region tumors. *Neurology* 1984; 34(Suppl 1):185 (abstr.).
4. Krause F. Operative Frielegung der Vierhügel, nebst Beobachtungen über Hirndruck und Dekompression. *Zentralbl Chir* 1926; 53:2812–2819.
5. Lazar ML, Clark K. Direct surgical management of masses in the region of the vein of Galen. *Surg Neurol* 1974; 2:17–21.
6. Neuwelt EA. The challenge of pineal region tumors. In: Neuwelt EA (ed.), *The Diagnosis and Treatment of Pineal Region Tumors*. Baltimore: Williams & Wilkins, 1984:1–30.
7. Page LK. The infratentorial-supracerebellar exposure of tumors in the pineal area. *Neurosurgery* 1977; 1:36–40.
8. Pecker J, Scarabin JM, Vallee B, et al. Treatment in tumours of the pineal region: value of stereotaxic biopsy. *Surg Neurol* 1979; 12:341–348.
9. Poppen JL. The right occipital approach to a pinealoma. *J Neurosurg* 1966; 25:706–710.
10. Reid WS, Clark WK. Comparison of the infratentorial and transtentorial approaches to the pineal region. *Neurosurgery* 1978; 3:1–8.
11. Sano K. Pineal region tumors: problems in pathology and treatment. *Clin Neurosurg* 1983; 30:59–91.
12. Stein BM. The infratentorial supracerebellar approach to pineal lesions. *J Neurosurg* 1971; 35:197–202.
13. Stein BM. Supracerebellar approach for pineal region neoplasms. In: Schmidek HH, Sweet WH (eds.), *Operative Neurosurgical Techniques: Indications, Methods, and Results*. New York: Grune & Stratton, 1983:599–607.
14. Stein BM, Fetell MR. Therapeutic modalities for pineal region tumors. *Clin Neurosurg* 1985; 32:445–455.
15. Sung DI, Harisliadis L, Chang CH. Midline pineal tumors and suprasellar germinomas: highly curable by irradiation. *Radiology* 1978; 128:745–751.
16. Van Wagenen WP. A surgical approach for the removal of certain pineal tumors: report of a case. *Surg Gynecol Obstet* 1931; 53:216–220.
17. Yamamoto I, Kageyama N. Microsurgical anatomy of the pineal region. *J Neurosurg* 1980; 53:205–221.

42

Surgical Approaches to Tentorial Meningiomas

Leonard I. Malis

Categorization of tentorial meningiomas depends to a large extent on the somewhat arbitrary choices of the authors.[1,3-6] I have chosen to limit the groups to those tumors with their largest attachment on the tentorium. This would apparently put one angle meningioma in the tentorial group, with another in the petrosal group on the basis of a centimeter or so of dural involvement, while both lesions have their total bulk in the cerebellopontine angle. One might count both tumors again in a review of angle meningiomas. As long as the factors are clear, this is presumably reasonable. With this acceptance of overlapping groups, I have divided tentorial meningiomas into six major groups.

Parasellar Tentorial Meningiomas

These tumors arise on the anterior extension of the tentorium along the cavernous sinus to the anterior clinoid. The evaluation of this group of tumors requires angiographic study of the carotid artery, which may be engulfed, and coronal thin-section computed tomography (CT) scanning with the bone algorithm to demonstrate the extent of hyperostosis. This may indicate bony reaction on the medial side of the cavernous sinus extending into the sphenoid sinus and show that the lesion is curable only by resecting the cavernous sinus and its neural structures. If the carotid is completely invaded but not occluded, the other carotid and the posterior communicating arteries are required to carry the circulation if the involved carotid is resected. In addition, a decision as to whether the patient is ready to accept a complete ophthalmoplegia with a permanently closed, useless eye, even though vision is preserved, will determine the possibility of complete resection. If the anterior tentorial tumor involves only the lateral wall of the cavernous sinus and does not involve the medial dura, the problem is easier.[2]

I have preferred to operate upon these cases through a supine oblique position with the head rotated a little farther so that it approaches 60 degrees. A wide opening of the sylvian arachnoid is carried out with the dissection carried across to the opposite side over the chiasm. This allows free cerebrospinal fluid drainage, a good deal of room, and virtually no need for retraction. The dissection is then carried along the carotid artery anteriorly and posteriorly, and the tumor is cored progressively through this approach. As the cavernous sinus is opened, the interior is filled with Gelfoam to collapse the sinusoids and to control all bleeding as well as to preserve the neural structures. Following posteriorly, the tentorial margin is divided as the extension of the remainder of the tumor is lifted out, generally from its position against the third nerve and the superior cerebellar and posterior communicating arteries.

The fourth nerve will ordinarily be deviated medially by this tumor and may be preserved, but it also can be totally engulfed, in which case it will be virtually impossible to not resect the fourth and still achieve a complete tumor removal. An isolated fourth nerve deficit is usually of little disturbance to the patient, and it is usually compensated by an automatic tilting of the head to the side, of which the patient is generally unaware. For a few patients, the diplopia on downward gaze is annoying and for them muscle recession can usually provide adequate relief. Meningiomas of this group generally push the 5th nerve fibers downward and rarely involve the surface of Meckel's cave. When the meningioma has extended from the dura of the temporal floor to involve the upper layer of Meckel's cave, it too may be resected with preservation of the neural fibers. In a few cases, the tumor extension does not go all the way to the free margin of the tentorium, but it would appear that division at this point avoids the possibility of compression by the remaining band if there is any postoperative swelling.

Petroclivotentorial Meningiomas

These are a separate group, generally considered as petroclival although they virtually always involve a significant amount of the free margin of the tentorium and the medial part of the attachment of the leaf to the petrous bone.[2] I prefer to approach these lesions, which can be quite formidable, through a petrosal approach. An absolute requirement is the demonstration of patency of both transverse sinuses and the torcular (Figs. 42-1 to 42-3). Like the angle tumors, I have preferred to do these in the semisitting position. I still find this advantageous, although many surgeons have given up the semisitting position in favor of the supine oblique or park bench position. A posterior fossa lateral craniectomy including the mastoid process is carried across the sigmoid and lateral sinuses, and then a temporal flap is turned against the floor. The dura is opened in the posterior and middle fossae to the junction of the lateral and sigmoid sinus, and the junction is doubly ligated and divided. The tentorium is then divided along the line of the petrosal sinus parallel to the petrous ridge, and the free margin is divided medial to the fourth nerve. The tentorium can now be elevated with the broad self-retaining brain retractor, lifting the posterior temporal lobe with the vein of Labbé intact, draining into the medial part of the lateral

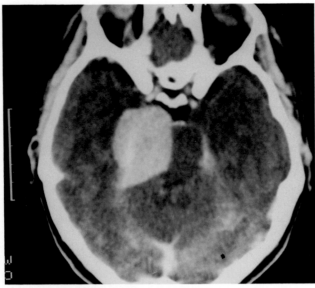

Figure 42-1 CT scan shows a tentorial meningioma extending up under the temporal lobe over the petrous apex. This type of tumor is usually best resected through a combined temporal and suboccipital petrosal approach.

sinus and through the torcular to the opposite lateral sinus and sigmoid and down through the opposite jugular vein. This prevents involvement or obstruction of the vein of Labbé, the one vein which virtually never can be safely resected.

The tentorial involvement in these tumors tends to be on the anterior medial margin, approaching the area where the previously discussed parasellar tentorial tumors involve the tentorial extension along the cavernous sinus to the carotid artery and anterior clinoid. After the exposure has been completed and the retractor placed under the tentorium, the posterior portion of the tentorial involvement is resected;

the major tumor lies against the clivus and medial petrous pyramid, where it may be progressively cored and resected, freeing it from the basilar artery and the clival dura (Figs. 42-4 and 42-5).

This part of the tumor generally receives a major blood supply from anteriorly through meningohypophyseal or tentoriomeningeal vessels, which can be readily coagulated when visualized after coring, surprisingly giving little problem during coring. For that portion extending upward into the cavernous sinus, the same considerations apply as discussed in the parasellar group. The entrance of the superior petrosal sinus to the cavernous sinus may require a clip at this point, particularly if it is widened. Inserting a piece of Gelfoam or Surgicel into the sinus opening so that a portion remains outside of the petrosal sinus gives a secure closure when the clip is then applied.

Angle Meningiomas

These tumors tend to arise from one of three locations: most common is the dural area and petrous bone between the entrance to Meckel's cave and the internal auditory meatus; next is the area superior to the internal auditory meatus; and least common is the area between the internal auditory meatus and the jugular foramen. This last group rarely involves the tentorium, though the first two groups almost invariably do.

I expose them by a laterally placed posterior fossa craniectomy, including the mastoid process and crossing the sigmoid sinus. The medially based semicircular dural incision is combined with two lateral relaxing incisions that are brought to the sigmoid sinus. Traction sutures through the lateral dural tab are sewn to the adjacent muscles, drawing the sigmoid sinus over the cut surface of the mastoid and providing a direct exposure along the petrous surface (Fig. 42-6). The facial, auditory, and vestibular nerves will regu-

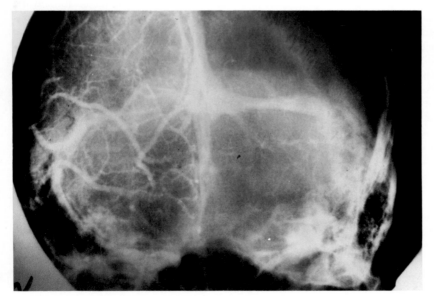

Figure 42-2 Same case as Fig. 42-1. The venous phase of the angiogram demonstrates absence of the drainage from the right transverse sinus to the torcular. For the petrosal approach with ligation of the transverse sinus at its junction with the sigmoid sinus, the vein of Labbé must be able to drain through the medial transverse sinus across the torcular and down the opposite side. This could not occur in this case, therefore precluding the approach with ligation.

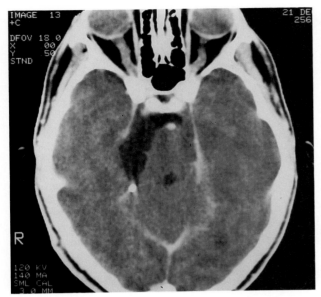

Figure 42-3 Same case as Figs. 42-1 and 42-2. CT scan 4 days after operation. Fortunately, complete removal could be achieved through a lateral suboccipital (angle) approach alone with resection of the tentorial leaf from below.

larly be pushed backward and downward by these tumors, depressed to contact the ninth and tenth nerves at the jugular foramen, with the anterior inferior cerebellar artery displaced tightly between the eighth and ninth nerves in those cases. Most of the blood supply will come from the petrous vessels, branches of the ascending pharyngeal and preauricular arteries. Coring of the tumor against the petrous bone will divide most of this blood supply and permit the tumor to be debulked and its capsule removed, clearing it to the surface of the invaded tentorium (Fig. 42-7). Hyperostotic

petrous bone below the tentorial attachment is carved away with a high speed diamond drill, avoiding the labyrinth if the patient is not already deaf, with particular care if the extension is anterior to protect the intrapetrous carotid artery. Any mastoid cells or middle ear connections opened in this drilling are closed with subcutaneous fat harvested from the lower end of the skin incision, which usually provides sufficient tissue. Of course, abdominal or other fat can be used in particularly thin individuals who have little subcutaneous fat in the neck.

After this has been accomplished, the tentorium may be divided around the margin of the tumor and bone from below. Extension of the tumor above the tentorium, usually quite small, can be separated from the undersurface of the occipital lobe and the tumor reflected downward along the line of the petrosal sinus. Here the petrosal sinus is fairly regularly involved with tumor and can be coagulated along the petrous ridge and stripped from this area up to pass the anterior extent of the tumor, which may cross over Meckel's cave to reach the cavernous sinus or may end anywhere in between. A single titanium clip may be necessary on the anterior part of the petrosal sinus after it has been divided. The petrosal vein and the vein of the lateral recess are virtually always part of the dissection of this tumor and are resected with it, although unlike the vein of Labbé, these veins have a very adequate collateral circulation and their sacrifice gives no problem (Fig. 42-8).

Tentorial Leaf Meningiomas

The meningiomas involving the tentorial leaf itself are the easiest to deal with. Depending upon their size and direction of extension they can be operated upon either from above or from below or both. Most of them appear to be somewhat larger in the posterior fossa than above the tentorium. Poste-

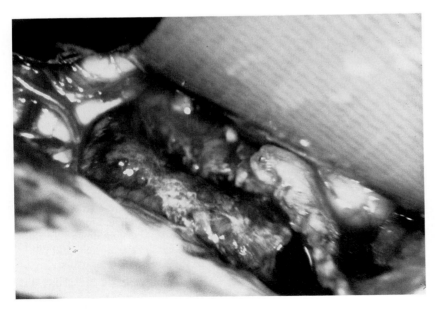

Figure 42-4 Right side, vertex up. Photographed field diameter, 2.4 cm. A petroclivotentorial meningioma involving the petrous apex and clivus on the right side has been approached with a combined suboccipital and subtemporal exposure with division of the lateral sinus at its junction with the sigmoid. The tentorium has been divided just medial to the superior petrosal sinus. The retractor supporting the temporal lobe and tentorium fills the right upper corner of the picture, while the cut edge of the tentorium is visible extending downward to the right from the middle of the retractor blade. The tumor fills the area to the left of the tentorium, whereas the upper surface of the cerebellum and remaining tentorium can be seen to the left lower corner. The upper pons is to the left upper corner.

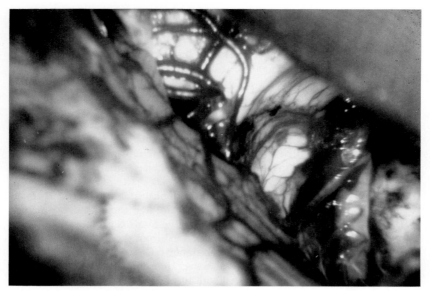

Figure 42-5 Same case as Fig. 42-4. The tumor has been removed. The basilar artery runs upward near the right lower corner of the photograph with the superior cerebellar artery curving downward and backward. The superior surface of the cerebellum fills the left lower half of the photograph. The fourth nerve crosses another branch of the superior cerebellar artery about the center of the photograph.

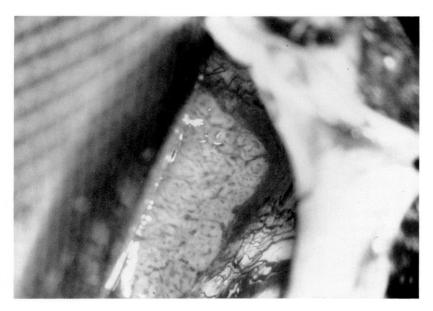

Figure 42-6 Vertex up; photographed field diameter, 2.4 cm. The right cerebellopontine angle has been exposed laterally. The retractor is to the left. The surface of a fungating meningioma fills the angle between the tentorium and the petrous dura with a congerie of small vessels on the dural and tentorial surfaces.

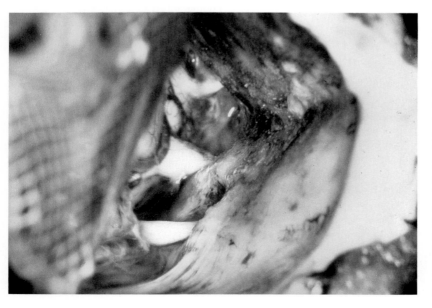

Figure 42-7 Same case as Fig. 42-6. The tumor has been removed, the facial and auditory nerves form a white band below the center of the picture entering the widely open internal auditory canal, from which a tongue of tumor has been removed. The seventh and eighth nerves are depressed against the arachnoid covering the anterior inferior cerebellar artery and the ninth nerve. Just anteriorly and superiorly, the fifth nerve can be seen entering Meckel's cave, where it also has been pushed downward. The fourth nerve can be seen just curving down past the tentorial edge. The tentorium and region of the superior petrosal sinus are covered with a thin layer of coagulated neoplasm.

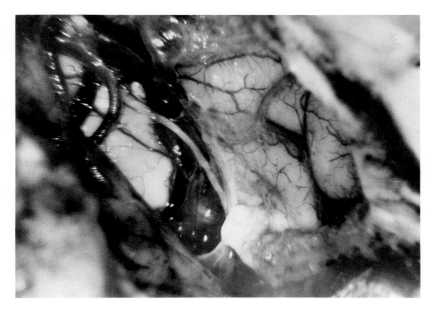

Figure 42-8 Vertex up; photographed field diameter, 2.4 cm. Right upper portion of the cerebellopontine angle. An angle meningioma has been resected. The retractor has been removed, and the cerebellum has dropped to the left and medially. The tentorial leaf has been resected through the free margin along the line of the superior petrosal sinus, which runs forward in the right lower corner. The undersurface of the temporo-occipital cortex is visible through the cut tentorium to the right, while the fourth nerve runs diagonally across between the cerebellum and the brain stem over the posterior cerebral and superior cerebellar arteries.

rior lesions may involve the lateral sinus, which may require resection. This is no problem if the sinus is totally occluded or even if patent though involved. If the torcular and the opposite lateral and sigmoid sinus are patent, resection of one lateral sinus is well tolerated (Fig. 42-9).

Tentorial Apex Meningiomas

Some of these tumors are relatively small, arising unilaterally at the apex of the tentorial notch, without involvement of any major venous structure. Such tumors may be resected quite readily from below after dividing the superior cerebellar veins bilaterally and allowing the cerebellum to drop

downward with the patient in the sitting position. The tumor and tentorial attachment may then be resected from below (Figs. 42-10 to 42-13).

These tumors are frequently bilateral and involve the junction of the falx and tentorium at the confluence of the vein of Galen and the straight sinus, often involving the precentral cerebellar veins and the veins of Rosenthal. Angiographic evaluation is required in order to demonstrate the patency of the various structures and the directions of the collateral, which determines what can or cannot be removed. Most often in these lesions, the straight sinus is completely occluded and drainage is through anterior collaterals.

I have preferred to approach such lesions with a bilateral occipital craniotomy. I have generally turned a unilateral free flap from the torcular upward, just lateral to the sagittal

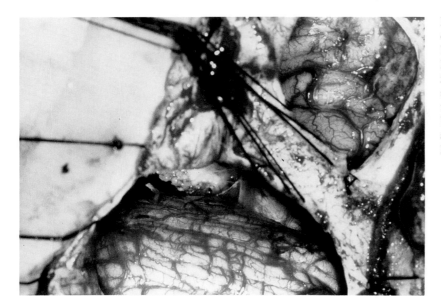

Figure 42-9 Photographed field diameter, 10 cm. A posterior exposure has been carried from the superior cerebellum up over the occipital lobe, and the invaded transverse sinus has traction sutures passed through it. The supratentorial portion of the meningioma has been resected. The transverse sinus and the involved posterolateral tentorial leaf will be resected.

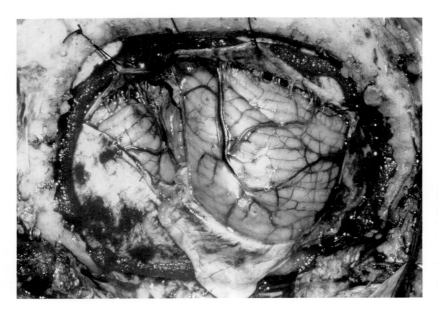

Figure 42-10 Photographed field diameter, 12 cm. Vertex up. The exposure of the posterior fossa craniectomy has been carried above the transverse sinus to permit elevation of the sinus with stay sutures and crosses the midline from the large right exposure to the modest left exposure.

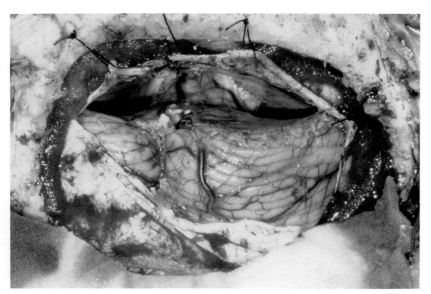

Figure 42-11 Same case as Fig. 42-10. The bridging veins have been coagulated and divided, permitting the cerebellum to fall away from the tentorium. Just to the right of the midline, well anteriorly on the tentorium, the lower edge of the tentorial margin meningioma can be seen.

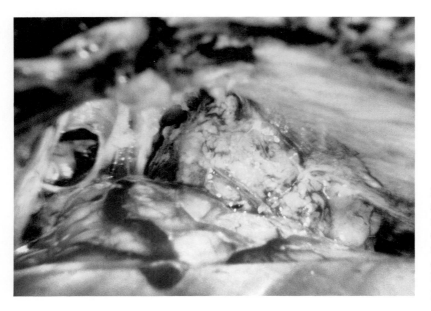

Figure 42-12 Same case as Figs. 42-10 and 42-11. Photographed field diameter, 2.4 cm. The meningioma coming down from the tentorium just posterior to its free margin and just to the right of the midline is now visible. The cerebellum fills the bottom third of the photograph to the left.

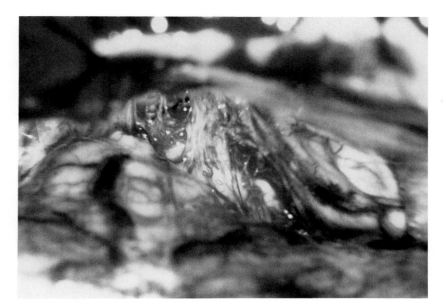

Figure 42-13 Same case as Figs. 42-10 to 42-12. The tentorium has been resected with the tumor through its free margin, exposing the undersurface of the medial portion of the temporo-occipital junction. More medially, the vein of Galen and the precentral cerebellar veins are exposed.

sinus. Under direct vision laterally the sagittal sinus dura is separated from the overlying calvarium and a free flap is cut across the midline for several centimeters on the other side. The larger flap is usually on the right side in right-handed individuals. The occipital pole is remarkable in that it has no major draining medial veins to the sagittal sinus and if a vein is present it can be interrupted without deficit. Separation along the medial side of the hemisphere from the falx is carried down to the straight sinus and out along the tentorial leaf. Two broad-bladed self-retaining retractors are then placed, one against the sagittal sinus and falx and the other against the medial surface of the occipital lobe. Deviating the sagittal sinus and falx a centimeter or so increases the available exposure if needed.

Depending upon the involvement of the straight sinus and the extent of the tumor above and below the tentorium, the supratentorial portion of the tumor may be cored, the falx divided, and dissection carried downward to the point where an occluded straight sinus can be divided and clipped and the attachment to the vein of Galen coagulated anteriorly and divided, preserving whatever collateral is present (Figs. 42-14 to 42-16). If the straight sinus is still patent and must be spared, it can be skeletonized with the removal of the falx and the tentorium on both sides of it with the recognition that either postoperative radiation will be required to possibly prevent recurrence or a secondary procedure may be necessary later, after the occlusion has been completed over the course of future years.

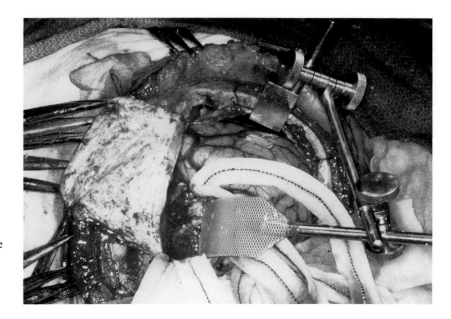

Figure 42-14 Photographed field diameter, 14 cm. A bilateral occipital supratentorial craniotomy, larger on the right, has been done. The right occipital lobe has been separated from the falx, exposing the falcotentorial meningioma.

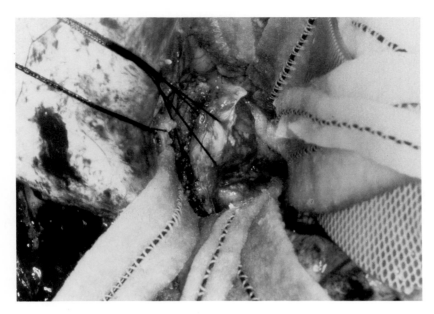

Figure 42-15 Same case as Fig. 42-14. Photographed field diameter, 6 cm. The meningioma has been partially cored, permitting excision through the tentorium lateral to the tumor and the placement of traction sutures in the cut tentorium, lifting the infratentorial portion of the tumor.

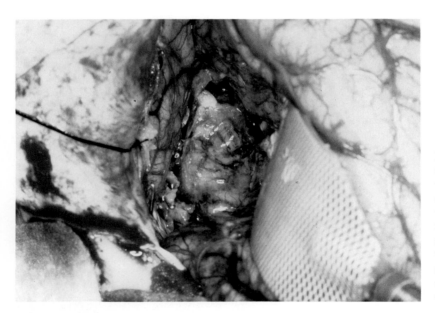

Figure 42-16 Same case as Figs. 42-14 and 42-15. Photographed field diameter, 6 cm. The falx, invaded straight sinus, and tentorium as well as the tumor have now been excised. The medial surface of the left hemisphere is seen through the area of falx resection, while the preserved arachnoid over the anterior cerebellum with the precentral cerebellar vein entering the vein of Galen is exposed anteriorly.

Torcular Meningiomas

At our present state of knowledge it would appear that unless a complete occlusion of the torcular area has occurred spontaneously and full collateral has developed, complete removal of these tumors cannot be achieved. They may present as hyperostotic lesions with rather large extension posteriorly, if bilateral, which is the true torcular meningioma. When unilateral, they are torcular meningiomas almost secondarily. These may attain large size without real invasion of the torcular, though they may be attached to the dura on one surface. After coring these unilateral tumors, the involved transverse sinus may be resected.

If bilateral, I have dissected them free from patent sinuses, but there are always segments of tumor attached along the surface of either the posterior sagittal sinus or the torcular itself (Figs. 42-17 to 42-19). Discretion may be the better part of valor here, with follow-up CT scans to determine recurrence and the need for reoperation or with radiation therapy as a possible prophylactic procedure.

I have on a few occasions made an opening in the sinus just large enough for one blade of the bipolar coagulator and then coagulated the sinus wall with through and through coagulation with one blade of the bipolar within the sinus and the other blade outside. I first carried out this procedure 10 years ago, and while recurrence has not yet taken place, one cannot be sure that it will not in the future. The high

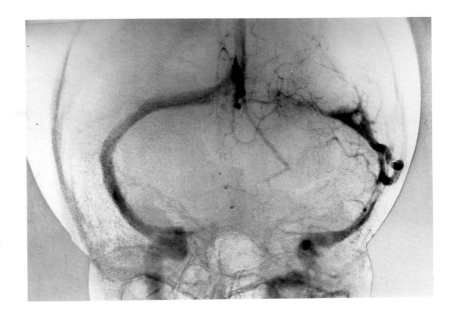

Figure 42-17 A meningioma involving and occluding the transverse sinus from the torcular laterally is demonstrated on the venous phase of the angiogram.

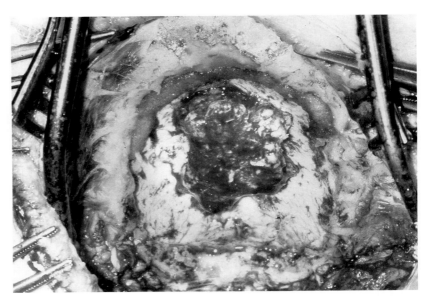

Figure 42-18 Same case as Fig. 42-17. Vertex up. Photographed field diameter, 10 cm. A paramedian suboccipital craniectomy has been carried out, going upward across the transverse sinus and exposing the surface of the transdural extension of the meningioma.

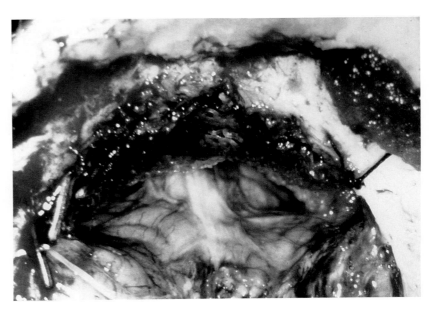

Figure 42-19 Same case as Figs. 42-17 and 42-18. Photographed field diameter, 5 cm. The tumor has been resected, including the involved part of the transverse sinus and the tentorial leaf, which has been covered with a sheet of Surgicel. The extension of the tumor across the midline did not invade the transverse sinus on the left, fortunately permitting preservation of the torcular and its drainage.

flow rate within the sinus has apparently protected the channel from thrombotic occlusion with this coagulation. I have not tried this technique in the more delicate structures such as the straight sinus. This group of tumors, because of their posterior hyperostosis, have had resection of the hyperostotic bone and cranioplasty ordinarily performed at the time of the original resection.

All in all, the tentorial meningiomas are a most challenging group of tumors. The advances in imaging and most particularly the development of microtechnique have vastly altered the previously dismal prognosis. We have not yet achieved but are certainly approaching the time when all benign tumors will be diagnosed earlier and treated well enough to result in a cured patient.

References

1. Guidetti B, Ciappetta P, Domenicucci M. Tentorial meningiomas: surgical experience with 61 cases and long term results. *J Neurosurg* 1988; 69:183–187.

2. Malis LI. Tumors of the parasellar region. *Adv Neurol* 1976; 15:281–299.

3. Malis LI. Surgical resection of tumors of the skull base. In: Wilkins RH, Rengachary SS (eds.), *Neurosurgery*. New York: McGraw-Hill, 1985:1011–1021.

4. Ojemann RG. Meningiomas: clinical features and surgical management. In: Wilkins RH, Rengachary SS (eds.), *Neurosurgery*. New York: McGraw-Hill, 1985:635–654.

5. Sekhar LN, Jannetta PJ, Maroon CJ. Tentorial meningiomas: surgical management and results. *Neurosurgery* 1984; 14:268–275.

6. Yasargil MG, Mortara RW, Curcic M. Meningiomas of basal posterior cranial fossa. In: Krayenbühl H, Brihaye J, Loew F, et al (eds.), *Advances and Technical Standards in Neurosurgery*. Vienna: Springer-Verlag, 1980; 7:3–115.

43
Surgical Exposure of Petroclival Tumors

Ossama Al-Mefty

Unlike other locations, surgical access to the clivus and petrous apex remains a formidable challenge. Despite numerous approaches designed to reach lesions at this deep-seated and vital location, the disappointments and shortcomings are still many and the perfect approach has yet to be developed. Detailed preoperative radiologic studies are crucial for surgical planning. Computed tomographic (CT) scanning and magnetic resonance imaging (MRI) not only reveal the presence of a lesion in this area but also depict the exact location of the mass, its extension, and, frequently, its nature. Coronal and sagittal imaging enhances the information obtained by these studies. The author still performs angiography to identify vascular lesions, depict tumor blood supply, demonstrate the location and displacement of the cerebral arteries, and determine the anatomy and patency of the dural venous sinuses.

Approaches to the posterior cranial base can be grouped into three main categories: intradural, anterior-extradural, and lateral (Fig. 43-1). The various extradural and lateral approaches are detailed in other chapters of this book. This chapter will briefly discuss approach selection for petroclival tumors and describe a petrosal approach for their removal.

The approach most suitable for a particular tumor is selected according to tumor location (intradural, extradural, or both), extension (upper, lower, or entire clivus), nature (benign, invasive, or malignant), and size. The transoral, transpalatal, or trans-sphenoidal approaches are used for midline extradural tumors. Intradural tumors at the petrous apex or the clivus are approached through the petrosal route, while large extra- and intradural tumors are accessed through a combined infratemporal approach with a suboccipital craniectomy.[1]

Intradural Approaches

Several conventional and combined intradural approaches have been used to reach petroclival tumors. These include the frontotemporal,[15] subtemporal transtentorial,[4] occipital transtentorial, suboccipital,[6] and combined subtemporal and suboccipital.[11,14] Most suited for a tumor located intradurally, the intradural approaches allow visualization of the neurovascular anatomy and its relation to the tumor. These approaches, however, have several disadvantages: (1) they require varying degrees of brain retraction, (2) the field is deep, (3) exposure of the ventrally located clival tumor is limited, (4) the exposure of neural and vascular structures around the brain stem is inadequate, and (5) the surgeon must work between cranial nerves and vessels in the posterior fossa and at the tentorial hiatus.

The *frontotemporal* approach, as it is used for clival and petroclival meningiomas, is elegantly described and illustrated by Yasargil et al.[15] Their results for these meningiomas are most impressive. Most neurosurgeons are familiar with the approach, the splitting of the sylvian fissure, and the clear exposure of the upper clivus. This approach is limited, however, to the upper clival area; dissection behind the dorsum sellae is carried out in an extremely narrow space between the carotid artery and the third nerve or the carotid artery and the optic nerve.

The *subtemporal* approach has been frequently used to remove tumors in the petroclival area. Opening the tentorium allows the surgeon to reach a tumor extending caudally into the posterior fossa. The temporal lobe is retracted, and the tentorium is incised parallel to the petrous ridge, from the free edge of the tentorium to the lateral sinus. The approach may be anterior or posterior, according to the part of the temporal lobe to be elevated. There are several advan-

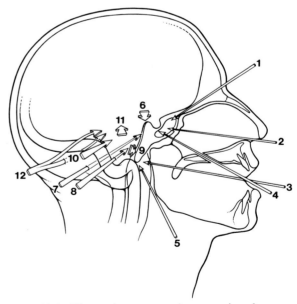

Figure 43-1 The various approaches targeting the petroclival area. The anterior extradural approaches include the transbasal (1), trans-sphenoidal (2), transoral (3), transpalatal (4), and transcervical (5). The intradural approaches include the pterional (6), retrosigmoid (7), subtemporal (11), and combined subtemporal and suboccipital (12). The lateral approaches include the infratemporal (9), translabyrinthine-transcochlear (8), and the petrosal (10).

tages to the subtemporal approach: (1) surgeons are familiar with the anatomy; (2) the superior pole of the tumor is clearly exposed; (3) the third and fourth cranial nerves are directly visualized upon exposing the tentorial hiatus; and (4) the fifth, seventh, and eighth cranial nerves, which are displaced superiorly or anteriorly, are visualized early. The major disadvantage is temporal lobe retraction, which frequently results in temporal lobe swelling. This occurs more often with a posterior subtemporal than the anterior approach and is particularly devastating on the dominant hemisphere. Sectioning of the zygomatic arch allows a more basal approach with less brain retraction.[1] There is considerable difficulty in reaching and exposing the inferior pole of the tumor when the tumor has a deep inferior extension. Since the upper cranial nerves (III, IV) are prominent in the field, injury to them is a potential risk.

The *suboccipital* approach is also a standard in neurosurgery but is more suitable for a tumor located in the cerebellopontine angle (CPA) than those which extend to the petrous apex or upper clivus.[13,15] It provides, however, access to the lower part of the clivus, and down to the foramen magnum. A very large tumor can be removed via this approach. The exposure requires some cerebellar retraction. The approach, which is posterior, provides poor access to a ventrally located lesion and is hindered by the requirement of working between the cranial nerves.

The *combined subtemporal and suboccipital* approach has also been used for many years to remove petroclival and tentorial tumors. In 1939, Bailey described an approach through a unilateral osteoplastic flap incorporating bone over the occipital lobe as well as over the posterior fossa.[3] The occipital lobe was then retracted superiorly and the tentorium was split following ligation of the transverse sinus. Subsequent to tumor removal, the sinus ends were reunited. Bailey believed that a well-developed sinus on the contralateral side was a prerequisite for this operation. A modification of this approach has been utilized by several authors. Malis extended the posterior fossa craniectomy with a lateral mastoidectomy.[11] He emphasized ligation of the transverse sinus with preservation of the vein of Labbé drainage through the opposite transverse sinus. This combined approach provides better exposure to clival and petroclival tumors which extend into the tentorial hiatus and the posterior fossa. Excessive brain retraction of the temporal lobe and the cerebellum, however, may still be required. Before undertaking this approach, angiographic confirmation of the patency of both sigmoid sinuses, and the connection of both through the torcular, is mandatory. Although many authors have stated that the sigmoid sinus can be ligated safely, complications due to sinus ligation do exist and have been reported. Sacrifice of the sinus is not necessary. The tumor can be dissected by alternating the field between the supra- and infratentorial avenues as described later.

Anterior Extradural Approaches

Anterior extradural approaches include the transoral (with or without glossotomy and mandibulectomy), transpalatal, transcervical, trans-sphenoidal, transmaxillary, and trans-

basal. An anterior extradural approach allows direct exposure of a lesion situated ventral to the brain stem, and obviates brain retraction, resection, or access obstruction of the lesion. Major disadvantages of these approaches are (1) septic sequelae may result from passing through the contaminated oral and nasal pharynx (transcervical is an exception); (2) the surgeon must work at considerable depth; (3) the exposure is restricted to the midline (transmaxillary is an exception); (4) the lateral extension cannot be visualized or dissected; (5) vascular control is not reliable; (6) obtaining a good dural repair is difficult; and (7) neurovascular structures in the posterior fossa are not visualized during the major portion of the dissection. Although these approaches have been utilized or suggested for intradural tumors, they are most suitable for extradural tumors.

Lateral Approaches

The lateral approaches evolved from the translabyrinthine approach. As early as 1904, Fraenkel and Hunt described an operation consisting of a wide suboccipital craniectomy with extension over the lateral sinus down to the point where the sinus enters the jugular bulb.[8] These authors thought that this approach to the CPA is more direct and the cerebellum incurs less pressure from retraction. In 1905, Borchardt reported a similar exposure.[5] He extended the bone removal over the lateral sinus and forward through the labyrinth, divided the sigmoid sinus, and exposed the CPA. House et al. have refined and popularized a similar exposure and further modified it to include the cochlea,[10] while Fisch has advocated the infratemporal approach, preserving the cochlea and the labyrinth with anterior transposition of the facial nerve.[7] Other modifications and combinations have been used by other authors.

A lateral approach shortens the distance to the clivus, provides excellent exposure to the middle and lower clivus with excellent visualization of the ipsilateral brain stem, and requires no brain retraction. Major septic spaces are not transgressed, and with good closure and obliteration of the eustachian tube, the risk of CSF leakage is minimal. Disadvantages of a lateral approach are hearing loss, either conductive or total; temporary paralysis of the seventh nerve following its mobilization or anterior transposition; poor exposure of the contralateral surface of the brain stem; and the sacrifice of the sigmoid sinus. A lateral approach can be tailored to suit the size and location of the lesion. The extent of the exposure can vary from a limited retrolabyrinthine space to a wide transtemporal exposure. These approaches are suitable for both extradural or intradural tumors with extension on the lower half of the clivus or tumors which extend both intra- and extradurally (large jugular foramen neuromas and giant glomus jugulare tumors).

A subtemporal exposure may also be added, with or without violation of the labyrinth.[2,9,12] This allows exposure of a lesion located at the petroclival junction or the upper half of the clivus, or even lesions extending from the middle fossa to the foramen magnum. This approach is most suitable for tumors located intradurally such as meningiomas, schwannomas, and epidermoid tumors. The following is a detailed description of this approach, which is centered on the petrous bone, creating several advantages: (1) the cerebellar and temporal lobes are minimally retracted; (2) the operative distance to the clivus is shortened by 3 cm; (3) the surgeon has a direct line of sight to the lesion and the anterior and lateral aspects of the brain stem; (4) the neural and otologic structures, including the cochlea, labyrinth, and facial nerve, are preserved; (5) the transverse and sigmoid sinuses, as well as the vein of Labbé and the basal occipital veins, are preserved; (6) the tumor's vascular supply is intercepted early in the procedure; and (7) multiple axes for dissection are provided.

Surgical Technique

The patient is placed supine with the head at the foot end of the operating table and the ipsilateral shoulder slightly elevated. The head is turned away from the side of the tumor, inclined toward the floor, and tilted toward the opposite side, making the petrous base the highest point of the operative field (Fig. 43-2). The head is fixed in a three-point Mayfield headrest. During the operation, the line of sight can be altered by rotating the table from side to side or up and down.

A reverse question-mark incision is made, starting at the zygoma in front of the ear, circling above the ear, and descending 1 cm medial to (behind) the mastoid process (Fig. 43-2). The temporalis muscle and the periosteum over the temporal and suboccipital areas are elevated and retracted anteriorly and inferiorly to the level of the external ear canal. Four burr holes are made, two on each side of the transverse sinus. A hole made just medial and inferior to the asterion opens into the posterior fossa below the transverse sigmoid sinus junction, while a hole located at the squamal and mastoid junction of the temporal bone, along the projection of

the superior temporal line, opens into the supratentorial compartment. A burr hole at each of these points will exactly flank the sigmoid sinus. The temporal bone and a portion of the occipital bone above the tentorium, as well as the occipital bone below the tentorium, are incised between burr holes with the craniotome (Fig. 43-3). The burr holes flanking the lateral sinus are then connected using a rongeur or high speed air drill. The single bone flap is elevated, exposing the transverse and sigmoid sinuses. The bone may be severely adherent to the dura where the sigmoid and transverse sinuses meet. An alternative to this method of skull bone removal is to perform a temporal craniotomy, followed by a posterior fossa craniectomy extending over the transverse sinus.

The second stage, drilling of the temporal bone, requires a thorough knowledge of the anatomy of the petrous bone and surrounding structures. The operative microscope, mounted on a Contraves stand and equipped with an adjustable-angle eyepiece (Zeiss, Inc., Thornwood, New York), is utilized. The angle of the eyepiece is changed as the field alternates between the subtemporal and suboccipital routes. The surgeon performs a complete mastoidectomy using a high speed air drill. A diamond bit should be used when drilling is close to vital anatomic structures. The sigmoid sinus is skeletonized down to the jugular bulb, and the sinodural angle, Citelli's angle, which identifies the position of the superior petrosal sinus, is exposed. The superficial mastoid air cells behind the posterior wall of the external ear canal, as well as the deep (retrofacial) air cells, are resected to identify the fallopian canal and the lateral and posterior semicircular canals. Drilling is continued along the pyramid to thin the petrous bone toward its apex. The facial canal as well as the middle and inner ear structures are kept intact, while opened air cells are obliterated with bone wax (Fig. 43-4).

When the surgeon needs a shorter and more lateral access to the petrous apex and clivus, the posterior fossa dura ante-

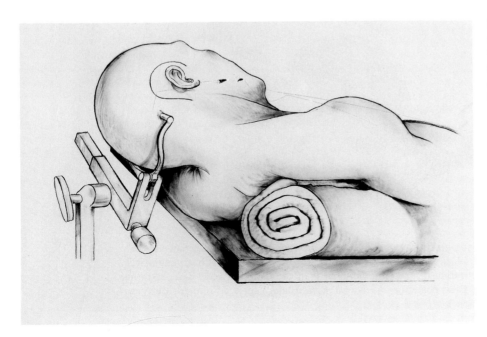

Figure 43-2 Artist's illustration of patient's position and the skin incision for a right-sided petrosal approach. (From Al-Mefty et al.,[2] with permission.)

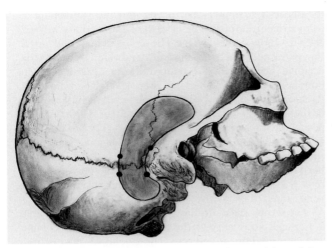

Figure 43-3 Artist's illustration depicting position of the burr holes and outlining the bone flap (right side).

When the lesion is large and extends significantly in both supra- and infratentorial compartments, the dura of the posterior and temporal fossae is then opened along both sides of the sigmoid sinus. The supratentorial incision is continued along the floor of the temporal fossa, while the infratentorial incision is extended to the jugular bulb. The dural flaps are left covering the cerebral cortex for protection. The posterior temporal lobe is gently retracted. The vein of Labbé is preserved by dissection from the cortical surface, allowing retraction of the temporal lobe without tension on the venous wall (Fig. 43-6). The cerebellar hemisphere, which naturally falls backward, needs little or no retraction. The author has found no need to transect the sigmoid sinus, since exposure may be obtained by alternating the visualized field above and below the tentorium.

Further relaxation is obtained by opening the arachnoid of the cerebellomedullary cistern and draining CSF. The tumor is devascularized by coagulating its insertion on the pyramid and the meningeal feeders over the tentorium. When the tumor is small or moderate in size, the seventh and eighth cranial nerves are usually stretched posteriorly and thus are easily identified. When the tumor reaches a large size, however, these cranial nerves may well be engulfed in the tumor.

A suitable area on the tumor surface is selected and the arachnoid over the tumor is opened. The tumor is then debulked with extreme caution since the seventh and eighth nerves, as well as the posterior inferior cerebellar artery (PICA) and anterior inferior cerebellar artery (AICA), may be embedded in the tumor. Debulking is performed using

rior to the sigmoid sinus is opened along the sigmoid sinus, the incision is extended upward toward a supratentorial dural incision, the superior petrosal sinus is clipped or coagulated and transected, and the incision is continued on the tentorium, parallel to the pyramid, and extended through the incisura. The retractor is then placed anteriorly, holding medially the sigmoid sinus, the cerebellum, and the cut edge of the tentorium (Fig. 43-5).

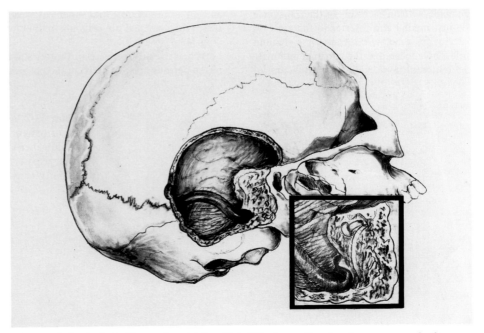

Figure 43-4 Artist's illustration (right side). The bone flap has been removed, the right sigmoid sinus has been skeletonized, and the petrous bone has been extensively drilled. *Inset:* Illustration of anatomic landmarks in the temporal bone demonstrating the facial canal and the posterior and lateral semicircular canals. (From Al-Mefty et al.,[2] with permission.)

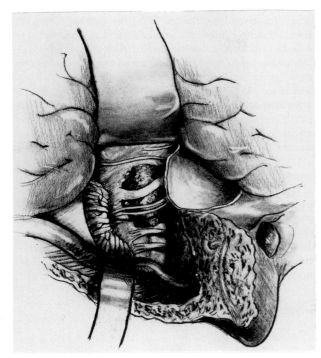

Figure 43-5 Artist's illustration (right side) demonstrating exposure of the tumor via a presigmoid sinus avenue. The sigmoid sinus and cerebellum are retracted medially, while the temporal lobe is retracted superiorly. The tentorium is incised along the pyramid through the incisura. The brain stem, cranial nerves, and tumor are visualized. (From Al-Mefty et al.,[2] with permission.)

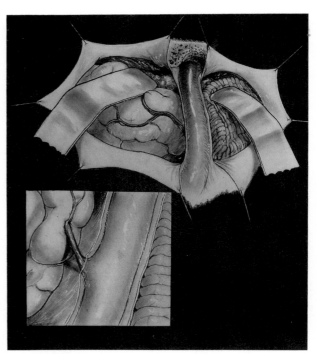

Figure 43-6 Artist's illustration (right side). The dura has been opened, leaving the transverse and sigmoid sinuses undisturbed. The cerebellar hemisphere and posterior temporal lobe are held by self-retaining retractors. *Inset:* Illustration of the dissection of the vein of Labbé from the temporal cortex to allow retraction of the temporal lobe without tension on the venous wall. (From Al-Mefty et al.,[2] with permission.)

suction, laser, the Cavitron ultrasonic aspirator (CUSA), and/or bipolar coagulation and microscissors. The supratentorial extension of the tumor, if present, is removed. The tentorium is then incised around the tumor, and if the tentorial notch has not been incised earlier, the incision is extended to it. During this maneuver, the surgeon must make every effort to preserve the trochlear nerve. Opening the tentorium allows excellent exposure to the upper pole of the tumor and the anterior and lateral aspects of the brain stem (Figs. 43-7 and 43-8). Trigeminal nerve rootlets are found under the tentorium, frequently stretched and separated by the tumor.

The tumor capsule is then dissected free from the surrounding structures. Maintaining dissection within the arachnoidal planes is crucial to preservation of the vital neural and vascular structures. Cranial nerves and the basilar artery and its branches may, however, be embedded in a large tumor, demanding meticulous and tedious dissection. A cut edge of the tumor should not be allowed to slip away lest the plane of cleavage be lost. Further hollowing of the tumor may be necessary before dissection of the thinned-out capsule can be continued.

The lower cranial nerves are dissected off the inferior pole of the tumor via the infratentorial avenue. Gentle dissection is required to avoid hypotension and bradycardia from vagal stimulation. The seventh and eighth cranial

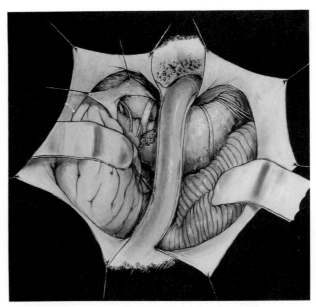

Figure 43-7 Artist's illustration (right side). The supratentorial extension of the tumor has been removed, and the tentorium has been split open. The relationship of the tumor to the cranial nerves (III through XI) and brain stem is demonstrated.

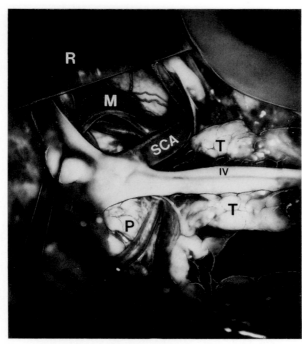

Figure 43-8 Enhanced operative photograph. Surgeon's view during removal of a tumor via the supratentorial avenue with an incised tentorium. The debulked tumor (T) lies in front of the midbrain (M) and pons (P). The IV nerve is seen on the lateral surface of the brain stem and tumor. SCA = Superior cerebellar artery; R = Retractor on temporal lobe.

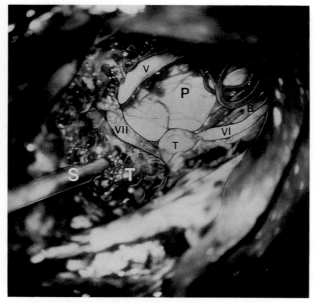

Figure 43-9 Enhanced operative photograph (right side) during the dissection of a meningioma via the infratentorial avenue. The upper portion of the tumor has been dissected from the brain stem, basilar artery (B), and cranial nerves V, VI, and VII. The lower part of the tumor (T) is still present. P = Pons; S = Suction device.

nerves are carefully dissected from the tumor. The sixth nerve, stretched anteriorly and inferiorly, is dissected free from the tumor and followed distally. Alternating the visualized field between the supra- and infratentorial routes allows the tumor capsule to be dissected carefully from the brain stem (Figs. 43-8 and 43-9). If it is not embedded in the tumor, the basilar artery is usually displaced to the opposite side. The preservation and careful dissection of the main and small branches of the basilar artery cannot be overemphasized.

Once the tumor has been excised, all neurovascular structures in the posterior fossa are covered with wet surgical patties, and the area of tumor insertion is vaporized extensively with the laser. If the tumor has extended into the internal auditory meatus, the meatus wall is drilled and the tumor removed. Extension through the jugular foramen is likewise removed. The dura is closed watertight, the periosteum is turned over the petrous bone to avoid a CSF leak, and the soft tissues are closed in multiple layers.

References

1. Al-Mefty O. *Surgery of the Cranial Base.* Boston: Kluwer Academic Publishers, 1989:239–258.
2. Al-Mefty O, Fox JL, Smith RR. Petrosal approach for petroclival meningiomas. *Neurosurgery* 1988; 22:510–517.
3. Bailey P. Concerning the technic of operation for acoustic neurinoma. *Zentralbl Neurochir* 1939; 4:1–5.
4. Bonnal J, Louis R, Combalbert A. L'abord temporal transtentorial de l'angle ponto-cérébelleux et du clivus. *Neurochirurgie* 1964; 10:3–12.
5. Borchardt M. Zur Operation der Tumoren des Kleinhirn-Brückenwinkels. *Berl Klin Wochenschr* 1905; 42:1033–1035.
6. Cushing HW, Eisenhardt L. *Meningiomas: Their Classification, Regional Behaviour, Life History, and Surgical End Results.* Springfield, IL: Charles C Thomas, 1938:169–223.
7. Fisch U, Pillsbury HC. Infratemporal fossa approach to lesions in the temporal bone and base of the skull. *Arch Otolaryngol Head Neck Surg* 1979; 105:99–107.
8. Fraenkel J, Hunt JR. Contribution to the surgery of neurofibroma of the acoustic nerve. *Ann Surg* 1904; 40:293–319.
9. Hakuba A, Nishimura S, Tanaka K, et al. Clivus meningioma: six cases of total removal. *Neurol Med Chir (Tokyo)* 1977; 17: 63–77.
10. House WF, Hitselberger WE, Horn KL. The middle fossa transpetrous approach to the anterior-superior cerebellopontine angle. *Am J Otol* 1986; 7:1–4.
11. Malis LI. Surgical resection of tumors of the skull base. In: Wilkins RH, Rengachary SS (eds.), *Neurosurgery.* New York: McGraw-Hill, 1985:1011–1021.
12. Morrison AW, King TT. Experiences with a translabyrinthine-transtentorial approach to the cerebellopontine angle: technical note. *J Neurosurg* 1973; 38:382–390.
13. Ojemann RG. Meningiomas: clinical features and surgical management. In: Wilkins RH, Rengachary SS (eds.), *Neurosurgery.* New York: McGraw-Hill, 1985:635–654.
14. Symon L. Surgical approaches to the tentorial hiatus. In: Krayenbühl H, Brihaye J, Loew F, et al (eds.), *Advances and Technical Standards in Neurosurgery.* New York: Springer-Verlag, 1982; 9:69–112.
15. Yasargil MG, Mortara RW, Curcic M. Meningiomas of basal posterior cranial fossa. In: Krayenbühl H, Brihaye J, Loew F, et al (eds.), *Advances and Technical Standards in Neurosurgery.* New York: Springer-Verlag, 1980; 7:1–115.

44

The Translabyrinthine Approach to Cerebellopontine Angle Tumors

John T. McElveen, Jr.

The translabyrinthine approach to the cerebellopontine angle was first suggested by Panse in 1904,[14] first performed by Quix of Utrecht in 1911,[16] and later used by Schmiegelow[17] and others to remove acoustic tumors. The approach fell into disfavor after it was condemned by Cushing in 1921 when he wrote, "There is no possible route more dangerous or difficult than this one".[3]

Benefiting from improved instrumentation and magnification, House and Hitselberger, in the 1960s, revived the translabyrinthine approach to lesions in the cerebellopontine angle.[8,11] Since its resurgence, teams of neurotologists and neurosurgeons have made this approach a mainstay of their surgical armamentarium and have expanded its indications.

Indications

The translabyrinthine approach is a direct anatomic route to lesions in and around the internal auditory canal (IAC). Exposure is facilitated by bone removal and not cerebellar retraction, and the facial nerve is identified distal to the tumor before the tumor is encountered.

Traversing the labyrinth destroys all residual hearing in the operated ear; consequently, this approach should be limited to cerebellopontine angle lesions not amenable to hearing conservation procedures. The decision is based on radiographic findings, vestibular testing, and audiologic information. In the author's experience, findings not favorable to hearing conservation include acoustic neurinomas greater than 1.5 cm to 2.0 cm. in diameter, neurofibromas of any size, tumors extending to the lateral end of the IAC [this is particularly well seen with gadolinium-enhanced

magnetic resonance imaging (MRI)], a normal caloric response on vestibular testing (indicating a possible inferior vestibular nerve origin), a speech reception threshold (SRT) worse than 50 dB, a speech discrimination score less than 80 percent, and markedly distorted or absent waveforms on evoked auditory brain stem response (ABR) testing.

Because of concerns regarding limited exposure, the translabyrinthine approach was restricted initially to lesions less than 2.5 to 3.0 cm in diameter. With increased experience, the translabyrinthine approach has been demonstrated to be particularly useful in larger tumors where there is no possibility of hearing preservation.[1,18] Intracapsular debulking effectively converts larger schwannomas to smaller, more manageable lesions, without the need for prolonged cerebellar retraction.

The usefulness of the translabyrinthine approach is not limited to removing tumors of the cerebellopontine angle. In patients with a transection of the facial nerve, and a total loss of hearing and vestibular function on the involved side, the translabyrinthine approach is the most direct means of exploring the entire course of the facial nerve.[7] Incapacitating, ear-related vertigo in a nonhearing ear is effectively treated with a translabyrinthine vestibular neurectomy.[15] In addition, modifications and extensions of the standard translabyrinthine approach afford access to the anterior part of the posterior fossa and the clivus (translabyrinthine-transcochlear approach),[12] and improve exposure of the inferior aspect of the posterior fossa (translabyrinthine-retrosigmoid approach).[5]

Anatomic Overview

A knowledge of temporal bone anatomy and the relationship between key structures within the temporal bone is essential to performing translabyrinthine surgery.

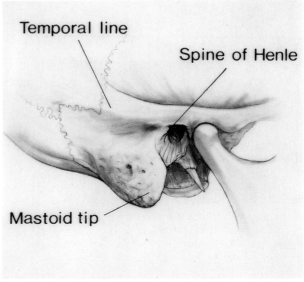

Figure 44-1 Right temporal bone (lateral view).

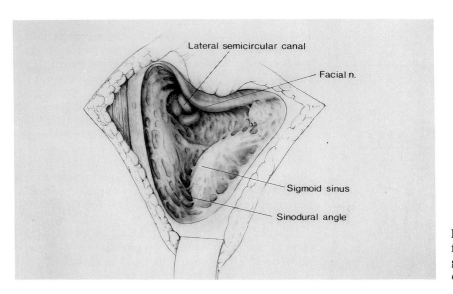

Figure 44-2 Right mastoid cavity following cortical mastoidectomy (surgeon's view). Anterior direction, *top;* caudal direction, *right.*

Surface Features

The key surface features include the temporal line, the suprameatal spine of Henle, and the mastoid tip (Fig. 44-1). The temporal line is a raised area that projects posteriorly from the zygomatic process and roughly corresponds to the floor of the middle fossa. It is used by the surgeon to determine the approximate location of the middle fossa plate. The suprameatal spine of Henle lies slightly posterior and superior to the external auditory canal and orients the surgeon to the location of the external auditory canal as well as the deeper lying aditus and lateral semicircular canal. The mastoid tip delimits the mastoid from the neck musculature.

Mastoid Features

Once the cortical bone has been removed from the mastoid, it is important that the surgeon identify and understand the relationships among the middle fossa plate, the sigmoid sinus, the sinodural angle, the lateral semicircular canal, and the facial nerve (Fig. 44-2). Projecting anteromedially from the sinodural angle is the superior petrosal sinus, which marks the junction between the middle fossa dural and the posterior fossa dural surfaces. The lateral semicircular canal is a key landmark to the mastoid segment of the facial nerve, which is at a similar depth within the temporal bone and is situated just inferior to the canal.

Labyrinthine Features

The hard endochondral bone that forms the osseous covering of the semicircular canals is often referred to as labyrinthine bone. In order to reach the IAC, the surgeon must traverse these canals, and the vestibule. The orientation of the semicircular canals is seen in Fig. 44-3. The ampullated ends of the canals, particularly the superior and posterior

Figure 44-3 Right temporal bone anatomy following mastoidectomy. The orientation of the semicircular canals is demonstrated.

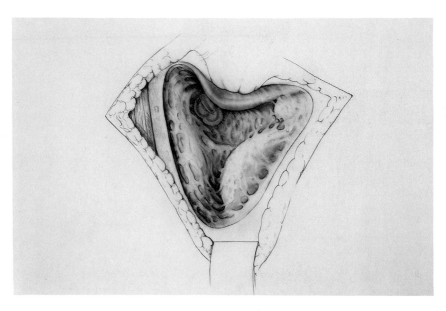

canals, serve as key surgical landmarks. Just medial to the superior semicircular canal ampulla lies the labyrinthine segment of the facial nerve. Consequently, careful dissection is essential when drilling anterior to this ampulla. Inferior to the ampullated portion of the posterior semicircular canal, and never superior to it, lies the jugular bulb. Occasionally the jugular bulb may abut the canal. Again, careful dissection inferior to the posterior canal is essential to avoid inadvertent injury to the jugular bulb.

The last labyrinthine landmark is the vestibule, a cavity situated at the convergence of the ampullated portions of the semicircular canals. The floor of the vestibule is the lateral extent of the IAC and is useful in the initial location of the IAC. In addition, it is important to recognize the relationship between the crus of the lateral semicircular canal and the tympanic portion of the facial nerve to avoid injury to the nerve.

Internal Auditory Canal Features

There are six key anatomic structures that assist in dissecting in and around the canal: the cochlear aqueduct, the jugular bulb, the transverse crest, the vertical crest (Bill's bar), the superior petrosal sinus, and the IAC itself (Fig. 44-4). The cochlear aqueduct lies inferior to the IAC and just superior and lateral to the glossopharyngeal nerve, marking the anteroinferior extent of the dissection. The jugular bulb, situated inferior to the IAC, marks the inferior limit of the dissection. The superior petrosal sinus runs superior to the internal auditory meatus and forms the superior extent of the dissection, with the anterior wall of the IAC forming the anterior extent of the dissection. The transverse crest, situated in the lateral aspect of the IAC, separates the superior from the inferior vestibular nerve. The most important landmark is the vertical crest (Bill's bar), which allows the surgeon to positively identify the facial nerve just as it enters the lateral aspect of the IAC.

Surgical Technique

Positioning

The operation is performed with the patient in the supine position and the surgeon seated. This position minimizes the likelihood of the patient developing venous air emboli and is more comfortable for the surgeon. The operating room table is reversed (patient's head at the foot of the table), allowing the surgeon adequate leg room and the anesthesiologist access to the table controls. The scrub nurse is positioned opposite the surgeon, and the microscope is brought in from the head of the table (Fig. 44-5).

Instrumentation and Equipment

Proper instrumentation facilitates dissection and minimizes the risk of inadvertent neural or vascular injury. Although it is beyond the scope of this chapter to review all of the instrumentation used in translabyrinthine surgery, there are certain instruments that are particularly useful. The operative microscope should be fitted with a 200-mm or a 250-mm objective lens and a fiber-optic light source. A suction-irrigation system minimizes thermal injury during drilling, and the specially designed Brackmann suction-irrigator (N0607; Storz Instrument Co, St. Louis, MO) prevents excessive suction from being applied to delicate neural structures. The neural dissector (Storz N1706) is very useful in lysing adhesions between the facial nerve and the tumor. Lastly, facial nerve monitoring equipment and use of the bipolar cautery further minimize injury to the facial nerve.

Operative Steps

The postauricular area and the left lower quadrant of the abdomen are prepped for surgery. The operative procedure

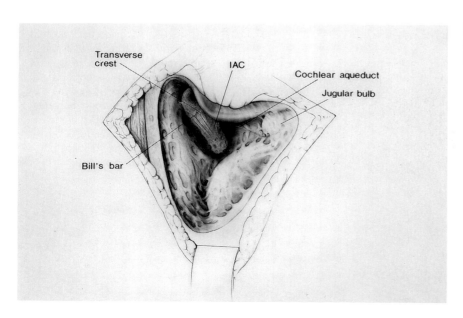

Figure 44-4 Right temporal bone anatomy following labyrinthectomy. IAC = internal auditory canal.

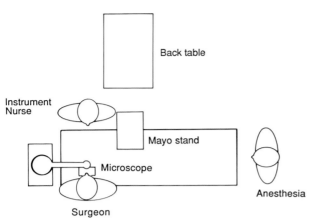

Figure 44-5 Operating room setup for otologic and neurotologic procedures.

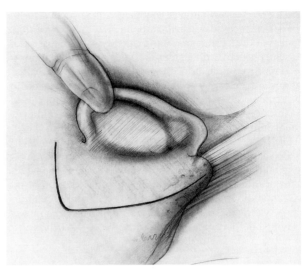

Figure 44-6 Incision for a right translabyrinthine approach. The patient is supine, with the face turned to the left.

begins with a curved postauricular incision approximately 2 to 3 cm behind the postauricular crease (Fig. 44-6). The incision extends down to the level of the temporalis fascia and muscle superiorly, and to the mastoid cortex inferiorly. The ear is reflected anteriorly and the soft tissue attachments to the mastoid cortex are separated with a Lempert periosteal elevator. To avoid transection of the external auditory canal, the dissection proceeds only to the suprameatal spine of Henle.

The cortex of the mastoid is removed with a cutting burr, revealing the middle fossa plate and the sigmoid sinus. Additional bone is removed from the retrosigmoid region. The operative microscope is used to more accurately define the structures within the temporal bone and facilitate bone removal. A thin layer of bone is left over the anterior aspect of the sigmoid sinus, and the sinus is depressed (Fig. 44-7). This facilitates exposure anteriorly and minimizes the risk of tearing the wall of the sigmoid sinus with the shaft of the burr later in the procedure. The remaining mastoid air cells

are removed with a cutting burr to the level of the lateral semicircular canal. Using a diamond burr, the mastoid portion of the facial nerve is delineated, being careful to leave a thin protecting layer of bone over the nerve. Once the cortical mastoidectomy has been performed, the sigmoid sinus decompressed, and the mastoid portion of the facial nerve defined, the first phase of the operation is complete.

The second phase involves opening the semicircular canals, removing bone from the posterior fossa dura and superior petrosal sinus, and identifying the jugular bulb and IAC (Fig. 44-8). When exteriorizing the semicircular canals, it is important to leave the superior canal ampulla and the posterior canal ampulla as landmarks for later dissection. The labyrinthine segment of the facial nerve runs just anterior

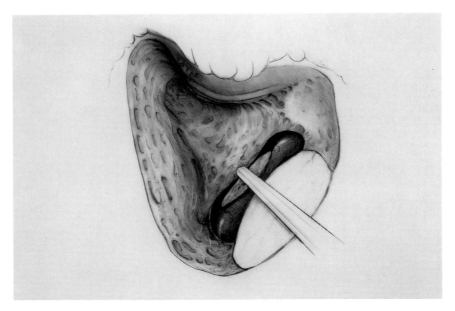

Figure 44-7 Right cortical mastoidectomy with bone removal in the retrosigmoid region. A thin layer of bone (Bill's island) has been left over the anterior portion of the sigmoid sinus as protection; the sinus is being depressed by the suction-irrigator. The posterior fossa dura (*white oval*) has been exposed behind the sigmoid sinus.

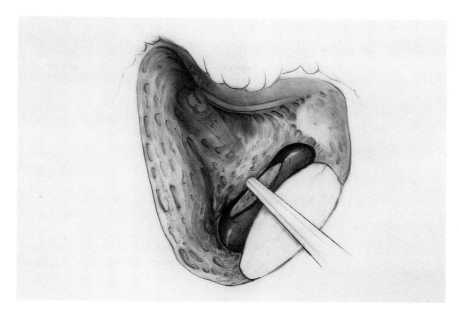

Figure 44-8 Identification of key structures in and around the IAC (right ear).

and superior to the superior canal ampulla, and the jugular bulb can be found anywhere inferior to the posterior semicircular canal ampulla.

The third phase of the operation involves skeletonizing the IAC; identifying the transverse crest, the vertical crest (Bill's bar), and the cochlear aqueduct; and maximizing the limits of the exposure by removing as much bone as possible superior, inferior, and posterior to the IAC (Fig. 44-9). The limits of exposure extend to the middle fossa dura superiorly, the facial nerve anteriorly, the cochlear aqueduct and jugular bulb inferiorly, and the posterior fossa dura posteriorly. At this point the facial nerve can be followed from its mastoid and tympanic segments around the geniculate ganglion and into the IAC. If the facial nerve is intentionally (as with a facial nerve neurinoma) or inadvertently transected during tumor removal, the facial nerve can be displaced from its fallopian canal and a primary anastomosis per-

formed (Fig. 44-10). Mobilizing the facial nerve by severing its greater superficial petrosal branch and its attachments to the stapedius muscle provides additional length, allowing a primary repair of the facial nerve with minimal tension on the anastomosis.

Entering the cerebellopontine angle and removing the tumor make up the fourth phase of the operative procedure. The dura is incised just inferior to the superior petrosal sinus and just superior to the jugular bulb. These two incisions are connected at the porus acusticus. The dura of the IAC is opened and the tumor is separated from the facial nerve, minimizing the lateral-to-medial traction on the facial nerve. A plane is developed between the capsule of the tumor and the surrounding arachnoid sheath. The tumor is then gutted, the eighth nerve is divided distally and proximally, and the tumor capsule is removed (Fig. 44-11).

Once the tumor has been completely removed and bleed-

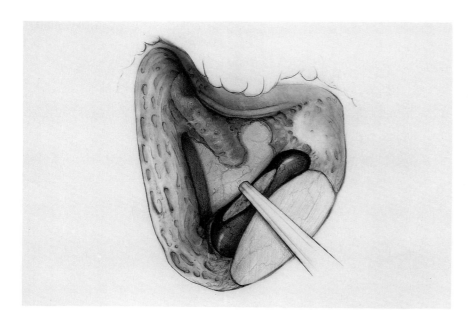

Figure 44-9 Exposure of the right IAC. The dura anterior to the sigmoid sinus has been exposed. The superior petrosal sinus is shown on the *left*, forming the superior boundary of this dural exposure.

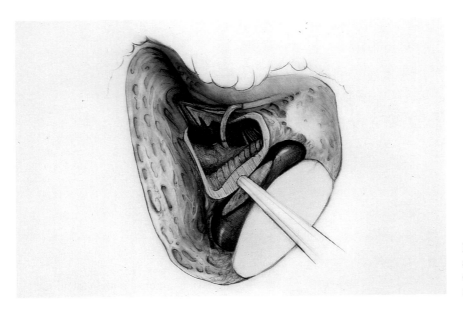

Figure 44-10 Primary facial nerve anastomosis following the resection of a facial nerve neurinoma via a right translabyrinthine approach.

ing controlled, one begins the last phase of the translabyrinthine procedure, the blockage of the dural defect with strips of autogenous abdominal fat. The fat is taken from the patient's left lower quadrant to minimize future confusion regarding an appendectomy. The fat is cut into 3-cm by 0.5-cm strips, soaked in a solution of streptomycin sulfate (50 mg/liter of lactated Ringer's solution) and then placed lengthwise into the dural defect. These strips of fat extend into the defect approximately a centimeter. By tightly packing the strips of fat into the dural defect, a tight seal is formed and the strips are unable to slip further into the posterior fossa. If this step is performed properly, the incidence of postoperative CSF leakage should be less than 2 to 5 percent.

The usefulness of an implantable bone conduction hearing device (Audiant implant; Xomed, Inc., Jacksonville, FL) is presently being evaluated at our medical center. Be-

fore closing the postauricular incision, the internal portion of the hearing device is implanted into the squama of the temporal bone. Six weeks after the operation, the patient is fitted with the external component of the implant, allowing him or her to hear sounds coming to the operated ear.

Limitations

Exposure of the cerebellopontine angle using the translabyrinthine approach can be limited. The region anterior to the porus acusticus, the area inferior to the jugular bulb, and the superior extent of the tentorium cannot be viewed directly with the standard translabyrinthine approach. This view may be further constricted by a small mastoid cavity, a low middle fossa plate, an anteriorly placed sigmoid sinus, or a

Figure 44-11 Right acoustic neurinoma removal via a translabyrinthine approach.

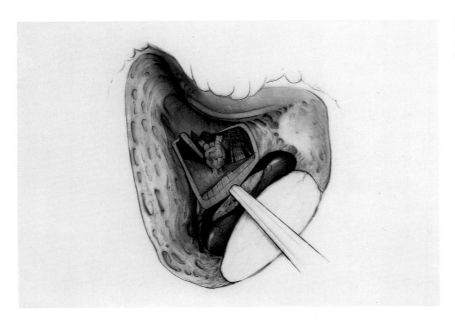

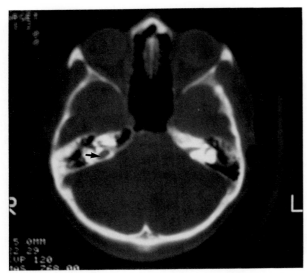

Figure 44-12 CT scan of a patient with a high jugular bulb (*arrow*).

high jugular bulb (Fig. 44-12). In such cases, it is particularly important that the surgeon remove bone extensively from the middle fossa, the retrosigmoid region, and the jugular bulb. If these measures are inadequate, the surgeon may need to modify or combine approaches to maximize the exposure. The transcochlear approach is particularly useful in exposing tumors of the petrous tip and clivus,[12] whereas the translabyrinthine-retrosigmoid approach facilitates exposure of the area inferior to the jugular bulb and the superior extent of the tentorium.[5]

Results

Complete tumor removal with preservation of the facial nerve and hearing remain the goals of acoustic neurinoma surgery. The ability to achieve these goals without inducing neurologic deficits, hydrocephalus, or CSF leakage, is dependent on the surgical approach, the size of the lesion, the instrumentation, and the experience and expertise of the surgical team.

The complete loss of hearing inherent in translabyrinthine surgery remains a disadvantage for this procedure. However, "useful" hearing preservation is rare in lesions greater than 15 mm in diameter, even with hearing conservation techniques.[18] The trade-offs and major advantages of the translabyrinthine approach are that the surgeon is able to identify the facial nerve before it becomes enmeshed in tumor and is able to remove the lateral-most aspect of the tumor under direct vision, thus facilitating preservation of the facial nerve and complete tumor removal.

A review by Brackmann et al. of 216 patients, 1 year following acoustic tumor removal, revealed normal facial function in 83 percent, partial paralysis in 16 percent, and total paralysis in 1 percent.[1] Normal facial function was preserved in 100 percent of the patients with small tumors (0.5 cm or less), in 85 percent of those with medium tumors

(0.5 to 2.0 cm), in 81 percent of those with large tumors (2.0 to 4.0 cm), and in 63 percent of those with giant tumors (>4.0 cm). In a review of 437 cerebellopontine angle lesions, Glasscock et al. reported that facial nerve function was preserved in 86 percent of the patients.[6] Facial function was preserved in 91 percent of those with small tumors (<1.5 cm), in 92 percent of those with medium tumors (1.5 to 2.9 cm), and in 56 percent of those with large tumors (≥3.0 cm). The facial nerve was kept anatomically intact in 93 percent of the 200 translabyrinthine cases reported by Tos and Thomsen.[19] In 65 percent, the function was completely normal; in 16.5 percent, there was minor weakness; in 8.5 percent, there was moderate to severe weakness; and in the remaining 9.5 percent, there was a complete loss of facial function. In reviewing any results, one must take into account the size of the tumors reported. In the Tos and Thomsen series, 77 of the 200 tumors (38.5 percent) were greater than 4.0 cm, and 48 of the 200 (24 percent) were between 2 and 4 cm. Among 50 patients with tumors, all greater than 2 cm in diameter, reported by Whittaker and Luetje, 84 percent had some facial nerve function postoperatively—52 percent had completely normal function, and an additional 28 percent had good function in repose with good eye closure.[20]

It is difficult to accurately compare the postoperative facial nerve function among series due to the lack of a standardized system to assess and report facial nerve function. However, recently the House-Brackmann grading system has been adopted to categorize the various degrees of facial palsy.[10] Hopefully, this system will gain widespread acceptance by both neurosurgeons and neurotologists, allowing a more accurate assessment and reporting of facial nerve function following acoustic neurinoma surgery.

Regardless of the approach, the complete removal of the acoustic tumor without risk to the patient's life is essential. In the series reported by Brackmann et al., all tumors were completely resected, with only one death (<0.4 percent).[1] In the series of Glasscock et al., a total resection was accomplished in 99 percent of the patients and the mortality rate was less than 1 percent.[6] In Whittaker and Luetje's series of 50 patients, the tumor was completely removed in all but six.[20] Four of the six operations were planned partial removals due to the patients' ages, and the remaining two partial resections were related to difficulties of tumor removal. There were no deaths in their series. In Tos and Thomsen's series of 200 patients, all but nine tumors were totally resected using a translabyrinthine approach.[19] Although five deaths occurred, only one was related to the translabyrinthine procedure. This was a 39-year-old woman with a 5-cm acoustic neurinoma who died from a postoperative hemorrhage.

Complications

Complications inevitably occur, even in the best of hands and regardless of the surgical approach. Translabyrinthine surgery is no exception. Bleeding into the posterior fossa following acoustic tumor surgery is life-threatening and requires immediate intervention. One advantage of the translabyrinthine operation is that a rapid decompression of the posterior fossa can be achieved by opening the incision and removing the strips of adipose tissue and the clot. Optimally, this is performed in the operating room, but if circumstances require, this can be performed at the patient's bedside.

Obstructive hydrocephalus can also be a life-threatening complication. Once the diagnosis is made, the clotted blood in the cerebellopontine angle should be removed immediately and a ventriculostomy placed. Fortunately, the incidence of postoperative hydrocephalus following translabyrinthine tumor removal is less than 1 percent.[4]

The incidence of CSF leakage following translabyrinthine acoustic tumor removal varies with the technique utilized to close the defect. In an early series reported by Brow (251 consecutive tumors from 1968 to 1975), CSF leakage following obliteration with one large piece of adipose tissue occurred in 20 percent of the patients.[2] This problem was largely resolved by using 0.5-cm by 3.0-cm strips of fat, as opposed to one large piece. In a report of 230 consecutive translabyrinthine procedures between 1971 and 1981, persistent CSF leakage that required operative closure was reduced to only one patient (<0.5 percent).[9]

Injury to the anterior inferior cerebellar artery during tumor removal can result in infarction of the brain stem and a severe neurologic deficit or death. In gutting the tumor using the translabyrinthine approach, one must be particularly careful to stay within the tumor capsule. Penetration through the capsule before adequately debulking the tumor may result in inadvertent injury to the anterior inferior cerebellar artery. Only on rare occasions is the artery within the tumor mass. This occurs when the vessel is tethered between the involuting walls of the tumor capsule. This can occasionally be seen on a high-resolution computed tomography (CT) scan (Fig. 44-13). Of the 13 fatalities reported by House and Hitselberger in their early series of 500 cerebellopontine angle tumors, 4 were the direct result of thrombosis of the anterior inferior cerebellar artery.[13]

Conclusions

The use of the translabyrinthine approach in the treatment of acoustic neurinomas should be reserved for those lesions not amenable to hearing conservation procedures. This decision should be based on objective radiographic and audiometric data, as well as the experience of the particular surgeon or surgical team, and not on an emotional bias. Innovations in bone implant hearing devices, implanted at the time of translabyrinthine surgery, may minimize the disability caused by the unilateral loss of hearing inherent in this approach.

Despite improvements in facial nerve monitoring techniques, the identification of the facial nerve within the temporal bone before it enters the tumor mass, as provided by the translabyrinthine approach, is preferable to attempting to identify it on the surface of the tumor, at the brain stem, or within the internal auditory canal. The reported rates of preservation of facial nerve function are good for the translabyrinthine approach, and this is one of its main advantages.

Although the translabyrinthine approach is a direct approach to the cerebellopontine angle that requires minimal cerebellar retraction, the exposure can be limited. If the exposure is too restricted, combining the translabyrinthine approach with the retrosigmoid approach or the transotic approach may improve the exposure and facilitate tumor removal.

Lastly, the translabyrinthine approach should be considered in selected cases of facial nerve tumors or injuries, because it facilitates facial nerve anastomosis or grafting. It should also be considered for the surgical approach to ear-related vestibular disorders.

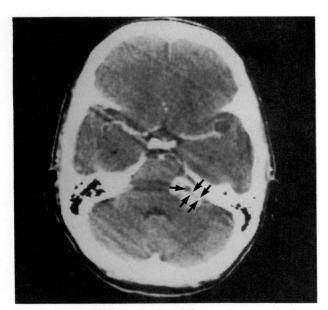

Figure 44-13 High resolution CT scan that reveals the anterior inferior cerebellar artery coursing through the acoustic tumor (*arrows*).

References

1. Brackmann DE, Hitselberger WE, Beneke JE, et al. Acoustic neuromas: middle fossa and translabyrinthine removal. In: Rand RW (ed.), *Microneurosurgery*, 3d ed. St Louis: Mosby, 1985: 311–334.
2. Brow RE. Pre- and postoperative management of the acoustic tumor patient. In: House WF, Luetje CM (eds.), *Acoustic Tumors*. Baltimore: University Park Press, 1979; 2:153–173
3. Cushing H. Further concerning the acoustic neuromas. *Laryngoscope* 1921; 31:209–228.
4. Glasscock ME III, Dickins JRE. Complications of acoustic tumor surgery. *Otolaryngol Clin North Am* 1982; 15:883–895.
5. Glasscock ME III, Hays JW, Jackson CG, et al. A one-stage combined approach for the management of large cerebellopontine angle tumors. *Laryngoscope* 1978; 88:1563–1576.
6. Glasscock ME III, Kveton JF, Jackson CG, et al. A systematic approach to the surgical management of acoustic neuroma. *Laryngoscope* 1986; 96:1088–1094.
7. Graham MD. Surgical exposure of the facial nerve: indications and techniques. *J Laryngol Otol* 1975; 89:557–575.

8. Hitselberger WE, House WF. Surgical approaches to acoustic tumors. *Arch Otolaryngol* 1966; 84:286–291.

9. House JL, Hitselberger WE, House WF. Wound closure and cerebrospinal fluid leak after translabyrinthine surgery. *Am J Otology* 1982; 4:126–128.

10. House JW, Brackmann DE. Facial nerve grading system. *Bull Am Acad Otolaryngol Head Neck Surg* 1985; 4:4.

11. House WF. Evolution of transtemporal bone removal of acoustic tumors. *Arch Otolaryngol* 1964; 80:731–742.

12. House WF, Hitselberger WE. The transcochlear approach to the skull base. *Arch Otolaryngol* 1976; 102:334–342.

13. House WF, Hitselberger WE. Fatalities in acoustic tumor surgery. In: House WF, Luetje CM (eds.), *Acoustic Tumors*. Baltimore: University Park Press, 1979; 2:235–264.

14. Panse R. Ein Gliom des Akustikus. *Arch Ohrenheilk* 1904; 61:251–255.

15. Pulec JL. Labyrinthectomy: indications, technique and results. *Laryngoscope* 1974; 84:1552–1573.

16. Quix F. Ein Fall von translabyrintharisch operiertem Tumor acusticus. *Ver Dtsch Otol Ges* 1912; 21:245–255.

17. Schmiegelow E. Beitrag zur translabyrinthären Entfernung der Akustikustumoren. *Z Ohrenheilk* 1915; 83:1–21.

18. Smith MF. Conservation of hearing in acoustic schwannoma surgery. *Am J Otol* 1985; Suppl:161–163.

19. Tos M, Thomsen J. "How I do it"—otology and neurotology: a specific issue and its solution. Cerebrospinal fluid leak after translabyrinthine surgery for acoustic neuroma. *Laryngoscope* 1985; 95:351–354.

20. Whittaker CK, Luetje CM. Translabyrinthine removal of large acoustic tumors. *Am J Otol* 1985; Suppl:155–160.

45

Strategies to Preserve Hearing during Resection of Acoustic Neurinomas

Robert G. Ojemann

The purpose of this chapter is to review the clinical features and technical details that contribute to preservation of hearing during resection of an acoustic neurinoma. Our previous publications present details related to this problem.[6,8-10] Selected reviews and reports emphasizing particular aspects of this subject are included in the references.[1-14]

When Can Useful Hearing Be Saved?

The chance of saving useful hearing in the patient with a unilateral acoustic neurinoma and no evidence of neurofibromatosis has a direct relationship to the size of the tumor and the preoperative level of hearing. In reports of patients in whom it has been possible to preserve some hearing, the tumor has usually been less than 2 cm in diameter.[2,3,9,10,12,14] This would not be unexpected from the observation that in larger tumors the cochlear nerve usually merges into the tumor.[5] In our series of patients with unilateral acoustic neurinomas, we have found that if the preoperative speech discrimination is 35 percent or more and the tumor is intracanalicular or extends up to 0.5 cm into the posterior fossa, the chance of saving useful hearing is 73 percent; 0.5 to 1.5 cm, 35 percent; and 1.5 to 2.5 cm, 15 percent.[8,10] When the tumor is 3.0 cm or larger, only a few cases of preserved hearing have been reported.[2,10]

The findings on preoperative audiometric studies that would indicate a higher probability of preserving hearing have been reviewed, and several surgeons have selected patients for attempted hearing preservation only when there is at least a 50-dB pure tone average and the speech discrimination score is 50 percent or better.[2,12,14] Most of our patients had preoperative discrimination scores of greater than 50 percent and all had a speech reception threshold of 45 dB

or less. When the preoperative discrimination score was less than 50 percent, useful hearing was preserved in only 1 of 7 patients.[8]

When useful hearing is preserved, the postoperative discrimination score is usually similar to or somewhat less than the preoperative score. It is a rare patient who shows dramatic improvement in speech discrimination, but some patients benefit from a low level of hearing preserved by the surgery.[1,2,8,10,14] For this reason we have defined postoperative useful hearing as a speech reception threshold no poorer than 70 dB and a discrimination score of at least 15 percent, although most patients have a discrimination score of 35 percent or better.[8]

In general, we use intraoperative monitoring to help to preserve hearing when there is at least a 35 percent discrimination score and the tumor is less than 2.0 cm in diameter. When the tumor is 2.0 cm or larger and there is good hearing, it is probably worthwhile to use intraoperative monitoring only in the rare circumstances where the patient has severely impaired hearing in the opposite ear.

Etiology of Hearing Loss during Tumor Removal

When the acoustic neurinoma is intracanalicular or the extension into the posterior fossa is 1.5 cm or less, the cochlear nerve is usually found on the tumor capsule as a separate bundle, allowing the possibility of nerve preservation. As the tumor enlarges, the cochlear nerve tends to be incorporated into the tumor so that in large tumors no more than 10 percent have a cochlear nerve that is on the tumor capsule.[5]

Even when the cochlear nerve can be saved, there are several mechanisms that still may contribute to loss of hearing. These include mechanical trauma to the nerve, ischemia to the nerve or cochlea, injury to the labyrinth, and extension of the tumor into the cochlea.

The ability to maintain the vascular supply to the nerve and cochlea is one of the most difficult problems in preserving hearing.[6,10,14] The location of the internal auditory artery is variable, and there may be more than one arterial vessel entering the internal auditory meatus. When the artery is on the anterior aspect of the nerve complex and does not need to be extensively dissected, the chances of saving hearing are better. In an occasional patient, we have found that an artery within the tumor or a small apparently insignificant vessel in the arachnoid going to the internal auditory meatus area seems to be the important blood supply for hearing. We have not found angiography to be of help in determining the relationship of the internal auditory artery to the tumor.

During exposure of the tumor and dissection of the cochlear nerve, fibrous attachments are cut and great care is taken to avoid excessive pressure or tension on the nerve. One area of particular concern will be found in the patient whose tumor extends far laterally into the internal auditory canal and may invade the cochlea. In this situation, complete removal of the tumor cannot be done without destroying hearing. The use of gadolinium-enhanced MRI may allow a more precise preoperative assessment of the lateral extension of the tumor.

Intraoperative Monitoring

The rationale for monitoring intraoperative auditory evoked potentials is that a change in hearing sufficient to make a detectable change in the evoked potentials would result in either minor disturbances in the hearing or one that is reversible. By its nature, monitoring requires a disturbance in hearing before the surgeon can be alerted. In some patients, even when feedback occurs within seconds, it may be too late to rectify the situation such as when there is sudden loss related to blood vessel occlusion. In other situations, the lack of change reassures the surgeon about the dissection. There are operations where changes occur that are reversible and recovery is seen after stopping or altering the dissection.

Our system of intraoperative monitoring has been reported in detail.[6,8-10] It involves the use of click-evoked potentials recorded by a needle electrode placed through the inferior part of the tympanic membrane on the cochlear promontory (electrocochleography) and by electrodes in the scalp (brain stem auditory evoked potentials; BAEPs). Electrocochleography allows monitoring of activity from both the auditory nerve (N1 component) and the vascular supply to the cochlea hair cells (cochlea microphonics), giving the surgeon information about the two important components in maintaining hearing. The recorded potentials are so much larger than the BAEPs that only a few seconds of trials are required to obtain a satisfactory recording. The BAEPs provide information concerning auditory activity within the brain stem (usually as Wave V).

We have also recorded directly from the cochlear nerve but this can present technical problems—recording cannot be made until the nerve is exposed, and it may be difficult to maintain the electrode in continuous contact with the nerve. On the other hand, this recording may give more precise information about direct trauma to the nerve.[14] The use of this type of recording has been described.[3,4,7,14]

In general, if both the auditory nerve potential and Wave V are preserved, there will be some postoperative hearing and if they are both lost, there will be no hearing.[8] The postoperative result is indeterminate when Wave V is lost and the auditory potential retained, but many patients have retained some hearing.

We have found the waveforms of the electrocochleogram to be stable and reproducible in most patients. There has been no problem with the eardrum. The potential problems with the recording include dislodgment of the electrode in the ear, blood or fluid entering the middle ear and blocking sound transmission (either from the electrode trauma or from opening the mastoid air cells), the inability to recognize the cochlea microphonic waveforms in some patients because of their small amplitude, the possibility that direct trauma to the cochlear nerve may not cause immediate changes in the electrocochleogram, and the theoretical possibility that potentials will be generated from a site distal to the tumor. Others have described the use of this system.[7,12]

The recording system is a sensitive indicator of cochlear nerve function and gives nearly an instantaneous feedback to the surgeon about the status of the hearing. It has given us information about the problems encountered in trying to preserve hearing. We believe the system has helped in the ability to save hearing, but to what extent its value has been in preventing hearing loss has not been documented.

Operative Technique

Our technique has been described and illustrated in detail in previous publications.[9,10] Recent modifications are included in this description.

Selection of Approach

Hearing may be preserved with either a middle fossa or suboccipital transmeatal approach to the tumor.[1,9,10] We have used the posterior fossa approach because the middle fossa exposure provided limited access to the posterior fossa, was associated with greater technical difficulty in removing the tumor, and was reported to be associated with a higher incidence of facial weakness.

Preoperative Medication and Anesthesia

Patients receive steroids for 48 h prior to operation. After induction of anesthesia, the patients are usually maintained with a combination of oxygen–nitrous oxide, sufentanil, and pancuronium. Muscle relaxants are kept to a minimum so facial nerve function can be monitored. Intravenous antibiotics are given, and the patient receives 20 mg of furosemide. During the exposure, 100 g of mannitol as a 20% solution is given.

Position and Placement of Monitoring Equipment

The patient is placed in a supine position with the ipsilateral shoulder slightly elevated and the head turned nearly parallel to the floor and elevated and held with a skeletal fixation headrest. During the operation the line of sight to the brain stem may be changed by moving the microscope and/or rotating the operating table from side to side, and hence the position has been called the supine-oblique position.[9-11]

Before preparation and draping of the surgical field, the monitoring equipment is placed. The function of the facial nerve is monitored continuously by using fine needle electrodes placed in the orbicularis oculi and orbicularis oris muscles and a motion sensor on the face to record mechanical activity during bipolar coagulation. This system allows detection of spontaneous activity when dissecting near the facial nerve and records the results of monopolar stimulation, which is used to locate and confirm the position of the nerve. The equipment is then placed for monitoring of auditory evoked potentials.

Incision and Exposure

A vertical incision is centered approximately 2.0 cm medial to the mastoid process. A graft of pericranial tissue, 3 to 4 cm in diameter, is taken from the occipital region and used in closing the cerebellar convexity dura at the conclusion of the operation. Suboccipital muscles are incised in line with the excision. The lateral two-thirds of the suboccipital bone is exposed.

A burr hole is made, the dura separated, and a craniotomy flap cut. Further bone is removed to bring the exposure to the transverse sinus and the lateral wall and floor of the posterior fossa. If the mastoid air cells are entered, they are occluded immediately with bone wax. If fluid enters these cells and gets into the middle ear, there may be interference with the intraoperative monitoring.

The dura is opened to expose the cerebellum over the lateral one-half to two-thirds of the craniotomy opening, leaving an area of medial dura intact under which the cerebellum may be retracted. The cerebellum is often quite relaxed because of the furosemide and mannitol administration, but usually it is gently elevated from the floor of the posterior fossa, the arachnoid is opened, and spinal fluid is allowed to drain. This is important because this allows exploration of the cerebellopontine angle with as little retraction as possible on the cerebellum. This must be done slowly and carefully because, on occasion, this retraction has altered the evoked response.[4,9] Changing the direction or degree of retraction usually causes the potentials to recover. Any bridging veins from the cerebellum to the dura are carefully divided. The Greenberg self-retaining retractors are then placed, and the operating microscope positioned.

Microsurgical Removal of the Tumor

The anatomy in the area of the tumor has been beautifully illustrated by Rhoton.[11] The arachnoid over the posterior capsule of the tumor is opened. The petrosal vein is usually divided. If the seventh and eighth nerve complex is not immediately visible, the cerebellar tissue next to the tumor may be shrunk with bipolar coagulation or a small amount of cerebellar tissue may be removed to expose the inferior medial aspect of the tumor and the nerve complex. If the nerve complex is still not seen, the posterior capsule of the tumor is stimulated. In almost all patients with small tumors and in over 80 percent with medium and large tumors, the facial and cochlear nerves will be on the anterior surface of the tumor and there will be no response to the stimulation of the posterior capsule. The next most common location for the facial nerve is to be compressed against the brain stem and then on the anterior superior surface of the capsule. On rare occasions, the facial nerve and the cochlear nerve are displaced posteriorly rather than in the usual anterior location. When stimulation is completed, the posterior capsule of the tumor is opened and an internal decompression is done. In smaller tumors, bipolar coagulation and sharp instruments are utilized; in large tumors, the ultrasonic aspirator is used. The tumor capsule can now be reflected laterally and superiorly to bring into view the vestibular nerves.

The surgeon has a choice of beginning the dissection medially or removing the dura over the internal auditory canal, drilling the bone and starting the dissection laterally. The preservation of hearing does not seem to relate to whether the dissection is carried along the nerve in a medial or lateral direction.[4] An attempt is made to preserve any arterial vessels going into the auditory meatus. The surgeon may need to alternate the dissection from different directions, continuing the dissection in an area where it seems to be going well and moving to another area if the dissection becomes difficult.

Medial dissection begins on the inferior medial aspect of the tumor capsule. The cochlear portion of the eighth nerve is not clearly seen at this stage because it is covered by the proximal superior vestibular nerve. The plane between the capsule and the eighth nerve is opened by sharp dissection with division of those vestibular fibers that are entering the tumor. We use a fine suction to retract the tumor capsule and clear the field and microdissectors and sharp dissection along the seventh and eighth nerves. The importance of sharp dissection to reduce trauma to the nerves has also been stressed by Jannetta et al.[4] Small vessels entering the tumor must be coagulated and divided with fine bipolar forceps at low power, but every effort is made to preserve any arteries running along the nerve complex. The facial nerve is often identified by its slightly grayish-white color in contrast to the more pale yellow color of the eighth nerve. The position is confirmed using monopolar stimulation.

When the bone over the internal auditory canal begins to interfere with the ability to reflect the tumor capsule laterally, or the dissection is difficult along the nerves, or there are transient changes in the monitored potentials, attention is directed to the exposure of the internal auditory canal.

To expose the internal auditory canal, the dura is removed over the region of the canal and the bone is carefully removed with an air drill, using constant suction and irrigation for cooling. Removal should extend for a distance of no more than 10 mm, since more lateral bone removal runs the risk of entering the semicircular canals. In the drilling of the canal, we pause at frequent intervals to check the potentials and to allow further cooling and irrigation of the area. After exposing the tumor in the canal, further internal decompression of the tumor is done. The lateral extent of the tumor is carefully defined. The vestibular nerves are sharply divided. One must be careful not to put traction on these nerves. Arterial vessels are preserved and the tumor carefully reflected medially. The attachments to the superior and inferior margins of the internal auditory meatus are divided. If dissection proves difficult, attention is again turned medially and the tumor is dissected from medial to lateral. The facial nerve is often most adherent in the region of the internal auditory meatus.

Great care is taken in the lateral dissection of the tumor, particularly if it extends beyond the limits of the bone exposure. We, as well as others, have encountered sudden hearing loss with removal of this lateral extension of tumor.[9,12] It is known that acoustic neurinomas may invade the cochlea, and removal of the last fragment of tumor may open the labyrinth or may damage the internal auditory artery. This dissection is difficult because of the limited exposure caused by the need to avoid the posterior semicircular canal.

Closure

After removal of the tumor, any mastoid air cells that have been entered while drilling to expose the internal auditory canal are occluded with bone wax and an adipose tissue graft is placed in the area where the bone was removed. After careful inspection of the hemostasis, the dura is closed with the graft of pericranial tissue and the bone flap is replaced.

Long-Term Results

In patients with unilateral tumors in whom we have saved hearing, we believe a total removal of the tumor has been accomplished.[8–10] Silverstein et al. have summarized the histologic studies that indicate that a microscopic complete removal of tumor may not be possible without removal of the eighth nerve.[14] However, to date we have not seen a recurrence of tumor in follow-up computed tomography and magnetic resonance images in our patients. This has also been the experience of others.[3,9,10,14]

In most patients where hearing has been retained, subsequent audiograms have remained stable. We, as well as others, have noted a small number of patients who have a delayed deterioration in hearing days to weeks after the operation. The reason for this is unknown.[4,9,13]

The attempt to save hearing does not change the ability to save facial nerve function. This function also relates to tumor size, as it does when no attempt is being made to save hearing.

Bilateral Acoustic Neurinomas

Surgery for bilateral acoustic neurinomas occurring in a patient with little or no expression of neurofibromatosis is similar to that for unilateral tumors. The tumor usually has a smooth capsule and displaces the facial and cochlear nerves, allowing the possibility of preserving function in these nerves with removal of the tumor. In contrast, the bilateral acoustic tumors associated with extensive expression of neurofibromatosis are often multilobulated, suggesting that such a tumor may form from multiple sites, or that there may be multiple separate tumors in the cerebellopontine angle (neurofibroma or meningioma).

When the patient has bilateral acoustic neurinomas with useful hearing in both ears, complete removal should be considered on one side if one or both tumors are small. This will give the best opportunity to preserve hearing.

The patient who is already deaf in one ear and shows progressive hearing loss in the only hearing ear presents a difficult problem. In several patients, we have done a planned subtotal removal of the tumor using intraoperative monitoring with internal decompression of the tumor and decompression of the internal auditory canal to try to stabilize hearing for as long as possible.

If both tumors are already of medium or large size when the patient is first seen, treatment is guided by the clinical symptoms. Usually one tumor will need to be removed. The extent of removal of the second tumor is based on evaluations of the clinical status. Patients who have no symptoms or have only mild symptoms that seem to be stable, are carefully followed with periodic audiometric and radiographic studies.

References

1. Gantz BJ, Parnes LS, Harker LA, et al. Middle cranial fossa acoustic neuroma excision: results and complications. *Ann Otol Rhinol Laryngol* 1986; 95:454–459.
2. Gardner G, Robertson JH. Hearing preservation in unilateral acoustic neuroma surgery. *Ann Otol Rhinol Laryngol* 1988; 97:55–66.
3. Harner SG, Laws ER Jr, Onofrio BM. Hearing preservation after removal of acoustic neurinoma. *Laryngoscope* 1984; 94:1431–1434.
4. Jannetta PJ, Møller AR, Møller MB. Technique of hearing preservation in small acoustic neuromas. *Ann Surg* 1984; 200:513–523.
5. Koos WT, Perneczky A. Suboccipital approach to acoustic neurinomas with emphasis on preservation of facial nerve and cochlear nerve function. In: Rand RW (ed.), *Microneurosurgery*. St. Louis: Mosby, 1985:335–365.
6. Levine RA, Ojemann RG, Montgomery WW, et al. Monitoring auditory evoked potentials during acoustic neuroma surgery: insights into the mechanism of the hearing loss. *Ann Otol Rhinol Laryngol* 1984; 93:116–123.
7. Linden RD, Tator CH, Benedict C, et al. Electrophysiological monitoring during acoustic neuroma and other posterior fossa surgery. *Can J Neurol Sci* 1988; 15:73–81.
8. Nadol JB Jr, Levine R, Ojemann RG, et al. Preservation of hearing in surgical removal of acoustic neuromas of the internal auditory canal and cerebellar pontine angle. *Laryngoscope* 1987; 97:1287–1294.
9. Ojemann RG, Levine RA, Montgomery WW, et al. Use of intraoperative auditory evoked potentials to preserve hearing in unilateral acoustic neuroma removal. *J Neurosurg* 1984; 61:938–948.
10. Ojemann RG, Martuza RL. Acoustic neuroma. In: Youmans JR (ed.), *Neurological Surgery*, 3d ed. Philadelphia: Saunders, 1990:3316–3350.
11. Rhoton AL Jr. Microsurgical anatomy of the brainstem surface facing an acoustic neuroma. *Surg Neurol* 1986; 25:326–339.
12. Sabin HI, Bentivoglio P, Symon L, et al. Intra-operative electrocochleography to monitor cochlear potentials during acoustic neuroma excision. *Acta Neurochir (Wien)* 1987; 85:110–116.
13. Samii M. Microsurgery of acoustic neurinomas with special emphasis on preservation of seventh and eighth nerves and the scope of facial nerve grafting. In: Rand RW (ed.), *Microneurosurgery*. St. Louis: Mosby, 1985:366–388.
14. Silverstein H, McDaniel AB, Norrell H. Hearing preservation after acoustic neuroma surgery using intraoperative direct eighth cranial nerve monitoring. *Am J Otol* 1985; Nov Suppl:99–106.

46

Peritorcular Meningiomas

Griffith R. Harsh IV
Charles B. Wilson

> Whether in relation to the torcular they start in the NE, NW, SW or SE corners, [peritorcular meningiomas] may come in time to box the entire regional compass; and when they have done so, there are few more formidable lesions surgically to encounter.
>
> *H. Cushing, 1938*

> The one good thing about torcular meningiomas is their rarity.
>
> *L. Malis, 1988*

Peritorcular meningiomas, although rare, have a special place in neurosurgical history. As noted by Cushing and Eisenhardt, the tendency of these tumors to produce visual field defects facilitated their preoperative localization, and such precise localization encouraged neurosurgical pioneers to attempt to remove them.[4] Birdsall and Weir in 1887 reported the first effort at removal of a peritorcular meningioma; their case was one of the earliest intracranial operations for tumor, and it ended in fatal postoperative hemorrhage.[2] One of the first successful operations for brain tumor was the removal of a parasagittal and peritorcular meningioma, as reported by Oppenheim and Krause in 1906.[10] The first case in Dandy's initial description of ventriculography was a peritorcular meningioma.[5]

Cushing and Eisenhardt first differentiated the peritorcular meningiomas as a distinct entity.[4] They identified 12 tumors among 77 parasagittal meningiomas that, because of involvement with the tentorium and lateral sinuses as well as the superior sagittal sinus and falx, presented the surgeon with difficulties of exposure and removal that increased the hazards of surgery. Torcular meningiomas have, as part of their dural base, dura forming the torcular; i.e., they arise from, invade, or are attached to a wall of the torcular itself. Peritorcular meningiomas arise from the dura of the posterior falx cerebri, posteromedial tentorium cerebelli, or su-

peroposterior falx cerebelli and, by virtue of compression or invasion of the superior sagittal, straight, transverse, and/or occipital sinuses, threaten dural venous sinus flow at the torcular Herophili. The relationship of peritorcular meningiomas to the posterior dural venous sinuses is paramount in the definition of this entity because of the profound implications of the tumor to venous sinus anatomic relationships for the clinical presentation, diagnosis, treatment, and outcome of patients with these tumors.

Pathologic Anatomy

The torcular Herophili, the site of confluence of the superior sagittal, straight, occipital, and both transverse sinuses, varies greatly from individual to individual. Rarely is there symmetrical intersection of these five sinuses at a central point beneath the internal occipital protuberance. Rather, peritorcular venous channels are usually asymmetrical and septate (Fig. 46-1). The distal superior sagittal sinus often has a double lumen. The right transverse sinus, which frequently carries most of the superior sagittal sinus outflow, is often larger than the left transverse sinus, which frequently carries most of the straight sinus flow. Occasionally, one transverse sinus may be congenitally atretic or even absent; distal outflow may be occluded as a result of sigmoid sinus or jugular vein occlusion by prior tympanic disease. The extent of communication of the superior sagittal flow with each transverse sinus and of one transverse sinus with the other is often critical to the clinical pathophysiology and surgical resectability of peritorcular meningiomas.

Peritorcular meningiomas arise from arachnoidal cap cells in the region of the torcular Herophili. Castellano and Ruggerio reported that there is a relative abundance of such cells along the posterior margin of the tentorium.[3] Cushing and Eisenhardt noted a predominance of angioblastic meningiomas in their group of peritorcular meningiomas; of the 12 tumors, 6 were angioblastic, 5 of which showed malignant histologic and clinical features.[4] Three of 12 tumors

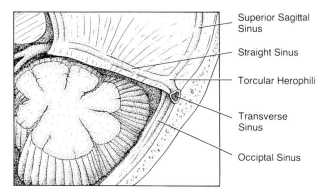

Figure 46-1. Peritorcular venous anatomy. The interrelations of the five venous sinuses in the region vary from individual to individual. The sinuses as well as the torcular Herophili itself may be septate. Often a true confluence may not exist.

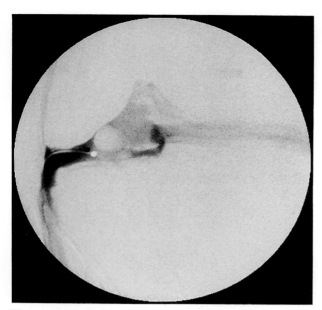

Figure 46-2. Intraluminal tumor growth. Selective retrograde venogram of the peritorcular venous sinuses depicts a spherical meningioma within the right transverse sinus obstructing venous outflow from the torcular Herophili.

were of the fibroblastic "whorl" type, 1 was psammomatous, 1 was fibrotic, and 1 was mesothelial. Such a skewed distribution of histologic subtypes has not been noted in the peritorcular tumors of other series of meningiomas. Interesting variants of peritorcular meningiomas include those associated with extensive hyperostosis in the region of the internal occipital protuberance (e.g., Cushing's Case 8, in which there was hyperostosis from the lambda to the foramen magnum) and those with *en plaque* extension of tumor along the venous sinuses (e.g., also Cushing's Case 8, in which tumor extended along the transverse sinus to involve three of the four peritorcular quadrants).[4] The dura is a poor barrier to tumor extension; there are numerous examples of tumors perforating the distal falx or posterior tentorium to reach an adjacent quadrant. Although meningiomas of benign histology may have such extension, it occurs with greater frequency among tumors with malignant histologic characteristics.

Except in cases of malignant histology, tumor growth is slow. Tumor expansion progressively displaces the adjacent occipital lobe or cerebellar hemisphere and compresses proximate sinuses. The clinical syndromes produced thus reflect occipital lobe or cerebellar dysfunction or manifest elevated intracranial venous pressure. The latter may produce generalized intracranial hypertension, which may be augmented by the mass of the tumor itself, and either focal or generalized cortical dysfunction. The development of clinical symptoms is usually insidious, and the tumor may become very large before symptoms become clinically evident. An exception to this tendency is the tumor that arises in the wall of a dural sinus and extends inwardly rather than outwardly; in such a case, florid clinical symptoms can be produced by a small tumor obliterating a venous sinus lumen (Fig. 46-2).

Clinical Presentations

The rarity of meningiomas in this region and the imprecision with which the term *peritorcular meningioma* has been used make estimation of a true incidence difficult. In addition to the 12 peritorcular meningiomas Cushing and Eisenhardt found in their series of 77 parasagittal meningiomas,[4] three series of posterior fossa menigiomas combined contained 4.9 percent (4 of 82) peritorcular tumors.[8,9,11] Three series of tentorial meningiomas combined contained 13 percent (14 of 109) peritorcular tumors,[3,6,12] and if the relative incidences of parasagittal, tentorial, and posterior fossa tumors are 10 percent, 5 percent, and 10 percent, respectively, of all intracranial meningiomas, peritorcular tumors represent about 1 percent of intracranial meningiomas.[7] Because of this low incidence, peritorcular tumors have not been distinguished from other meningiomas in reported series other than that of Cushing and Eisenhardt.[4]

In that series, seven patients were male and five were female.[4] The average age at presentation was 35.5 years. These patients uniformly had large tumors causing severe neurologic deficits. The median interval between symptom onset and diagnosis was 1 year; the mean interval was 1.5 years. Predictably, the presenting symptoms and signs reflected either occipital or cerebellar compression or intracranial hypertension secondary to venous outflow obstruction (Table 46-1). All patients had papilledema; at least half also had homonymous field cuts suggestive of an occipital contribution to their visual loss and the supratentorial presence of tumor. Headache was global in half of the patients who noted it; this most likely reflects increased intracranial pressure. Occipital and suboccipital pain, probably resulting from deformation of surrounding dura, was described by the other half. Neck pain and stiffness may have indicated incipient tonsillar herniation. Cerebellar signs, indicative of infratentorial tumor extension, included nystagmus, dysmetria, hypotonia, and ataxia. Notably, there was no case of acute neurologic deterioration that might result from sudden thrombosis of a partially occluded dominant sinus. Presumably, the slow growth of these tumors permits the development of sufficient collateral flow to preclude such a catastrophe.

TABLE 46-1 Clinical presentation of patients with peritorcular meningiomas ($n = 12$)*

Symptoms		Signs	
Visual loss	11	Papilledema	12
Headache	10	Homonymous field cut	7
Neck pain/stiffness	4	Cerebellar deficits	5
Gait difficulty	3	Scotoma/atrophic blindness	3
Memory problems	2	Cortical sensorimotor loss	3

*Reported by Cushing and Eisenhardt.[4]

Diagnostic Studies

Gadolinium-enhanced magnetic resonance (MR) imaging and multiprojection subtraction angiography are the most valuable neurodiagnostic tools for assessing peritorcular meningiomas. Formerly, neurosurgeons relied on signs of increased intracranial pressure and peritorcular calcification observed on plain skull roentgenograms for diagnosis and on the ventriculographic pattern of aqueductal deformation for localization of these tumors. Computed tomography greatly facilitated the preoperative diagnosis of these tumors and still is valuable in defining bone detail, especially if there is hyperostosis and intratumoral calcification.

Multiplanar MR imaging, however, offers far superior anatomic detail of the tumor and its relation to both surrounding brain and adjacent venous sinuses. On T1-weighted images, most meningiomas are isointense with brain. Large parenchymal or tumor vessels are apparent as cylindrical areas of signal void. There is some increase in relative intensity of tumor on T2-weighted images, but this is usually less marked than is the case with neurofibromas. Intratumoral calcification appears as a signal void on MR T1- and T2-weighted scans. Peritumoral edema shifts from hypointense on T1-weighted images to hyperintense with T2 weighting. Gadolinium enhances the contrast between tumor and brain (Figs. 46-3 and 46-4). The distinctiveness of the margin between tumor capsule and cortex may correlate with the ease of maintenance of a plane of surgical dissection and with benign rather than invasive malignant histology.

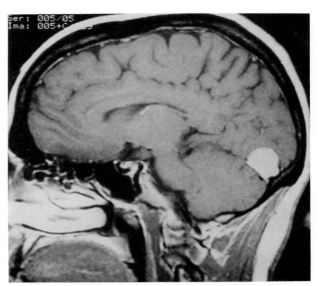

Figure 46-4. T1-weighted gadolinium-enhanced MR image in a parasagittal plane. Multiplanar imaging of this peritorcular meningioma depicts the tumor's relation to the torcular Herophili, greatly facilitating the planning of the surgical approach.

The multiplanar capacities of MR permit depiction of the tumor's relation to the sinuses and tentorium, valuable information in preoperative planning. The midsagittal and medial parasagittal views show the relation of the tumor to the falx cerebri and the falx cerebelli, and the coronal view clearly demonstrates the relation of the tumor to the transverse sinuses (Figs. 46-3 and 46-4). The degree of extension above and below the tentorium is readily apparent. Tumor extension is evident as thickening of dural leaves that becomes more intense with gadolinium; enhancement without thickening represents only dural hyperemia along the course of the tumor's blood supply. The MR image also helps predict the status of the sinuses. A patent sinus has a signal void characteristic of flowing blood; this is especially evident on T2-weighted scans, in which contrast with the higher intensity of CSF is maximized. A partially occluded sinus is heterogeneous in intensity; regions of signal void corresponding to normal flow are interrupted by regions of increased intensity indicative of stasis. A uniformly intense sinus suggests occlusion; occasionally, however, a sinus with very slow flow appears bright and falsely appears to be completely occluded.

Equally essential to preoperative planning is multiplanar angiography. The diagnosis of meningioma is confirmed by the appearance of the tumor's dense capillary blush in the late venous phase. Displacement of normal blood vessels or their involvement with tumor is shown by angiography. The feeding arteries—usually the middle meningeal and occipital branches from the external carotid artery, meningeal branches of the vertebral artery, and the tentorial branches of the cavernous internal carotid artery—should be identified and, as often as is possible, embolized. An effort should be made to embolize vessels within the tumor itself. Large feeding arteries should be filled with embolic material and

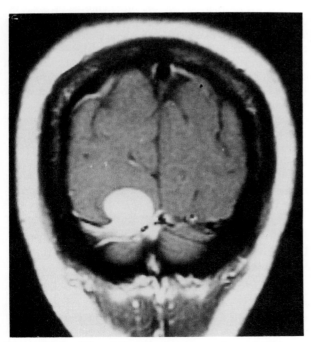

Figure 46-3. T1-weighted gadolinium-enhanced MR image in a coronal plane. This peritorcular meningioma envelopes the right transverse sinus at the torcular Herophili.

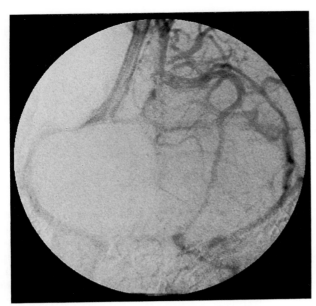

Figure 46-5. Anterior-posterior projection of the venous phase of an internal carotid angiogram. Incomplete filling of the distal superior sagittal sinus, torcular Herophili, and right transverse sinus are suggestive of a tumor compressing the proximal right transverse sinus. The left transverse sinus is congenitally atretic. Inadequacy of venous outflow resulted in elevated intracranial pressure.

occluded more proximally by a detachable balloon after embolization is completed.

Even more critical is precise delineation of the peritorcular venous anatomy. The pattern of flow in each sinus should be carefully studied. Sinus occlusion is manifest by absence of filling and collateral flow of blood away from the torcular Herophili (Fig. 46-5). The details of site and cause of venous sinus obstruction are best seen on retrograde dural sinus venography (Fig. 46-2). Direct endovascular cannulation of the transverse sinus also permits trials of sinus obliteration; clinical tolerance of sinus occlusion and intraluminal pressure proximal to the blockage are assessed during balloon inflation. Such information is invaluable to the surgeon planning operative excision of a peritorcular meningioma.

Treatment

The goal of treatment of patients with torcular meningiomas is the relief of neurologic manifestations and the prevention of further tumor growth. This is best accomplished by total surgical resection. Efforts at total removal, however, must be tempered by the following: (1) the patient's age, medical condition, and type of neurologic deficit; (2) the probability that a catastrophic outcome will follow occlusion of a sinus on which the brain is reliant; and (3) the favorable long-term results achievable by subtotal resection followed by radiation therapy. Clearly a more aggressive surgical stance is warranted for the otherwise healthy young female patient

with a large tumor causing progressive focal neurologic deficits than for the elderly male patient with an apparently slowly growing tumor discovered incidentally. Temporizing surgical measures such as optic nerve sheath fenestration, designed to relieve visual deficits arising from elevated intracranial venous pressure, or ventriculoperitoneal shunting of obstructive hydrocephalus may be indicated in cases where a patient's medical condition or the tumor's anatomic geometry precludes tumor resection by craniotomy. Such procedures, if they relieve neurologic deficits, may also permit delay of an operation on a tumor incompletely occluding a major sinus until further tumor growth completely occludes the sinus such that it can be divided and resected. Ventriculoperitoneal shunting is not indicated if removal of tumor is anticipated; intraoperative ventricular drainage of an expanded ventricle facilitates occipital lobe retraction in supratentorial approaches to peritorcular tumors, and tumor removal may relieve the aqueductal and fourth ventricular compression responsible for the hydrocephalus.

The choice of operative approach depends on the tumor's size and location, the nature of sinus involvement, and the goals of surgery. The extent of peritorcular exposure needed depends on the number of peritorcular quadrants containing tumor and the tumor's geometry. A unilateral occipital craniotomy or suboccipital craniectomy may suffice for tumors occupying only a single quadrant. Exclusively supratentorial tumors that penetrate the falx cerebri but not the tentorium may be exposed by a bilateral occipital craniotomy. In the case of large bilateral supratentorial extensions, the risk of inducing cortical blindness from bilateral calcarine injury may be reduced by monitoring visual evoked potentials or staging sequential unilateral procedures. Similarly, exclusively infratentorial tumors perforating the falx cerebelli can be removed through a bilateral suboccipital craniectomy. For unilateral tumors extending through the tentorium, a combined supratentorial and infratentorial approach is often justified. In many cases, however, the portion of the tumor extending across the tentorium can be removed through a unilateral occipital craniotomy or suboccipital craniectomy alone. The supratentorial approach has the advantage of the extensive exposure gained by wide lateral retraction of the occipital lobe; few cortical veins drain medially from the occipital lobe, and those that exist can be sacrificed without risk of neurologic deficit. The infratentorial approach, however, averts the risk of retraction-induced injury to the visual cortex. In either case, wide transtentorial exposure can be obtained by dividing the tentorium from the incisura to the anterior margin of the transverse sinus. In the removal of tumors that arise directly from the torcular wall, exposure of all four quadrants of the peritorcular region is advisable because it permits control of all venous inflow and outflow to the region.

The position of the patient is a matter of surgeon's preference. The sitting, Concorde, and 45-degree prone oblique positions all afford adequate access in unilateral approaches. Either the sitting or Concorde position is preferred for bilateral exposures. A horseshoe incision with its apex at lambda and its base between the mastoid processes is excellent for bilateral combined exposures. It may be narrowed and/or shortened if less exposure is required. Bone removal is usually accomplished by free occipital flap craniotomy and/or suboccipital craniectomy. Piecemeal rongeuring of bone is the safest method of removal when traversing the superior sagittal sinus, transverse sinuses, or the torcular Herophili itself. Dural adhesion to bone that results from hyperostosis or age greatly increases the risk of tearing a feeding artery or unroofing a venous sinus. The danger of the former can be reduced by performing a strip craniectomy at the margins of the bone flap and interrupting dural vessels before removal of the bone flap. The incidence of the latter can be reduced by performing a unilateral free-flap craniotomy to the edge of the superior sagittal sinus and torcular Herophili on one side and then, under direct vision, freeing the superficial surface of the sinuses from overlying bone before removing the contralateral craniotomy plate (L. Malis, personal communication, 1988). When dural adhesion to bone is unlikely because the patient is young, the tumor small, and hyperostosis absent, a single craniotomy flap can be used to expose all four quadrants of the peritorcular region. Infiltrated or hyperostotic bone should be removed and discarded.

Dura should be incised at a distance of at least 2 cm from the tumor's margin. It should be hinged so as to maximize the view of peritorcular tumor. Drainage of CSF supratentorially by ventriculostomy of the lateral ventricle or infratentorially by opening the cisterna magna facilitates subsequent retraction. Tumor distant from the venous sinuses should be separated from occipital or cerebellar cortex by microsurgical dissection and truncated.

The likelihood of achieving the goal of total resection depends on the nature of sinus involvement by the tumor; only rarely is tumor resection precluded by tumor attachment to eloquent cortex or critical arteries. The portion of a venous sinus completely occluded by tumor can be resected safely. When removing an occluded superior sagittal sinus, special care must be taken to preserve the anterior and lateral collaterals carrying the hemispheric flow. An involved transverse sinus can be divided and resected if preoperative venography has shown that (1) the sinus is occluded by tumor or is congenitally atretic, (2) its proximal portion communicates completely with a patent contralateral transverse sinus of adequate caliber, or (3) the superior sagittal sinus and straight sinus are fully confluent with a patent contralateral transverse sinus of adequate caliber. Interruption of a transverse sinus should be proximal to the inflow of the vein of Labbé. If preoperative venography has not clearly demonstrated the adequacy of the contralateral sinus, trial occlusion of the involved sinus by temporary intraoperative clamping may help assess the compensatory capacity of the contralateral sinus. The occipital sinus is of little importance unless, as a hypertrophied collateral of an obstructed transverse sinus, it carries substantial superior sagittal or straight sinus outflow to the jugular bulb.

When the venous anatomy dictates preservation of the flow through a sinus involved with tumor, the possibility of removal of the tumor from the sinus depends on the extent of sinus involvement. If the tumor merely abuts or is attached to the sinus by arachnoidal adhesions, it can be peeled from the sinus wall. The external sinus surface should then be coagulated with the bipolar cautery. Laser fulguration of the sinus wall should be avoided, because it may cause endothelial damage that subsequently induces catastrophic sinus thrombosis (J. Ransohoff, personal com-

munication, 1988). When the tumor is frankly invasive of one wall of a critical sinus, tumor external to the sinus should be truncated. The invaded wall and intrasinus extension of the tumor can often be removed, and the resultant defect closed by direct suture or with a patch graft. This is best done by sequentially opening and closing small segments of the sinus as the tumor is progressively removed from within the sinus. The walls of the partially opened sinus can be grasped by vascular forceps or small clamps such that they can be released to permit removal of the tumor or approximated to allow closure (Fig. 46-6). Transient opening of the sinus in such a controlled fashion permits removal of an intrasinus tumor with relatively little blood loss.

Attempts to remove a tumor involving more than one wall of the sinus are much more hazardous. Sinus flow must be interrupted during the resection of two walls. Construction of a patch graft that will maintain patency when sinus venous pressure is low is difficult. There have been isolated reports of tumor removal and patch graft repair of the more proximal portions of the superior sagittal sinus using a diversionary shunt. An analogous approach using a superior sagittal sinus to transverse sinus shunt during isolation and repair of a tumor-invaded torcular Herophili is conceptually intriguing but extremely hazardous. Removal of such a tumor might necessitate shunting flow from the superior sagittal, straight, and occipital sinuses and replacement of the torcular Herophili by a four-limbed prosthesis.

The risks concomitant with interruption or diversion of venous sinus flow and reconstruction of the torcular Herophili in an attempt to achieve complete resection of a peritorcular tumor are unwarranted (L. Malis, J. Ransohoff,

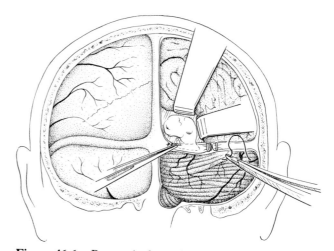

Figure 46-6. Removal of a peritorcular meningioma extending within the transverse sinus into the torcular. With the right occipital lobe elevated superiorly and laterally, the right transverse sinus, occluded by tumor, has been divided distally. Proximally, the dural leaves of the torcular-transverse sinus junction are alternately opened, closed, and sutured as tumor extending into the torcular is progressively removed. This permits subsequent proximal ligation and division of the transverse sinus, leaving the torcular-transverse sinus junction free of tumor.

R. Ojemann, personal communication, 1988). Although incomplete resection of meningiomas is frequently followed by recurrent tumor growth,[13] excellent results have accrued from subtotal resection of tumor external to the sinus and irradiation of the residual lesion. Malis obtained complete removal of 2 of 20 torcular meningiomas and reports that the 18 patients with residual tumor have done well after receiving postoperative irradiation (L. Malis, personal communication, 1988).

Focal external cobalt beam irradiation (50 to 60 Gy) of the residual tumor is recommended.[1,14] Focused high-energy irradiation from the gamma knife or linear accelerator may carry a greater risk of unwanted dural sinus thrombosis. Intraoperative marking of tumor margins by nonmagnetic metal clips facilitates planning of radiation therapy. Chemotherapy should be considered only if the tumor has malignant histologic characteristics. Postoperative follow-up review should consist of a periodic neurologic examination and gadolinium-enhanced MR imaging.

References

1. Barbaro NM, Gutin PH, Wilson CB, et al. Radiation therapy in the treatment of partially resected meningiomas. *Neurosurgery* 1987; 20:525–528.
2. Birdsall WR, Weir RF. Brain surgery: removal of a large sarcoma, causing hemianopsia, from the occipital lobe. *Med News (Phila)* 1887; 50:421–428.
3. Castellano F, Ruggiero G. Meningiomas of the posterior fossa. *Acta Radiol (Suppl) [Stockh]* 1953; 104:1–177 (see pp 26–69).
4. Cushing H, Eisenhardt L. *Meningiomas: Their Classification, Regional Behaviour, Life History, and Surgical End Results.* Springfield: Charles C Thomas, 1938.
5. Dandy WE. Localization or elimination of cerebral tumors by ventriculography. *Surg Gynecol Obstet* 1920; 30:329–342.
6. Guidetti B, Ciappetta P, Domenicucci M. Tentorial meningiomas: surgical experience with 61 cases and long-term results. *J Neurosurg* 1988; 69:183–187.
7. MacCarty CS, Taylor WF. Intracranial meningiomas: experiences at the Mayo Clinic. *Neurol Med Chir (Tokyo)* 1979; 19:569–574.
8. Markham JW, Fager CA, Horrax G, et al. Meningiomas of the posterior fossa: their diagnosis, clinical features, and surgical treatment. *Arch Neurol Psychiatry* 1955; 74:163–170.
9. Martinez R, Vaquero J, Areitio E, et al. Meningiomas of the posterior fossa. *Surg Neurol* 1983; 19:237–243.
10. Oppenheim H, Krause F. Ein operativ geheilter Tumor des Occipitallappens des Gehirns. *Berl Klin Wochenschr* 1906; 43:1616–1619.
11. Russell JR, Bucy PC. Meningiomas of the posterior fossa. *Surg Gynecol Obstet* 1953; 96:183–192.
12. Sekhar LN, Jannetta PJ, Maroon JC. Tentorial meningiomas: surgical management and results. *Neurosurgery* 1984; 14:268–275.
13. Simpson D. The recurrence of intracranial meningiomas after surgical treatment. *J Neurol Neurosurg Psychiatry* 1957; 20:22–39.
14. Wara WM, Sheline GE, Newman H, et al. Radiation therapy of meningiomas. *AJR* 1975; 123:453–458.

47

Microsurgical Anatomy of the Region of the Foramen Magnum

Albert L. Rhoton, Jr.
Evandro de Oliveira

Lesions in the region of the foramen magnum present special problems in operative management because of the many structures involved. The structures which must be considered in planning an operative approach to the region include the brain stem and spinal cord; the lower cranial and upper spinal nerves; the vertebral artery and its branches; and the ligaments uniting the atlas, axis, and occipital bone.[2,4]

Osseous Relationships

The osseous structures in the region of the foramen magnum are the occipital bone, the atlas, and the axis. The occipital bone surrounds the foramen magnum (Fig. 47-1). The foraminal opening is oval shaped and is wider posteriorly than anteriorly. The wider posterior part transmits the medulla, and the narrower anterior part sits above the odontoid process. The occipital bone is divided into a squamosal part located above and behind the foramen magnum, a basal part situated in front of the foramen magnum, and paired condylar parts located lateral to the foramen magnum. The squamous part is an internally concave plate located above and behind the foramen magnum. The internal surface has a prominent ridge, the internal occipital crest, which descends in the midline and serves as the attachment for the falx cerebelli. This crest bifurcates to form paired lower limbs which extend along each side of the posterior margin of the foramen magnum.

The basilar part, which is also referred to as the clivus, is a thick plate of bone which extends forward and upward, at an angle of about 45 degrees from the foramen magnum to join the sphenoid bone. The superior surface of the clivus is concave from side to side and is separated on each side from

the petrous part of the temporal bone by the petro-occipital fissure. The inferior surface has a small elevation, the pharyngeal tubercle, which gives attachment to the raphe of the pharynx.

The paired condylar parts are situated at the sides of the foramen magnum. The occipital condyles, which articulate with the atlas, are located lateral to the anterior half of the foramen magnum. A tubercle which gives attachment to the alar ligament of the odontoid process is situated on the medial side of each condyle. The hypoglossal canal, which transmits the hypoglossal nerve, is situated above and forward of the condyle. The condylar fossa, a depression located on the external surface behind the condyle, is often perforated to form a canal, through which an emissary vein passes.

The atlas, the first cervical vertebra, differs from the other cervical vertebrae by being ring shaped and by lacking a vertebral body and a spinous process (Fig. 47-2). It consists of two thick lateral masses which are connected in front by a short anterior arch and behind by a longer curved posterior arch. The position of the usual vertebral body is occupied by the odontoid process (dens). The posterior arch has a groove on the lateral part of its upper outer surface in which the vertebral artery courses. The groove may be partly or fully converted into a foramen by a bridge of bone which arches backward from the superior articular facet to the posterior arch. The upper and lower surfaces of each lateral mass have oval facets which articulate with the occipital condyles and the superior articular facets of the axis. The medial aspect of each lateral mass has a small tubercle for the attachment of the transverse ligament of the atlas. The transverse processes are unusually long and can be felt through the overlying tissues. Each transverse foramen, which transmits a vertebral artery, is situated between the lateral mass and the transverse process.

The axis, the second cervical vertebra, more closely resembles the typical vertebra than the atlas but is distinguished by the odontoid process, which projects upward from the body (Fig. 47-2). On the front of the dens is an articular facet which forms a joint with the facet on the back of the anterior arch of the atlas. The dens has a pointed apex which is joined by the apical ligament, a flattened side where the alar ligaments are attached, and a groove at the base of its posterior surface where the transverse ligament of the atlas passes. The dens and body are flanked by a pair of large oval facets which extend laterally from the body onto the adjoining parts of the pedicles and articulate with the inferior facets of the atlas. The superior facets do not form an articular pillar with the inferior facets but are anterior to the latter. The transverse processes are small. Each transverse foramen faces superolaterally, thus permitting the lateral deviation of the vertebral artery as it passes up to the more widely separated foramina in the atlas.

Ligamentous and Articular Relationships

The ligaments and articulations important in planning operative approaches are those joining the atlas, axis, and occipital bone (Fig. 47-3). The articulation of the atlas and axis

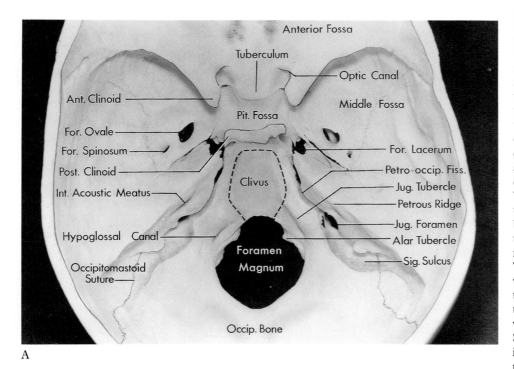

Figure 47-1 Osseous relationships, base of skull. *A.* Superior view. *B.* Inferior view. *A, B.* The occipital bone (Occip. Bone) surrounds the oval-shaped foramen magnum, which is wider posteriorly than anteriorly. The narrower anterior part sits above the odontoid process and is encroached on from laterally by the occipital condyles (Occip. Condyle). The wider posterior part transmits the medulla. The basilar part (Bas. Part) of the occipital bone is also referred to as the clivus. The part of the clivus which can be removed through an anterior operative approach is shown with an interrupted line. Structures in the exposure include the jugular foramen (Jug. Foramen); jugular tubercle (Jug. Tubercle); sulcus of the sigmoid sinus (Sig. Sulcus); carotid canal (Car. Canal); foramen lacerum (For. Lacerum), ovale (For. Ovale), and spinosum (For. Spinosum); anterior (Ant. Clinoid) and posterior clinoid processes (Post. Clinoid); pituitary fossa (Pit. Fossa); stylomastoid foramen (Stylomastoid For.); internal acoustic meatus (Int. Acoustic Meatus); external occipital protuberance (Ext. Occip. Protuberance); external occipital crest (Ext. Occip. Crest); inferior nuchal line (Inf. Nuchal Line); petro-occipital fissure (Petro-occip. Fiss.); and condylar fossa (Cond. Fossa). (From de Oliveira et al.,[4] with permission.)

comprises four synovial joints; two median ones on the front and back of the dens and paired lateral ones between the opposing articular facets on the lateral masses of the atlas and axis. Each joint on the front and back of the dens has its own capsule and synovial cavity. The anterior one is situated between the anterior surface of the dens and the posterior aspect of the anterior arch of the atlas. The posterior one lies between the cartilage-covered anterior surface of the transverse ligament of the atlas and the posterior surface of the dens.

The atlas and axis are united by the cruciform and the anterior and posterior longitudinal ligaments and the articular capsules surrounding the joints between the opposing articular facets on the lateral masses. The cruciform ligament has transverse and vertical parts which form a cross behind the dens. The transverse part, called the transverse

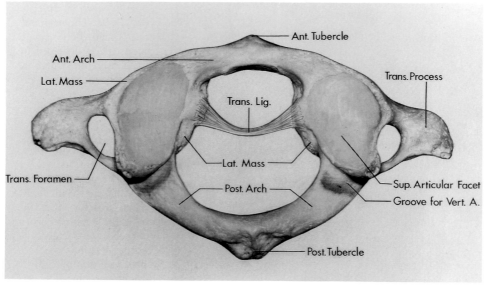

A

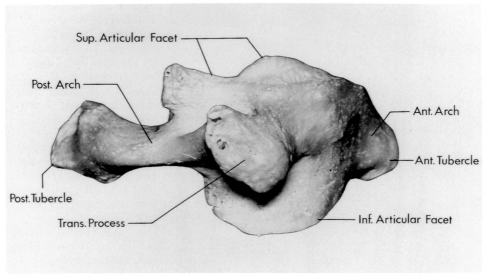

B

Figure 47-2 Atlas and axis. *A, B.* The atlas. *A.* Superior view. *B.* Lateral view. The atlas consists of two thick lateral masses (Lat. Mass) which are connected in front by a short anterior arch (Ant. Arch) and posteriorly by a longer posterior arch (Post. Arch). The medial aspect of each lateral mass has a small tubercle for the attachment of the transverse ligament (Trans. Lig.) of the atlas. The transverse foramina (Trans. Foramen) transmit the vertebral arteries. The upper surface of the posterior arch adjacent to the lateral masses has paired grooves in which the vertebral arteries (Vert. A.) course. Other structures include the anterior (Ant. Tubercle) and posterior tubercles (Post. Tubercle), transverse processes (Trans. Process), and the superior (Sup. Articular Facet) and inferior articular facets (Inf. Articular Facet). *C, D.* The axis. *C.* Lateral view. *D.* Anterior view. The axis is distinguished by the odontoid process (Dens). On the front of the dens is an articular facet which forms a joint with the facet on the back of the anterior arch of the atlas. The dens is grooved at the base of its posterior surface where the transverse ligament of the atlas passes. The superior articular facets are anterior to the inferior facets. The transverse foramina are directed superolaterally, thus permitting the lateral deviation of the vertebral arteries as they pass up to the more widely separated foramina in the atlas. (From de Oliveira et al.,[4] with permission.)

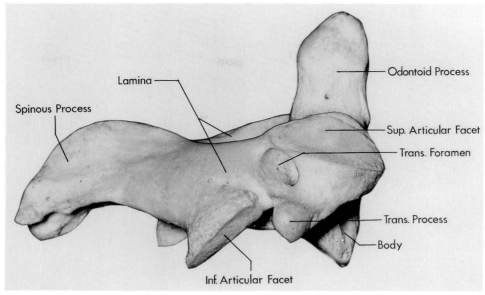

C

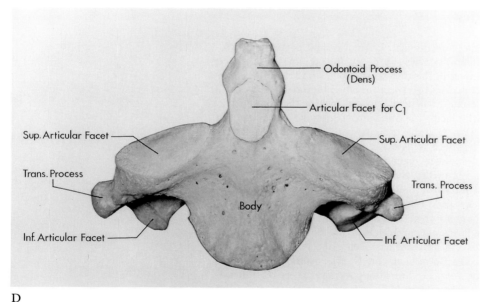

D

Figure 47-2 Continued

ligament, arches across the ring of the atlas behind the dens and is broader behind the dens than where it is attached to a tubercle on the medial side of the lateral masses of the atlas. As it crosses the dens, small longitudinal bands are directed upward and downward. The cranial extension is attached to the upper surface of the clivus between the apical ligament of the dens and the tectorial membrane. The lower band is attached to the posterior surface of the body of the axis.

In front, the atlas and axis are connected by the anterior longitudinal ligament, a wide band, fixed to the anterior arch of the atlas and the front body of the axis. The posterior longitudinal ligament is attached above to the transverse

part of the cruciform ligament and the clivus. Posterior to the spinal canal, the atlas and axis are joined by a broad, thin membrane that extends from the posterior arch of the atlas to the laminae of the axis.

The atlas and the occipital bone are united by the articular capsules surrounding the atlanto-occipital joints and by the anterior and posterior atlanto-occipital membranes (Fig. 47-3). The anterior atlanto-occipital membrane extends from the anterior edge of the foramen magnum to the anterior arch of the atlas. The posterior atlanto-occipital membrane extends from the posterior margin of the foramen magnum to the posterior arch of the atlas. The lateral border

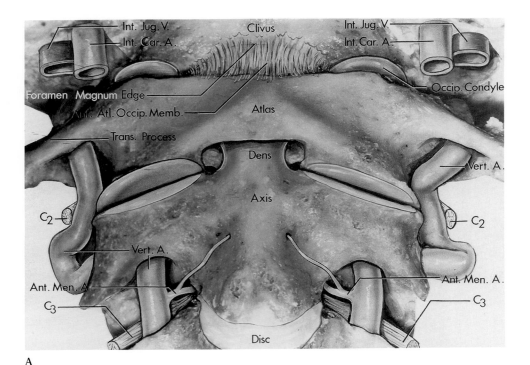

A

Figure 47-3 Osseous and ligamentous relationships. Anterior and posterior views. *A–C.* Anterior views. *A.* The vertebral arteries (Vert. A.) ascend anterior to the cervical nerve roots through the foramina in the transverse processes (Trans. Process). The anterior meningeal arteries (Ant. Men. A.) send one branch into the axis and another to the dura in the spinal canal. Structures exposed include the anterior atlanto-occipital membrane (Ant. Atl. Occip. Memb.), internal jugular veins (Int. Jug. V.), internal carotid arteries (Int. Car. A.), and occipital condyles (Occip. Condyle). *B.* The anterior arch of the atlas has been removed to expose the apical (Apical Lig.), cruciform (Cruciform Lig.), and alar ligaments (Alar Lig.). The horizontal part (Horiz. Part) of the cruciform ligament, which is also called the transverse ligament (Trans. Lig.), passes behind the dens, and the vertical part (Vert. Part) is seen above the dens. The body of C-2 has been removed. The anterior meningeal arteries form an arterial arch above the odontoid process. *C.* The odontoid process has been removed. The cruciform ligament forms a synovial joint with the odontoid process. The articular cartilage on the cruciform ligament has been preserved. The alar and apical ligaments lie anterior to the cruciform ligament. *D, E.* Posterior views of the anterior margin of the foramen magnum. *D.* The dura covering the tectorial membrane has been removed. This membrane extends downward from the clivus to insert on the upper cervical vertebrae. Structures in the exposure include the abducens (VI), facial (VII), vestibulocochlear (VIII), glossopharyngeal (IX), vagus (X), accessory (XI), and hypoglossal nerves (XII); internal acoustic meatus (Int. Acoustic Meatus); dentate ligament (Dentate Lig.); and jugular foramen (Jug. Foramen). *E.* Part of the tectorial membrane has been removed to expose the alar and the vertical and horizontal parts of the cruciform ligament. (From de Oliveira et al.,[4] with permission.)

of this membrane arches behind the vertebral artery and the first cervical nerve root and may be ossified in the area where it arches behind the vertebral artery.

Four fibrous bands—the tectorial membrane, the paired alar ligaments, and the apical ligament—connect the axis and the occipital bone (Fig. 47-3). The tectorial membrane is a cephalic extension of the posterior longitudinal ligament which covers the dens and cruciform ligament. It is attached

below to the posterior surface of the body of the axis and above to the upper surface of the occipital bone in front of the foramen magnum. The alar ligaments arise on each side of the upper part of the dens and attach to the medial surfaces of the occipital condyles. The apical ligament extends from the tip of the dens to the anterior margin of the foramen magnum and is situated between the anterior atlanto-occipital membrane and the cruciform ligament.

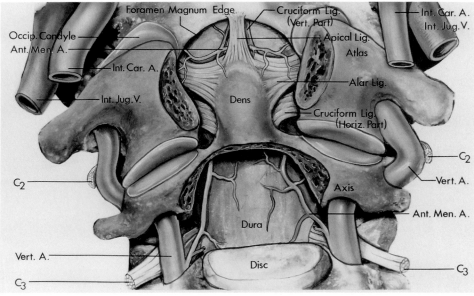

B

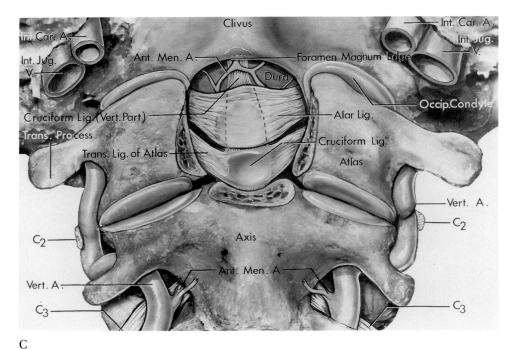

C

Figure 47-3 Continued

Neural Relationships

The neural structures situated in the region of the foramen magnum are the caudal part of the brain stem, cerebellum, and fourth ventricle; the rostral part of the spinal cord; and the lower cranial and upper cervical nerves (Figs. 47-4 and 47-5). The spinal cord blends indistinguishably into the medulla at a level arbitarily set to be at the upper limit of the dorsal and ventral rootlets forming the first cervical nerve. It is easier to differentiate this level on the ventral than on the dorsal surface because the ventral rootlets of the first cervical nerve are always present, and the dorsal rootlets are absent in many cases. The fact that the junction of the spinal cord and medulla is situated at the rostral margin of the first cervical root means that the medulla, and not the spinal

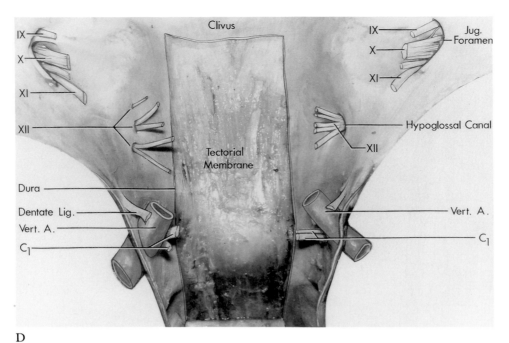

D

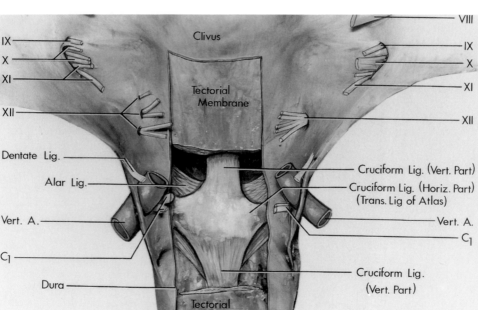

E

Figure 47-3 Continued

cord, occupies the foramen magnum. In the upper cervical region the rootlets which unite to form the spinal part of the accessory nerve emerge through the lateral funiculus in front of the dorsal roots.

The dentate ligament is a white fibrous sheet that is attached to the spinal cord medially and to the dura laterally (Fig. 47-4). Its medial border has a continuous linear attachment to the cord midway between the dorsal and ventral roots. Its lateral border is attached at intervals by fibrous triangular processes to the dura. The most rostral triangular process is attached to the dura at the level of the foramen magnum, and the second one is attached posterior and infe-

rior to the initial intradural segment of the vertebral artery. The lateral border of the dentate ligament between the two most rostral triangular processes is attached to the vertebral and posterior spinal arteries and to the C1 root, making separation of these structures difficult.

The upper spinal cord blends indistinguishably into the lower medulla (Figs 47-4 and 47-5). The anterior surface of the medulla is formed by the medullary pyramids, which face the clivus, the anterior edges of the foramen magnum, and the rostral part of the odontoid process. The anterior median sulcus divides the upper medulla in the anterior midline between the pyramids, disappears on the lower

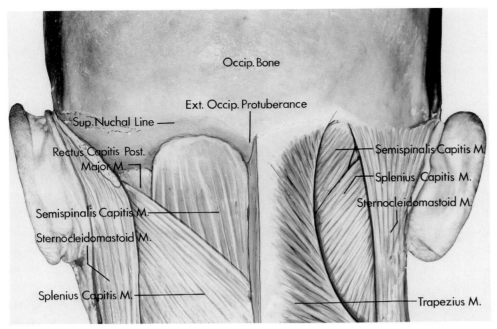

A

Figure 47-4 Posterior views. *A.* The superficial muscles which attach to the occipital bone (Occip. Bone) are preserved on the right side and have been removed on the left side. The superficial muscles which are attached to the superior nuchal line (Sup. Nuchal Line) and the external occipital protuberance (Ext. Occip. Protuberance) are the trapezius and sternocleidomastoid muscles (M.). On the left side, the trapezius muscle has been removed, and the upper part of the splenius capitis and sternocleidomastoid muscles have been reflected laterally to expose the semispinalis capitis and rectus capitis posterior (Post.) major muscles. *B.* The sternocleidomastoid, trapezius, and splenius capitis muscles have been removed on both sides, and the semispinalis and longissimus capitis muscles have been removed on the left side to expose the deep suboccipital muscles. The rectus capitis posterior minor arises on the occipital bone above the foramen magnum and inserts on the atlas. The rectus capitis posterior major extends from the occipital bone to the spinous process of the axis. The inferior (Inf.) oblique muscle extends from the spinous process of the axis to the transverse process of the atlas, and the superior (Sup.) oblique muscle extends from the transverse process of the atlas to the occipital bone. The vertebral artery (Vert. A.) and the C-1 nerve root are seen in the suboccipital triangle, which is situated between the superior and inferior oblique and the rectus capitis posterior major muscles. *C.* The semispinalis capitis and rectus capitis posterior major muscles have been removed on both sides. The posterior atlanto-occipital membrane (Post. Atl. Occip. Memb.) extends from the arch of the atlas to the posterior margin of the foramen magnum. The vertebral arter-

ies and C-1 nerve roots pass anterior to the lateral margin of this membrane. *D.* The muscles and bone above the foramen magnum have been removed. The posterior meningeal arteries (Post. Men. A.) arise below the occipital condyles (Occip. Condyle) and ascend on the dura. The occipital (Occip. A.) and ascending pharyngeal arteries (Ascend. Pharyngeal A.) also give rise to meningeal branches (Men. A.). The left vertebral artery passes through a complete ring of bone on the arch of the atlas before entering the dura. Radiculomuscular branches (Rad. Musc. A.) arise from the vertebral artery. *E.* The dura has just been opened. Structures exposed include the posterior spinal artery (Post. Sp. A.), accessory nerve (XI), sigmoid sinus (Sig. Sinus), posterior condylar foramen (Post. Cond. For.), dentate ligament (Dentate Lig.), and posterolateral sulcus (Post. Lat. Sulc.). *F.* Relationships of the dentate ligament and accessory and cervical nerves. Enlarged view of another specimen. Right side. The spinal portion of the accessory nerve arises from the dorsolateral margin of the spinal cord and ascends between the dorsal roots and the dentate ligament. The accessory nerve anastomoses with the C-1 and C-2 dorsal rootlets. The spinal cord does not contribute a dorsal root to the C-1 nerve. The C-1 nerve root passes through the dura with the vertebral artery. The most rostral triangular process of the dentate ligament is attached to the dura at the level of the foramen magnum. The posterior spinal artery splits into ascending (Ascend. Br.) and descending branches (Descend. Br.). There is a small ganglion in the anastomosis between the accessory nerve and the C-1 nerve root. (From de Oliveira et al.,[4] with permission.)

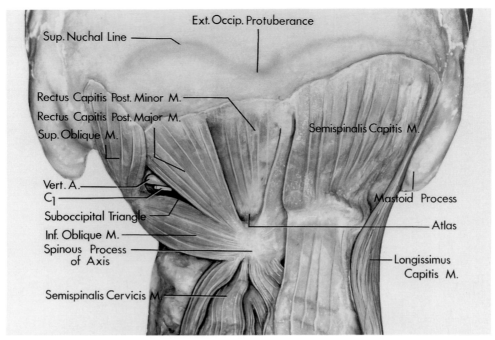

B

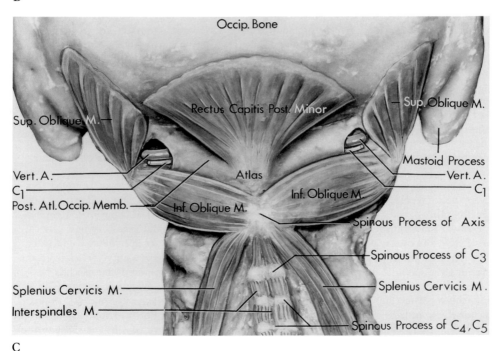

C

Figure 47-4   Continued

medulla at the level of the decussation of the pyramids, but reappears below the decussation and is continuous caudally with the anterior median fissure of the spinal cord. The lateral surface of the medulla is formed predominantly by the inferior olives. The posterior surface of the medulla is formed by the inferior cerebellar peduncles, the gracile fasciculus and tubercle medially, and the cuneate fasciculus and tubercle laterally. The belly of the pons which sits on

the clivus is convex from side to side as well as from top to bottom.

The cerebellum rests above the posterior and lateral edges of the foramen magnum. Only the lower part of the hemispheres formed by the tonsils and the biventral lobules and the lower part of the vermis formed by the nodule, uvula, and pyramid are related to the foramen magnum. The biventral lobule sits above the lateral part of the fora-

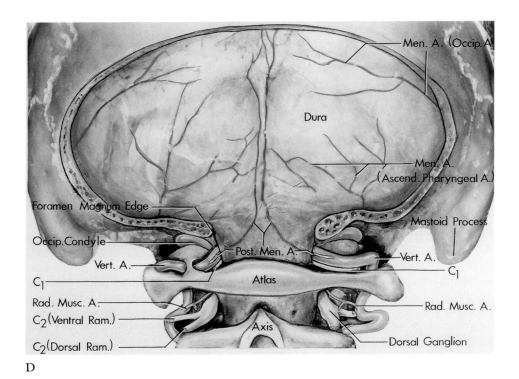

D

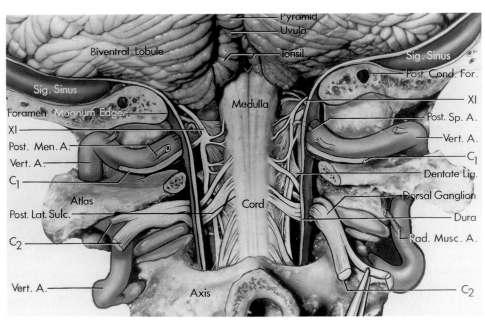

E

Figure 47-4 Continued

men magnum, and the tonsils rest above the level of the posterior edge.

The cerebellar surface above the posterior part of the foramen magnum has a deep vertical depression, the posterior cerebellar incisura, which contains the falx cerebelli and extends inferiorly toward the foramen magnum. The vermis is folded into and forms the cortical surface within this incisura. The vermian surface within the incisura has a diamond

shape. The upper half of the diamond-shaped formation has a pyramidal shape; thus, it is called the pyramid. The lower half of the diamond-shaped formation, the uvula, projects downward between the tonsils, thus mimicking the situation in the oropharynx. Inferiorly, the posterior cerebellar incisura is continuous with the vallecula cerebelli, an opening between the tonsils that extends upward through the foramen of Magendie into the fourth ventricle.

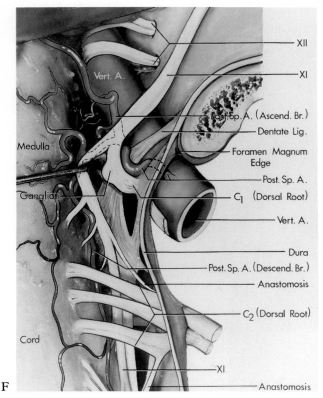

F

Figure 47-4 Continued

Cranial Nerves

The lower four cranial nerves are sufficiently close to the foramen magnum that they may be involved by lesions arising there. The rootlets forming the hypoglossal nerve arise from the medulla along a line that is continuous inferiorly with the line along which the ventral spinal roots arise (Figs. 47-4 and 47-5). These rootlets exit the medulla along the anterior margin of the olive and pass behind the vertebral artery to reach the hypoglossal canal. The vertebral artery may stretch the hypoglossal rootlets posteriorly over its dorsal surface. The hypoglossal canal may be divided by a bony septum which separates the nerve into two bundles as it exits the skull.

The glossopharyngeal, vagus, and accessory nerves are considered together because they are formed by a series of rootlets which arise in a continuous line along the medulla and spinal cord and exit the skull through the jugular foramen (Figs. 47-4 and 47-5). The glossopharyngeal and vagus nerves arise from the medulla along the posterior margin of the olive. The only location where the glossopharyngeal nerve may consistently be distinguished from the vagus nerve is just proximal to a dural septum which separates these nerves as they penetrate the dura to enter the jugular foramen.[4,14]

The accessory nerve is the only cranial nerve that passes through the foramen magnum (Figs. 47-4 and 47-5). It has a cranial part composed of the rootlets which arise from the medulla and join the vagus nerve, and a spinal portion formed by the union of a series of rootlets which arise from the lower medulla and upper spinal cord. In the posterior fossa, the accessory nerve is composed of one main trunk from the spinal cord and three to six small rootlets which emerge from the medulla. The most rostral medullary rootlets are functionally inferior vagal rootlets since they arise from the vagal nuclei. The lower medullary rootlets join the spinal portion of the nerve. The spinal contribution arises as a series of rootlets situated midway between the ventral and dorsal rootlets. The rootlets contributing to the accessory nerves may arise as low as the C-7 root level.[4] These rootlets unite to form a trunk having a diameter of approximately 1.0 mm, which ascends through the foramen magnum between the dentate ligament and the dorsal roots.

All of the 50 accessory nerves examined in our study had connections with the dorsal roots of the upper cervical nerves.[4] The most common and largest anastomosis was with the dorsal root of the first cervical nerve. The C-1 dorsal roots frequently arose solely from the accessory nerve without there being a contribution from the C-1 level of the spinal cord. About one-third of C-1 dorsal roots received rootlets that arose from the spinal cord at the C-1 level, but these also had anastomotic fibers from the accessory nerve. The accessory nerves may also have an anastomotic connection with the C-2 to C-5 dorsal roots.[4,13]

Spinal Nerve Roots

The spinal rootlets in the region of the foramen magnum pass directly lateral to reach their dural foramina (Figs. 47-3 to 47-5). The first cervical nerve is located just below the

The tonsils, which sit above the posterior edge of the foramen magnum, are commonly involved in herniations through the foramen magnum. Each tonsil is an ovoid structure which is attached along its superolateral border to the remainder of the cerebellum. The inferior pole and posterior surface of the tonsils face the cisterna magna and are visible from the suboccipital operative exposure. The lateral surface of each tonsil is covered by the biventral lobule. The medial and anterior surfaces and the superior pole of each tonsil all face, but are separated from, other neural structures by narrow clefts. The anterior surface of each tonsil faces, and is separated from, the posterior surface of the medulla by the cerebellomedullary fissure. The medial surfaces of the tonsils face each other across the vallecula. The ventral aspect of the superior pole faces the inferior half of the roof of the fourth ventricle.

The cerebellomedullary fissure, which extends superiorly between the cerebellum and the medulla, is situated rostral to the dorsal margin of the foramen magnum. This fissure extends superiorly to the level of the roof and the lateral recesses of the fourth ventricle. The dorsal wall of the fissure is formed by the uvula in the midline and the tonsils and biventral lobules laterally. The ventral wall, formed by the inferior medullary velum and tela choroidea, is exposed by removing the tonsils. The inferior medullary velum is a thin bilateral semitranslucent butterfly-shaped sheet of neural tissue that blends into the ventricular surface of the nodule medially and stretches laterally across the superior pole of the tonsil. The tela choroidea, from which the choroid plexus projects, forms the lowest part of the roof of the fourth ventricle.

foramen magnum and differs from the other cervical nerves in the consistency and origin of the dorsal rootlets forming the nerve. The C-1 ventral root is composed of 4 to 8 rootlets which join and course laterally. Before entering the dural foramen, the C-1 ventral root and the corresponding dorsal root, if present, attach to the posterior inferior surface of the initial intradural part of the vertebral artery. They then pass through the funnel-shaped dural foramen around the verte-

bral artery. The ventral root joins the dorsal root in or external to the dural foramen.

The dorsal root of the first cervical nerve is more complicated than the ventral root because of the variations in its composition and its connections with the accessory nerve. In our study of the 25 spinal cords in which one would expect to find 50 C-1 dorsal roots arising from the cord, only 15 were found.[4] The accessory nerve contributed a root to

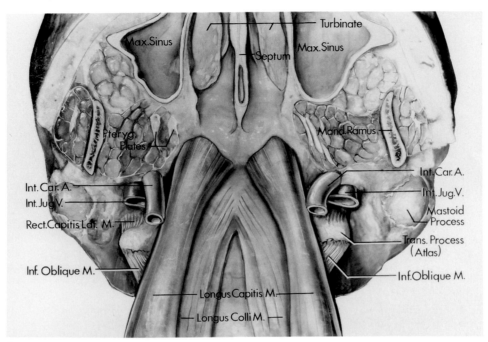

A

Figure 47-5 Anterior views. *A*. The structures anterior to the prevertebral muscles have been removed. Structures exposed include maxillary sinuses (Max. Sinus), ramus of the mandible (Mand. Ramus), inferior oblique (Inf. Oblique M.) and rectus capitis lateralis muscles (Rect. Capitus Lat. M.), transverse process (Trans. Process), internal carotid artery (Int. Car. A.), and internal jugular vein (Int. Jug. V.). *B*. The muscles have been removed. The clivus has been opened above the foramen magnum. The dorsal meningeal branches (Dorsal Men. A.) of the meningohypophyseal trunks descend to anastomose with branches of the ascending pharyngeal arteries (Ascend. Pharyngeal A.). Structures in the exposure include the medial (Med. Pteryg. M.) and lateral pterygoid muscles (Lat. Pteryg. M.); medial (Med. Pteryg. Plate) and lateral pterygoid plates (Lat. Pteryg. Plate); glossopharyngeal (IX), vagus (X), accessory (XI), and hypoglossal nerves (XII); and jugular foramen (Jug. Foramen). *C*. The clivus, the anterior arch of the atlas, and the dens have been removed. Structures exposed include the abducens (VI), facial (VII), and vestibulocochlear nerves (VIII); anterior median (Ant. Med. Sulc.) and pontomedullary sulci (Pon. Med. Sulc.); choroid plexus (Chor. Plex.); foramen of Luschka (F. Luschka); pyramidal decussation (Pyramid Decuss.); dentate ligament (Dentate Lig.); and occipital condyle (Occip. Condyle). *D–F*. Exposure of the clivus through the pharynx in a cadaver. *D*. The mucosa on the ventral surface of the hard palate and the adjacent part of the soft palate have been removed to expose the pharyngeal mucosa on the clivus. *E*. The lower part of the clivus has been removed to expose the vertebral and basilar arteries (Bas. A.) and the origins of the posterior inferior cerebellar (P.I.C.A.), anterior inferior cerebellar (A.I.C.A.), anterior spinal (Ant. Sp. A.), and direct perforating arteries (Dir. Perf. A.). *F*. The vomer has been removed to expose the sphenoid sinus and sellar floor. *G*. Another specimen. The opening in the clivus exposes tortuous vertebral and basilar arteries. (From de Oliveira et al.,[4] with permission.)

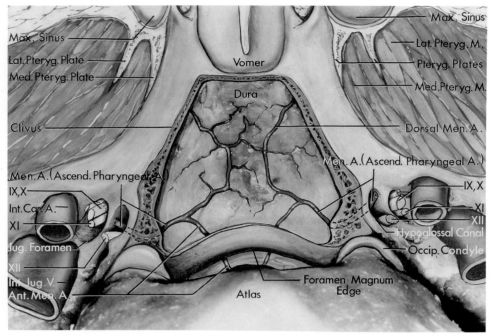

B

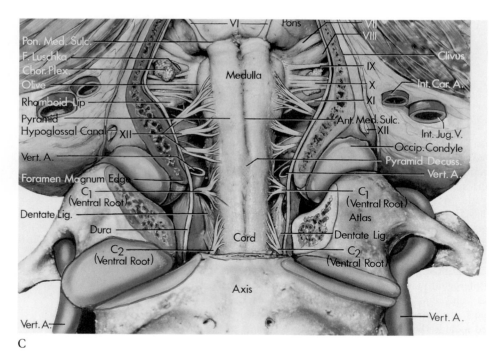

C

Figure 47-5   Continued

the first cervical nerve in 28 of the 35 roots lacking a dorsal root which arose from the spinal cord. In the remaining seven cases, the C-1 dorsal root was absent. Each of the 15 dorsal roots which arose from the spinal cord also had a contribution from the accessory nerve.[4]

Arterial Relationships

The major arteries related to the foramen magnum are the vertebral and posterior inferior cerebellar arteries, and the

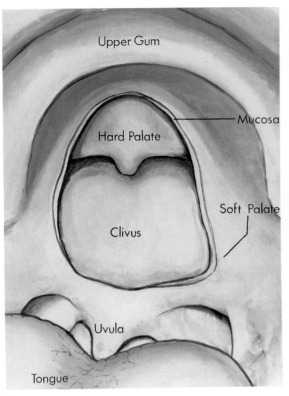

D

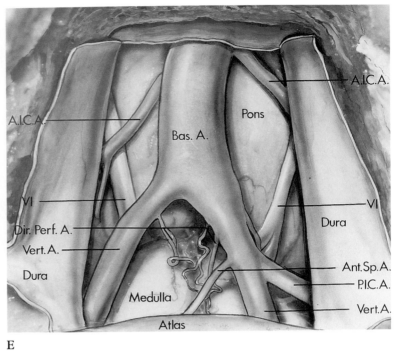

E

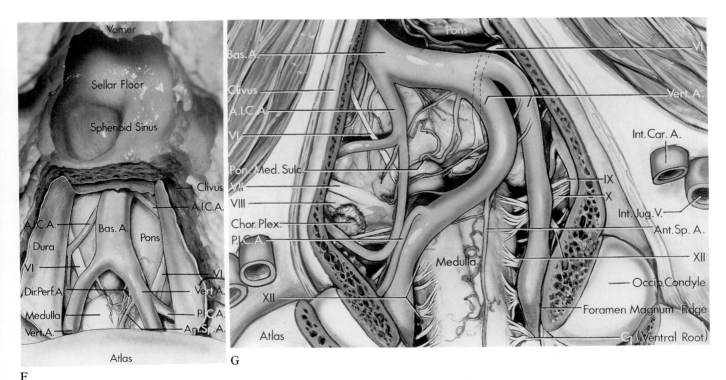

F

G

Figure 47-5 Continued

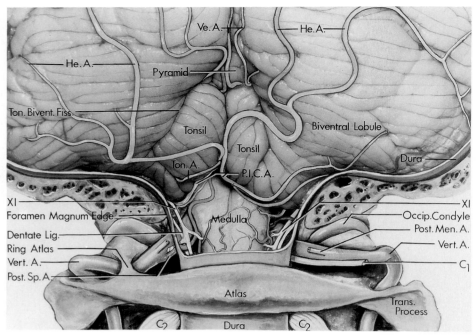

A

Figure 47-6 Arterial relationships. Posterior views. *A.* The vertebral arteries (Vert. A.) ascend through the foramina in the transverse processes (Trans. Process), course below the occipital condyles (Occip. Condyle), and give rise to the posterior spinal (Post. Sp. A.) and posterior meningeal arteries (Post. Men. A.) before entering the dura. The posterior inferior cerebellar arteries (P.I.C.A.) course around the tonsils and divide into tonsillar (Ton. A.), vermian (Ve. A.), and hemispheric arteries (He. A.). Structures exposed include the tonsillobiventral fissure (Ton. Bivent. Fiss.), dentate ligament (Dentate Lig.), and accessory nerve (XI). *B.* The tonsils and adjacent part of the biventral lobule have been removed to show the relationship of the posterior inferior cerebellar arteries to the foramen magnum and roof of the fourth ventricle. The posterior spinal artery splits into ascending (Ascend. Br.) and descending branches (Descend. Br.). The structures forming the inferior half of the roof of the fourth ventricle (4V) are the tela choroidea (Tela) and the inferior medullary velum (Inf. Med. Vel.). Structures exposed include the peduncles (Ped.) of the flocculi, inferior cerebellar peduncles (Inf. Cer. Ped.), choroidal arteries (Chor. A.), marginal sinus (Marg. Sinus), lateral recesses (Lat. Recess), and foramina of Luschka (F. Luschka) and Magendie (F. Magendie). *C.* The structures forming the inferior half of the roof of the fourth ventricle, except for the most caudal strip of the tela have been removed in another specimen. The left posterior inferior cerebellar artery passes posteriorly between the rootlets of the hypoglossal and accessory nerves, and dips below the level of the foramen magnum to form a caudal loop before ascending behind the roof of the fourth ventricle. The right posterior inferior cerebellar artery ascends from its origin without forming a caudal loop. Both posterior inferior cerebellar arteries split into medial (Med. Tr.) and lateral trunks (Lat. Tr.). Structures exposed include the facial (VII), vestibulocochlear (VIII), glossopharyngeal (IX), vagus (X), and hypoglossal nerves (XII); middle (Mid. Cer. Ped.) and inferior cerebellar peduncles; choroid plexus (Chor. Plex.); and jugular foramen (Jug. Foramen). (From de Oliveira et al.,[4] with permission.)

meningeal branches of the vertebral and external and internal carotid arteries (Figs. 47-4 to 47-6).[4,8,11,12] The paired vertebral arteries ascend through the transverse processes of the upper six cervical vertebrae, enter the dura behind the occipital condyles, and ascend through the foramen magnum to reach the front of the medulla. The segment most intimately related to the foramen magnum passes medially behind the lateral mass of the atlas and across the groove on the upper surface of the lateral part of the posterior arch of the atlas. This bony groove is frequently transformed into a bony canal which completely surrounds a short segment of the artery (Fig. 47-4).

The intradural segment begins at the dural foramen just inferior to the lateral edge of the foramen magnum. The

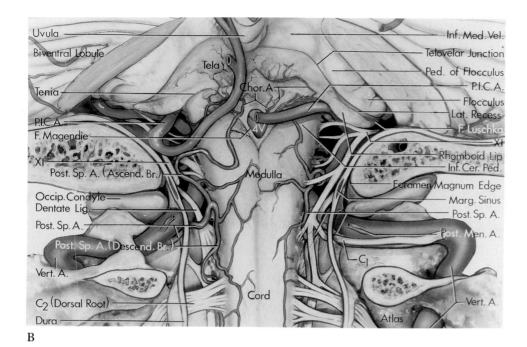

B

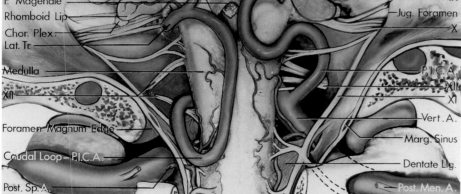

C

Figure 47-6 Continued

dura in this region forms a funnel-shaped foramen around a 4- to 6-mm length of the artery. The first cervical nerve exits the spinal canal, and the posterior spinal artery enters the spinal canal through this dural foramen with the vertebral artery. These three structures are bound together at the foramen by fibrous dural bands (Fig. 47-4). The initial intradural segment of the vertebral artery passes just superior to the dorsal and ventral roots of the first cervical nerve and just anterior to the posterior spinal artery, the dentate ligament, and the spinal portion of the accessory nerve.

The branches arising from the vertebral artery in the re-

gion of the foramen magnum are the posterior spinal, anterior spinal, posterior inferior cerebellar, and anterior and posterior meningeal arteries. The paired posterior spinal arteries usually arise from the vertebral arteries, just outside the dura, but they may also arise inside the dura or from the posterior inferior cerebellar arteries (Figs. 47-4 and 47-6). In the subarachnoid space, they course medially behind the rostralmost attachments of the dentate ligament and divide into an ascending branch to the medulla and a descending branch to the spinal cord.

The posterior inferior cerebellar artery usually originates

within the dura, but it may infrequently originate from the terminal extradural part of the vertebral artery.[8,10] It may arise at, above, or below the level of the foramen magnum; of the 42 arteries found in 50 cerebella in our study, 35 arose above and 7 arose below the foramen.[4] In its course around the antereolateral surface of the medulla, it passes rostral or caudal to or between the rootlets of the hypoglossal nerve, and in its course around the posterolateral medulla it passes above, below, or between the rootlets of the glossopharyngeal, vagus, and accessory nerves. As it passes between the latter nerves, it may be ascending, descending, or passing laterally or medially, or may be involved in a complex loop that stretches and distorts these nerves. Of the 42 arteries, 16 passed between the rootlets of the accessory nerve, 10 passed between the rootlets of the vagus nerve, 13 passed between the vagus and accessory nerves, 2 passed above the glossopharyngeal nerve between the latter nerve and the vestibulocochlear nerve, and 1 passed between the glossopharyngeal and vagus nerves.[4,8] After reaching the area dorsal to the glossopharyngeal, vagus, and accessory nerves, it passes around the cerebellar tonsil near the roof of the fourth ventricle and bifurcates into a medial and lateral trunk. The medial trunk supplies the vermis and the adjacent part of the hemisphere, and the lateral trunk supplies the tonsil and the hemispheres.

The anterior spinal artery is formed by the union of the paired anterior ventral spinal arteries, which originate from the vertebral arteries (Fig. 47-5). One of the anterior ventral spinal arteries may continue inferiorly as the anterior spinal artery, and the other may terminate on the medulla. The anterior spinal artery descends through the foramen magnum on the anterior surface of the medulla and the spinal cord in or near the anterior median fissure.

The dura around the foramen magnum is supplied by the meningeal branches of the ascending pharyngeal and occipital arteries, the anterior and posterior meningeal branches of the vertebral artery, and the dorsal meningeal branch of the meningohypophyseal trunk of the intracavernous segment of the internal carotid artery (Figs. 47-4, 47-5, and 47-6). Infrequently, the posterior inferior cerebellar and posterior spinal arteries and the intradural part of the vertebral artery give rise to meningeal branches. The anterior meningeal branch of the vertebral artery enters the spinal canal through the C2-3 intervertebral foramen and ascends between the posterior longitudinal ligament and the dura (Fig. 47-3). At the level of the apex of the dens, these paired arteries join to form an arch over the apex of the dens. The posterior meningeal artery arises from the vertebral artery as it courses around the lateral mass of the atlas and ascends in the dura near the falx cerebelli. The ascending pharyngeal branch of the external carotid artery sends branches through the hypoglossal canal and jugular foramen to the dura above the foramen magnum (Fig. 47-5). The meningeal branch of the occipital artery is inconstant. It penetrates the cranium through a mastoid emissary foramen.

Venous Relationships

The venous structures in the region of the foramen magnum are divided into three groups: one composed of the extradu-

ral veins, another formed by the intradural (neural) veins, and a third constituted by dural venous sinuses (Fig. 47-7).[9] The three groups anastomose through bridging and emissary veins.

The extradural veins are divided into an extraspinal part, the vertebral venous plexus, which is formed by the veins draining the deep muscles surrounding the cervical vertebrae, and an intraspinal component, the epidural venous plexus, which courses in the epidural space, primarily laterally, with some connections anterior and posterior on the outer surface of the dura. There are anastomotic connections between the epidural and vertebral venous plexus which surrounds the terminal extradural segment of the vertebral artery.

The venous channels in the dura surrounding the foramen magnum are the marginal and occipital sinuses and the basilar venous plexus (Fig. 47-7). The marginal sinus is located in the dura lining the rim of the foramen magnum. The occipital sinus courses in the cerebellar falx. Its lower end divides into paired limbs, each of which courses anteriorly around the foramen magnum to join the sigmoid sinus or the jugular bulb. The basilar venous plexus is located between the layers of the dura on the clivus and extends from the dorsum sellae to the anterior rim of the foramen magnum. It is formed by interconnecting venous channels which anastomose with the inferior petrosal sinuses laterally, the cavernous sinuses superiorly, and the marginal sinus and epidural venous plexus inferiorly.

The intradural veins in the region of the foramen magnum drain the lower part of the cerebellum and brain stem, the upper part of the spinal cord, and the cerebellomedullary fissure. The veins of the medulla and spinal cord form longitudinal plexiform channels which anastomose at the foramen magnum. The main vein on the posterior surface of the medulla is the median posterior medullary vein. It courses along the posterior median medullary sulcus and divides superiorly, near the obex, into the paired veins of the inferior cerebellar peduncle, each of which courses on the surface of the inferior cerebellar peduncle parallel to and below the lower edge of the fourth ventricle to join veins on the lateral surface of the medulla. The median posterior medullary vein is continuous below with the median posterior spinal vein. Bridging veins connect these veins to the dural sinus in the region of the foramen magnum. The veins draining the tonsils and adjacent part of the cerebellum and brain stem ascend along the vermis to terminate in the sinuses in the region of the torcular. The veins on the anterior and lateral surface of the medulla drain into the veins in the cerebellopontine angle, which form the superior petrosal veins and empty into the superior petrosal sinus.

Herniations

Herniation of cerebellar tissue into the foramen magnum may cause neural compression and even death. These herniations are commonly referred to as tonsillar herniations; however, the herniation usually involves the tonsils and biventral lobules, both of which are deeply grooved by the edge of the foramen magnum.[4,6] The herniation may compress the medulla and be so severe that the herniated tissue

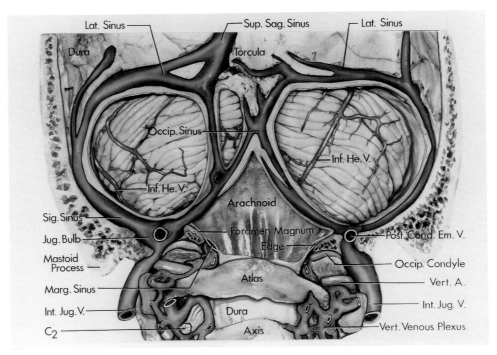

A

Figure 47-7 Venous relationships. Posterior views. *A.* The dura over the cerebellum has been removed except in the area of the venous sinuses. The occipital sinuses (Occip. Sinus) join the torcular above and the jugular bulbs (Jug. Bulb) below. The vertebral venous plexus (Vert. Venous Plexus) anastamoses with the posterior condylar emissary (Post. Cond. Em. V.) and internal jugular veins (Int. Jug. V.). The marginal sinus (Marg. Sinus) courses in the dura at the level of the foramen magnum. Structures exposed include the superior sagittal (Sup. Sag. Sinus), lateral (Lat. Sinus), and sigmoid sinuses (Sig. Sinus); vertebral artery (Vert. A.); inferior hemispheric veins (Inf. He. V.); and occipital condyles (Occip. Condyle). *B.* The dura below the lateral and sigmoid sinuses has been removed. The median posterior medullary vein (Med. Post. Med. V.) splits below the fourth ventricle (4V) to form the paired veins of the inferior cerebellar peduncle (V. of Inf. Cer. Ped.). Structures exposed include the accessory (XI) and hypoglossal nerves (XII); dentate ligament (Dentate Lig.); cerebellomedullary (Cer. Med. Fiss.) and tonsillobiventral fissures (Ton. Bevent. Fiss.); and bridging (Br. V.), inferior retrotonsillar (Inf. Retroton. V.), and median posterior spinal veins (Med. Post. Sp. V.). *C.* The tonsils have been removed to expose the inferior medullary velum (Inf. Med. Vel.) and tela choroidea (Tela). Structures exposed include the choroid plexus (Chor. Plex.), foramina of Luschka (F. Luschka) and Magendie (F. Magendie), vein of the cerebellomedullary fissure (V. of Cer. Med. Fiss.), glossopharyngeal (IX) and vagus nerves (X), and the inferior cerebellar peduncles (Inf. Cer. Ped.). *D.* The front of the brain stem has been exposed. The veins which cross the front of the brain stem are the median anterior pontomesencephalic (Med. Ant. Pon. Mes. V.), median anterior medullary (Med. Ant. Med. V.), median anterior spinal (Med. Ant. Sp. V.), lateral anterior medullary (Lat. Ant. Med. V.), lateral anterior spinal (Lat. Ant. Sp. V.), transverse pontine (Trans. Pon. V.), and transverse medullary veins (Trans. Med. V.) and the vein of the pontomedullary sulcus (V. of Pon. Med. Sulc.). Other structures in the exposure include the carotid artery (Int. Car. A.); abducens (VI), facial (VII), and vestibulocochlear nerves (VIII); jugular foramen (Jug. Foramen); and pontomedullary sulcus (Pon. Med. Sulc.). *E.* Superior view. Venous sinuses surrounding the foramen magnum. There are diffuse anastomoses between the venous sinuses around the foramen magnum. Structures exposed include the basilar venous plexus (Bas. Plexus); superior (Sup. Petrosal Sinus), inferior petrosal (Inf. Petrosal Sinus), and cavernous sinuses (Cav. Sinus); vertical (Vert. Part) and horizontal parts (Horiz. Part) of the occipital sinus (Occip. Sinus); superior petrosal veins (Sup. Pet. V.); oculomotor (III), trochlear (IV), and trigeminal nerves (V); internal acoustic meatus (Int. Acoustic Meatus); meningeal arteries (Men. A.); and tentorium (Tent.). Small dural sinuses (*dotted lines*) connect the jugular bulbs with the veins in the hypoglossal canals. (From de Oliveira et al.,[4] with permission.)

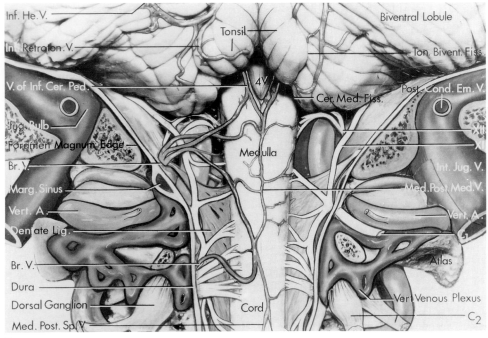

B

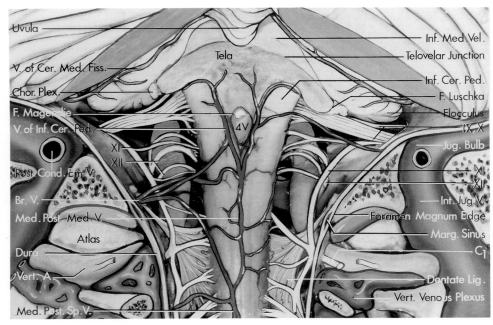

C

Figure 47-7 Continued

undergoes necrosis. Patients with herniation at the foramen magnum may be asymptomatic or present with pain, signs of neural compression, increased intracranial pressure, and sudden unexpected death. Symptoms caused by dysfunction of the cerebellum, brain stem, and lower cranial and upper spinal nerves include pain in the neck and upper arms, dizziness, ataxia, disturbances of gait, diplopia, dysphagia, tinnitus, decreased hearing, nystagmus, weakness up to the degree of quadriparesis, and sensory deficit in the extremi-

ties. Coughing or sneezing may aggravate the symptoms and cause syncope. Some patients without prior symptoms who die suddenly are found to have herniations through the foramen magnum at autopsy. The occurrence of sudden death in these patients means that herniation at the foramen magnum is a precarious situation which can be aggravated by minor stresses. The common denominator in these cases of sudden death is herniation of the tonsils and adjacent part of the biventral lobule into the foramen magnum.[6] The herniation

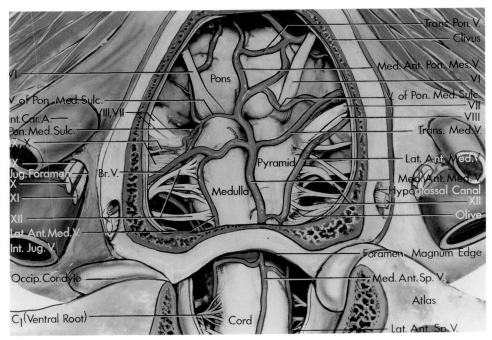

D

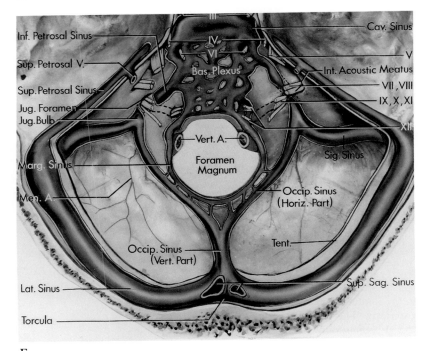

E

Figure 47-7 Continued

may be bilateral and symmetrical, though more commonly there is not strict symmetry, and it may be unilateral. The herniated tonsils are tightly pressed against the medulla. Acute or chronic herniations may be seen with space-occupying lesions, such as cerebellar astrocytomas or cystic tumors. Chronic herniation is seen with the Chiari Type I malformation.

Tumors

Foramen magnum tumors have frequently eluded early diagnosis because they cause bizarre symptoms simulating cervical spondylosis, multiple sclerosis, or degenerative disease.[1] Tumors arising in the region of the foramen magnum were divided by Cushing and Eisenhardt into a craniospinal group, tumors which arise above and grow downward toward the foramen magnum, and a spinocranial group, tumors which arise below and grow upward toward the foramen magnum.[3] The intradural extramedullary tumors in this region are usually benign, with meningiomas and schwannomas being the most frequent.[3,15] The frequency rate of meningioma to schwannoma is 26:4.[3,4,15] Craniospinal menigiomas tend to originate anteriorly or anterolaterally, and spinocranial meningiomas tend to arise laterally or posterolaterally, close to the initial part of the intradural segment of the vertebral artery. The intramedullary tumors are represented mainly by astrocytomas and ependymomas. Cerebellar tumors, especially those originating in the fourth ventricle, such as ependymomas, medulloblastomas, and choroid plexus papillomas, and those arising in the lower part of the cerebellar hemisphere or vermis, may extend into or through the foramen magnum into the upper spinal canal. Chordomas and metastases are the most common extradural tumors. The chordomas usually arise at the level of the clivus and may extend caudally into the foramen magnum.

Surgical Approaches

The foramen magnum may be approached anteriorly or posteriorly. A posterior operative approach is commonly selected for intradural lesions, and an anterior approach is frequently selected for extradural lesions situated anterior to the foramen magnum (Fig. 47-8).

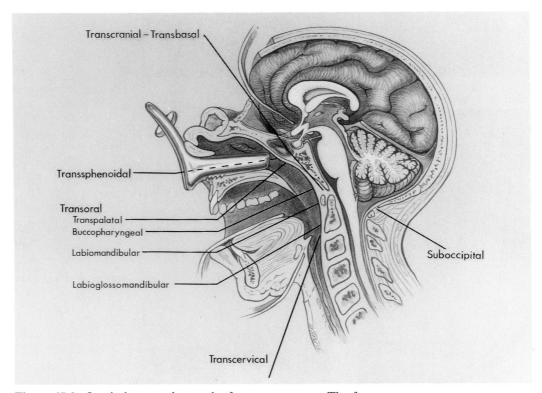

Figure 47-8 Surgical approaches to the foramen magnum. The foramen magnum may be approached anteriorly or posteriorly. The posterior approach through a suboccipital craniectomy and upper cervical laminectomy is commonly selected for intradural lesions, and an anterior approach is most frequently selected for extradural lesions situated anterior to the foramen magnum. The transoral approach through the mouth and the posterior pharyngeal wall is referred to as the buccopharyngeal approach. The basic transoral approach may be modified to include the transpalatal approach, in which the soft palate or both the soft and hard palates are opened, and the labiomandibular or labioglossomandibular approaches, in which lip, chin, mandible, and possibly the tongue and floor of the mouth are split to increase the exposure. Other types of anterior approaches are the transcervical approach directed through the submandibular area along the anterior border of the sternocleidomastoid muscle; the transcranial-transbasal approach, in which the clivus is reached through a bifrontal craniotomy following resection of the sphenoid and ethmoid sinuses; and the trans-sphenoidal approach directed through the sphenoid sinus to the upper part of the clivus. (From de Oliveira et al.,[4] with permission.)

Anterior Operative Approaches

Anterior approaches are used to reach tumors of the atlas, axis, and clivus; for the resection and fixation of the odontoid process following ligamentous and osseous injury; for decompressing bony malformations of the craniovertebral junction such as basilar invagination; and for approaching aneurysms of the vertebral and basilar arteries. The greatest advantage of the anterior approach is the direct route to the lesion, and the major disadvantages are the frequency of cerebrospinal fluid leak, pseudomeningocele, and meningitis following the exposure of intradural lesions by this approach.

The transoral route through the mouth and the posterior pharyngeal wall, referred to as the buccopharyngeal approach, is the anterior approach most commonly selected. The basic transoral approach may be modified to include a transpalatine approach, in which the soft palate or both the soft and hard palates are opened, and the labiomandibular or labioglossomandibular approach, in which the lip, mandible, and possibly the tongue and floor of the mouth are split to increase the exposure. Other types of anterior approach are the transcervical approach directed through the submandibular area along the anterior border of the sternocleidomastoid muscle; the transcranial-transbasal approach, in which the clivus is reached through a bifrontal craniotomy; and the trans-sphenoidal approach, in which the clivus is reached through the sphenoid sinus. The details of the transoral and transcervical approaches are reviewed elsewhere in this volume.

Subfrontal-Transbasal Approach

The subfrontal-transbasal approach may be used to approach tumors of the anterior side of the foramen magnum if the tumor also involves and requires resection of part of the ethmoid and sphenoid bones and the clivus (Fig. 47-9). [5] The transbasal approach is done through a Souttar scalp incision and a bifrontal free bone flap situated strictly supraorbital without regard for the frontal sinuses. The subfrontal dura is separated from the orbital roofs, the olfactory nerves are divided at the cribriform plates, and the extradural dissection is carried posteriorly to the lesser wings of the sphenoid bone, the tuberculum sellae, and the base of the anterior clinoid processes. The clivus is reached after resecting the posterior part of the floor of the anterior cranial fossa, the upper walls of the ethmoid and sphenoid sinuses, and the floor of the sella. Proceeding downward from the sellar floor, the clivus is removed to open the anterior margin of the foramen magnum. Separation of the pharyngeal mucosa from the front of the spine permits exposure of the anterior arch of the atlas and even the C-2 and C-3 vertebral bodies. The nasal and pharyngeal mucosa should not be opened. Dural defects are closed with a leakproof dural substitute more than twice the size of the defect, which is sutured to the dura at the most remote margins of the exposure. The orbital roofs, cranial base, and clivus are reconstructed using autologous bone grafts. The transbasal approach may be combined with a transnasal-trans-sphenoidal route to gain access to the sella and to remove all of the clivus below the

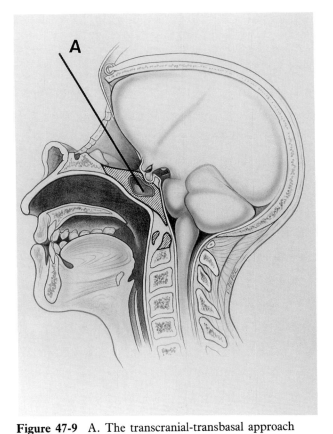

Figure 47-9 A. The transcranial-transbasal approach may be used to approach tumors of the anterior edge of the foramen magnum if the tumor also involves and requires resection of part of the ethmoid and sphenoid bones (*oblique lines*). B. Upper left. The Souttar scalp incision is situated behind the hairline, and the bifrontal craniotomy (*interrupted lines*) is placed strictly supraorbital without regard for the frontal sinuses (*oblique lines*). Lower right. The subfrontal dura is separated from the orbital roofs, the olfactory nerves are divided at the cribriform plates, and the extradural dissection is carried to the lesser wings of the sphenoid bone, the tuberculum sellae, and the base of the anterior clinoid processes (Ant. Clinoid). The clivus is reached after resecting the posterior part of the floor of the anterior cranial fossa, the upper part of the walls of the ethmoid and sphenoid sinuses, and the floor of the sella. Proceeding downward, the clivus is removed to open the anterior margin of the foramen magnum. Separation of the pharyngeal mucosa from the front of the spine exposes the anterior arch of the atlas and even the front of the C-2 and C-3 vertebral bodies. The nasal and pharyngeal mucosa should not be opened. Dural defects are closed with a leakproof dural graft after dealing with the lesion. C. The orbital roof and the remainder of the cranial base are reconstructed using bone grafts. If the clivus has been removed, the graft above the ethmosphenoidal space is fitted into the edge of a vertical graft extending from the anterior margin of the foramen magnum or the anterior arch of the atlas to the floor of the sella. (From de Oliveira et al.,[4] with permission.)

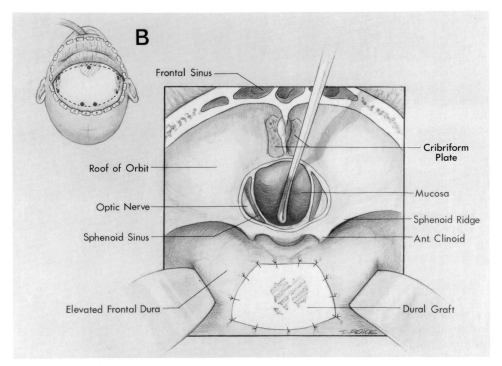

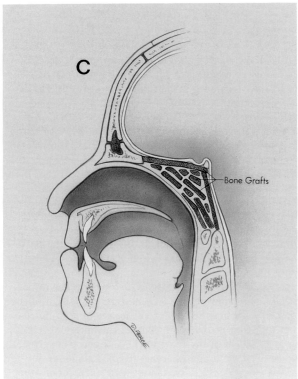

Figure 47-9 Continued

level of the dorsum sellae. The most frequent complications are cerebrospinal fluid leaks, meningitis, and pseudomeningoceles.

Trans-sphenoidal Approach

The trans-sphenoidal approach may be used to expose the upper third of the clivus (Fig. 47-10).[7] In approaching the clivus, the floor of the sella is removed and the bony opening is extended downward on the clivus to the inferior margin of the sphenoid sinus. Lesions extending to the upper third of the clivus may be biopsied or partially removed through this approach. The sellar and clival openings are closed with fat or muscle and nasal septal cartilage. The advantage of this approach is the low complication rate, and the disadvantage is the small operative field limited to the superior third of the clivus.

Posterior Approaches

The posterior approaches are preferred for most intradural lesions (Fig. 47-11). The patient is most commonly placed in the semisitting position. The prone or three-quarter prone ("park bench") position is used for adults having occlusive cerebrovascular disease and infants. Either a vertical midline or hockey-stick suboccipital incision is used. The vertical midline incision is used for lesions situated in the upper spinal canal and posterior or posterolateral in the area at the level of, or above, the foramen magnum. The upper limbs of the Y-shaped muscle incision begin at the level of the superior nuchal line, lateral to the external occipital protuberance, and join several centimeters below the inion, leaving a musculofascial flap along the superior nuchal line for closure. The major extracranial hazard is injury to the vertebral artery as it courses along the lateral part of the posterior arch of the atlas.

The hockey-stick incision is selected if the lesion extends anterior or anterolateral to the brain stem toward the jugular foramen or the cerebellopontine angle. A muscular cuff is left attached along the superior nuchal line to facilitate the closure. This incision permits removal of the full posterior rim of the foramen magnum and the posterior elements of the atlas and axis and, in addition, the completion of a unilateral suboccipital craniectomy of sufficient size to expose

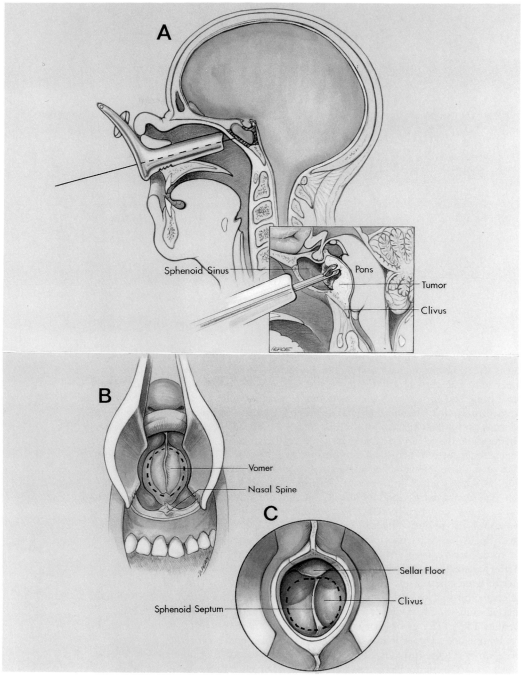

Figure 47-10 Trans-sphenoidal approach. *A*. Upper left. This approach directed beneath the upper lip, along the nasal septum, and through the sphenoid sinus may be used to expose the upper third of the clivus. The resectable area *(oblique lines)* includes the floor and anterior wall of the sella, the vomer, and the upper one-third of the clivus. This approach is suitable for biopsying some tumors which extend upward on the clivus from the foramen magnum. Lower right. A cup forceps biopsies a clival tumor. *B*. View through a nasal speculum. The anterior nasal spine is preserved, and the anterior part of the septal cartilage remains attached to the septal mucosa on one side. The nasal speculum is inserted between the left side of the nasal septum and its mucosa. The nasal septum and the mucosa on the right side of the septum are pushed to the right by the speculum, and the mucosa on the left side of the septum is pushed to the left. The keel on the vomer is exposed. *C*. Magnified view. The vomer has been removed to open the sphenoid sinus. The sellar floor is above the midline septum. In approaching the clivus, the floor of the sella is removed, and the opening in the bone is extended downward on the clivus *(interrupted lines)* to the inferior margin of the sphenoid sinus. (From de Oliveira et al.,[4] with permission.)

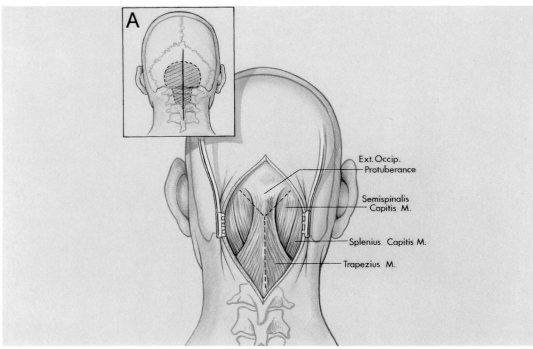

Labels in figure:
- Ext. Occip. Protuberance
- Semispinalis Capitis M.
- Splenius Capitis M.
- Trapezius M.

Figure 47-11 Suboccipital approaches. Either a vertical midline or hockey-stick incision is used. The patient is most commonly placed in the semisitting position. *A.* Upper left. The vertical midline incision is selected for lesions situated in the upper spinal canal and for those located posterior or posterolateral in the area above the foramen magnum. The incision is of sufficient length to complete a suboccipital craniectomy and a laminectomy of the axis and atlas *(oblique lines)*. Lower right. The subcutaneous tissues are separated from the underlying fascia near the inion in order to gain room for a Y-shaped incision in the muscles (M.). The upper limbs of the Y begin at the level of the superior nuchal line and join several centimeters below the inion. *B.* Upper left. Dural incision *(interrupted lines)*. Lower right. Intradural exposure. The major extracranial hazard is injury to the vertebral artery (Vert. A.) as it courses along the lateral part of the posterior arch of the atlas. The vertebral arteries give rise to the posterior inferior cerebellar (P.I.C.A.) and posterior spinal arteries (Post. Sp. A.). The median posterior spinal (Med. Post. Sp. V.) and median posterior medullary veins (Med. Post. Med. V.) course in the midline. The vein of the inferior cerebellar peduncle (V. of Inf. Cer. Ped.) courses below the fourth ventricle. Inferior hemispheric (Inf. He. V.) and inferior vermian veins (Inf. Ve. V.) course on the cerebellar surface. Bridging veins (Br. V.) pass from the neural surfaces to the adjacent sinuses. The accessory nerve (XI) ascends behind the dentate ligament (Dentate Lig.). The glossopharyngeal (IX) and vagus nerves (X) pass toward the jugular foramen. *C.* Upper left. Skin incision *(solid line)* and bone removal *(oblique lines)*. Lower right. Intradural exposure. The hockey-stick incision extends superomedial from the mastoid process along the superior nuchal line to the inion and downward in the midline. This incision is selected if the lesion extends anterolateral or anterior to the brain stem toward the jugular foramen or cerebellopontine angle. This exposure permits the removal of the full posterior rim of the foramen magnum and the posterior elements of the atlas and axis and, in addition, completion of a unilateral suboccipital craniectomy of sufficient size to expose the anterolateral surface of the brain stem and the nerves in the cerebellopontine angle. Tumors in this area may extend upward through the cerebellomedullary fissure to be attached to the roof or floor of the fourth ventricle (4V). Resection of one tonsil may facilitate the exposure. Laterally situated tumors may be attached to the initial intradural segment of the vertebral artery and the thick dural cuff around the artery, which also incorporates the posterior spinal arteries and the C-1 nerve root in fibrous tissue. As one moves superiorly along the lateral surface of the medulla, the origin of the posterior inferior cerebellar arteries and the glossopharyngeal, vagus, accessory, facial (VII), vestibulocochlear (VIII), and trigeminal nerves (V) are encountered. The dura is closed with a dural substitute if closure of the patient's dura constricts the cerebellar tonsils or the cervicomedullary junction. The sigmoid sinus (Sig. Sinus) is in the lateral margin of the exposure. (From de Oliveira et al.,[4] with permission.)

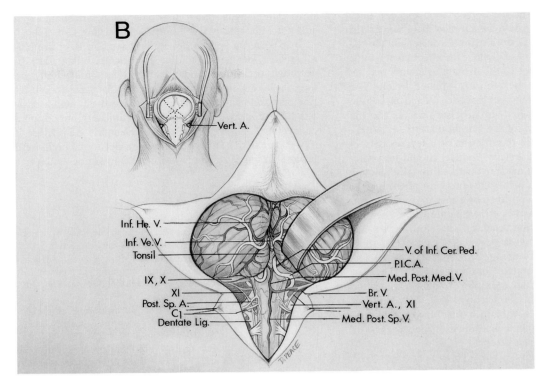

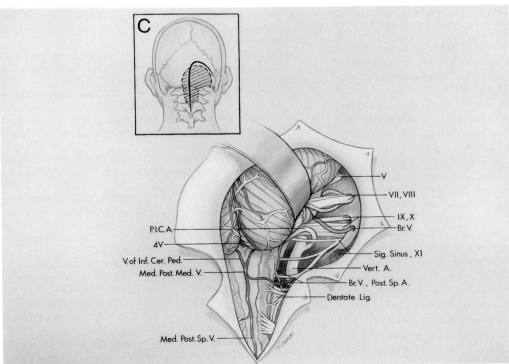

Figure 47-11 Continued

the anterolateral surface of the brain stem and the nerves in the cerebellopontine angle.

The marginal and occipital sinuses are encountered in opening the dura. Posterior intradural lesions may separate easily from the surface of the brain and spinal cord. On the other hand, they may be attached to the nerve roots and spinal cord, or they may extend upward through the cerebellomedullary fissure to be attached to the inferior medullary velum, choroid plexus, or the floor of the fourth ventricle. Resection of one tonsil may facilitate the exposure of tumors in this area. Care is required to avoid injury to the posterior inferior cerebellar artery as it courses around the tonsil.

Laterally situated tumors may be attached to the initial

intradural segment of the vertebral artery and the thick dural cuff around the artery, which also incorporates the posterior meningeal and posterior spinal arteries and the C-1 nerve root in fibrous tissue. Dividing the attachments of the upper triangular processes of the dentate ligaments may facilitate the exposure of an anteriorly situated lesion. The most difficult lesions to remove are those situated anterior to the glossopharyngeal, vagus, and accessory nerves and the lateral medullary segment of the vertebral artery. Exposing these lesions may require the division of a few rootlets of these nerves, but first the nerve rootlets should be gently separated and an attempt made to operate through the interval between the rootlets before dividing any of them. Another route through which it may be easier to reach a lesion anterior to the medulla and pons is the interval between the lower margin of the vestibulocochlear and facial nerves and the upper margin of the glossopharyngeal nerve. The intracapsular contents of the tumor are removed, and the remaining tumor capsule is separated from the surface of the brain stem and nerves rather than attempting to deliver the whole intact tumor through the limited exposure. Extreme care should be utilized when cutting into tumors, especially meningiomas, which may encase a segment of the vertebral or posterior inferior cerebellar artery.

Selection of Operative Approach

Anterior extradural lesions of the clivus or upper cervical vertebrae are best reached by one of the anterior approaches. The transoral approach is selected for most anterior extradural lesions because it provides a midline exposure and is the most direct route to the pathology. Before selecting an anterior approach, which would require that the dura be opened through the oropharynx, one should consider choosing a posterior approach since the incidence of cerebrospinal fluid leak, and meningitis, is high if the dura is opened through the oropharynx. The transcervical approach has the advantage of reaching the foramen magnum through the deep fascial planes of the neck rather than through the oropharynx; however, the depth of the exposure, the length of the time required to complete the dissection, and the fact that the foramen magnum is not approached from the midline have prevented it from gaining common usage. The transcranial-transbasal approach offers another anterior route for reaching the foramen magnum; however, this approach should not be considered for a tumor strictly localized in the region of the foramen magnum but might be used for an extensive lesion involving the ethmoid and sphenoid sinuses as well as the clivus and foramen magnum. The trans-sphenoidal approach provides an easy route for biopsying lesions in the region of the foramen magnum if they extend to the upper third of the clivus, but it does not provide adequate exposure for removing larger lesions of the region.

The posterior approaches are preferred for most intradural lesions. The vertical midline incision and a bilateral suboccipital craniectomy and upper cervical laminectomy are used for lesions situated in the upper spinal canal and posterior or posterolateral in the area above the foramen magnum. The hockey-stick incision and a unilateral suboccipital craniectomy and upper cervical laminectomy are selected if the lesion extends anterolateral or anterior to the brain stem toward the jugular foramen or cerebellopontine angle.

References

1. Abbott KH. Foramen magnum and high cervical cord lesions simulating degenerative disease of the nervous system. *Ohio State Med J* 1950; 46:645–651.
2. Coin CG, Malkasian DR. Foramen magnum. In: Newton TH, Potts DG (eds.), *Radiology of the Skull and Brain: The Skull*, Vol 1, book 1. St. Louis: Mosby, 1971:275–286.
3. Cushing HW, Eisenhardt L. *Meningiomas: Their Classification, Regional Behaviour, Life History, and Surgical End Results.* Springfield, IL: Charles C Thomas, 1938:169–180.
4. de Oliveira E, Rhoton AL Jr, Peace D. Microsurgical anatomy of the region of the foramen magnum. *Surg Neurol* 1985; 24:293–352.
5. Derome P. The transbasal approach to tumors invading the base of the skull. In: Schmidek HH, Sweet WH (eds.), *Current Techniques in Operative Neurosurgery.* New York: Grune & Stratton, 1977:223–245.
6. Friede RL, Roessmann U. Chronic tonsillar herniation: an attempt at classifying chronic herniations at the foramen magnum. *Acta Neuropathol (Berl)* 1976; 34:219–235.
7. Hardy J, Grisoli F, Leclercq TA, et al. L'abord trans-sphénoidal des tumeurs du clivus. *Neurochirurgie* 1977; 23:287–297.
8. Lister JR, Rhoton AL Jr, Matsushima T, et al. Microsurgical anatomy of the posterior inferior cerebellar artery. *Neurosurgery* 1982; 10:170–199.
9. Matsushima T, Rhoton AL Jr, de Oliveira E, et al. Microsurgical anatomy of the veins of the posterior fossa. *J Neurosurg* 1983; 59:63–105.
10. Matsushima T, Rhoton AL Jr, Lenkey C. Microsurgery of the fourth ventricle: Part 1. Microsurgical anatomy. *Neurosurgery* 1982; 11:631–667.
11. Newton TH. The anterior and posterior meningeal branches of the vertebral artery. *Radiology* 1968; 91:271–279.
12. Newton TH, Mani RL. The vertebral artery. In: Newton TH, Potts DG (eds.), *Radiology of the Skull and Brain: Angiography*, Vol 2, book 2. St. Louis: Mosby, 1974:1659–1709.
13. Ouaknine G, Nathan H. Anastomotic connections between the eleventh nerve and the posterior root of the first cervical nerve in humans. *J Neurosurg* 1973; 38:189–197.
14. Rhoton AL Jr, Buza R. Microsurgical anatomy of the jugular foramen. *J Neurosurg* 1975; 42:541–550.
15. Stein BM, Leeds NE, Taveras JM, et al. Meningiomas of the foramen magnum. *J Neurosurg* 1963; 20:740–751.

48
Gangliogliomas

Leslie N. Sutton
Roger J. Packer
Luis Schut

Gangliogliomas are unusual central nervous system tumors of children and young adults which are composed of both differentiated neurons and a background stroma of glial cells. The term was originally introduced by Courville in 1930; he thought that the tumor arose from undifferentiated cells that became neoplastic yet eventually differentiated along both glial and neuronal lines to achieve the mature forms of the cells.[1] Because differentiation was complete, he thought that the tumor must be essentially benign (Fig. 48-1). In the past, some authors have suggested that gangliogliomas are hamartomatous with limited growth potential. Most modern workers agree, however, that these are true neoplasms.

Pathologically, the diagnosis requires both astrocytic and neuronal cell populations to be present, although in most cases the astrocytic cell line will predominate.[3] Some tumors will show foci of oligodendroglioma as well. In most instances, the appearance of neurons is abnormal for the location in which they are found, although in some areas such as

the thalamus and basal ganglia it may be difficult to ascertain whether the neurons are part of the neoplastic process or are simply normal neurons surrounded by neoplastic astrocytes. To be considered neoplastic, neurons must be either clearly heterotopic (located away from gray matter) or atypical, showing disorientation, bizarre shapes or sizes, or binucleation. Within a ganglioglioma, calcification is frequent, as are cystic areas. Malignant gangliogliomas are unusual, and when they occur, the malignant features are virtually always in the glial component. It is not known whether histologic evidence of malignancy in the astroglial component carries the usual poor outlook of the malignant glioma.[10]

Several series have been reported,[5,8–10] with an incidence ranging from 0.4 percent in a large series of brain tumors[12] to 7.6 percent in a series of pediatric brain neoplasms.[4] The incidence seems to be increasing, as computed tomography (CT) scanning and more recently magnetic resonance imaging (MRI) have allowed earlier diagnosis.

Clinical Presentation

The mean age at presentation is 12 years, with a predominance between 7 and 18 years.[9,10] Adult patients are occasionally reported.[11] A male predominance has been noted in one series.[10]

The presenting symptoms are usually of long duration (average, 1.5 years), although more recent patients are being diagnosed earlier as radiologic studies become more easily obtainable. Patients almost invariably present with seizures when the lesion is supratentorial.[7–10] The seizures themselves are not particularly characteristic, and the specific type depends upon the site of the lesion. Temporal lobe convulsions are frequent, as gangliogliomas frequently occur in the temporal lobe,[7,10] but grand mal, focal motor, and

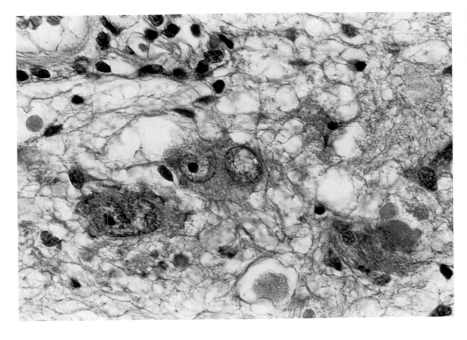

Figure 48-1 Histology of ganglioglioma. Neoplastic ganglion cells with double nuclei are seen with mature glial cells (HSE × 400).

461

mixed types can occur. Seizures tend to worsen with time, and the diagnosis of a brain tumor is established when they become uncontrollable even with appropriate anticonvulsant medication. Focal neurologic deficits are unusual, even when the lesion is located in an eloquent area, such as the motor cortex. Symptoms and signs of increased intracranial pressure such as headache, papilledema, or alteration in consciousness are rare. Patients may have evidence of a diffuse cerebral disturbance such as poor school performance or behavioral disturbances, but this may reflect frequent seizures or the effects of anticonvulsant medication. The predominance of seizures is probably a function of the slow-growing nature of this tumor, which also explains the lack of focal neurologic symptoms and signs of increased intracranial pressure.

Although gangliogliomas typically occur in the cerebral hemispheres, the tumor may arise in other locations. Courville presented several patients with a tumor arising from the region of the tuber cinereum who presented with hypothalamic symptoms or hydrocephalus.[1] Other authors have described gangliogliomas arising in the cerebellum, brain stem, or spinal cord.[1,3,4,6]

Radiologic Investigations

The radiologic manifestations of gangliogliomas were examined during the pre-CT era.[5] The major features described were calcification on plain skull films (10 percent) and an avascular mass seen on angiography or pneumoencephalography. The appearance on CT scan is variable; gangliogliomas may be isodense, of increased density, or hypodense to the degree that they may be confused with CSF-containing arachnoid cysts or porencephalies.[8,11] There are frequently areas of calcification.[8,10,11] Many tumors will involve the cortical surface, and these tend to indent the inner table of the skull (Fig. 48-2). Contrast enhancement, if it occurs, is minimal.

MR images have proved useful in the diagnosis of ganglioglioma, and in some cases the diagnosis can be predicted preoperatively.[9] The low-density tumors seen on CT have a decreased signal on T1-weighted images and are readily distinguished from CSF (Fig. 48-3). On T2-weighted images, the lesions appear as discrete areas of increased signal intensity, and the appearance of swollen gyri can be seen on the cortical margin (Fig. 48-4). With calcified lesions, MRI may be helpful in excluding vascular malformations. Sagittal and coronal images are helpful in identifying the relationship of the lesion to areas of eloquent cortex and in planning the operative exposure.

Treatment and Outcome

The mainstay of treatment is surgical excision, and gross total removal is possible in the majority. Despite the CT appearance of low density, the tumor is usually solid, although cystic areas may be present. Lesions which appear on the surface have the appearance of pale, swollen gyri

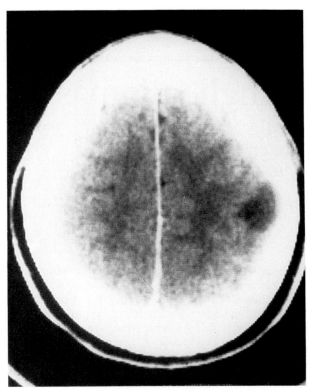

Figure 48-2 Typical appearance of a peripherally located ganglioglioma on CT scan. The lesion is of low density and did not enhance with contrast material. There is mass effect as evidenced by indentation of the inner table of the skull. This appearance may suggest an arachnoid cyst. (From Sutton et al.,[9] with permission.)

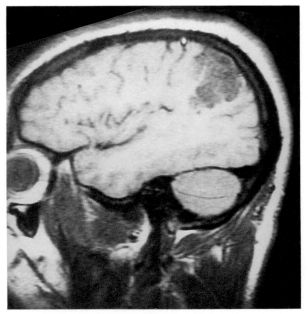

Figure 48-3 T1-weighted MR image of a ganglioglioma showing decreased signal intensity in an area involving the cortex. This image was obtained on a 1.5T instrument (TR 600 TE 25, first echo). (From Sutton et al.,[9] with permission.)

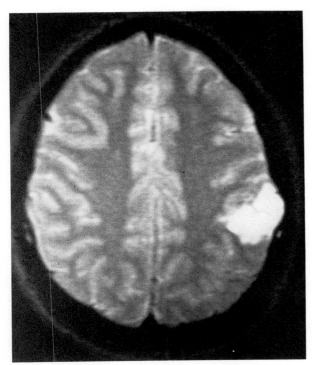

Figure 48-4 T2-weighted MR image of the same patient as shown in Figs. 48-2 and 48-3. The lesion is of increased signal intensity (TR 2500, TE 80, second echo). (From Sutton et al.,[9] with permission.)

which are readily separable from the adjacent normal brain at the intervening sulci. They tend to be avascular, and lumps of calcium may be evident. At the depths of the lesion the plane is often obscure, and it is advisable to be conservative in this part of the dissection, as these lesions may not recur, even if subtotally removed. Gangliogliomas may grow in inconvenient locations, such as the interhemispheric fissure, motor cortex, visual areas, or speech areas. The neoplasm itself subserves no neurologic function and can be removed safely even from these areas, although one must expect transient neurologic deficit from retraction. Subcortical lesions are best localized intraoperatively using real-time ultrasound to minimize the size of the cortical incision and to ensure an adequate removal. Gangliogliomas of the medial temporal lobe are treated by formal temporal lobectomy as for a seizure disorder.[10]

Postoperative radiologic evaluations of these patients have been a problem. The postoperative CT scan may appear indistinguishable from the preoperative study despite a total tumor excision, since the tumor cavity fills with CSF. Studies performed a year or more after tumor removal, however, will show the area of the operation to be much smaller, as brain tissue gradually fills in the cavity.[2] Subsequent enlargement of this low-density area bespeaks recurrence and should lead to consideration of reexploration, especially if seizure control is failing. MRI is useful in evaluating the completeness of excision, in that residual or recurrent tumor will have different signal characteristics than CSF.

The outlook for this tumor is excellent if radical surgical excision can be accomplished.[3,8–10] Seizure control tends to improve after surgery, sometimes dramatically, and it is often possible to reduce or even discontinue anticonvulsant medication.[10] Most modern authorities reserve radiation therapy for gangliogliomas with frankly malignant features or those which recur and in whom reoperation is not practical.

References

1. Courville CB. Ganglioglioma: tumor of the central nervous system: review of the literature and report of two cases. *Arch Neurol Psychiatry* 1930; 24:438–491.
2. Cox JD, Zimmerman HM, Haughton VM. Microcystic ganglioglioma treated by partial removal and radiation therapy. *Cancer* 1982; 50:473–477.
3. Garrido E, Becker LF, Hoffman HJ, et al. Gangliogliomas in children: a clinicopathologic study. *Childs Brain* 1978; 4:339–346.
4. Johannsson JH, Rekate HL, Roessmann U. Gangliogliomas: pathological and clinical correlation. *J Neurosurg* 1981; 54:58–63.
5. Katz MC, Kier EL, Schechter MM. The radiology of gangliogliomas and ganglioneuromas of the central nervous system. *Neuroradiology* 1972; 4:69–73.
6. Mizuno J, Nishio S, Barrow DL, et al. Ganglioglioma of the cerebellum: case report. *Neurosurgery* 1987; 21:584–587.
7. Steegmann AT, Winer B. Temporal lobe epilepsy resulting from ganglioglioma: report of an unusual case in an adolescent boy. *Neurology* 1961; 11:406–412.
8. Sutton LN, Packer RJ, Rorke LB, et al. Cerebral gangliogliomas during childhood. *Neurosurgery* 1983; 13:124–128.
9. Sutton LN, Packer RJ, Zimmerman RA, et al. Cerebral gangliogliomas of childhood. *Prog Exp Tumor Res* 1987; 30:239–246.
10. Ventureyra E, Herder S, Mallya BK, et al. Temporal lobe gangliogliomas in children. *Childs Nerv Syst* 1986; 2:63–66.
11. Zimmerman RA, Bilaniuk LT. Computed tomography of intracerebral gangliogliomas. *J Comput Tomogr* 1979; 3:24–30.
12. Zülch KJ. *Brain Tumors: Their Biology and Pathology.* New York: Springer-Verlag, 1965.

49
Subependymomas

Setti S. Rengachary

Subependymomas are indolent, slow-growing benign neoplasms originating from the subependymal glial matrix, consisting of a mixture of astrocytic, ependymal, and transitional cell clusters surrounded by their fibers.[23] They generally project into the ventricular lumen rather than into the brain parenchyma. Many are asymptomatic, found incidentally at autopsy. In contrast, spinal subependymomas arising in relation to the central canal of the spinal cord compress the cord substance early, invariably produce symptoms, and behave like other primary intrinsic neoplasms of the spinal cord.[21] Likewise, tumors arising from the septum pellucidum, the region of the foramen of Monro, or the aqueduct invariably produce symptoms, principally because of early occlusion of midline cerebrospinal fluid pathways.[8,12] Others compress certain critical diencephalic structures, causing impairment of cognitive functions and memory. About a fourth of the symptomatic intracranial tumors have mixed tumor cell populations, and consist of a mixture of ependymoma and subependymoma. The prognosis in such instances is much less favorable, approximating that of a pure ependymoma. The size of the neoplasm is another factor that affects the prognosis. Symptomatic tumors, regardless of their location, tend to be large. Although the neoplasm is known to occur in either sex, it is more common in men, and those harboring asymptomatic lesions tend to be older, in their seventh to ninth decades. The tumor has been reported in all decades of life; the mean age of occurrence of symptomatic tumors is 39 years, compared to 59 for asymptomatic lesions. To this date, subependymomas have not been detected in children under 2 years of age.

Scheinker[22] is generally credited as being the first to report this neoplasm as a distinct entity (in 1945), although there are other earlier series of astrocytic and ependymal neoplasms, some of which contained tumors that can be classified as subependymomas by currently accepted histologic criteria. Fewer than 200 authentic cases have been reported to date, but increasing numbers of asymptomatic lesions are likely to be detected with the widespread use of computed tomography (CT) and magnetic resonance imaging (MRI).

Although the subependymoma is generally considered to be a neoplasm, there is some suggestive evidence to indicate that subependymomas may represent hamartomas from maldevelopment. Subependymomas of the fourth ventricle have been associated with heterotopic neuroglial tissue in the leptomeninges.[13] There is also an isolated case report of subependymomas presenting at the same time in identical twins.[6] Rubinstein considers that in some instances the lesions may be reactive in nature; he quotes one instance of chronic granular cryptococcal ependymitis and meningitis associated with subependymoma.

Pathology

The lesion originates immediately beneath the ependymal surface. As it grows, it almost invariably projects into the ventricular lumen, lifting the ependymal surface. Exceptionally, a subependymoma originating along the lateral ventricle may grow out into the brain parenchyma rather than into the ventricle, resembling a primary frontal lobe neoplasm.[16] Typically, there is a well-defined demarcation between the deeper surface of the lesion and the adjacent brain parenchyma. It does not have a true capsule, but it grows by expansion rather than infiltration. The surface of the mass is very smooth because it is covered by an ependymal lining. Larger lesions may be lobulated. The common sites of occurrence are the lateral ventricles, the septum pellucidum area, the foramen of Monro region, the third ventricle, the aqueduct, and the fourth ventricle. In the fourth ventricle it may be attached to the floor, roof, or lateral recess or recesses. The distribution of the tumor in the various areas of the ventricular system is presumably related to the amount of subependymal glial matrix, which varies from region to region.[25] The size of the neoplasm ranges from a few millimeters to several centimeters across. Although the tumor occurs as a single mass, as many as eight nodules have been recorded in a single patient.[5] On occasion, the tumor arises concurrently with other primary neoplasms, such as glioblastoma or choroid plexus papilloma, but this is probably coincidental.[5]

Attachment of the neoplasm to the underlying brain parenchyma through a broad base is the rule, but a few pedunculated subependymomas have been reported.[14,27] The latter float free in the ventricular fluid, tethered to the ventricular wall through a narrow pedicle. Large masses may have multiple secondary sites of attachment to the ventricular surface;[5] in such cases it may be difficult to ascertain the primary site of origin during surgical exploration.

The consistency varies from soft to rubbery, presumably depending upon the proportion of glial fibers within the lesion. The cut surface is smooth, with a very light tan color. Gross calcification and cystic changes have been observed.[24] The tumor is generally avascular; hemorrhage within the lesion is exceptional.[4]

Obstructive ventriculomegaly is to be expected with subependymomas in certain strategic locations along the midline cerebrospinal fluid pathways. A lesion originating from the septum pellucidum may occlude one or both foramina of Monro,[8,19] and a mesencephalic lesion, the aqueduct. A large fourth ventricular lesion may entirely fill that cavity.[22] A tumor originating in the lateral recess of the fourth ventricle may extend out into the cerebellopontine angle, erode the petrous bone, and simulate a primary neoplasm in that location, such as an acoustic neurinoma or meningioma.[1] A tumor arising from the roof or the floor of the fourth ventricle may encroach rostrally into the cerebral aqueduct or caudally into the cervical spinal canal.[3]

Microscopically, the tumor typically consists of nests of glial cells separated by glial fibers. This characteristic appearance has led some pathologists to coin the term "subependymal glomerate astrocytoma."[3,11] Critical histologic studies have shown that some of the cells within these glomerate nests have attributes of ependymal cells (blepharoplasts, microvilli, cilia, and characteristic junctional complexes) and others, of astrocytes; still others are transitional between the two. Indeed, a peculiar type of primitive cell called the "tanycyte," which has attributes of an ependymal cell in one pole and of a glial cell in its opposite pole, has been noted in ependymal neoplasms.[9] These cells are normally found in the ependymal lining of lower mammals. Although the term *subependymal mixed glioma* is more accurate,[5] the simpler alternative *subependymoma* as originally described by Scheinker is well established in the literature; it is doubtful that other terms will replace the latter.

The tumor is sparsely cellular and mitotic figures are extremely rare, confirming the slow nature of tumor growth. The fibers between the cells stain positively for glial fibrillary acidic protein by the immunoperoxidase technique. Microcystic degeneration may occur within the glial fibrous matrix, giving it a spongy appearance (Fig. 49-1). These microcysts may coalesce to form larger cysts. Variably scattered foci of calcification may appear within the glial matrix. Hemorrhage and hemosiderin deposition within the neoplasm are extremely rare.[4]

The tumor in about 25 percent of individuals contains areas of cellular ependymoma.[7] The latter areas show the features expected of classic ependymomas such as true or pseudorosettes, increased vascularity, frequent mitotic figures, areas of necrosis, and increased cellularity.[10]

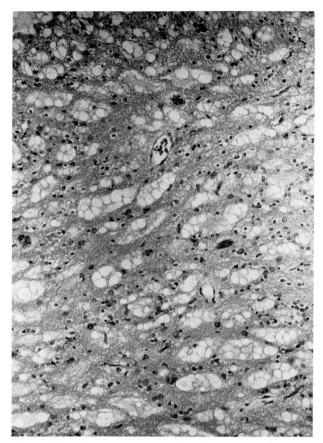

Figure 49-1 Subependymoma showing microcystic degeneration (H & E, ×100).

Symptoms and Signs

Headache and vomiting, an indication of raised intracranial pressure, are the most common initial presenting symptoms. Papilledema with transient obscurations of vision may be present in individuals with long-standing raised intracranial pressure. Ataxia in itself is a nonspecific sign. It may be related to ventriculomegaly with stretching of the corticospinal tract fibers, or it may be a sign of tumor arising from the floor of the fourth ventricle, especially if associated with vertiginous spells, vomiting, horizontal, vertical, or rotary nystagmus, bilateral spasticity, hyperactive reflexes, and Babinski's signs. Lesions arising from the septum pellucidum may induce a personality disorder, impairment of recent and remote memory, episodes of transient loss of consciousness, and generalized convulsions.[8] Some may exhibit parkinsonian features such as bradykinesia, cogwheel rigidity, and rhythmic tremor.[19,20] Alteration of mood, apathy, and lack of initiative may suggest impairment of limbic structures. Diplopia and cranial nerve impairment are seen in brain stem lesions. In late or extreme obstructive hydrocephalus, patients may present in coma with no focal localizing signs. Occasionally, an asymptomatic subependymoma

is discovered by CT or MRI during the evaluation of a patient with an unrelated neurologic disorder or unrelated symptoms.

Diagnostic Imaging

The majority of subependymomas are isodense with brain parenchyma on CT scans without contrast administration; with contrast, they generally do not enhance.[26] Although diffuse and uniform enhancement has been reported with authentic subependymomas,[24] intense diffuse enhancement associated with parenchymal edema should arouse suspicion of a mixed ependymoma-subependymoma. Calcification and cystic changes within the tumor can be readily discerned on CT as hyperdense and hypodense areas, respectively. Rare instances of hemorrhage into the tumor may be diagnosed as well.

MRI is a very helpful test, especially in instances where the tumor is isodense on CT scan and does not enhance with a contrast agent. The tumor outline appears as a hyperintense signal in T1- and T2-weighted images (Fig. 49-2). Because these tumors are avascular, cerebral angiography is the least useful diagnostic test.

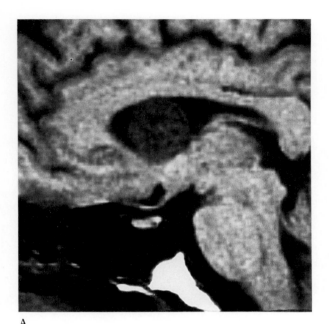

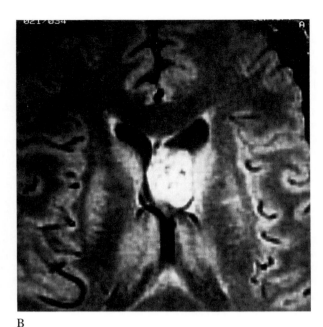

A   B

Figure 49-2   Sagittal (*A*) and axial (*B*) views (T1-weighted MR images) of a subependymoma arising from the septum pellucidum.

Therapy and Prognosis

Septum pellucidum lesions may be approached either through a transcallosal or a transfrontal, transventricular approach. Removal of the tumor is technically simple because of avascularity. Fourth ventricular lesions are ordinarily exposed through a standard midline posterior fossa approach, with splitting of the vermis.

Tumors attached to the floor of the fourth ventricle carry the worst prognosis because of location. A mixed ependymoma-subependymoma carries a worse prognosis than a pure subependymoma. Recurrences do not occur unless the initial tumor resection is incomplete or the original tumor was a mixed tumor. Radiation therapy or other adjunctive therapies are unjustified in pure subependymomas.

Spinal Subependymomas

Spinal subependymomas are extremely rare. Only about eight cases have been reported to date.[2,3,15,17,18,21] All reported patients have been symptomatic. The symptoms and signs and radiologic features are indistinguishable from those of other primary intrinsic neoplasms of the spinal cord. Most occur in the cervical cord or at the cervicothoracic junction. Unlike ependymomas, which arise occasionally from the filum terminale, subependymomas have not been reported in that location. In one rare instance, the entire spinal cord was involved with tumor.[18] In another, the cervical tumor was an extension of an intracranial medullary neoplasm.[3]

The technique of removal of the neoplasm is no different from that used for other primary neoplasms of the spinal cord. After a median myelotomy and application of fine pial stay sutures, a plane of cleavage between the neoplasm and the cord is defined and the tumor is excised under magnification using customary surgical adjuncts such as the ultrasonic aspirator or laser. The histologic appearances of spinal subependymomas are indistinguishable from those of intracranial lesions. However, it may be difficult to arrive at the correct diagnosis based upon frozen section examination. If only a partial resection is accomplished during an initial operation because of an incorrect frozen section report, one should not hesitate to consider a second attempt at complete resection and cure.

References

1. Azzarelli B, Rekate HL, Roessmann U. Subependymoma: a case report with ultrastructural study. *Acta Neuropathol (Berl)* 1977; 40:279–282.
2. Bardella L, Artico M, Nucci F. Intramedullary subependymoma of the cervical spinal cord. *Surg Neurol* 1988; 29:326–329.
3. Boykin FC, Cowen D, Iannucci CAJ, et al. Subependymal glomerate astrocytomas. *J Neuropathol Exp Neurol* 1954; 13:30–49.
4. Changaris DG, Powers JM, Perot PL Jr, et al. Subependymoma presenting as subarachnoid hemorrhage: case report. *J Neurosurg* 1981; 55:643–645.
5. Chason JL. Subependymal mixed gliomas. *J Neuropathol Exp Neurol* 1956; 15:461–470.
6. Clarenbach P, Kleihues P, Metzel E, et al. Simultaneous clini-

cal manifestation of subependymoma of the fourth ventricle in identical twins: case report. *J Neurosurg* 1979; 50:655–659.

7. Fokes EC Jr, Earle KM. Ependymomas: clinical and pathological aspects. *J Neurosurg* 1969; 30:585–594.

8. French JD, Bucy PC. Tumors of the septum pellucidum. *J Neurosurg* 1948; 5:433–449.

9. Friede RL, Pollak A. The cytogenetic basis for classifying ependymomas. *J Neuropathol Exp Neurol* 1978; 37:103–118.

10. Fu YS, Chen ATL, Kay S, et al. Is subependymoma (subependymal glomerate astrocytoma) an astrocytoma or ependymoma? A comparative ultrastructural and tissue culture study. *Cancer* 1974; 34:1992–2008.

11. Godwin JT. Subependymal glomerate astrocytoma: report of two cases. *J Neurosurg* 1959; 16:385–389.

12. Hehman K, Norrell H, Howieson J. Subependymomas of the septum pellucidum: report of two cases. *J Neurosurg* 1968; 29:640–644.

13. Ho KL. Concurrence of subependymoma and heterotopic leptomeningeal neuroglial tissue. *Arch Pathol Lab Med* 1983; 107:136–140.

14. Kunicki A. Pedunculated gliomas in the lateral ventricle. *J Neurol Neurosurg Psychiatry* 1965; 28:548–551.

15. Lee KS, Angelo JN, McWhorter JM, et al. Symptomatic subependymoma of the cervical spinal cord: report of two cases. *J Neurosurg* 1987; 67:128–131.

16. Lobato RD, Sarabia M, Castro S, et al. Symptomatic subependymoma: report of four new cases studied with computed tomography and review of the literature. *Neurosurgery* 1986; 19:594–598.

17. Matsumura A, Hori A, Spoerri O. Spinal subependymoma presenting as an extramedullary tumor: case report. *Neurosurgery* 1988; 23:115–117.

18. Pluchino F, Lodrini S, Lasio G, et al. Complete removal of holocord subependymoma: case report. *Acta Neurochir (Wien)* 1984; 73:243–250.

19. Riskaer N. Cysts and tumors of the septum pellucidum. *Acta Psychiatr Neurol* 1944; 19:331–346.

20. Rushing CM, Hathaway BM. Subependymal glomerate astrocytoma. *South Med J* 1965; 58:1137–1139.

21. Salcman M, Mayer R. Intramedullary subependymoma of the cervical spinal cord: case report. *Neurosurgery* 1984; 14:608–611.

22. Scheinker IM. Subependymoma: a newly recognized tumor of subependymoral derivation. *J Neurosurg* 1945; 2:232–240.

23. Scheithauer BW. Symptomatic subependymoma: report of 21 cases with review of the literature. *J Neurosurg* 1978; 49:689–696.

24. Stevens JM, Kendall BE, Love S. Radiological features of subependymoma with emhasis on computed tomography. *Neuroradiology* 1984; 26:223–228.

25. Tennyson VM, Pappas GD. Ependyma. In: Minckler J (ed.), *Pathology of the Nervous System*. New York: McGraw-Hill, 1968; 1:518–531.

26. Vaquero J, Cabezudo JM, Nombela L. CT scan in subependymomas. *Br J Radiol* 1983; 56:425–427.

27. Vaquero J, Herrero J, Cabezudo JM, et al. Symptomatic subependymomas of the lateral ventricles. *Acta Neurochir (Wien)* 1980; 53:99–105.

50

Meningeal Hemangio-pericytomas

Michael J. Ebersold
Bernd Scheithauer
Barton L. Guthrie

The first description of hemangiopericytoma was that of a tumor outside the central nervous system, frequently involving the soft tissues of the thigh, buttock, and retroperitoneum. Stout and Murrary developed the concept of hemangiopericytoma, a vascular tumor featuring Zimmerman's pericytes; only one of Stout's 25 subsequently reported cases was stated to involve the meninges.[27] A review of the literature, however, reveals that Bailey et al. had already described three "angioblastic meningiomas" in 1928.[1] Although strong opinions have been expressed as to whether they represent separate entities, many now consider the angioblastic meningioma and the hemangiopericytoma to be one and the same, an opinion with which we concur.[10] The clinicopathologic features of these morphologically identical tumors have been confused not only because authors have long referred to them as distinct lesions but also because some have reported the existence of tumors with intermediate features.[23] It is nonetheless probable that most reports and reviews of angioblastic meningiomas refer to a tumor synonymous with hemangiopericytoma of the central nervous system.[4]

There are a number of excellent clinicopathologic reviews of meningeal hemangiopericytomas.[5,6,9,21,22,24,28] Much of our present understanding and the views expressed herein are based upon these reviews, other sources,[13,15,18] and a recently completed review of 44 patients with meningeal hemangiopericytoma seen at our institution.

Incidence and Behavior

Much of the confusion between angioblastic meningioma and hemangiopericytoma has its basis in semantics. Most important is the understanding that the latter is distinct from ordinary meningiomas. Grossly, both have a similar topographic distribution, arising preferentially from the falx, tentorium, dural sinuses, and skull base. In addition, both meningioma and hemangiopericytoma are dural-based, compress rather than invade the brain, and are frequently found to be very vascular at the time of surgery. In many instances, these tumors seem to involve the leptomeninges, making difficult the maintenance of an avascular surgical plane. Total resection may also be complicated by the tendency of both types of tumors to be irregular at their interface with adjoining tissue.

The meningeal hemangiopericytoma is a rare tumor. In a review of our own data based upon 1,976 patients who had undergone surgery for meningioma between 1960 and 1980, 24 hemangiopericytomas were encountered; their incidence, therefore, is 2.4 percent of the meningiomas. This is in agreement with other authors who have found the incidence to be less than 4 percent of meningiomas[2,6,11,12,21,22,25,29] and approximately 0.5 percent of all tumors of the central nervous system. Hemangiopericytoma in tissue outside the brain is a well-established entity, with several large series having been reported.[5,19]

These publications stress frequent recurrence, and metastasis rates approaching 50 percent. Long-term follow-up is mandatory, because recurrence or metastasis may be delayed for years. In a previously published series of 26 patients from this institution, it was found that the aggressive nature of the hemangiopericytoma resulted in a recurrence rate of 80 percent and a rate of metastasis of 23 percent.[9] More recently, we had the opportunity of enlarging the study group and extended the duration of follow-up; it was observed that the patients who had undergone surgery between the years 1938 and 1987 experienced 1-, 5-, and 10-year recurrence rates of 15, 65, and 76 percent, respectively, and that the rate of metastasis at 10 and 15 years was 33 percent and 64 percent, respectively (Fig. 50-1).[10]

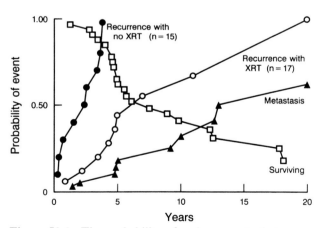

Figure 50-1 The probability of various events that were observed in 44 patients seen at our institution between 1938 and 1987. Details of the initial operation were known for 38 of these 44 patients, and 21 of the 38 were thought to have no gross residual tumor. Seventeen had gross residual tumor after the initial surgery. Seven of the above patients died of other causes, and seven died of their tumor after developing metastases. Although some of the deaths obviously occurred from recurrence of the primary tumor, the presence of metastases was a very bad prognostic sign. XRT = radiation therapy.

The meningioma is much less likely to recur following surgical removal, and metastases are very rare. For patients whose tumors were grossly totally removed, Simpson found the recurrence rate to be only 9 percent.[25] Simpson reported a 19 percent recurrence rate for meningiomas that were totally removed but in which cauterization of the dural attachment site was required.

Pathology

Light Microscopy

Light microscopy shows a hemangiopericytoma to consist of plump to spindle-shaped cells (Fig. 50-2). Occasional zones of hypocellularity are found, but microcysts are uncommon. Mitotic figures are frequent; in the 1978 review, these ranged from 1 to 5 per 10 high-power fields,[9] and in our current review, averaged 7 per 20 high-power fields.[10]

Nuclei are generally delicate, round to fusiform, and demonstrate neither coarse chromatin nor nucleolar prominence. Binucleation or multinucleation of tumor cells is very infrequent; however, cellularity is generally high and may be either dense and patternless or show some fibrogenesis. Vascularity is quite variable, with some of these tumors demonstrating abundant thin-walled vascular networks likened to "staghorns" in configuration with lined flat inconspicuous endothelial cells. Some cells or groups of cells are surrounded by fine reticulin-staining fibers. The reticulin stain often, but not invariably, shows a typical pattern of fine fibers surrounding individual or small groups of tumor cells.

Interestingly, no significant tendency to increasing anaplasia was demonstrated when comparing recurrent or metastatic lesions to the original or primary tumor.[10] Neverthe-less, 3 of 11 cases in the 1978 review demonstrated "dedifferentiation," with plumper cells, more prominent nucleoli, and less reticulin among tumor cells in later specimens.[9]

Immunocytology

Winek et al., in a recent study of immunohistochemical characteristics of 9 peripheral and 13 central nervous system (CNS) hemangiopericytomas as well as 40 ordinary meningiomas, noted similar immunoprofiles for the hemangiopericytoma regardless of site [vimentin, positive; epithelial membrane antigen (EMA), negative]. In contrast, both EMA and vimentin reactivity was observed in all ordinary meningiomas studied.[30] These results support the concept that hemangiopericytoma and meningioma are distinct neoplasms.

Electron Microscopy

Electron microscopic studies of ordinary meningiomas have demonstrated their ultrastructural similarity to normal arachnoid membrane. The cells are cohesive, show intricate interdigitation of their membranes with those of adjoining cells, demonstrate numerous intercellular desmosomes, and are devoid of pericellular basement membrane. Their cytoplasm contains varying numbers of intermediate filaments, the basis of the vimentin reaction noted above. In contrast, the cells in a hemangiopericytoma are often less cohesive, show few and structurally simpler intercellular junctions, and contain fewer as well as less dispersed cytoplasmic microfilaments. The intercellular space often contains deposits of basement membrane–like material which is apparent on reticulin stains (Fig. 50-2).[4]

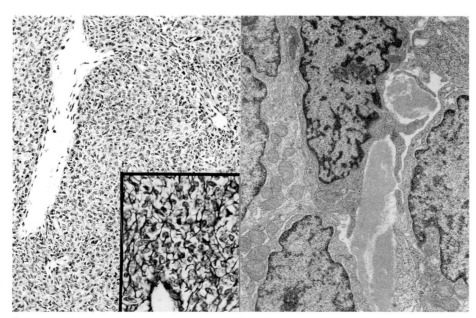

A   B

Figure 50-2 Microscopic appearance of a hemangiopericytoma. *A*. The typical light microscopic appearance of a hemangiopericytoma composed of small ovoid to elongated cells associated with staghorn vascular channels. (Hematoxylin and eosin stain, ×160). *Inset:* A reticulin stain demonstrating a dense intercellular reticulin pattern (×400). *B*. An electron micrograph demonstrating cohesion of elongated tumor cells with scant processes; note the lack of frequent intercellular junctions, a feature prominent in meningiomas. Note the intercellular basement membrane-like material, the basis of the reticulin reaction (×9000).

Location

Although the hemangiopericytoma has been reported to arise at both extra- and intracranial sites, those involving the CNS often, but not invariably, originate in the meninges. Some series have reported 10 to 30 percent of CNS lesions to involve the spinal cord,[22,24] whereas in our most recent review, only 2 of 44 tumors were spinal.[10] The intracranial distribution of hemangiopericytomas is similar to that reported for ordinary meningiomas. In our 44 cases, 27 patients (62 percent) presented with supratentorial tumors, their favored locations including the parasagittal region, tentorium, and sphenoid wing.

Clinical Presentation

In contrast to patients with meningiomas, among whom two-thirds are found to be female, 55 to 70 percent of hemangiopericytomas occur in males.[2,3,12,21] In addition, hemangiopericytomas occur in a slightly younger age group, averaging 38 to 42 years,[11,22,24] unlike patients with meningiomas, who have a mean age in the early 50s.[2,12,21,26] As reported by others, we confirmed the finding that patients with a hemangiopericytoma are often symptomatic for less than a year before diagnosis.[6,22,24,28] This contrasts to similar reviews of meningiomas, wherein most patients exhibit symptoms for 1 to 2 years.[21] In our series, the average symptomatic interval for hemangiopericytoma was only 99.75 months during the computed tomography (CT) era.[10]

Not surprisingly, the clinical presentation of hemangiopericytomas reflects the location of the tumor. Sixty-eight percent of our 44 patients presented with headaches, and 16 percent with seizures. Patients with posterior fossa lesions were most likely to demonstrate gait disturbance and dysequilibrium.[10]

Radiographic Diagnosis

Plain x-ray films are generally not revealing. At the present time, the diagnosis will almost always be established before radiographic evidence of increased intracranial pressure. Although ordinary meningiomas may at times be associated with hyperostosis, it has not been reported with a hemangiopericytoma. One of our 44 cases of hemangiopericytoma was accompanied by a lytic lesion on skull films.

The CT scan and magnetic resonance imaging (MRI) appearances of a hemangiopericytoma are usually indistinguishable from those of an ordinary meningioma (Fig. 50-3). Indeed, a diagnosis of meningioma is most often rendered. The finding of calcium within a tumor, however, is strong evidence against the diagnosis of hemangiopericytoma.

The angiographic appearance of a hemangiopericytoma likewise resembles that of a meningioma. Of the 20 most recent angiograms in our patients with hemangiopericytoma, 9 showed vascular lesions with the typical tumor blush, and 11 demonstrated avascular masses. The blood supply may be intradural, extradural, or a combination of both.

Surgical Treatment

The surgical treatment of a hemangiopericytoma is essentially that of a meningioma. Preoperative embolization may be considered for a small proportion of tumors which are both highly vascular and derive their major blood supply from vessels appropriate for embolization. Because of the significant tendency of these tumors to recur locally and to eventually metastasize, aggressive and thorough resection is the goal.

Despite efforts at achieving complete removal whenever possible, local recurrence and, to a lesser extent, metastases are all too often noted. Among the last 32 patients who had their initial surgery at our institution, slightly over half (17) developed local recurrence at an average of 47 months after the initial operation (Fig. 50-1). Ten of the 32 also developed at least one metastasis within 2 to 20 years after the initial operation (lung, 4; bone, 4; soft tissue, 2; liver, 1; retroperitoneum, 1; diffuse in meninges, 1). Multiple metastases were noted in two cases.

The tendency of recurrence reflects the fact that it is often impossible to be sure that complete removal has been accomplished. In our own review, the mean survival of the patients having had gross total tumor removal was 91 months, whereas subtotal removal was associated with an average survival of 65 months. For technical reasons, it seems particularly difficult to achieve gross total removal in cases wherein the posterior fossa and tentorium are involved; our own data support this conclusion and highlight the surgical challenge. In addition to the technical difficulties encountered in the resection of posterior fossa tumors, patients do not tolerate posterior fossa tumor recurrence as well as supratentorial recurrence. The difficulties and limitations inherent in repeat posterior fossa surgery no doubt negatively affect survival statistics. In our experience, for instance, the average survival of patients undergoing gross total removal of tentorial or posterior fossa tumors versus that of patients undergoing subtotal removal was 76 and 53 months, respectively, whereas patients with similarly treated supratentorial tumors survived 110 and 75 months, respectively. The operative mortality rate in our series of 44 patients was found to be 9 percent, but there have been no surgical deaths in the last 15 years.[10]

Postoperative Radiation Therapy

The impressive recurrence rate of hemangiopericytoma coupled with its potential for metastasis despite apparent total removal make it clear that surgery alone cannot be considered the sole solution to the treatment of hemangiopericytoma. As early as 1949, Stout reported the reduction in tumor volume with radiation therapy in an 11-year-old girl with a rectal hemangiopericytoma.[27] The response of peripheral hemangiopericytoma to radiation therapy has also

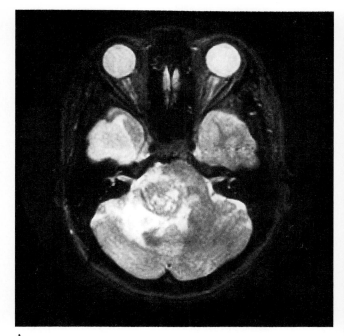

A

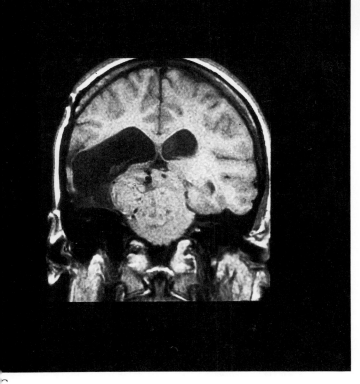

C

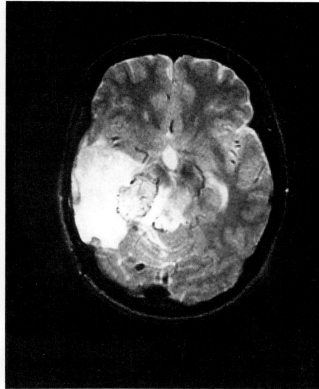

B

Figure 50-3 *A.* A T2-weighted axial MR image through the posterior fossa demonstrates a lobulated tumor mass with mixed signal intensities in the right cerebellopontine angle. Note the marked displacement of the brain stem and the surrounding edema in the cerebellum. *B.* A T2-weighted axial image at a higher level demonstrates the mass extending through the tentorial notch. The high-intensity area in the middle cranial fossa is secondary to previous surgery. *C.* A T1-weighted coronal image shows the predominantly isointense mass, with focal areas of hypointensity consistent with cyst formation or areas of necrosis, involving the posterior and middle cranial fossae. Note the marked indentation and displacement of the brain stem.

been reported by others.[5–7] In addition, several authors have suggested that radiation is beneficial in the treatment of meningeal hemangiopericytomas.[8,9,14,16,17,20,29] For instance, Fukui et al. documented the reduction in size of meningeal hemangiopericytomas 6 months after 4000 to 6000 cGy.[8]

Our own review of the effects of radiation therapy upon hemangiopericytomas demonstrated definite benefits. Even though we were more likely to recommend radiation therapy in cases wherein incomplete tumor removal was likely, patients receiving radiation therapy did better than those treated by surgery alone. In our most recent review of 32 patients, 17 underwent radiation therapy and 15 did not. In this heterogeneous group, radiation therapy increased the recurrence-free interval from 34 months to 75 months ($p < 0.05$) (Fig. 50-1). It was our observation that doses in excess of 4500 cGy, especially doses above 5100 cGy, were more likely to prevent local recurrence.[10] In the three patients who received 5130, 5200, and 5600 cGy, respectively, there was no recurrence. In addition, we noted that patients receiving radiation therapy after their first operation survived an average of 2.5 years longer than those who did not. This observation, however, was not statistically significant because of the small numbers of such patients.[10]

Despite the beneficial effects of radiation therapy, it is of interest that all intracranial recurrences following radiation lay within the treatment field. It is our opinion, therefore, that little is to be gained from whole brain or spinal axis irradiation.

Conclusions

The meningeal hemangiopericytoma is a rare and aggressive lesion which is considered synonymous with angioblastic meningioma. Unlike the classical meningiomas, which are more common in females, hemangiopericytomas occur with greater frequency in males. Typically, meningeal hemangiopericytomas occur in a somewhat younger age group than do meningiomas. In our patients, such factors as tumor cellularity, cytologic atypia, and mitotic activity were of little or no prognostic significance. The same was true of patient sex and age at the time of diagnosis.

Recurrence and, to a lesser extent, metastases are common and mandate an aggressive approach with complete surgical removal if possible. Postoperative radiation treatment to the operative site should be seriously considered for tentorial or posterior fossa tumors as well as in instances wherein gross total removal could not be achieved. Doses in the range of 5400 to 5700 cGy directed to the primary tumor bed and surrounding margin are suggested by our recent review.[10] Long-term follow-up, at least up to 15 years, is necessary in that late recurrence and late metastases to lung, bone, and soft tissue are not uncommon.

References

1. Bailey P, Cushing H, Eisenhardt L. Angioblastic meningiomas. *Arch Pathol Lab Med* 1928; 6:953–990.
2. Chan RC, Thompson GB. Morbidity, mortality, and quality of life following surgery for intracranial meningiomas: a retrospective study in 257 cases. *J Neurosurg* 1984; 60:52–60.
3. Cushing H, Eisenhardt L. *Meningiomas: Their Classification, Regional Behaviour, Life History and Surgical End Results.* Springfield, IL: Charles C Thomas, 1938.
4. Dardick I, Hammar SP, Sheithauer BW. Ultrastructural spectrum of hemangiopericytoma: a comparative study of fetal, adult and neoplastic pericytes. *Ultrastruct Pathol* 1989; 13:111–154.
5. Enzinger FM, Smith BH. Hemangiopericytoma: an analysis of 106 cases. *Hum Pathol* 1976; 7:61–82.
6. Fabiani A, Favero M, Trebini F. On the primary meningeal tumors with special concern to the hemangiopericytoma pathology and biology. *Zentralbl Neurochir* 1980; 41:273–284.
7. Friedman M, Egan JW. Irradiation of hemangiopericytoma of Stout. *Radiology* 1960; 74:721–730.
8. Fukui M, Kitamura K, Nakagaki H, et al. Irradiated meningiomas: a clinical evaluation. *Acta Neurochir (Wien)* 1980; 54:33–43.
9. Goellner JR, Laws ER Jr, Soule EH, et al. Hemangiopericytoma of the meninges: Mayo Clinic experience. *Am J Clin Pathol* 1978; 70:375–380.
10. Guthrie BL, Ebersold MJ, Scheithauer BW, et al. Meningeal hemangiopericytoma: histopathological features, treatment, and long-term follow-up of 44 cases. *Neurosurgery* 1989; 25:514–522.
11. Jääskeläinen J, Servo A, Haltia M, et al. Intracranial hemangiopericytoma: radiology, surgery, radiotherapy, and outcome in 21 patients. *Surg Neurol* 1985; 23:227–236.
12. Jellinger K, Slowik F. Histological subtypes and prognostic problems in meningiomas. *J Neurol* 1975; 208:279–298.
13. Kernohan JW, Uihlein A. *Sarcomas of the Brain.* Springfield, IL: Charles C Thomas, 1962.
14. King DL, Chang CH, Pool JL. Radiotherapy in the management of meningiomas. *Acta Radiol Ther Phys Biol* 1966; 5:26–33.
15. Kochanek S, Schröder R, Firsching R. Hemangiopericytoma of meninges. I. Histopathological variability and differential diagnosis. *Zentralbl Neurochir* 1986; 47:183–190.
16. Lal H, Sanyal B, Pant GC, et al. Hemangiopericytoma: report of three cases regarding role of radiation therapy. *AJR* 1976; 126:887–891.
17. Lesoin F, Bouchez B, Krivosic I, et al. Hemangiopericytic meningioma of the pineal region: case report. *Eur Neurol* 1984; 23:274–277.
18. Lolova I, Kamenova M. Hemangiopericytoma of the brain: histological and histochemical study of four cases. *J Neurosurg* 1973; 39:636–641.
19. McMaster MJ, Soule EH, Ivins JC. Hemangiopericytoma: a clinicopathologic study and long-term follow-up of 60 patients. *Cancer* 1975; 36:2232–2244.
20. Mira JG, Chu FCH, Fortner JG. The role of radiotherapy in the management of malignant hemangiopericytoma: report of eleven new cases and review of the literature. *Cancer* 1977; 39:1254–1259.
21. Mirimannoff RO, Dosoretz DE, Linggood RM, et al. Meningioma: analysis of recurrence and progression following neurosurgical resection. *J Neurosurg* 1985; 62:18–24.
22. Pitkethly DT, Hardman JM, Kempe LG, et al. Angioblastic meningiomas: clinicopathologic study of 81 cases. *J Neurosurg* 1970; 32:539–544.
23. Russell DS, Rubinstein LJ. *Pathology of Tumours of the Nervous System,* 4th ed. Baltimore: Williams & Wilkins, 1977:74–79.
24. Schröder R, Firsching R, Kochanek S. Hemangiopericytoma of meninges. II. General and clinical data. *Zentralbl Neurochir* 1986; 47:191–199.
25. Simpson D. The recurrence of intracranial meningiomas after surgical treatment. *J Neurol Neurosurg Psychiatry* 1957; 20:22–39.
26. Skullerud K, Löken AC. The prognosis in meningiomas. *Acta Neuropathol (Berl)* 1974; 29:337–344.
27. Stout AP. Hemangiopericytoma: a study of twenty-five new cases. *Cancer* 1949; 2:1027–1035.
28. Thomas HG, Dolman CL, Berry K. Malignant meningioma: clinical and pathologic features. *J Neurosurg* 1981; 55:929–934.
29. Wara WM, Sheline GE, Newman H, et al. Radiation therapy of meningiomas. *AJR* 1980; 123:453–458.
30. Winek RR, Scheithauer BW, Wick MR. Meningioma, meningeal hemangiopericytoma (angioblastic meningioma), peripheral hemangiopericytoma and acoustic schwannoma: a comparative immunohistochemical study. *Am J Surg Pathol* 1989; 13:251–261.

51

Surgery for a Single Brain Metastasis

Byron Young
Roy A. Patchell

Factors Influencing Prognosis and Treatment

Metastases to the brain make up approximately half of all intracranial tumors and occur in 20 to 40 percent of patients with systemic cancer.[5] Brain metastases are single in about 50 percent of cases.[7] The term *single brain metastasis* is applied to patients with one metastasis in the brain but makes no inference about the presence or absence of cancer elsewhere in the body. The term *solitary brain metastasis* refers to a rare subgroup of patients with a single brain metastasis in whom the brain metastasis is the only known cancer in the body.

The occurrence of brain metastasis is usually associated with a poor prognosis regardless of therapy. Untreated patients with brain metastases have a median survival of only about 1 month.[16,20] Virtually all untreated patients die as a direct result of the brain tumor. With corticosteroid treatment alone, the median survival is increased to approximately 2 months. As is true for untreated patients, most patients treated with corticosteroids alone die as a direct result of the brain metastases.[10,21] Whole brain radiation therapy (WBRT) increases median survival to 3 to 6 months.[2–6,10,15–17,29] Large retrospective studies have shown that most patients treated with WBRT ultimately die from progressive systemic cancer and not as a direct result of the brain metastases.[4,5,29] However, the WBRT survival data were derived from studies containing large numbers of patients with extensive systemic disease and relatively short expected survivals. In the subgroup of patients whose only metastases are to the brain, death is more likely to be due to the brain metastasis than to progressive systemic disease.[29] Therefore, in patients with controlled systemic cancer who develop brain metastases, the treatment of the brain lesion or lesions is the factor that will most likely determine length of survival.

From a theoretical standpoint, the combination of surgery followed by postoperative radiation therapy should be more effective at eradicating brain metastases than radiation or surgery alone. Radiation therapy is most effective where cells are relatively small in number and are well oxygenated. In the center of the tumor, where tumor cells are more numerous and hypoxic conditions usually exist, radiation may fail to completely destroy tumor cells.[1] Although sterilization of brain metastases by radiation therapy alone is documented, in most cases, residual tumor remains despite irradiation. Surgery can completely remove all tumor cells; however, residual tumor remains in about one-third of patients,[12–14,22] even after "complete" surgical resection. Rational treatment plans combining surgical debulking and radiation therapy have been developed to overcome the deficiencies of both types of treatment.

Despite the theoretical advantages of combined surgical and radiation treatment, the role of surgery remains unclear due to an absence of any prospective randomized trials showing the efficacy of surgical treatment. Many uncontrolled surgical series have shown longer survivals of surgically treated patients when compared with historical controls treated with WBRT alone.[12,23,26,28] Retrospective reports of uncontrolled studies of patients treated with WBRT (and containing small numbers treated with surgery plus postoperative WBRT) have also generally shown an increased survival in the surgically treated patients.[2,4,8,15,16,29] However, neither historical controls nor controls consisting of concurrent unselected patients treated with WBRT alone are appropriate for comparing the efficacy of surgery plus WBRT versus WBRT alone. Patients who receive surgical treatment are usually selected from among patients with controlled or no known systemic disease (and consequently longer expected survivals), whereas patients treated with WBRT alone include patients with more extensive disease and generally much poorer prognoses. Patchell et al. used matched control groups to compare surgery and WBRT with WBRT alone.[18] Although this study suggested that surgery was effective, the study was retrospective and did not use randomized assignment to treatment groups. The effectiveness of surgical treatment (if any) can only be tested by a prospective randomized trial.

Two randomized prospective studies have been performed to determine the effectiveness of surgery. In a recently completed study at our institution, patients with single brain metastases were randomly assigned to one of two treatment groups: (1) the Surgical Group had complete surgical removal of the brain metastasis followed by WBRT, and (2) the Radiation-alone Group had a stereotactic needle biopsy of the brain lesion followed by WBRT. All patients received 3600 cGy WBRT. Fifty-four patients were entered into the study; however, six (11 percent) were found not to have metastatic brain tumors after resection or biopsy. Of the remaining 48 patients, 25 were in the Surgical Group, and 23 were in the Radiation-alone Group. Local recurrence of the brain metastasis was more common in the Radiation-alone Group, 52 percent versus 20 percent ($p < 0.02$). Overall survival was significantly longer ($p < 0.03$) in the Surgical Group (median 40 weeks versus 15 weeks). Quality of life (based on the time that the Karnofsky score[11] remained $\geq$ 70 percent) was also significantly ($p < 0.006$) better in the Surgical Group. The 30-day mortality rates were 4 percent in both the Surgical Group and the Radiation-alone Group.

A Dutch study is currently near completion, and preliminary results also show an advantage to surgery (personal communication). From our study, we concluded that surgery reduces the local tumor recurrence rate, and this results in a subsequent reduction of morbidity and mortality due to neurologic causes. Therefore, patients with single brain metastases treated with surgical resection plus WBRT live longer and have a better quality of life than patients treated with WBRT alone.

With any surgical procedure, operative mortality has to be weighed against any possible benefit from surgery. In older series of patients with single brain metastases who were treated with surgery, operative mortality rates were in the range of 10 to 34 percent.[3,9,13,14,19,20,22,25] However, with improvement in surgical technique (particularly the introduction of microsurgery), computer-assisted stereotactic surgery, intraoperative ultrasonography, and the widespread use of steroids, mortality rates in most series reported during the last 10 years have been under 10 percent.[12,15,18,23,26,28] The 4 percent rate in our study was well within the acceptable range and was identical to the 30-day mortality rate in the Radiation-alone Group. Other recent surgical series report no excess mortality due to surgery when compared with radiation alone. Kelly et al. reported no mortality in a series of 45 patients using computer-assisted stereotactic techniques.[12] Sundaresan et al. reported a 3 percent mortality.[23]

Although the results of our randomized trial show that surgery plus WBRT is superior to WBRT alone in the treatment of single brain metastases, WBRT alone will remain the treatment of choice for most patients with brain metastases. Only about 50 percent of brain metastases are single, and the general consensus among neuro-oncologists and neurosurgeons is that resection of multiple lesions is not justified, except in rare circumstances. Moreover, nearly half of the patients with single metastases are not surgical candidates due to inaccessibility of the tumor, uncontrolled or extensive systemic disease, and other factors.[18] Thus, approximately 25 percent of patients with brain metastases could benefit from surgical resection. The rest should be treated with WBRT alone.

Standard practice has been to assume that patients with systemic cancer developing an intracranial lesion have a brain metastasis. An interesting finding in our study was the high percentage of patients who proved not to have metastatic brain tumors after surgery or biopsy. All patients had tissue-proven primary tumors diagnosed prior to entry into the study. Despite having computed tomography (CT) and magnetic resonance imaging (MRI) findings consistent with single brain metastases, 11 percent of the total (6/54) did not have metastatic tumors. Due to the relatively high rate of misdiagnosis of metastatic lesions with CT scans,[24] even when surgical resection is not recommended, a stereotactic needle biopsy should usually be done to confirm the diagnosis. This practice should especially be followed in patients with controlled systemic cancer whose survival is likely to be dependent on the treatment of the brain lesion. Half of our patients who were proved not to have brain metastases had potentially treatable intracranial infectious or inflammatory processes.

Surgical Indications

The patients with brain metastases who are most likely to benefit from surgical resection are patients with (1) a single surgically accessible lesion, (2) either no remaining systemic disease (true solitary metastasis) or with controlled systemic cancer limited to the primary site only, and (3) a life expectancy of at least 2 months. Because the median time that Karnofsky scores remain ≥70 percent is about 2 months in patients treated with WBRT alone, patients with life expectancies less than that receive adequate palliation from radiation alone and are unlikely to gain any benefit from surgery. A therapeutic approach to brain metastasis is given in Fig. 51-1.

Patients with metastasis from systemic lesions that are highly radiosensitive, such as lymphoma, germ-cell tumors, or leukemia, should have WBRT as the primary treatment. However, even those patients with very radiosensitive cancers with a single brain lesion should be offered diagnostic stereotactic biopsy before treatment of the brain lesion. Between 5 and 10 percent of brain lesions in patients with known systemic cancer are not metastases, so tissue confirmation of cerebral metastasis is necessary for accurate treatment planning.

The best treatment of the locally recurrent metastatic lesion after surgical resection and radiation therapy requires considerable judgment. If the lesion is presumed to be ra-

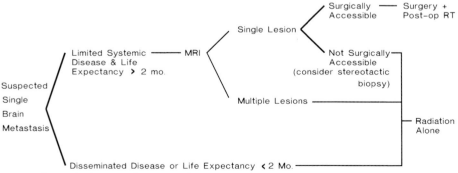

Figure 51-1 A therapeutic approach to brain metastasis. Mo. = months; MRI = magnetic resonance imaging; RT = radiation therapy.

dioresistant (such as a metastasis of kidney, melanoma, or lung origin), and the recurrent lesion remains a single metastasis, repeat surgical resection is the best option when the patient's Karnofsky rating is above 60 and the systemic disease is controlled. The efficacy of interstitial brachytherapy in this circumstance is being determined in clinical trials.

Surgery is ordinarily contraindicated when multiple intracranial lesions are present. Situations in which the authors very rarely offer surgical treatment to patients with multiple metastatic lesions include (1) removal of a cerebellar lesion judged to be life-threatening by mass effect on the brain stem (associated with an asymptomatic or relatively radiosensitive supratentorial lesion), (2) a large radiosensitive supratentorial life-threatening lesion associated with multiple lesions, and (3) two metastatic lesions that can be removed through the same cranial opening.

Surgical Treatment

The microsurgical removal of a cerebral metastasis is performed following the same general techniques of craniotomy and microsurgery that are used for the removal of other intracranial lesions.[27] However, in planning the surgical procedure, two features of a cerebral metastasis must be anticipated: (1) the propensity of a cerebral metastasis to cause substantial cerebral edema and (2) the small size of many metastatic lesions at the time of surgical resection. Administering corticosteroids preoperatively for at least 48 h to patients with considerable mass effect will help prevent transdural herniation at the time of tumor exposure.

Metastatic lesions are often removed when they are quite small because the extensive cerebral edema associated with the lesion rather than the lesion per se has caused early neurologic symptoms. Likewise, asymptomatic tumors discovered as part of the survey evaluation of patients with a newly discovered systemic cancer may be very small. These small lesions, if not superficial, may be quite difficult to locate under a normal-appearing cortical surface. Computer-assisted stereotactic techniques are very helpful to precisely place the bone flap over the tumor. Because most of the patients will receive postoperative radiation therapy, a linear scalp incision is preferred in order to decrease the chance of complications caused by poor wound healing. To lessen the possibility of a postoperative deficit, stereotactic or intraoperative ultrasound techniques should be used to precisely locate small subcortical tumors before making any cortical incision. Intraoperative ultrasound or direct localization of the lesion with the stereotactic probe or needle should be used during exposure of the lesion through a small cortical incision; these techniques provide a direct route to the tumor and a means of avoiding elegant areas of the brain. These measures prevent the prolonged exploration for an elusive small lesion, which is the major cause of postoperative neurologic deficits. Microsurgical, laser, and ultrasonic aspiration techniques are invaluable adjuncts to these localizing devices for the safe removal of small metastatic lesions which are deep-seated or adjacent to elegant areas of the brain. Complication rates of less than 5 percent are reported in recent series. Very small lesions (less than 1 cm in diameter) are better localized stereotactically than with ultrasound. Subcortical tumors should be approached by a dissection plane through the sulcus. Only the most superficial tumors should be removed through an opening in the gyrus.

Complete tumor resection is accomplished in about two-thirds of cases.[12–14,22] In our randomized study, contrast CT scans done 1 to 5 days postoperatively showed removal in all cases. However, late local recurrence appeared in 20 percent of these patients. The potential for late local recurrence is the basis for administering radiation therapy after surgical resection. Kelly et al. reported no local recurrences in their series of 44 patients using very sophisticated computer-assisted stereotactic resection techniques.[12] They pointed out, however, that the postoperative radiation therapy that most of their patients received may have contributed to their excellent results. Based on currently available data, postoperative radiation should be administered even after apparently "complete" surgical resection.

References

1. Bergonié J, Tribondeau L. Interpretation of some results of radiotherapy and an attempt at determining a logical technique of treatment. *Radiat Res* 1959; 11:587–588.
2. Berry HC, Parker RG, Gerdes AJ. Irradiation of brain metastases. *Acta Radiol Ther Phys Biol* 1974; 13:535–544.
3. Black P. Brain metastasis: current status and recommended guidelines for management. *Neurosurgery* 1979; 5:617–631.
4. Cairncross JG, Kim JH, Posner JB. Radiation therapy for brain metastases. *Ann Neurol* 1980; 7:529–541.
5. Cairncross JG, Posner JB. The management of brain metastases. In: Walker MD (ed.), *Oncology of the Nervous System*. Boston: Martinus Nijhoff, 1983:341–377.
6. Deeley TJ, Edwards JMR. Radiotherapy in the management of cerebral secondaries from bronchial carcinoma. *Lancet* 1968; 1:1209–1213.
7. Delattre JY, Krol G, Thaler HT, et al. Distribution of brain metastases. *Arch Neurol* 1988; 45:741–744.
8. DiStefano A, Yap HY, Hortobagyi GN, et al. The natural history of breast cancer patients with brain metastases. *Cancer* 1979; 44:1913–1918.
9. Grant FC. Concerning intracranial malignant metastases: their frequency and the value of surgery in their treatment. *Ann Surg* 1926; 84:635–646.
10. Horton J, Baxter DH, Olson KB, et al. The management of metastases to the brain by irradiation and corticosteroids. *AJR* 1971; 111:334–336.
11. Karnofsky DA, Burchenal JH. The clinical evaluation of chemotherapeutic agents in cancer. In: MacLeod CM (ed.), *Evaluation of Chemotherapeutic Agents*. New York: Columbia University Press, 1949:191–205.
12. Kelly PJ, Kall BA, Goerss SJ. Results of computed tomography–based computer-assisted stereotactic resection of metastatic intracranial tumors. *Neurosurgery* 1988; 22:7–17.
13. Lang EF, Slater J. Metastatic brain tumors: results of surgical and neurosurgical treatment. *Surg Clin North Am* 1964; 44:865–872.
14. MacGee EE. Surgical treatment of cerebral metastases from lung cancer: the effect on quality and duration of survival. *J Neurosurg* 1971; 35:416–420.
15. Mandell L, Hilaris B, Sullivan M, et al. The treatment of single brain metastasis from non-oat cell lung carcinoma: surgery and radiation versus radiation therapy alone. *Cancer* 1986; 58:641–649.

16. Markesbery WR, Brooks WH, Gupta GD, et al. Treatment for patients with cerebral metastases. *Arch Neurol* 1978; 35: 754–756.

17. Order SE, Hellman S, Von Essen CF, et al. Improvement in quality of survival following whole-brain irradiation for brain metastasis. *Radiology* 1968; 91:149–153.

18. Patchell RA, Cirrincione C, Thaler HT, et al. Single brain metastases: surgery plus radiation or radiation alone. *Neurology* 1986; 36:447–453.

19. Ransohoff J. Surgical management of metastatic tumors. *Semin Oncol* 1975; 2:21–27.

20. Richards P, McKissock W. Intracranial metastases. *Br Med J* 1963; 1:15–18.

21. Ruderman NB, Hall TC. Use of glucocorticoids in the palliative treatment of metastatic brain tumors. *Cancer* 1965; 18: 298–306.

22. Störtebecker TP. Metastatic tumors of the brain from a neurosurgical point of view: a follow-up study of 158 cases. *J Neurosurg* 1954; 11:84–111.

23. Sundaresan N, Galicich JH, Beattie EJ Jr. Surgical treatment of brain metastases from lung cancer. *J Neurosurg* 1983; 58:666–671.

24. Todd NV, McDonagh T, Miller JD. What follows diagnosis by computed tomography of solitary brain tumour? Audit of one year's experience in southeast Scotland. *Lancet* 1987; 1: 611–612.

25. Vieth RG, Odom GL. Intracranial metastases and their neurosurgical treatment. *J Neurosurg* 1965; 23:375–383.

26. White KT, Fleming TR, Laws ER Jr. Single metastasis to the brain: surgical treatment in 122 consecutive patients. *Mayo Clin Proc* 1981; 56:424–428.

27. Wilkins RH. Principles of neurosurgical operative technique. In: Wilkins RH, Rengachary SS (eds.), *Neurosurgery*. New York: McGraw-Hill, 1985:427–438.

28. Winston KR, Walsh JW, Fischer EG. Results of operative treatment of intracranial metastatic tumors. *Cancer* 1980; 45:2639–2645.

29. Zimm S, Wampler GL, Stablein D, et al. Intracranial metastases in solid-tumor patients: natural history and results of treatment. *Cancer* 1981; 48:384–394.

Index

INDEX